──── **FIRST EDITION** ────

MANAGING PIG HEALTH AND THE TREATMENT OF DISEASE

A REFERENCE FOR THE FARM

Michael R. Muirhead

Thomas J. L. Alexander
Contributing Author and Editor

5M Enterprises Limited

Copyright © 5M Enterprises Ltd. 1997
Published by 5M Enterprises Ltd.
PO Box 233
Sheffield
S35 0PB
United Kingdom

All rights reserved. No reproduction, copy or transmission of this publication may be made without written permission.

ISBN 0 9530150 0 9

No part of this publication may be reproduced, copied or transmitted save with written permission or in accordance with the provisions of the Copyright Act 1956 (as amended), or under the terms of any licence permitting copying issued by the Copyright Licensing Agency, 33-34 Alfred Place, London, WC1E 7DP Tel: 0171 436 5931

Any person who does any unauthorised act in relation to this publication may be liable to criminal prosecution and civil claims for damages.

A CIP catalogue record for this book is available from the British Library.

Note to the Reader

The methods of treatment and control of conditions discussed in the book are guidelines only. Any recommendations given and so used are the responsibility of the producer, and the advice of his or her veterinarian should be sought in case of doubt. No responsibility is accepted by the authors or publishers for any application of the advice given in this book because each farm and region is different and responses cannot be predicted. Some trade names and their chemical compounds are used throughout. No endorsement is intended nor is any criticism implied of similar products not named.

5M Enterprises Ltd. would welcome your comments regarding this book. All feedback will be taken into account and hopefully help enhance subsequent editions.

Please write to us at: 5M Enterprises Ltd.
PO Box 233
Sheffield S35 0BP
United Kingdom

Alternatively e-mail us at **5m@fivementerprises.demon.co.uk**
You can also contact us via our web page at:

http://www.fivementerprises.demon.co.uk/

and view other products that are under development or for sale.

About the Authors

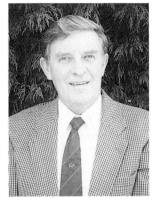

Michael R. Muirhead   BVM&S, FRCVS, DPM.

Mike Muirhead is the senior partner in the Garth Veterinary Group, a specialist pig practice in the UK. He is a past president of the Pig Veterinary Society, a Fellow of the Royal College of Veterinary Surgeons and a diplomate in Pig Medicine. For the past 30 years he has provided consultancy services to a number of breeding and large and small commercial operations both in Europe and North America. He has published over 63 papers on management and disease control and lectured extensively to many farming groups. He received the David Black award in 1980, the Bledesloe award from the National Agricultural Society of England in 1985 and the Dalrympe Champney's cup from the British Veterinary Association in 1989. He is a regular contributor to International Pig letter and he is also a partner in a large pig unit.

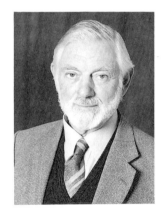

Thomas J. L. Alexander   PhD, MVSc, BSc, MRCVS, DPM.

Tom Alexander teaches pig husbandry, pig medicine and infectious diseases at the University of Cambridge where he has been deputy head of the veterinary school for six years. He is internationally known for his research on vomiting and wasting disease, swine dysentery, streptococcal meningitis and medicated early weaning which was his brainchild. He was one of the first veterinarians world-wide to take a post graduate degree in pig medicine, at Guelph, in Canada in 1960 and followed up with a PhD in enteric viruses of the pig in 1965. He has been international consultant veterinarian to the Pig Improvement Company since 1967. He was a partner in a 200 sow pig farm in the 1970s. He was also on the Board of Directors of a large mixed farming business which included 5,000 sows for 15 years, being chairman for six. He was a founding member of the British Pig Veterinarian Society and its president for two years and was the convenor of the organising committee of the first International Pig Veterinary Society Congress in 1969. He was a prime influence on the development of a National Diploma in Pig Medicine for the Royal College of Veterinary Surgeons and chaired its Pig Medicine Board. He has been invited to give papers and do consultancy work in most pig-rearing countries of the world.

ACKNOWLEDGEMENTS

The production of this book has been my intention for over 20 years following requests by many pig farmers and pig industry personnel for reading references relating to problems on the farm.

Many people in many ways have contributed to the contents and the management health and disease control information it contains.

It would be impossible to refer to everyone by name and it would be unfair to those people left out. Individual references therefore have been purposely omitted. However I would like to thank and acknowledge the contributions that many groups have made over the years including:

Members of the Garth Veterinary Group; Neville Kingston, Paul Thompson, Dr John Carr and associate veterinarians.

The authors of International Pig Letter. The late Al Lemon, Professor Richard Penny, Mike Wilson, Gary Dial and Frank Aherne and editors Neal Black and Grant McGinnis.

Members of the American Association of Swine Practitioners.

Pig Improvement Company, National Pig Development Company.

Newsham Hybrid and JSR Healthbred.

Cliff Johnson my farm manager who has helped put into practice many of the new control procedures (or rejected them!).

Mark Enright for his chapter on Health and Safety and Control of Substances Hazardous to Health.

The many pig farmers and veterinarians consulted with over the years.

Tom Alexander who has contributed significantly through his extensive knowledge and in particular with his red pen as editor by making the observations and comments more user friendly and scientifically correct.

This book would not have been completed without the continual devotion to the task by my secretary Pauline Tams and my son James of 5M Enterprises. Pauline has had to cope with the illegible writings of two veterinarians and numerous alterations and corrections.

Finally without the constant encouragement and help from my wife Louise who has endured long hours of silence I would not have finished the project.

No book is ever complete (or without fault) but we hope that this one will provide scope for debate, education, improvements in health and disease control and finally more profitable pig farming.

Michael R. Muirhead
May 1997

How to Get the Best Use Out of This Book.
IMPORTANT - PLEASE READ.

Managing Pig Health and the Treatment of Disease has been written with a clear objective - to help you the pig producer or advisor, to understand, identify, manage and treat disease problems that are specific to your farm, with advice as appropriate from your veterinarian.

It should also help to maximise production and profitability because as a practical manual it can be referred to during the working day.

The book is not meant to be a substitute for your veterinarian but to give you a clearer understanding of what should be done to counter disease and increase production and thus be able to interpret and implement veterinary advice more effectively. It also aims to promote communication between the veterinarian and the farmer.

It is designed for easy reference when you encounter a problem or have a query. For example if greasy pig disease is affecting weaners, you will find that the disease is discussed in chapter 9 "Managing and Treating Disease in the Weaner, Grower and Finishing Period". If the problem is in sucking pigs the salient points will be found in chapter 8 "The Farrowing and Sucking Period". You will also find it further illustrated under chapter 10 "Skin Conditions".

The Structure of the Book

About the Authors
Acknowledgements
How to get the best use out of this book
Contents
1. **An Introduction to the Anatomy and Physiology of the Pig**
2. **Understanding Disease**
3. **Managing Health and Disease**
4. **Treating Disease**
5. **Reproduction: Non Infectious Infertility**
6. **Reproduction: Infectious Infertility**
7. **Managing and Treating Disease in the Dry Period**
8. **Managing and Treating Disease in the Farrowing and Sucking Period**
9. **Managing and Treating Disease in the Weaner, Grower and Finishing Period**
10. **Skin Conditions**
11. **Parasites**
12. **Exotic Diseases**
13. **Poisons: Recognition, and Control**
14. **Nutrition and Disease**
15. **Surgical, Manipulative and Practical Procedures on the Farm**
16. **Welfare and Disease**
17. **Health and Safety**
    Appendix
    Index
    Abbreviations

It is essential you familiarise yourself with the layout before you use the book.

Chapter 1 clarifies the terminology used throughout the book and discusses the basic outline of the anatomy and physiology of the pig. For those of you who already have a good biological knowledge this will be elementary but for others it will be the basis for understanding the rest of the book. Abbreviations are listed at the end of the book.

Chapters 2 and 3 describe the fundamental causes of disease and how infectious organisms are spread and controlled.

The contents and specific problems are outlined at the beginning of each chapter in alphabetical order.

Relevant chapters open with an explanation of the factors that contribute to the management control of the diseases or conditions.

If you are unable to identify a disease refer to the "identifying problems" format in the relevant chapter. These can be used to relate the clinical signs you observe to common causes.

If in doubt consult your veterinarian.

At the end of relevant chapters a list of medicines is given as a guide to treatments and dose levels[*]. The last column in this guide is available for you to document the trade names of these drugs that are available in your country.

The book is extensively cross-referenced and in some cases duplicated - purposely - for ease of access and to give a wide understanding and appreciation of each problem area.

Metric measurements are used throughout the book. Imperial measurements methods of conversions and quick reference tables are given in the appendix

Treatment regimes are designated by the symbol ☐ and management control procedures by ◆

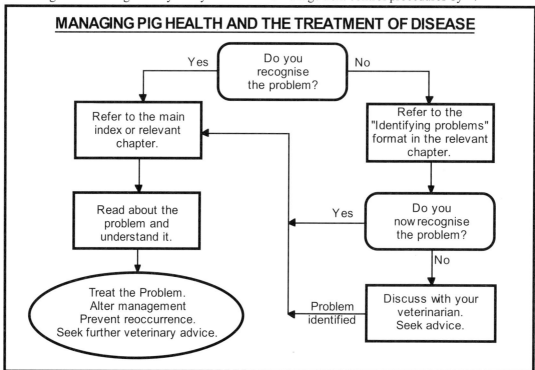

---

[*] *The authors are aware that regulations governing drug usage vary in different countries. In some countries many of the drugs listed may be obtained on prescription only or can be administered only by or under the supervision of a veterinarian. You should, of course, conform to your national regulations and whatever the regulations you are advised to consult your veterinarian regularly.*

CONTENTS

1. An Introduction to the Anatomy and Physiology of the Pig (and the Technical Terms used in the Book)

Terminology, anatomy and physiology 3
    Circulatory system 4
    Digestive system... 5
    Endocrine system 7
    Immune system 8
    Muscular system 9
    Nervous system 10
    Reproductive system...10
    Respiratory system..14
    Sensory systems 15
    Skeletal system..15
    Urinary system 17

2. Understanding Disease

Definition of health and disease...21
The causes of disease 21
Infectious agents..22
    Viruses...22
    Bacteria 24
    Fungi 26
    Parasites 27
Non infectious agents 27
    Trauma..27
    Hereditary and congenital defects (developmental abnormalities)....28
    Nutritional deficiencies and excesses..28
    Poisons - toxic agents 29
    Stress..29
How infectious agents are spread..31
    Direct contact between pigs..31
    Disease dissemination by vehicles 32
    Spread of infection between different ages of pig within a farm.....33
    Environmental contamination on the farm.....................................33
    Airborne transmission and other methods 34
    By people 37
    By pigs 38
    Maintaining freedom from disease - biosecurity 40
Selecting your source of breeding stock 40
Disinfection...44
The costs of disease 48
Depopulation and repopulation 50

3. Managing Health and Disease

Management components of health control 55
Immunity - how the pig responds to infection 56
    Innate (i.e. Inherited) and non-specific resistance 58

    Acquired specific immunity 60
    The role of passive immunity in the development of actively
        acquired immunity 62
    Serological tests 62
    Vaccination 63
    Immunosuppression 65
Medicinal control of disease 66
Eradicating disease 66
Recognising disease on the farm 66
    The use of sight 66
    Observation of the group 67
    Changes in behaviour 67
    The use of smell 67
    The use of touch 67
    The use of sound 67
Clinical examination of the herd 67
    Assessing health, management and disease in outdoor
        production 70
The management and treatment of the sick pig 74
    The design of the hospital pen 75
Disposal of dead pigs 76
The consultant or specialist veterinarian 76
Staff training and education 77
    An example of management failures and disease 81
The use of records 82
    Recording objectives 82
Planning for efficient production and disease control 88
    Management procedures for maximising the mating programme ... 88
Management of the environment 89
    Environmental factors affecting dry sows 90
    Environmental factors affecting lactating sows and sucking pigs ... 90
    Environmental factors affecting growing pigs 91
    Air quality 91
    Environmental temperatures 92
    Stocking densities 93
    Segregated weaning and disease control procedures 94
Nutrition and feeding 101
Water 102

4. Treating Disease

Understanding medicines 107
    Legal requirements 107
    How medicines are prescribed 107
Understanding dosage levels 108
    In-feed medications 108
    Injectable medicines 108
    Water medication 108
Controlling and storing medicines 109
    Disposing of medicines 109
Types of medicine and their application 110
Anti bacterial drugs and their uses 111
    Types of antibacterial drug 111
    Aminoglycosides 111
    Cephalosporins 111
    Macrolides 111

Penicillins 112
Quinalones...112
Sulphonamides 112
Tetracyclines 112
Other antibacterial drugs 112
Antibacterial sensitivity tests....................................112
Administrating medicines by injection 112
Using the syringe and needle................................... 113
Self inoculation 113
Sites of injection...113
Administrating medicines topically................................ 114
Administrating medicines in water................................. 115
Group treatment 115
Individual pig treatment 116
Administrating medicines in-feed.................................. 117
Factors to consider when using in-feed medication ... 117
Strategic medication... 118
Pulse medication 120
Continuous medication... 120
Medicated early weaning (MEW)................................. 120
Trade name of antibacterial drugs............................ 120
Anaesthetics, sedatives, analgesics................................ 121
Products available... 121
Parasecticides 122
Vaccines... 124
Hormones... 125
Hormones used to control the oestrus cycle 126
Growth promoters 126
Probiotics 127
Electrolytes.. 127
Rehydration by mouth.. 128
Examples of some pig vaccines available in the EU and
elsewhere 1997... 129

5. Reproduction: Non Infectious Infertility

The breeding female... 133
The use and interpretation of records 135
Understanding farrowing rates and production losses..... 136
Embryo and foetal losses 137
Group 1 losses - anoestrus 137
Acclimatisation of gilts 140
Light 142
Group 2 losses - ovulation and egg production 143
Group 3 losses - fertilisation 144
Group 4 losses - implantation................................... 145
Group 5 losses - foetal death and the mummified pig................ 147
Detecting pregnancy 148
Methods of pregnancy diagnosis (PD)..................... 148
A practical format for diagnosing pregnancy on the farm 149
Abortion and seasonal infertility 149
Non infectious causes... 150
Infectious causes 151
Group 6 losses - stillborn pigs 152
Low litter size 153
The boar... 154

    Anatomy and physiology 154
    Facts about semen 155
    Fertilisation 156
    Libido 157
Mating procedures 157
    Single service (supervised) 157
    Skip services 158
    Multiple services 159
    Key points to a successful mating 159
    Artificial insemination (AI) 160
    Fungal poisoning - mycotoxicosis 160

6. Reproduction: Infectious Infertility

Diseases affecting reproduction 165
Viral infertility 167
    Aujeszky's disease / pseudorabies virus (AD or PRV) 167
    Bovine viral diarrhoea virus (BVDV) and border disease
    virus (BDV) 168
    Classical swine fever virus (CSF) - hog cholera virus (HC) 168
    Encephalomyocarditis virus (EMCV) 169
    Enteroviruses (SMEDI) 169
    Porcine cytomegalovirus (PCMV) 170
    Porcine parvovirus (PPV) 170
    Porcine reproductive and respiratory syndrome (PRRS) 173
    Swine influenza virus (SI) 177
Bacterial infertility 178
    Abortion 178
    Brucellosis 179
    Endometritis and the vulval discharge syndrome 180
    Eperythrozoonosis (Epe) 184
    Erysipelas 185
    Leptospirosis 186

7. Managing and Treating Disease in the Dry Period

General clinical signs of disease 193
Management and disease 193
    Records 193
    Reasons for sow disposal 194
    Reasons for keeping sows beyond 6 litters 194
    Reasons for not keeping sows beyond 6 litters 194
    Key points to maintaining longevity in the breeding female 194
    Nutrition and feeding 195
    Housing 196
    Hygiene 196
    Temperature 196
    Ventilation 196
    Water 196
    Light 196
    Stockmanship 196
    Stress 196
    The boar 197
Diseases that may be seen in the dry period 197
Identifying problems in the dry sow 197

Abortion - see chapters 5 and 6 198
Abscesses 199
Anaemia 199
Anthrax 200
Atrophic rhinitis 200
Aujeszky's disease 200
Back muscle necrosis 201
Biotin deficiency 201
Brucellosis 201
Bursitis 202
Bush foot / foot rot 202
Clostridial diseases 203
Cystitis and pyelonephritis 203
Erysipelas 205
Fractures 207
Gastric ulcers 207
Glässers disease (*Haemophilus parasuis*) 209
Haematoma 209
Jaw and snout deviation 209
Lameness 209
Laminitis 211
Leg weakness (osteochondrosis - OCD) 211
Leptospirosis 214
Mange 214
Mastitis 214
Meningitis 215
Mortality 215
Muscle tearing 216
Mycoplasma arthritis (*Mycoplasma hyosynoviae* infection) .. 216
Peritonitis 217
Pneumonia 217
Porcine enteropathy (PE) 218
Porcine epidemic diarrhoea (PED) 218
Porcine parvovirus (PPV) 218
Porcine reproductive and respiratory syndrome (PRRS) 218
Porcine stress syndrome (PSS) 218
Prolapse of the rectum 219
Prolapse of the vagina and cervix 220
Salmonellosis 220
Salt poisoning - (water deprivation) 221
Shoulder sores 221
Streptococcal infections 221
Swine dysentery (SD) 221
Swine influenza or flu (SI) 222
Thin sow syndrome 222
Vice - abnormal behaviour 223
Vulval discharge 223
Medicines and other drugs for use in the dry sow 224

8. Managing and Treating Disease in the Farrowing and Sucking Period

How to achieve low pre-weaning mortality 227
Using records to identify problems 227
Understanding and maximising the role of the sow 229
      Breed and selection 229

Age	229
Parturition - farrowing	230
Controlled farrowings	233
Udder	234
Udder oedema and failure of milk let down	236
Mammary hypoplasia - undeveloped udder	237
Agalactia - no milk	237
Mastitis - inflammation of the mammary glands	237
Management at farrowing	239
Farrowing house design	239
Preparing the farrowing house	241
Preparing the sow	241
Maternity management - supervising the farrowings	241
Acclimatising the newborn piglet to the creep area	242
Maximising colostrum intake	242
Fostering piglets	242
The stillborn pig	244
Nutrition	246
Diseases of the farrowing and lactating sow	247
Identifying problems in the lactating sow	247
Atrophic rhinitis (AR)	248
Aujeszky's disease (AD)	248
Clostridial diseases	248
Cystitis / pyelonephritis	248
Eclampsia	249
Electrocution	249
Enzootic pneumonia (EP) - *Mycoplasma hyopneumoniae*	249
Erysipelas	250
Fever	250
Fractures	250
Gastric / intestinal torsion	251
Gastric ulcers	251
Leg weakness - osteochondrosis (OCD)	251
Osteomalacia (OM)	251
Metritis - inflammation of the womb	252
Porcine enteropathy (PE)	252
Porcine parvovirus (PPV)	252
Porcine reproductive and respiratory syndrome virus (PRRS)	253
Prolapse of the bladder	253
Prolapse of the rectum	253
Prolapse of the uterus (womb)	254
Prolapse of the vagina and cervix	254
Salt poisoning - (water deprivation)	255
Savaging of piglets (cannibalism)	255
Shoulder sores	256
Vulva haematoma	256
Diseases and problems in the sucking pig	257
Identifying problems in the piglet	257
Actinobacillosis	258
Anaemia - iron deficiency	259
Arthritis - joint infections	260
Atresia ani - (no anus or no rectum)	261
Atrophic rhinitis (AR)	261
Aujeszky's disease (AD)	262
Brucellosis	262
Bursitis	262
Clostridial diseases	263

Coccidiosis (coccidia) 263
Congenital tremor (CT) - shaking piglets 264
Cryptosporidiosis 265
Diarrhoea or scour 265
Enzootic pneumonia (EP) - (mycoplasma infections) 267
Eperythrozoonosis (Epe) 267
Epitheliogenesis imperfecta - (imperfect skin) 269
Erysipelas 269
Glässers disease (*Haemophilus parasuis* HPS) 269
Greasy pig disease - (exudative epidermitis) 270
Hypoglycaemia - low blood sugar level 271
Leptospirosis 272
Mange mites (*Sarcoptes scabiei*) 272
Middle ear infections 272
Navel bleeding / pale pig syndrome 272
Porcine epidemic diarrhoea (PED) - scour 273
Porcine reproductive and respiratory syndrome (PRRS) 273
Porcine respiratory corona virus infection (PRCV) 274
Rotavirus diarrhoea 274
Salmonellosis 275
Splaylegs 275
Streptococcal meningitis 276
Swine dysentery (SD) 276
Swine influenza (SI) 276
Teat necrosis 276
Tetanus 277
Thrombocytopaenic purpura - bleeding 277
Transmissible gastro-enteritis (TGE) 277
Vomiting and wasting disease / ontario encephalitis 279
Vitamin E deficiency and iron toxicity 279
Summary - 12 key points to piglet survival 279
Medicines and other drugs for use in lactating sows and
sucking pigs 280

9. Managing and Treating Disease in the Weaner, Grower and Finishing Period

Managing the weaner for health and maximum productivity 285
Managing the growing pig for health and efficient production 288
Diseases of the weaned and growing pig 295
Identifying problems in the post-weaning period - 5-20kg weight 296
Identifying problems in the growing period - 20-110kg weight 298
    Abscesses 299
    Actinobacillus pleuropneumonia (APP) 299
    Anthrax 301
    Arthritis 301
    Atrophic rhinitis (AR) - progressive disease (PAR) 301
    Aujeszky's disease (AD) or pseudorabies (PR) 303
    Back muscle necrosis 304
    Bordetellosis 304
    Bursitis 304
    Bush foot / foot rot 304
    Classical swine fever (hog cholera), African swine fever ... 305
    Clostridial diseases 305
    Coccidiosis 305
    Coliform infections and post-weaning diarrhoea 306

Colitis 307
Enteric diseases 308
Enzootic pneumonia (EP) or *Mycoplasma hyopneumoniae*
infection 308
Eperythrozoonosis (Epe) 311
Erysipelas 312
Foot-and-mouth disease (FMD) 313
Fractures 313
Gastric ulcers 314
Glässers disease (*Haemophilus parasuis* HPS) 315
Greasy pig disease - (exudative epidermitis) 316
Haematoma 317
Lameness 317
Leg weakness - osteochondrosis (OCD) 318
Leptospirosis 319
Mange mites (*Sarcoptes scabiei*) 319
Middle ear infection 319
Mortality 319
Mulberry heart disease (vitamin E / selenium) 320
Mycoplasma arthritis (*Mycoplasma hyosynoviae* infection) 321
Oedema disease (OD) - bowel oedema 322
Parasites 323
Pasteurellosis 323
Porcine epidemic diarrhoea (PED) 323
Porcine enteropathy (PE) 324
Porcine reproductive and respiratory syndrome (PRRS) 325
Porcine respiratory corona virus infection (PRCV) 326
Porcine stress syndrome (PSS) 326
Prolapse of the rectum 327
Rectal stricture 328
Respiratory diseases and control strategies 328
Rotavirus 333
Ruptures or hernias 334
Salmonellosis 334
Salt poisoning - (water deprivation) 336
Spirochaetal diarrhoea 336
Streptococcal infections 336
Swine dysentery (SD) 338
Swine influenza (SI) 341
Torsion of the stomach and intestines 341
Transmissible gastro-enteritis (TGE) 342
Tuberculosis 342
Vice - abnormal behaviour (tail biting, flank chewing,
ear biting) 342
Yersinia infection 344
Medicines and other drugs for use in weaned and finishing pigs 344

10. Skin Conditions

Structure and appearance of the skin 349
How to recognise skin conditions 349
Identifying the causes of skin conditions 351
    Abscesses 352
    Anaemia 353
    Aujeszky's disease (AD) - pseudorabies (PR) 354
    Bursitis 354
    Cyanosis 354

Epitheliogenesis imperfecta or defective skin 355
Erythema 355
Erysipelas 355
Flank biting 355
Granuloma 356
Greasy pig disease (exudative epidermitis) 356
Greasy skin 357
Haematoma 357
Haemorrhage 358
Hyperkeratinization 358
Insect bites 358
Jaundice 358
Lice 358
Mange (sarcoptic) 359
Necrosis of the skin 359
Parakeratosis 361
Photosensitisation 361
Pityriasis rosea 361
Porcine reproductive and respiratory syndrome - (PRRS) 361
Preputial ulcers 362
Pustular dermatitis 362
Ringworm 362
Shoulder sores 362
Swine pox 363
Sunburn 363
Tail biting 363
Thrombocytopaenic purpura - bleeding 363
Ulcerative spirochaetosis (ulcerative granuloma) 364
Vesicular diseases 364
Vulval oedema 365

11. Parasites

Internal parasites 369
    The direct life cycle 370
    The indirect life cycle 370
Recognising a worm problem 370
Management control and prevention 371
Treatment programmes for internal parasites 373
Round worms (nematodes) 373
    Kidney worms *(Stephanurus dentatus)* 373
    Large white worms or ascarids *(Ascaris suum)* 375
    Lungworms *(Metastrongylus apri)* 376
    Muscle worms *(Trichinella spiralis)* 376
    Nodular worms *(Oesophagostomum dentatum)* 376
    Red stomach worms *(Hyostrongylus rubidus)* 377
    Stomach hair worm *(Trichostrongylus axei)* 377
    Thick stomach worm *(Ascarops strongylina* and
        Physocephalus sesalatus) 377
    Thorny-headed worm *(Macracanthorhynchus hirudinaceus)* 377
    Thread worm *(Strongyloides ransomi)* 378
    Whipworm *(Trichuris suis)* 378
Tapeworms 378
    Pork bladder worm *(Cysticercus cellulosae)* 378
    Human tapeworm *(Taenia solium)* 378
Protozoan diseases 379
    Balantidium coli 379

    Coccidiosis (coccidia) 379
    Cryptosporidiosis *Cryptosporidium parvum*) 380
    Toxoplasmosis (toxoplasma) 381
Bacteria 381
    Eperythrozoonosis (Epe) 381
External parasites 382
    Flies 383
    Lice 385
    Mange - dermodectic (follicle mites) 385
    Mange (sarcoptic) 385
    Ticks 388

12. Exotic Diseases

Introduction 393
    What are exotic diseases? 393
    Why this chapter has been written 393
    Which countries are free from which diseases? 394
Diseases 394
    African swine fever (ASF) 394
    Aujeszky's disease (AD) - pseudorabies (PR) 396
    Blue eye disease (BE) 400
    Brucellosis 401
    Classical swine fever (CSF) - hog cholera (HC) 403
    Foot-and-mouth disease (FMD) 406
    Japanese B. encephalitis (JBE) 408
    Leptospirosis 408
    Porcine epidemic diarrhoea (PED) 410
    Porcine respiratory coronavirus (PRCV) 411
    Swine vesicular disease (SVD) 411
    Teschen disease 412
    Transmissible gastro-enteritis (TGE) 414
    Vesicular exanthema of swine (VES) 415
    Vesicular stomatitis (VS) 415
Protecting your herd against serious infectious diseases 417
    Vaccinate 417
    Biosecurity 417

13. Poisons: Recognition, Treatment and Control

Dose effect 423
Intake of poisons 423
Detoxification and excretion 423
Factors in the pig that influence the effects of a poison 423
How to recognise poisoning 423
Clinical signs of different poisons 425
Potential poisons 426
    Algae 426
    Arsenic 427
    Coal tars 427
    Copper 427
    Ethylene glycol 428
    Fluorine 428
    Herbicides 428
    Iron dextran 428
    Insecticides 429
        Carbamates 429

    Chlorinated hydrocarbons 429
    Pyrethrins 429
    Organophosphorus compounds (OPs) 429
  Lead 430
  Manganese 430
  Medicines 430
    Carbadox 430
    Furazolidone 430
    Monensin 430
    Olaquindox 431
    Penicillin 431
    Salinomycin 431
    Sulphonamides 431
    Tiamulin 431
  Mercury 431
  Metaldehyde 431
  Mycotoxins 431
    Aflatoxins 432
    Ergot toxins 433
    Fumonisins 433
    Ochratoxin and citrinin 433
    Trichothecenes 434
    Zearalenone 434
  Nitrates and nitrites 434
  Plants 435
    Bracken *(Pteridium aquilinum)* 435
    Cocklebur *(Xanthium)* 435
    Deadly nightshade *(Solanum)* 435
    Oak leaves and acorns 435
    Pigweed *(Amaranthus)* 435
    Pokeweed *Phytolacca)* 435
    Sorghum *(Sorghum)* 435
    Yellow jasmine *(Gelsemium)* 435
    Water hemlock *(Conium maculatum)* 435
  Salt (water deprivation) 435
  Selenium 436
  Toxic (slurry) gases 436
    Ammonia 436
    Carbon dioxide 437
    Carbon monoxide 437
    Hydrogen sulphide (H_2s) 437
    Methane 437
  Warfarin 438

14.   Nutrition and Disease

  The role of amino acids 446
  The role of energy 446
  Common diseases and conditions associated with nutrition 447
    Abortion and seasonal infertility 448
    Anaemia 450
    Colitis 450
    Diarrhoea 451
    Fractures 454
    Gastric ulcers 454
    Lameness 456
      Calcium and phosphorus 456
      Osteodystrophy 456
      Osteoporosis (OP) and osteomalacia (OM) 456
      Rickets 457
      Vitamin A 457
      Leg weakness or osteochondrosis 458
    Prolapse of the rectum 458

    Reproduction 459
    Respiratory diseases 461
    Salt poisoning - (water deprivation) 461
    Torsion of the stomach and intestines.................................. 462
    Udder oedema and failure of milk let down.......................... 462
    Water 463
Minerals and vitamins... 465
    Biotin 465
    Choline 465
    Copper 465
    Cyanocobalamin B_{12} 465
    Folic acid.. 465
    Iodine.. 465
    Iron 466
    Magnesium 466
    Manganese 466
    Nicotinamide.. 466
    Pantothenic acid 466
    Potassium.. 466
    Riboflavin B_2 466
    Sodium and chloride... 466
    Thiamine 467
    Vitamin E / selenium (mulberry heart disease) 467
    Vitamin K 468
    Zinc... 468
Non nutritional supplements 468
    Probiotics 469

15. Surgical, Manipulative and Practical Procedures

    Antibiotic administration into the anterior vagina post-service 474
    Blood sampling methods available... 475
    Castration of the normal pig 478
    Castration of the ruptured pig 480
    Cleaning and disinfection of buildings - see also water 481
    De-tusking a boar... 482
    Docking (tail clipping) piglets... 483
    Epidectomy... 484
    Feedback 485
    Flutter valve and its use 486
    Fumigation of houses using formaldehyde vapour 487
    Hysterectomy - emergency or planned 488
    Identification - tattooing, slap marking, tagging, transponders, implants, ear notching 491
    Injecting piglets with iron 493
    Lancing an abscess or a haematoma... 495
    Libido checking - training boars to use a stool............................ 496
    Local anaesthesia 496
    Lime washing concrete floors.. 497
    Mating the sow with the boar... 498
    Pregnancy diagnosis 499
    Penis - examination.. 500
    Prolapse of the rectum 501
    Prolapse of the cervix 503
    Prolapse of the uterus (womb)... 504
    Prostaglandin injections to initiate farrowing.............................. 505
    Recording air movement temperature and humidity in a house 506

Restraining the pig 507
Sampling air for dust levels 508
Sampling feeds for laboratory testing 509
Sampling milk from a mammary gland with mastitis 509
Sampling the air for toxic levels of gases 510
Semen collection and artificial insemination on the farm 511
Slaughter - humane destruction 515
Stomach tube - How to use one 517
Suturing skin and muscle 518
Swabbing the nose and tonsils for toxigenic pasteurella or
other bacteria 521
Syringes and needles and their use 523
Teeth clipping 525
Temperature recording from the rectum 526
Udder - methods of examination 527
Umbilical cord applying a clamp 528
Vasectomy 529
Vulval haematoma- treating a haematoma 530
Water - cleaning and sterilising a system 531

16. Welfare and Disease

Guidelines to good welfare practices 535
The 5 freedoms 535
Factors responsible for good welfare 536
Disease & welfare problems associated with indoor housing 539
    Sow stalls and confinement 539
    Cubicles or free access stalls 540
    Group sow housing 543
    Yards and individual feeders 544
The health and welfare of lactating sows and sucking piglets 546
The health and welfare of newly weaned sows indoors 546
The health and welfare of weaned and growing pigs 548
The health and welfare of sows outdoors 550

17. Health and Safety

Introduction 555
The management of health and safety 555
The cost benefits 557
How to develop a health and safety management system
for your farm 558
    Step 1 - Identify the people involved on your farm 558
    Step 2 - Understand your national regulations 560
Policy statements and policy organisation 561
    Step 3 - Produce your policy statements 561
    Step 4 - Assign responsibilities for health and safety 561
Risk assessments 562
    Step 5 - Plan your risk assessments 562
    Step 6 - Carry out your risk assessments 568
    Step 7 - Devise and apply your control measures 570
    Records 572
Safe systems of work (SSW's) 572
    Step 8 - Document your safe systems of work (SSW's) 572
    Step 9 - Document your accident, first aid, fire and emergency
    procedures 573
    Step 10 - Review your system periodically 575

APPENDIX   Quick References and Useful Information

Further reading - references and information..................................580
Product references..582
Equipment, materials, medicines and chemicals you may require
on the farm for maintaining health and controlling disease 583
    Equipment and materials..583
    Chemicals..583
    Antibiotics and antibacterial substances 584
    Sedatives 584
    Anti-inflammatory injections...584
    Anthelmintics...584
    Coccidiostats...584
    Hormones 584
    Action on the uterus 584
    Nutrition and metabolism 585
    Parasecticides - topical use 585
    Miscellaneous substances..585
    Mating to farrowing date indicator 585
Physiological data..586
    Blood sampling requirements for serological tests....................586
    Semen..586
    Urine 586
    Haematology SI (standard international)................................586
    Temperature, respiration, pulse rates 586
    Enzyme tests in serum or plasma International units (i.u.) 586
    Biochemistry..586
    Sampling herds to detect evidence of infection.........................587
        95% confidence limit 587
        99% confidence limit 587
Units of measurement used in biological science..........................587
    Metric units and relative values...587
    How to convert units of measurements................................588
Quick conversion tables 588
    Length - inches - millimetres - centimetres.............................588
    Length - miles - kilometres...589
    Length - feet - yards - metres 589
    Weight - pounds - kilograms 589
    Area - square feet - square metres 589
    Volume - pints - gallons - litres..590
    Temperature conversion °C - °F...590
Growth 591
    Calculating days to slaughter (growth rate unknown)...............591
    Effect of variable growth rate on days to slaughter 591
    The possible effects of feed changes on the growing pig............591

INDEX 595

ABBREVIATIONS .... Inside back cover

1 An Introduction to the Anatomy and Physiology of the Pig

(and the Technical Terms used in the Book)

Terminology, anatomy and physiology 3
    Circulatory system 3
    Digestive system 5
    Endocrine system 7
    Immune system 8
    Muscular system 9
    Nervous system 10
    Reproductive system 10
    Respiratory system 14
    Sensory systems 15
    Skeletal system 15
    Urinary system 17

2 Managing Pig Health and the Treatment of Disease

Chapter 1

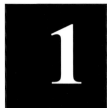 An Introduction to the Anatomy and Physiology of the Pig

(and the Technical Terms used in the Book)

Terminology, Anatomy and Physiology

An understanding of disease processes can be difficult if the reader has little scientific background. For those who have not had training in biological subjects this chapter looks at the basic areas of knowledge necessary to appreciate and understand the information given in this book. All the diseases and conditions mentioned briefly in this chapter are discussed in detail later.

The anatomy and physiology of the pig can be broadly grouped into eleven interrelated systems:
- Circulatory system.
- Digestive system.
- Endocrine system.
- Immune system.
- Muscular system.
- Nervous system.
- Reproductive system - Male
                       - Female
- Respiratory system.
- Sensory systems.
- Skeletal system.
- Urinary system.

Circulatory System

First, study Fig.1-1, then read the following while still referring to the figure. The circulatory system consists of the heart which is a four chamber suction and pressure pump that moves blood through two separate systems, one to and from the lungs and the other around the body. The blood returns to the heart from the body through a series of veins, which terminate in two large veins called the anterior and posterior vena cava. Blood returns from the lungs through the pulmonary veins. The top two chambers or auricles receive the blood from the veins and pass it into the strong muscular bottom chambers called the ventricles. Oxygen depleted blood from the body enters the right auricle, where it is then pumped into the right ventricle leaving by two pulmonary arteries that deliver the still un-oxygenated blood to the lungs. Oxygenated blood from the lungs is then returned through the pulmonary veins to the left auricle, where it is pumped to the left ventricle and finally out through the main artery, the aorta, to be transported around the body. If the lungs are damaged by disease such as pneumonia, they cannot oxygenate the blood efficiently, the tissues become starved of oxygen and cannot function properly.

When the pig walks or runs its skin may then become blue and it has difficulty breathing. Chronic pneumonia may also hold back the blood supply causing congestion and heart problems.

Arteries are the muscular tubes that carry the blood away from the heart. These branch off into smaller arteries like the branch of a tree eventually becoming very fine arterioles. The arterioles branch further into microscopic tubes called capillaries which exchange fluid through their walls. This enables the cells of the body to receive both oxygen and nutrients and eliminate carbon dioxide. The capillaries then combine to form first small veins, which in turn lead to larger ones. The blood now contains carbon dioxide and reduced levels of oxygen and returns to the heart via the anterior and posterior vena cava to recommence its circulation around the lung.

There is an important subsidiary circulatory system called the hepatic (i.e. liver) portal system. You will see in Fig.1-1 that two arteries provide oxygen to the stomach and intestines (and also the pancreas and spleen). They keep branching until they form capillaries which then join together to form the portal vein which carries the blood to the liver. There the portal vein breaks up into another capillary-type network, where the blood comes into direct contact with the liver cells. The vessels then join together again to form the hepatic veins which discharge the blood into the posterior vena cava. The blood from the intestines carries nutrients from the food eaten and also sometimes harmful substances (toxins). The liver cells are able to modify some of the nutrients for use elsewhere and also to store some. They also detoxify harmful substances. The liver is supplied with oxygen via a separate artery, the hepatic artery.

The internal linings of the heart are covered by a smooth shiny tissue called the endocardium. The rate of contraction is known as the pulse rate. This can be felt either at the base of the ear or under the tail and varies from 200 beats per minute in the young piglet to 70 in the adult.

The blood consists of two main parts, a fluid called plasma and cells. Nutrients such as proteins, sugars and fats are circulated throughout the body in the plasma and waste products are collected to be detoxified in the liver and excreted via the kidneys. The plasma also carries hormones which are produced in one part of the body and

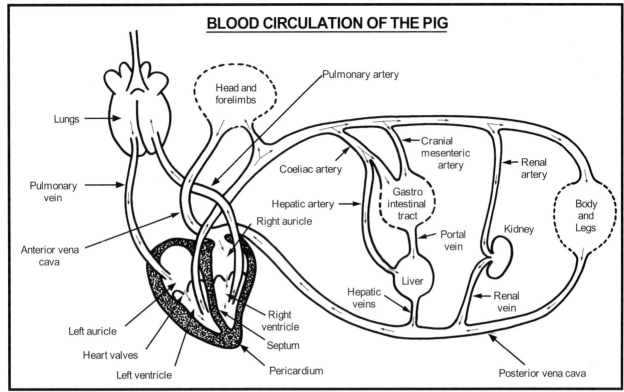
(Fig.1-1)

act on another. It also carries antibodies to combat infection. The plasma also supports red blood cells (erythrocytes) which contain the substance haemoglobin whose main function is to transport oxygen around the body and bring back carbon dioxide to be expelled from the lungs. The next largest group in the plasma are the white cells (leucocytes) which are the first line of defence against infectious agents. The third type of cells are blood platelets. These are really small fragments of cells which are associated with the clotting mechanisms of blood. When blood clots the liquid that remains outside the clot is serum and this contains the antibodies. Serum may be used to inject into pigs to provide an immediate source of immunity.

Failure of blood to clot and subsequent loss of red cells into the tissues is not uncommon in pigs and occurs in thrombocytopaenic purpura - a clotting defect disease - and warfarin poisoning.

Terminology

Albumin - The most abundant protein in the blood.
Anaemia - Any reduction in the number of red cells or in the haemoglobin they contain is described as anaemia and the extent of this is measured either by determining the number of red cells or the level of haemoglobin in the blood .
The causes of anaemia include:
- Bowel haemorrhage (porcine haemorrhagic enteropathy, fungal toxins, acute bowel infection associated with E. coli infection of piglets, salmonella infections or swine dysentery).
- Damage to bone marrow.
- *Eperythrozoonosis suis*. This is a blood borne bacterium that can destroy red blood cells.
- Gastric ulcers and bleeding - or any other cause of haemorrhage.
- Heavy parasite burdens.
- Iron, copper or vitamin deficiencies.

Anoxia - Lack of oxygen. Tissues begin to die after a few minutes.
Antibody - The protective proteins produced in response to the antigenic stimulation. They fight infections.
Antigen - This is the foreign protein contained in viruses, bacteria, fungi or toxins. The body responds by producing an antibody.
Antiserum - This is serum containing higher than normal amounts of antibody against a specific antigen. It is used by injection to give an immediate temporary immunity.
Blood count - A laboratory test that determines the numbers of red and white cells and platelets in the blood.
Blood volume - Approximately 8% of body weight expressed as litres .
Blood platelets (thrombocytes) - These are cell fragments involved in blood clotting.
Blood poisoning - A common term used to describe large numbers of pathogenic bacteria in the blood.
Capillaries - Very tiny tubes about the diameter of a red

cell. These allow water oxygen and nutrients to diffuse out to the tissues.

Cyanosis - Blueing of the skin and extremities due either to anoxia, toxaemia (toxins in the blood) or septicaemia (pathogenic bacteria in the blood).

Endocardium - This is the surface tissue lining the inside of the heart. Endocarditis is the end result of the invasion of this tissue by bacteria, in particular erysipelothrix (which causes erysipelas) and streptococci. Both organisms often cause growths on the heart valves called valvular endocarditis. This makes the valves leaky and less effective.

Erythrocytes - These are the red blood cells. In the normal pig there are approximately 7 million per mm^3.

Globulins - The proteins that make up the antibodies. They are called gamma globulins.

Granulocytes - These consist of specialised cells called neutrophils, eosinophils and basophils that engulf and destroy bacteria and viruses. They are also called macrophages.

Haematuria - Blood in the urine often seen in cystitis - inflammation of the bladder.

Haemoglobin - This is the chemical substance in the red cells that is involved in the transport of oxygen.

Haemoglobinuria - Free haemoglobulin in the urine resulting from the breakdown of blood cells.

Haemolysis - This is the process by which haemoglobin is released from the red cells when the cell envelope is damaged.

Hydropericardium - Excess fluid around the heart. It is often seen in bacterial infections and shock reactions.

Hypoglycaemia - A low level of sugar in the blood. Common in newborn piglets.

Leucocytes - These are the white blood cells of which there are two types, granulocytes and agranulocytes. The granulocytes contain granules in the cell and depending on how they stain they are called neutrophils, eosinophils and basophils. Neutrophils engulf bacteria (phagocytosis), eosinophils increase in chronic disease particularly parasitic disease. Basophils produce a substance called histamine during allergic reactions. Agranulocytes consist of monocytes and lymphocytes.

Lymph - Excessive tissue fluid drained by the lymphatic system. It is similar to plasma.

Lymphatics - A drainage system that removes fluids from tissues and the lymph nodes.

Lymph nodes - These act as filters for lymph and are one of the body's first defences against infection.

Lymphocytes - These are important cells of the immune system producing immunoglobulins. They are of two types, T and B. The total leucocytes in a normal pig are approximately 15,000 per mm^3 and numbers increase markedly with bacterial infections. However in some viral diseases their numbers can be significantly reduced.

Macrophages - These take in and usually destroy foreign materials including bacteria and viruses. See granulocytes and monocytes.

Monocytes - These cells engulf bacteria. When they migrate into tissues they become localised tissue macrophages.

Myocardium - Heart muscle.

Myocarditis - Inflammation of the heart muscle. Any scientific term ending with the term "itis" implies inflammation. Inflammation is the body's response to tissue damage and is associated with swelling, poor circulation, reddening, pressure and pain.

Diseases causing myocarditis include streptococcal infections, certain virus infections and deficiencies of Vitamin E or iron. Poisons such as selenium and monensin and the porcine stress syndrome can also cause marked changes to heart muscle.

Oedema - Swelling of tissues due to excess fluid. Common in the udder of the newly farrowed sow.

Oxyhaemoglobin - This is haemoglobin combined with oxygen. It is the vehicle by which oxygen is carried around the body.

Pericarditis - The pericardium is the clear sac-like membrane that encloses the heart. Pericarditis occurs as a result of infectious agents which cause respiratory diseases. These include pasteurella, mycoplasma, haemophilus, actinobacillus, streptococci and salmonella bacteria and viruses such as flu and porcine respiratory reproductive virus.

Plasma - Unclotted blood without the blood cells.

Septicaemia - Pathogenic bacteria in the blood stream.

Serum - The liquid left after the blood has clotted. It contains large quantities of antibodies which can be used in the laboratory to test for evidence of exposure to diseases or in the field to provide temporary quick protection.

Thrombocyte (blood platelet) - This is responsible for blood clotting.

Thrombosis - The formation of a blood clot in an artery or a vein.

Toxaemia - Toxins in the blood stream

Spleen - This organ acts as a reservoir for blood.

Vasiculitis - This describes inflammation of either veins or arteries and it is often a consequence of diseases such as swine fever, erysipelas, *Actinobacillus pleuropneumoniae*, *Haemophilus parasuis* and salmonellosis.

Viraemia - Viruses in the blood stream

Digestive System

The digestive tract can be considered as a tube that starts at the mouth and finishes at the rectum (Fig.1-2). In some respect its contents can be considered as outside the body. The back of the mouth opens into the pharynx which is the common area for the passage of both food and air. A valve or flap of tissue called the soft palate automatically moves to protect the opening into the trachea or windpipe when swallowing. The tonsils of the pig are situated on the surface of the soft palate. The oesophagus is the tube that leads from the pharynx to the

6 Managing Pig Health and the Treatment of Disease

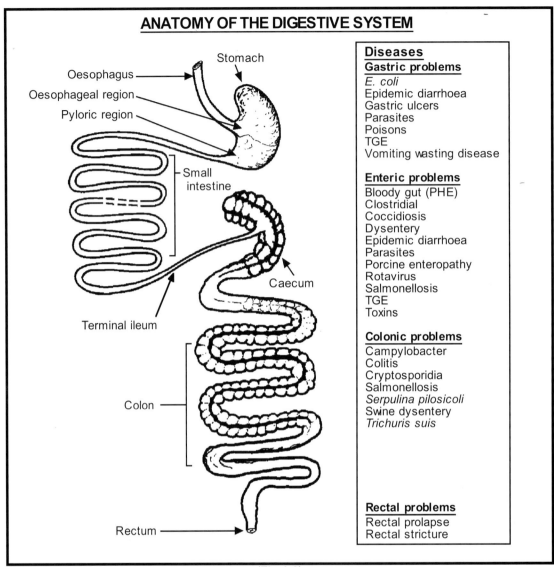

(Fig.1-2)

stomach, down which food is propelled.

The main infectious diseases of the mouth are the vesicular ones including foot-and-mouth disease and swine vesicular disease, although occasionally lesions on the skin around the mouth may be seen in aujeszky's disease and porcine reproductive and respiratory syndrome PRRS. Infection of both the gums and bones are common following faulty teeth clipping.

The digestive system of the pig has the ability to convert vegetable and animal materials into highly digestible nutrients. Its anatomy and physiology are similar to that of humans. In the stomach the major disease problems are associated with inflammation of its lining called gastritis which may result in vomiting. Vomiting also occurs in systemic disease where the organism has spread throughout the body (in infections such as erysipelas), and from toxins produced by bacteria or during high fevers.

Gastric ulceration is common in growing pigs occurring in the area where the oesophagus enters the stomach (oesophageal region).

The intestine has two distinctive parts, the small and the large intestine. Inflammation of the former is called enteritis (although sometimes enteritis may mean inflammation of both parts) and the latter colitis. Enteritis is very common and caused by specific viral, bacterial or parasitic infections. The small intestine in cross section contains millions of finger like projections called villi. (Fig.1-3). These increase the absorptive area enormously and thus the efficiency of the digestive process. The large bowel or colon commences with the caecum, the area of the intestinal tract responsible for the digestion of

Chapter 1

cellulose. Two diseases are commonly seen in the rectum particularly in growing pigs, rectal stricture and rectal prolapse, both of which are discussed in chapter 9.

Terminology

Ascites - Fluid in the abdomen.
Atrophy - A loss of tissue due to disease or malfunction. Atrophy of the villi in the intestine occurs at weaning time causing malabsorption.
Bloody gut - A descriptive term applied to haemorrhage in the lower part of the small intestine or the complete digestive tract. The latter is seen where there is complete torsion of the intestines. Porcine enteropathy is a common cause. (See chapter 9).
Carbohydrates - These consist of two types, crude fibre and soluble carbohydrates. Crude fibre is a mixture of cellulose. Cellulose digestion takes place in the large intestine.
Caecum - A blind sac, at the beginning of the large intestine.
Colitis - Inflammation of the colon or first part of the large bowel. The caecum is often inflamed at the same time (typhlitis). This is a common condition in young growing pigs from 20-60kg weight, caused by nutritional factors and/or infectious agents.
Colon - The spiral part of the large intestine.
Crypts - The bases of the villi.
Duodenum - This is the first part of the small intestine.
Enteritis - Inflammation of the small intestine. This leads to diarrhoea which is common in sucking pigs, weaners and growers.
Enterocytes - Cells at the base or crypts of the villi in the intestine. They multiply and maintain the length of the villi.
Gall bladder - An organ attached to the liver which produces bile that helps in the digestion and absorption of fats.
Gastric ulcers - Erosions of the mucous lining of the stomach occurring mainly in the oesophageal region. Very common and if severe they result in haemorrhage and death.
Gastritis - Inflammation of the stomach lining. Often causes vomiting.
Gingivitis - Inflammation of the gums.
Glossitis - Inflammation of the tongue.
Hepatitis - Inflammation of the liver.
Ileitis - Inflammation of the ileum.
Ileum - The terminal part of the small intestine.
Jejunum - The middle part of the small intestine.
Liver - This organ is the main factory of the body, building new materials and degrading old ones.
Lignin - See carbohydrates.
Lumen - The open space of the small intestine.
Mucosa - The internal lining of the digestive tract. The cells produce mucus which lubricates the surface and also protects against many pathogenic organisms.
Oesophagus - The muscular tube from the pharynx to the stomach.
Omentum - A reflected net-like membrane from the peritoneum that covers the stomach and intestine.
Pancreas - A gland attached to the duodenum by a tube, which produces digestive enzymes and insulin.
Pars oesophagus - The area of the stomach near the entrance of the oesophagus. A common site for the development of ulcers.
Peritoneum - This is the smooth shiny membrane that covers all the surfaces of the abdomen and its contents.
Peritonitis - Inflammation of the peritoneum.
Pharynx - The common passage for food and air at the back of the throat.
Proteins - These are composed of amino acids which contain carbon, hydrogen, oxygen, sulphur, nitrogen and phosphorus. Combinations of different amino acids produce different proteins.
Soft palate - The flap of tissue that separates the trachea and the oesophagus. It contains the tonsils.
Salivary glands - There are three of these called the parotid, mandibular and sublingual glands. They secrete saliva into the mouth.
Tonsillitis - Inflammation of the tonsils.
Tonsils - Two patches of lymphatic tissue at the back of the throat on the soft palate.
Villi - Finger like projections into the lumen of the small intestine. (Fig.1-3).

CROSS SECTION OF THE SMALL INTESTINE

Labels: Muscle coat, Submucosa, Mucosal surfaces, Villi, Lumen, Crypts, Enterocytes, Intestinal wall

(Fig.1-3)

Endocrine System

Endocrines or hormones are the substances produced

Managing Pig Health and the Treatment of Disease

by various glands, which are carried by blood or other body fluids to influence and control the pigs metabolism. There are nine main glands (Fig.1-4) in the pig which are responsible for controlling a variety of vital functions

Generally the diseases associated with the failure of the endocrine glands are not important in the pig. However when the regulatory and stimulatory mechanisms between the hypothalamus, the anterior pituitary gland and the ovaries fail, anoestrus (not coming on heat) or reproductive malfunction result, including cystic ovaries. In the male testicular function is affected. The hypothalamus stimulates the anterior part of the pituitary gland to release the follicle stimulating and luteinising hormones (FSH and LH). These in turn act upon the ovaries and the testes to regulate their function. (See chapter 5).

Terminology

Follicle stimulating hormone (FSH) - Produced by the anterior pituitary gland. It stimulates the formation of follicles in the ovaries,
Growth hormone - Responsible for promoting growth of most tissues throughout the body. It is produced by the pituitary gland in association with the hypothalamus.
Hypothalamus - An area in the brain responsible for providing both nervous and hormonal control over most other hormone producing glands.
Luteinising hormone (LH) - Stimulates ovulation and is produced by the pituitary gland.
Oestrogen - The female hormone responsible for all the female sexual characteristics. It is produced by the ovary.
Oxytocin - Produced by the pituitary gland. This stimulates uterine contractions during farrowing and causes milk let down. It also aids in the movement of sperms and eggs.
Progesterone - The hormone that maintains pregnancy. It is produced by the corpus luteum in the ovary.
Prolactin - This is produced by the pituitary gland and controls milk production.
Prostaglandins - These are produced by the uterus and the placenta and are associated with the initiation of farrowing or abortion.
Testosterone - The male hormone responsible for all the male sexual characteristics. It also controls the development of sperm.

Immune System

The various mechanisms that protect the pig from infectious agents can be considered in six groups:
- **Complement system** - This is a non specific protective mechanism that acts on any foreign cells or viruses that do not possess certain pig proteins on their surface. It consists of a number of chemicals found in the plasma which act together as a cascade to remove or destroy organisms.
- **Chemical factors** - These include non specific enzymes (such as lysozyme in saliva) and acids which may be found in mucus, saliva and gastric juices. These immobilise or kill pathogens.
- **Mechanical factors** - These include the skin, mucus, sweat, lining of the nose, mouth, oesophagus, intestine, colon, vagina, flow of urine and the passage of faeces.
- **Macrophage cells** - These are found throughout the body in tissues and in the blood stream where they are called monocytes. They engulf and digest bacteria. They also have an important role in controlling viral and fungal diseases. The cells are of two types called leucocytes and monocytes.
- **Specific acquired immunity** - This is of two types; that which is activated by cells and called cell mediated immunity and antibodies present in the blood called humoral immunity. Cell mediated immunity arises when T type lymphocytes come into contact with antigens and they are stimulated to produce antibodies. It takes 7-14 days for these to develop. Humoral immunity is produced from B lymphocytes which have met the antigen previously and their response is immediate. Some lymphocytes also kill other cells that contain antigens or they may act immediately against antigens.
- **Immunoglobulins** - Specific antibodies of which there are different types namely immunoglobulins, IgG, IgM and IgA. They are found in blood, in milk and particularly in colostrum. All internal surfaces of the body also contain them.

Certain infectious agents can suppress the immune system sufficiently to make the animal more susceptible to other infections. Examples are *Mycoplasma hyopneumoniae*, aujeszky's disease virus, pasteurella bacteria, swine influenza and porcine reproductive respiratory syndrome virus (PRRS) all of which cause pneumonia.

GLANDS AND HORMONE PRODUCTION	
Glands	Function
Adrenal	These are attached to the kidney surface. Their hormones control growth, sugar metabolism, kidney function and stress.
Hypothalamus	Found at the base of the brain. The main controlling gland. Its hormones control most body functions and all other glands, together with sexual activity.
Ovaries	Produce the female hormones oestrogen and progesterone.
Pancreas	Located in a fold of the duodenum. Produces insulin to control sugar metabolism.
Parathyroids	Located near the thyroid glands in the neck. Control calcium and phosphorus deposition.
Pituitary	Found at the base of the brain. Hormones control growth, reproduction, lactation and stress.
Placenta	Afterbirth membranes that cover the foetus. Maintains pregnancy and produce female hormone.
Testicles	Produce the male hormone testosterone.
Thyroid	Controls metabolism and growth.

(Fig.1-4)

Terminology

Adjuvant - A substance added to an inactivated vaccine to make it more effective.

Antibodies - Complex large proteins (called gamma-globulins) which are produced by specialised cells in response to invading antigens. These stick specifically to the invading antigen neutralising it or triggering off a destructive reaction.

Antigen - Foreign invading substance (i.e. a substance which is not normally part of the pig's body), usually consisting of protein or part of a protein, which stimulates the body to produce antibodies. Antigens exist on the surfaces of bacteria, viruses and parasites.

Antiserum - Serum with high antibody levels against a specific infection. It has usually been produced experimentally in laboratory animals by injecting the infection into them.

Blood sample - Whole blood sample taken hygienically with a syringe into a bottle or by a pin prick through the skin absorbing the droplet of blood with blotting paper.

Commensal bacteria - Bacteria that live permanently in or on the body without causing disease.

Epithelium - Cellular membrane (e.g. mucous membranes) containing epithelial and other cells.

Hyperimmune antiserum - The same as antiserum above but emphasising its high titre.

Lymphocytes - Specialised defence cells in lymph nodes, other lymphatic tissue and the blood which produce antibodies or take part in cellular immunity.

Mucous membranes - Cellular membranes (e.g. those lining the gut) which secrete a sticky substance called mucus on to their surfaces.

Mucus - A clear sticky semi-liquid secreted by cells in mucous membranes.

Pathogenic infection - An infectious organism which has the potential to cause disease. This is in contrast to the many organisms that live normally in or on the body which never cause disease and are called commensals.

Phagocytes - Cells of the body whose special task is to engulf bacteria, viruses, or parasites in an attempt to destroy them. They are also called macrophages.

Phagocytosis - The process whereby the specialised cells of the body engulf bacteria, viruses or parasites in an attempt to destroy them.

Plasma sample - A whole blood sample taken hygienically with a syringe and mixed with an anti-clotting agent so that it remains liquid. The sample is spun fast in a centrifuge and the red and white blood cells sediment to a firm pellet at the bottom leaving a clear liquid - the plasma.

Serology - Tests done in the laboratory to detect the level of specific antibodies in serum samples. ("ology" means study of - so literally serology means "study of serum").

Serum sample - A whole blood sample taken hygienically with a syringe and allowed to clot. The serum is the clear straw-coloured liquid which can be drawn off with a pipette. It contains the antibodies.

Titre - The concentration of a specific antibody in a serum sample. It is expressed as the amount by which the serum has to be diluted before a serological test goes negative.

Virulence - How pathogenic an organism is. Organisms with a high capability of causing disease are called highly virulent.

Muscular System

There are three types of muscle in the pig:

- **Involuntary or smooth muscle** - Found in the digestive and genital systems and the blood vessel walls.
- **Cardiac muscle** - The heart consists largely of this muscle. It is involuntary.
- **Voluntary or skeletal muscle** - This is the main muscle mass forming the muscular-skeletal system. These muscles are attached to the surface membrane covering bones called the periosteum. Inflammation of this covering is called periostitis.

Disease of the muscles in the pig are common and the symptoms seen depend upon which muscle groups are involved. The failure of muscle development may also be due to nerve or bone diseases. The common clinical signs include swelling, pain, wasting or trembling of the muscles. In some diseases there is death of muscle cells. Porcine stress syndrome (PSS) is a common heritable condition (recessive gene) associated with the sudden onset of prolonged muscle spasms which causes failure of the normal metabolism and the development of acid conditions throughout the body. It frequently ends in death.

Terminology

Asymmetric hind quarter syndrome - One hind leg muscle mass appears less than the other. It can arise where poor quality iron injections are given or it may be a congenital condition. It may be part of the porcine stress syndrome (PSS).

Back muscle necrosis - Sudden acute lameness and swellings of the lumber muscle often associated with PSS.

Congenital muscle hypertrophy - A breeding defect with excessive muscle formations.

Dark firm dry muscle (DFDM) - Describes the appearance of abnormal muscle at slaughter. Considered part of the PSS condition.

Mulberry heart disease (MHD) - Heart muscle failure associated with unavailability of vitamin E and or selenium.

Muscle necrosis - Dead muscle tissue. This can arise due to loss of blood supply caused by bacterial thrombosis (bacteria clogging up the blood vessels), physical damage or toxic damage. Iron toxicity, vitamin E or selenium deficiency are further examples.

Myodegeneration - Loss of function of muscle due to muscle fibres degenerating. Common problems are associated with deficiencies of vitamin E and or selenium.
Myopathy - This term describes any muscle disease.
Myositis - Inflammation of muscle often caused by trauma or infection.
Pale soft exudative muscle (PSE) - Describes the appearance of abnormal muscle at slaughter. Part of the PSS condition.
Pietrain creeper syndrome - Progressive muscle weakness in pigs from 3-12 weeks old. Considered to have a hereditary basis.
Porcine stress syndrome (PSS) - A heritable condition involving defective muscle metabolism.

Nervous System

The nervous system of the pig consists of four basic parts.

- **The brain** - The nervous tissue enclosed by the skull. Part of the central nervous system (CNS). It is covered completely by clear membranes called the meninges.
- **Spinal cord** - The other part of the CNS. It extends from the brain as a narrowed bore tube, through the spinal canal to the tail. Between each of the vertebra, which make up the spine itself, it sends branches out to different parts of the body. The spinal cord is responsible for transmitting the electrical impulses from the brain to these branches.
- **Peripheral nervous system** - Nerves leave the brain and the spinal cord and transmit the electrical impulses throughout the body. This system is the voluntary one that is under the pig's control.
- **Autonomic nervous system** - This is the involuntary nervous system of the pig with separate nerves controlling a wide range of involuntary functions. This system partly controls the heart beat, movement of the muscular walls of the digestive system, the hormonal systems and the excretory systems.

There are a number of important bacterial and viral diseases that cause clinical nervous signs in the pig. Such signs arise by infection of the brain, the brain covering, the spinal cord or any of the peripheral nerves.

Some common diseases associated with nervous signs include:

- African swine fever (ASF).
- Aujeszky's disease (AD) Pseudorabies (PR).
- Classical swine fever (CSF) - Hog cholera (HC).
- Congenital tremor - caused by an as yet unidentified virus (possibly a circovirus), swine fever or congenital defects.
- Haemagglutinating encephalomyelitis virus (HEV) infection.
- Iron toxicity.
- Middle ear infection.
- Oedema disease (bowel oedema).
- Poisons - Arsenic.
  Mercury.
  Monensin.
  Organophosphorus compounds.
- Salt - water deprivation
- Porcine stress syndrome (PSS).
- Splay leg - a disease of piglets at birth.
- Streptococcal meningitis (SM).
- Teschen or Talfan diseases.
- Tetanus.

Terminology

Cerebrospinal fluid - Fluid that circulates around within the brain and spinal cord. Samples of this fluid can be obtained by needle and syringe for laboratory tests to diagnose nervous disease.
Congenital tremor - A condition in newborn piglets characterised by muscle tremors and shaking. (See chapter 8).
Encephalitis - Inflammation of the brain.
Encephalomyelitis - Inflammation of the brain and spinal cord. Viruses multiplying in the central nervous system primarily cause encephalitis and encephalomyelitis although they may cause meningitis as well. Such viruses include aujeszky's (pseudorabies), rabies, teschen / talfan, haemagglutinating encephalitis (vomiting and wasting disease), classical swine fever, African swine fever, blue eye disease in Mexico, encephalomyocarditis in the US, Caribbean and some other countries, and Japanese B. encephalitis in S.E. Asia.
Meninges - Clear membranes covering the surface of the brain.
Meningitis - Inflammation of the meninges which is extremely painful and often results in dramatic clinical signs. Bacterial infections causing meningitis include *Streptococcus suis* (mainly type 2), salmonella, *Haemophilus parasuis*, *E. coli* and any bacteria gaining access to the meninges from a septicaemia. Viruses may also cause meningitis. Middle ear infection may be mistaken for meningitis.

Reproductive System

Fig.1-5 and Fig.1-6 show the anatomy of the reproductive tracts of the sow and the boar.

Terminology

Abortion - The production of a premature non-viable litter, 111 days or less after mating.
Agalactia - Failure of milk let down or shortage of milk or no milk. The udder may be congested with or without mastitis. In certain conditions, such as mild ergot poisoning, mammary glands fail to develop.
Cervix - The neck of the womb. Inflammation of the cervix is called cervicitis. Cervicitis is not common in the pig, but erosion of the thick folds occurs in old sows and can cause infertility.

Conception rate - As a % this is calculated by:

$$\frac{\text{No. of females which conceived}}{\text{No. of females mated or inseminated}} \times 100$$

The calculation is based on a given period of time. Often pig farmers calculate this over the same period of time for both. The top and bottom numbers should be calculated over equivalent periods of time so that the same sows are being counted.

The number conceived can be assessed by the number that did not return to heat or by the numbers judged to be pregnant at the first pregnancy test. Note that the conception rate is generally higher than the farrowing rate because of later embryo / foetus loss. Rolling one month, three month and six month averages of conception rates give an early indication of any developing infertility problems.

Conceptus - Fertilised ovum and embryo.
Corpora haemorrhagica - When the follicle ruptures to release the egg there is a small amount of haemorrhage. This is the name given to the bloody tissues that remain.
Corpus albucans - After pregnancy or after the animal has been in oestrus the corpus luteum disappears and shrinks to a small white body called the corpus albucans.
Corpus luteum - The corpora haemorrhagica becomes consolidated and forms the corpus luteum. This is the body that produces progesterone, the female hormone that maintains pregnancy.
Cryptorchid - A male pig whose testes have not descended through the inguinal canals. Normally, the testes develop in the abdomen and descend through the inguinal canal to the scrotum before birth. Sperm production in the testes require a cooler environment than that of the abdomen.
Embryo - The multicellular organism that develops in the uterus from the fertilised egg up to about 20-30 days when it becomes a foetus.
Endometritis - Inflammation and infection of the lining of the womb (the endometrium).
Epididymis - A coiled tube attached to the upper surface of the testicle where the sperm is stored. The sperm leaving it enters the vas deferens. It has a head and a tail. The tail can be cut off (epidectomy) to sterilise the boar. (See chapter 15).
Erythema - Reddening of the skin that is often seen when one or more mammary glands have mastitis.
Farrowing rate (%) This equals

$$\frac{\text{No. females farrowed}}{\text{No. females mated}} \times 100$$

Female - Breeding female including gilts and sows. A gilt becomes a breeding female either from an arbitrary time before mating (e.g. when first brought into the mating area) or, more commonly, when she is first mated. Some pig farmers only include her from the time she farrows but this results in high and less useful indications of herd fertility when farrowing rates and numbers of pigs per female per year are calculated.
N.B. Many people use the term pigs per sow per year but this must include gilts.
Fertilised ovum - The egg as it multiplies and grows to approximately day seven post fertilisation.
Foetus - This describes the developing piglet from approximately 30 days through to maturity.
Inguinal canal - Gap between the muscles of the abdomen in the groin through which the spermatic cord passes from the abdomen to the testicle.
Implantation - The attachment of the embryo to the uterine wall by establishment of the placenta commencing 12 to 14 days post-mating.
Inverted nipples - These are shown in Fig.1-7. If the teat sphincter cannot be seen at eye level it is likely that such a teat will remain inverted and will not be functional. This is important to appreciate when selecting or receiving a gilt for breeding. Some inverted nipples will become more normal and be functional when the mammary gland develops but when selecting you cannot take the chance.
Note that each teat has two orifices and teat ducts which drain two quite separate mammary glands, front (anterior) and back (posterior).
Irregular return - A return to oestrus more than 23 days after the previous one.
Lactation length - The period from farrowing to weaning in days.
Litters/per female/per year is calculated by:

$$\frac{\text{No. of farrowings over 3 months}}{\text{Average No. breeding females in the herd}} \times 4$$

In large herds this can also be calculated on rolling one month, three month and six month averages which gives a historical indication of rising or falling fertility. Thus for a three month average

$$\frac{\text{Average No. females in the herd over last 3 months}}{\text{Number of farrowings over last 3 months}} \times 4$$

Mammary oedema - Mammary tissues may contain excess amounts of fluid at farrowing. This fluid can either be under the skin when it can be easily seen and palpated, or deep in the actual tissue itself. Both these conditions can lead to agalactia, mastitis and poor availability of colostrum.
Mammary system - The udder of the sow consists of two parallel rows of 5 to 7 teats inter-spaced on each side.
Mastitis - Inflammation of the mammary gland is invariably associated with infection. Bacteria causing it include klebsiella, streptococci, staphylococci and *E. coli*.
Mastitis metritis agalactia syndrome (MMA) - This syndrome is most commonly associated with mastitis usually coliform mastitis i.e. caused by *E. coli* or klebsiella but it is also associated with endometritis. The sow is usually sick, running a high temperature and

producing little milk. Other terms are sometime used for this syndrome including periparturient hypogalactia syndrome, puerperal toxaemia, and farrowing fever.

Mating - The complete act of copulation involving one or more services.

Mummified pigs - Piglets which died in the uterus and in which the tissues and fluids have been reabsorbed leaving black shrunken skeletal remains.

Non productive days (NPD) - These include all the days when the sows and gilts are either not pregnant or suckling.

It therefore always includes:
- Entry of the gilt into the herd to point of mating.
- Time from weaning to mating.
- Time from mating to remating if the female is found not to be pregnant and returns to heat.
- Time after a female has been culled until the time it is slaughtered.

NPD is a useful calculation because if it lengthens it may indicate a number of serious problems, including increases in the fail-to-farrow females (not in pig at term - NIP), females dying during pregnancy, and gilts with delayed puberty.

Oestrus (or heat) - The period during which the sow is receptive to the boar (i.e. will stand to be mated). Usually 1-3 days.

Oestrus cycle - The period from one oestrus to another. 19-22 days interval is normal.

Orchitis - Inflammation of the testicle. A specific example is infection by *Brucella suis* bacteria. Non infectious orchitis can arise from trauma to one or both testicles. Occasionally there may be a haemorrhage developing into a haematoma (a pocket of blood).

Ovaries - Two small structures which control the oestrus cycle and from which the follicles are produced and the eggs released.

Oxytocin - A hormone produced by the anterior pituitary gland. Its function is to release milk from the glands and at the same time cause the uterus to contract.

Parity - Used to describe the number of times a female has farrowed.

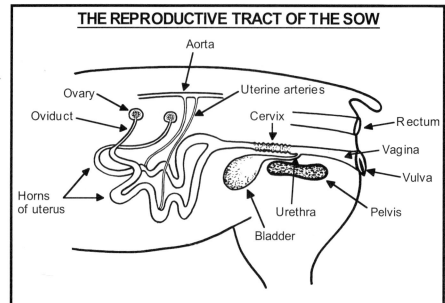

(Fig.1-5)

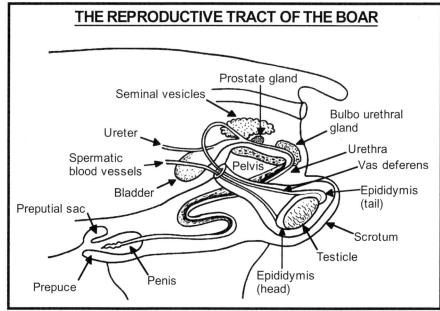

(Fig.1-6)

e.g. Pregnant gilt = Parity 0
Gilt farrowed for the first time = Parity 1
Sow which has had two litters = Parity 2

(NB. Some people get confused and use the term parity when they mean pregnancy).

Pigs weaned per sow per year - The number of pigs produced in any 12 month period. In a large herd this is usually calculated as a one month, three month and six month rolling average of the whole herd.

Prepucial sac - This is a sac inside the prepuce, the size of a golf ball, that contains a foul smelling fluid with a high bacterial content. Do not squeeze its contents into

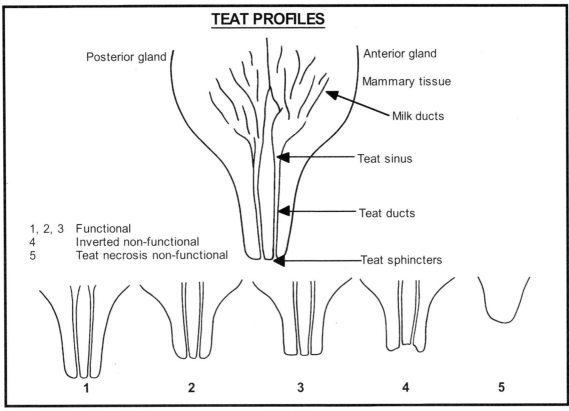

(Fig.1-7)

the vagina at service or you may precipitate an endometritis or cystitis and nephritis. Similarly if you are collecting semen by gloved hand for on-farm artificial insemination you must not contaminate it with prepucial sac contents.

Prolactin - A hormone from the pituitary gland involved in the initiation and maintenance of milk production.

Pyometra - Accumulation of pus in the womb following infection. It is also called pyometritis. This is common when heavy vulva discharges are seen or a retained foetus or placenta are present.

Regular return - A return to oestrus usually 19-22 days after previous one.

Salpingitis - Inflammation of the oviducts (fallopian tubes) that carry the eggs from the ovary down towards the womb.

Scrotum - This is a sack made of relatively thin pliable skin which has a muscular inner fibro-elastic layer which contracts in a cold environment and relaxes in a hot environment.

Seminal vesicles - These are glands which together with the prostate and bulbo-urethral glands provide fluid and nourishment for the sperm, the fluids being passed out during ejaculation.

Spermatic cord - Fibrous cord, containing the vas deferens and blood vessels, by which the testicles are suspended.

Stillborn pigs - Piglets observed dead behind the sow at birth.

Teat necrosis - Damage to the end of the teat can result in death and sloughing of tissues. This is called necrosis. It is caused by abrasive floor surfaces in the first 18-24 hours of birth and can be an important reason for rejecting gilts for breeding.

Testicle - The gland in which the sperm is produced.

Urethritis - inflammation of the urethra, the tube which carries both sperm and urine down the penis in the boar or urine from the bladder to the vagina in the sow. Urethritis is uncommon in the boar but can occasionally be caused by small calculi or stones formed in the kidneys. The urethra of the sow is much more likely to become contaminated and infected because its opening is so close to the vulva. Urethritis and cystitis are therefore common in the sow.

Uterus (womb) - Consists of two horns up to 1.5m in length that contain the foetuses.

Vagina - The passageway from the exterior to the cervix. Vaginitis (inflammation) occurs following trauma, infection or multiple matings.

Vas deferens - The muscular tube that at ejaculation propels the sperm from the tail of the epididymis on the testes up through the inguinal canal and into the urethra where it joins just below the neck of the bladder. Vasectomising a boar involves cutting the vas deferens

midway between the tail of the epididymis and its entry to the abdomen, removing 30-50mm of it. (See cptr 15).
Vulva - The vagina opens to the exterior through the fleshy lips of the vulva. Oedema of the vulva (swelling containing fluid) occurs in late pregnancy and trauma is very common in loose-housed sows. The tissues contain many blood vessels and are prone to haemorrhage. Haemorrhage (haematoma) is also seen in the gilt post farrowing. Such animals can bleed to death. (See chapter 15).

Respiratory System

The respiratory system of the pig commences at the nostrils which lead into two nasal passages. These contain the dorsal and ventral turbinate bones. (Fig.1-8). The ventral turbinates consist of four thin main bones, two on each side separated by a cartilaginous septum. You can imagine these as four hair curlers placed inside the nose. The respiratory tract is lined by a smooth membrane called a mucous membrane because it is bathed in a sticky mucus. It is also covered with minute hair like structures which are able to brush the mucus across the surface by their wavy motion. They move the mucus in the nose, bronchial tree and trachea to the throat where it is swallowed. The air breathed in through the nose is warmed by the turbinate bones which, because of their scroll-like shape, cause turbulence. This throws out the larger of the small particles so that they stick to the mucus and are swept to the throat. The many branches of the bronchi as they decrease in diameter have a similar effect on more minute particles. The mucus elevator then carries them to the throat. Only the vary smallest particles reach the alveoli where the alveolar macrophages engulf and remove them. Internally, the nasal passages open into the pharynx (throat) which is a common passage for food and air. The food is swallowed down the oesophagus and the air is sucked into the larynx at the back of the throat. The larynx (voice box) controls inspiration and expiration. It opens into the trachea which passes down into the chest where it divides into two bronchi. The bronchi branch into smaller bronchi and continue to branch gradually reducing in size to become bronchioles which terminate in very tiny air sacs called alveoli. Oxygen is passed from the alveoli into the blood stream and carbon dioxide is passed out. The lungs are divided into seven lobes as shown in Fig.1-8.

Terminology

Abscess - Area of pneumonia containing pus where the infection has been sealed off from the remainder of the lung tissue by a fibrous capsule.
Actinobacillus pleuropneumoniae - Originally called haemophilus. A bacterium that produces a severe haemorrhagic and necrotising pneumonia with pleurisy.
Alveolar macrophages - These cells which are located in the alveoli engulf bacteria and viruses. They are destroyed by some viruses e.g. the porcine respiratory reproductive syndrome (PRRS) virus.

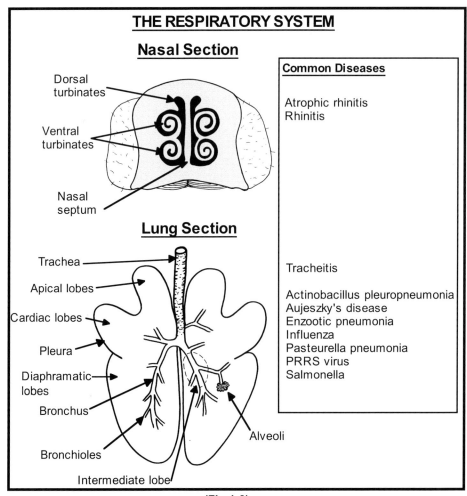

(Fig.1-8)

Atrophic rhinitis - Rhinitis caused by toxigenic (toxin producing) strains of *Pasteurella multocida*, in which the turbinates loses their tissues (atrophy) irreversibly. This is now called progressive atrophic rhinitis to distinguish it from non-progressive atrophic rhinitis caused by *Bordetella bronchiseptica* (with the addition of other organisms) and/or environmental contaminants, which is less severe and heals when the infection is stopped by the immune response.
Bronchitis - Inflammation of the bronchi or bronchioles in the lung.
Consolidating pneumonia - The lung tissue has collapsed and become solid. A common example is infection by *Mycoplasma hyopneumoniae* (enzootic pneumonia) which causes inflammation of the anterior lobes of the lungs.
Enzootic pneumonia - Also called mycoplasmal pneumonia. Caused by *Mycoplasma hyopneumoniae,* which produces a consolidating pneumonia of the lower parts of the anterior lobes of the lungs.
Glässers disease - Caused by *Haemophilus parasuis*. It can produce a severe pneumonia and consolidation with fibrinous pleurisy.
Lung worms - Small thread-like worms causing a parasitic pneumonia.
Necrotising pneumonia - Necrosis means death of tissue within the living animal. Necrotising pneumonia occurs where the organism or its toxins kill lung tissue. An abscess may result. A common example is pneumonia caused by *Actinobacillus pleuropneumoniae*.
Pasteurella - Bacteria found as normal inhabitants of the upper respiratory tract. They often cause secondary infections, for example, following *Mycoplasma hyopneumoniae* infection. There are two common species *P. haemolytica* and *P. multocidia* the latter being the common one in pigs.
Pleurisy - Also called pleuritis. The shiny membranes that cover the surface of the lungs and the inside of the chest wall are called the pleura. Infection or inflammation of these surfaces is called pleurisy. This together with pericarditis is very common in the pig and accounts for considerable loss through condemnation at slaughter. Viruses such as flu, PRRS, swine fever and the bacteria *Actinobacillus pleuropneumoniae*, *Haemophilus parasuis* and *Pasteurella multocidia* can cause pleurisy.
Pneumonia - Inflammation in any part of the lung tissue. There are different types of pneumonia.
Pyaemic pneumonia - Multiple small abscesses scattered through the lungs that have been carried there via the blood stream. A common example is pyaemia from tail biting. The carcase is condemned at slaughter.
Respiratory rate - This varies from 20-40 breaths per minute in piglets and growing pigs and 15-20 per minute in sows.
Rhinitis - Describes any form of inflammation to the delicate mucous lining of the nose. Some agents such as dust and gases may cause it but there is no long-term damage to the nose structure. Sneezing always occurs with rhinitis.
Salmonella choleraesuis - A bacterium specific to the pig causing generalised salmonellosis and pneumonia.
Swine influenza (SI) - A virus infection which produces clearly demarcated dark purple red lesions in the lungs.
Tracheitis - Inflammation of the trachea (windpipe). Influenza may cause a very heavy "barking" cough.
Turbinate bones - Dorsal and ventral. Scrolls of bone inside the nasal passages. They warm and filter air as it passes through the nose.

Sensory Systems

The pig, like the human, experiences sound, sight, smell, taste, heat, cold, pain and balance. The way it responds to these assists us in the recognition of health and disease. For example, pain together with posture will often indicate a specific disease such as fracture of the vertebrae in the spine. Poor balance may be associated with infections of the middle part of the ear which is common in the young growing pig. Likewise the stockpersons own senses, particularly sight, smell and touch, are important in assessing whether the pig is healthy or ill and performing to its maximum biological efficiency.

Sight for example allows the stockperson to observe the lying patterns, any abnormal excretions, signs of disease and unevenness of growth. It also helps to appreciate the quality of the environment.

Smell allows the stockperson to detect toxic gases, blocked drains, putrefying tissue and humidity, important points to consider in respiratory disease. He or she may also learn to detect the smell of scour.

Chapter 3 discusses in detail how you can use these senses to manage disease.

Skeletal System

The structure of a bone and joint are shown in Fig.1-9. A joint consists of the ends of two bones held together by ligaments and muscles, surrounded by a strong membrane and covered with smooth cartilage which form what are known as the articular surfaces. Cartilage is dense material that is shock absorbing. The two articular surfaces are surrounded by a thin membrane called the joint capsule, the inner part of which is secretory and produces the joint fluid (synovial fluid). The muscles and ligaments surrounding the joint are attached to the periosteum, the membrane which covers bone. Beneath the periosteum is the layer of compact bone that provides the strength of the structure. The centre is composed of a spongy mass containing marrow, from which many of the cells circulating in the blood are produced. Near the ends of the bones are flattened areas of cartilage running at right angles to the bone called the epiphyseal plates, which by increasing their thickness cause bones to grow in length and width. The separation of bones at these plates is a common occurrence in leg weakness or osteochondrosis, particularly in young growing animals.

Bone is continually being broken down and rebuilt even in adults who have stopped growing. Thus they are able to repair fractures and respond to pressures. The main pressures are from muscle tone and exercise. Pigs that are able to exercise are likely to have stronger bones and joints than those that can not. Thus sows kept in total individual confinement have softer more brittle bones than sows kept in pens, yards, or outdoors.

In contrast, the articular cartilage when damaged and eroded cannot repair itself and is replaced by less effective fibrous tissue. This process can be progressive.

Terminology

Adventitious bursa - A soft swelling containing fluid, resulting from a callous. Often found over the hock and elbow.
Apophyseolysis - Separation of the growth plate at the point of attachment of the main muscle mass on the back of the pelvis. It is commonly seen in the second parity female. The hind leg cannot be pulled backwards because the muscle attachment has been lost.
Arthritis - Inflammation of the joint. This can occur as a result of damage, but in the pig most cases are caused by infection resulting in increased synovial fluid, inflammation of the synovial membrane, sometimes erosion of the articular cartilage and sometimes the formation of pus. It is an extremely painful condition and makes the pig lame. Common infections causing this include *Mycoplasma hyosynoviae*, *Haemophilus parasuis*, streptococci, staphylococci, *Coryne bacterium* and *Erysipelothrix rhusiopathiae*.
Bush foot - Infection of the hoof and the bones in the foot. It arises from trauma and damage to the solar surface of the hoof. The claw is often swollen.
Bursa - A true bursa is a sac containing lubricating fluid but in pigs the term is often used to describe a fibrous lump beneath the skin covering bony prominences, caused by constant pressure.
Callous - An outgrowth of bone due to trauma to or irritation of the periosteum.
Chondrocytes - Cells found in cartilage. They form future bone.
Crepitus - The broken ends of bone rubbing together.
Epiphyseolysis - Separation of the epiphyseal or growth plate. It occurs as part of the leg weakness syndrome and fractures can occur for example, in the ball and socket joint of the femur. In young growing animals separation of the plates in the vertebrae in the spine can result in spinal paralysis.
Foot rot - Infection involving the soft tissues between the two claws.
Laminitis - Inflammation of the soft sensitive tissues inside the hoof.

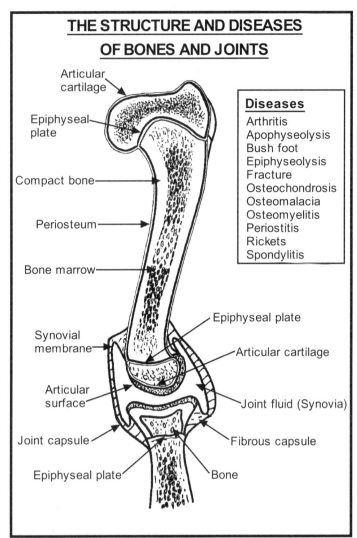

(Fig.1-9)

Leg weakness - A term used to describe conformation defects and abnormalities of gait in both fore and hind limbs. It is also used to describe osteochondrosis.
Osteomyelitis - Infection of the bone itself and the bone marrow in its spongy centre. It can occur after a septicaemia with organisms such as streptococci and erysipelas. It is often seen in the jaw bone after faulty teeth clipping.
Osteomalacia - This describes a softening of the bones and is caused by poor calcium and phosphorus deposition into the compact bone. This can be associated with the loss of these minerals during lactation or their unavailability in the diet.
Osteochondrosis (OCD) - This involves changes in the articular cartilage and the bone and it is very common. Most if not all modern pigs show such changes to bone structure at a microscopic level. Another term is leg weakness.
Periostitis - Inflammation of the periosteum. This is

extremely painful and can arise through trauma or occasionally infection. The most common causes are mechanical damage to knees in sucking pigs, swelling or leg calluses particularly on the hind legs, seen on many animals that are reared on concrete floors.
Rickets - Soft bones due to a shortage of phosphorus or deficiency of vitamin D.
Rig - Synonymous with cryptorchid - A boar in which one or more testicles have not descended into the scrotum.
Synovial fluid - Oily fluid in the joint.
Synovitis - Inflammation of tendon sheaths and joint capsules.
Tenosynovitis - Inflammation of tendons and tendon sheaths. Often caused by *Mycoplasma hyosynoviae*.

Urinary System

The kidneys are the organs in the body that filter out toxic and other waste materials from the bloodstream and maintain the body's fluid balance (Fig.1-10). Blood passes from the aorta into the kidney where it is filtered and returned back into the blood stream. The toxic products are then passed with fluid into the ureters which lead down to the bladder. Urine leaves the bladder via the urethra to the exterior.

Terminology

Calculi - These may be seen as powder like deposits on the vulva of sow or as small stones in the urine. They are due to the crystallisation of mineral deposits and are not usually of any clinical significance. They are particularly striking in the kidneys of piglets which have died of TGE or greasy pig disease and are exaggerated in mercury poisoning.
Cystitis - Inflammation usually due to infection of the lining of the bladder. The normal thickness of the bladder is approximately 10mm but in severe cases it may be up to 50mm. Haemorrhage often occurs and in such cases mortality in sows can be high.
Haematuria - Blood in urine. Always consider this as serious, a sign of severe cystitis / pyelonephritis.
Haemoglobinuria - Free haemoglobulin in the urine.
Nephritis - Inflammation of the kidney. It can be associated with several different bacteria that are transmitted either via the bloodstream (septicaemia) or reflux from the bladder. Bacteria or their toxins can damage the delicate filtering mechanism of the kidney. These include *Staphylococcus hyicus* (greasy pig disease), salmonella, streptococci and erysipelas. *Eubacterium suis* (*Corynebacterium suis*) is the commonest specific cause of ascending (i.e. reflux) nephritis and cystitis. Haemorrhage into the kidneys is common in the swine fevers. Fungal mycotoxins may also damage the kidneys but do not cause inflammation.
pH - Urine is normally slightly acid, pH5 to 6.6. (Neutral is pH7). After weaning however, urine becomes alkaline (>pH7) for up to 3 weeks. Sows with pH more

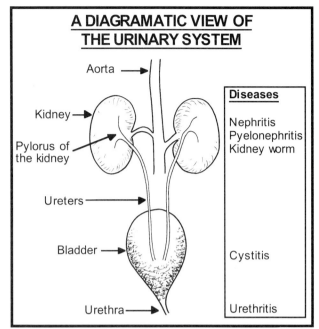

(Fig.1-10)

than 7.5 probably have pyelonephritis and mortality in such animals can be high particularly if it reaches a level of 8.
Proteinuria - Protein in the urine. Normal levels are 6-20mg/100 ml. Levels are elevated in kidney disease.
Pyelonephritis - The ureters arise from the cup-shaped pylorus or collecting area in the kidneys. Infection of this area together with the kidney is called pyelonephritis. It is a common disease in the sow. Bacteria associated with this include *E. coli,* streptococci and *Eubacterium suis* (*Corynebacterium suis*) the latter being the most common and important.
Pyuria - Pus in the urine.
Urethritis - Inflammation of the urethra.

18 Managing Pig Health and the Treatment of Disease

Chapter 1

2 Understanding Disease

Definition of health and disease...21
The causes of disease 21
Infectious agents 22
    Viruses...22
    Bacteria...24
    Fungi 26
    Parasites..27
Non infectious agents...27
    Trauma 27
    Hereditary and congenital defects (developmental abnormalities)...............28
    Nutritional deficiencies and excesses 28
    Poisons - toxic agents 29
    Stress...29
How infectious agents are spread...31
    Direct contact between pigs...31
    Disease dissemination by vehicles...32
    Spread of infection between different ages of pig within a farm...................33
    Environmental contamination on the farm..33
    Airborne transmission and other methods 34
    By people..37
    By pigs..38
    Maintaining freedom from disease - biosecurity 40
Selecting your source of breeding stock..40
Disinfection 44
The costs of disease..48
Depopulation and repopulation...50

Chapter 2

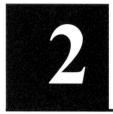

Understanding Disease

Definition of Health and Disease

The term "Health" means different things to different people. Absence of diseases is clearly a prerequisite but in pigs it means more than that. It is a state of physical and psychological well-beings that allows the pig to express its genetic potential for maximising productivity, reproductive performance and lean meat production.

> **The most important factor in preventing disease and maximising health and production is good husbandry**

The term "disease" means an unhealthy disorder of body and mind, sometimes with pain and unease, that is likely to prevent the pig from exploiting its genetic potential resulting in lowered productivity.

The level of clinical disease is described by the term morbidity.

Disease can be clinical (i.e. the affected pig shows clinical signs) or sub-clinical (the affected pig shows no obvious clinical signs). Sub-clinical disease can also have an adverse affect on productivity.

You should distinguish between sub-clinical disease and sub-clinical infection. Every healthy herd, without exception, carries a multitude of potentially pathogenic infections, mainly in the gut but also in the nose, throat, skin and genitals, which are not causing disease either clinical or sub-clinical.

There is a delicate balance between these potential pathogens and the pigs' immunity to them. Any physical or psychological disturbance of this immunity may render the pig susceptible.

Good husbandry, including good stockmanship aims to avoid such disturbances, provided the more virulent diseases are absent (e.g. atrophic rhinitis, TGE).

Good husbandry means good housing, good nutrition and good management.

Good stockmanship means care and attention to the pig's health and welfare.

This delicate balance between potential pathogens and the pigs immunity becomes even more precarious on a herd basis. By causing disease in small groups of pigs as a result of poor husbandry, the pathogenic organism multiplies up to a concentration that may overcome the more resistant pigs. The concentration again builds up and threatens to overwhelm the collective immunity of the herd (i.e. herd immunity).

The Causes of Disease

It is likely that when considering the causes of disease you think first of infectious micro-organisms. You would be right to do so in that infectious disease plays a much bigger role in pig herds, particularly large intensive pig herds, than in animals kept individually such as dogs and cats. Nevertheless there are other non-infectious causes of disease which may also be damaging to the herd and to productivity and profitability.

> **Most diseases in pig herds have multiple causes.**

Causes of disease are considered here under nine main headings:

Infectious agents
- Viruses
- Bacteria including
  - Chlamydia
  - Anaplasma
  - Mycoplasma
- Fungi
- Parasites

Non infectious agents
- Trauma
- Hereditary and congenital defects (developmental abnormalities)
- Nutritional deficiencies and excesses
- Toxic agents (poisons)
- Stress

There are other causes, such as tumours, which in pig herds are much less important and will not be dealt with here.

When you think of disease it is often only in terms of a single cause. In some cases this may be right (e.g. a poisoning or a highly virulent virus infection such as

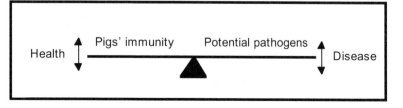

22   Managing Pig Health and the Treatment of Disease

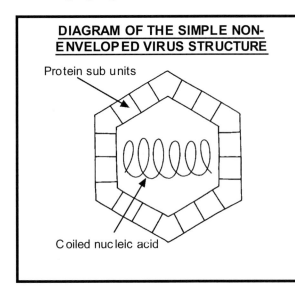
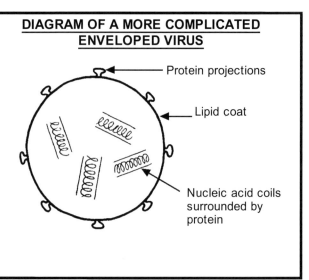

(Fig.2-1)

foot-and-mouth disease). In most cases you would be wrong however, because disease in pig herds usually results from the interplay between a number of predisposing, primary and contributory causes.

You should bear this in mind when you are thinking how to suppress disease.

Infectious Agents

VIRUSES

What are viruses?

Pathogenic organisms that infect pigs can be listed in order of decreasing size and complexity and viruses are the smallest of the infectious agents. They cannot be seen by the type of light microscope that is used for looking at bacteria. They can only be seen through an electron microscope.

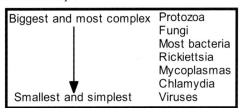

At their simplest they consist only of nucleic acid (i.e. their genes) and proteins which are arranged around the nucleic acid in a geometrical design and which protect the gene. (Fig.2-1). Some larger ones also have a loose outer coat (the envelope) which may contain lipids (fats) and carbohydrates which are derived from the hosts cell. They also contain proteins.

> *Viruses can only multiply inside the host cells.*
> *Viruses cannot multiply outside the host.*

Viruses contain a genetic code in the nucleic acid but they do not contain the full mechanisms for their own multiplication. They have no energy-generating systems and lack chemicals such as enzymes required for their own reproduction. They depend entirely on those of the host.

This is the first important point to be aware of. Outside the host viruses are inert. They have no metabolic activity. Inside the host's cell they behave like pirates. Their genes using the host's nucleus take over control of part or all of the cells mechanisms. They code these mechanisms to make many more viruses exactly like the ones that invaded. This activity usually damages or destroys the cells.

How do they get into cells?

The proteins on their surface stick specifically to receptors on the cells' surfaces. The cells then engulf them as if they were taking in particles of food but the particles are destructive invaders. They quickly loose their outer

DNA VIRUSES CAUSING DISEASES IN PIGS		
Family Name	Pig Diseases	Countries in Which They Occur
Adeno virus	Pneumonia	World-wide (?) but little known.
Circovirus	Congenital tremor (?)	World-wide (?) but little known.
Herpes virus	Aujeszky's disease(AD) - pseudorabies (PR) Cytomegalovirus: Inclusion body rhinitis	World-wide except Denmark, UK. World-wide
Iridovirus	African swine fever	Sardinia, Africa.
Papovirus	Genital papilloma	Little known.
Parvovirus	Porcine parvovirus	World-wide and very common.
Pox virus	Swine pox	World-wide but uncommon.

(Fig.2-2)

envelopes and the proteins covering their genes, which then take over from the cells nucleus and direct the cell to make more viruses. Some viruses (RNA viruses) replicate in the cytoplasm and some (DNA viruses) in the nucleus

The classification of a virus

All animal, plant and bacterial genes are made of a nucleic acid called DNA (deoxyribonucleic acid) which is found in the central nucleus of the cells and a further one RNA (ribonucleic acid) found in the cytoplasm. Virus genes however only contain one or the other.

The first broad classification is therefore into DNA viruses and RNA viruses. Fig.2-2 and Fig.2-3. These are then classified into families based on their shape, size and structure. N.B. No prion diseases (equivalent to BSE in cattle) are known to occur in pigs.

Fig.2-4 illustrates the approximate survival times of viruses that cause pig diseases. Some are extremely fragile and survive only a matter of days whereas others can persist for months. The survival times given are only approximate because in any virus they vary widely depending on the material it is on (faeces, salvia, blood, water, dust etc.), the temperature, the humidity, sunlight, and relative acidity. In general viruses survive long periods if frozen, fairly long periods in damp overcast cold weather, but only short periods in hot sunny dry weather. This is why virus diseases are more common in winter than summer. This information clearly is important in their control. Most but not all viruses are destroyed by strong acid or alkaline solutions and those that have a fat coating are quickly inactivated by fat solvents.

Some viruses can multiply sub-clinically in a pig for long periods of time (a carrier state) as in the case of aujeszky's (pseudorabies) disease and the cytomegalovirus that causes inclusion body rhinitis. Others can be carried sub-clinically for intermediate periods of 2 to 3 months such as PRRS but others such as TGE are usually eliminated after a week or two. However they may also persist in herds for long periods by successions of pigs post-weaning maintaining the infection.

Virus may be shed in saliva, urine, faeces, milk or in expired air from the lungs, or from vesicles on the skin.

The transmission may be by direct pig to pig contact, or indirect contact on farm machinery, pig trucks, or by vectors such as the wind, birds, flies, or discarded human pig meat products.

Viruses contain either DNA or RNA. Never both.

RNA VIRUSES CAUSING DISEASES IN PIGS

Family Name	Pig Diseases	Countries in Which They Occur
Arbovirus	Japanese B. encephalitis	S.E. Asia
Aterivirus	Porcine reproductive and respiratory syndrome (PRRS)	North America, Asia and Europe
Calicivirus	Vesicular exanthema	USA (eradicated by slaughter).
Cardiovirus	Encephalomyocarditis	Virus is world-wide, disease in North America and Caribbean mainly.
Coronavirus	Vomiting wasting disease (HEV). Porcine respiratory corona virus (PRCV) Transmissible gastro-enteritis (TGE) Porcine epidemic diarrhoea (PED)	World-wide Europe and North America. Everywhere except Ireland, Australia. Europe mainly.
Orthomyxovirus	Influenza	World-wide.
Paramyxovirus	Pneumonia Blue eye disease	World-wide ? (Little known). Mexico only.
Pestivirus	Classical swine fever	Germany, South America, Asia.
Picornavirus	Foot-and-mouth disease Teschen/Talfan disease SMEDI Swine vesicular disease	South America, Africa, Asia. World-wide. Asia, Italy. World-wide.
Reovirus	Rotavirus enteritis	World-wide.
Rhabdovirus	Rabies Vesicular stomatitis	World-wide except UK, Ireland, Australasia, North America.

(Fig.2-3)

APPROXIMATE SURVIVAL TIMES OF PIG VIRUSES OUTSIDE THE PIG AND THEIR POTENTIAL AIRBORNE TRANSMISSION.

Diseases Caused by Viruses	Approximate Survival Time in Favourable Conditions	Airborne Spread up to
African swine fever	18 months	N
Aujeszky's disease (pseudorabies)	14 days	4000m
Influenza	A few days	T
Foot-and-mouth disease	8 weeks	300km
Parvovirus	2 - 6 months	N
PRRS	4 days	4000m
SVD	3 months	N
Swine fever, hog cholera	2 months	N
TGE	3 weeks	N
Diseases Caused by Bacteria / Mycoplasma		
Actinobacillus pleuropneumonia	2 weeks	T
Anthrax	Indefinitely	N
Brucellosis	3 weeks	N
Cystitis (*E. suis*)	7 days	N
E. coli scour	6 months	N
Enzootic pneumonia	3 days	2000m
Erysipelas	Up to 8 weeks	N
Greasy pig disease (*Staphylococcus*)	3 weeks	N
Mastitis (*Klebsiella*)	4 weeks	N
Rhinitis - pasteurella	7 days	T
Salmonella	6 months	10m
Streptococcal meningitis	5 days	10m
Swine dysentery	8 weeks	N
Tuberculosis	2-3 years	10m
Arthritis (*Mycoplasma hyosynoviae*)	2 days?	10m

N = Not known to occur   T = Thought to occur but not proven

(Fig.2-4)

Clinical signs of disease

Viruses such as classical swine fever disseminate throughout the body and damage different organs thus producing a variety of clinical signs. Some such as TGE virus are more specific and disseminate sub-clinically initially to become concentrated in one or two target organs, which in this disease is the intestinal lining, causing diarrhoea. Some viruses can only multiply in one organ and swine influenza for example is generally only found in the lungs and respiratory tract.

Common pig viruses and their associated symptoms are shown in Fig.2-5.

The diseases marked by an asterisk (*) are the major ones that are notifiable in many countries and controlled by eradication policies. The diseases marked by a **T** are the most important at farm level.

Diagnosis of virus infections

It is more difficult and expensive to grow viruses than bacteria in the laboratory. They have to be grown in living cell-cultures artificially in tubes or bottles or in the living cells of embryos in hens eggs. Some cannot be grown by either of these methods. So until fairly recently virus diseases were diagnosed by their clinical signs and post-mortem lesions and confirmed by serology. Serology requires two blood samples to be taken from each animal 1 to 2 weeks apart so that rising antibody levels can be demonstrated. A single sample is less helpful because you do not know whether the antibody levels are rising from a recent infection or are persisting from an old infection.

Over recent years new techniques have speeded up and simplified laboratory diagnosis because the virus does not have to be cultured. The use of the electron microscope directly on to faeces or samples from lesions has assisted in diagnosis, further aided by the fluorescent antibody test (FAT) that again can be carried out directly on faeces or lesion samples. The ELISA test is now commonly used in many diseases (e.g. Foot-and-mouth disease) to provide a rapid accurate diagnosis. New techniques such as polymerise chain reactions (PCRs) have been developed to demonstrate the virus genetic material (i.e. the DNA or RNA) in samples, and such tests for PRRS virus are now available. Their advantage is that they can accurately detect tiny amounts of the DNA or RNA. Unfortunately they are expensive if done in small numbers.

Treatment

☐ Some new drugs are available for the treatment of a few viral infections in human beings but they are expensive and not available for use in pig diseases.

VIRUS DISEASES OF THE PIG AND MAIN CLINICAL SIGNS	L	D	R	N	I	M
* Aujeszky's disease (AD) - Pseudorabies (PR)			✓	✓	✓	
* Classical swine fever (CSF)	✓	✓	✓	✓	✓	
Congenital tremors (CT)				✓		
Cytomegalovirus			✓	✓		
Encephalo-myocarditis (EMC)				✓	✓	✓
Enterovirus (SMEDI)					✓	
* Foot-and-mouth disease (FMD)	✓		✓			✓
(T) Porcine epidemic diarrhoea (PED)		✓				
(T) Porcine parvovirus (PPV)					✓	
Porcine respiratory corona virus (PRCV)			✓			
(T) Porcine reproductive and respiratory syndrome (PRRS)			✓		✓	✓
(T) Rotavirus		✓				
(T) Swine influenza (SI)			✓		✓	
Swine pox						✓
* Swine vesicular disease (SVD)	✓					✓
(T) Transmissible gastro-enteritis (TGE)		✓				
Vomiting wasting disease				✓		

L = Lameness   D = Diarrhoea   R = Respiratory   N = Nervous
I = Infertility   M = Miscellaneous (Urinary, Mastitis, Skin, heart etc.)
* Notifiable in most countries.   T = Important at farm level.

(Fig.2-5)

> **Remember**
> *antibiotics have no effect on viruses only on the secondary bacteria.*

Since viruses have no cell wall and no metabolism of their own antibiotics will not destroy them, although they may help by preventing secondary bacterial infection. Hyper-immune antiserum might be helpful in some virus infections if given by injection, but in general they are not commercially available.

BACTERIA

Grouped under this heading are chlamydia, mycoplasma and other bacteria generally.

CHLAMYDIA

These and anaplasma used to be classified separately from bacteria but are now regarded as bacteria. Chlamydia are the first of the very small bacteria that live inside or on the surface of a host cell and they like viruses are obligatory parasites. They are relatively unimportant in the pig but can be associated with respiratory disease, heart sac infection and in the case of *Eperythrozoon suis*, anaemia and infertility. They are also associated with jaundice and poor growth although the bacteria can also be commensal parasites, in which case they cause little if any problems. Chlamydia can also cause abortion and may be responsible for a new emerging disease. In the pig they are mostly respiratory spread or in the case of

Eperythrozoon suis by biting insects or inoculation. Eperythrozoonosis can be diagnosed from blood smears examined under the microscope or more recently by PCRs.

MYCOPLASMA

Mycoplasma are very tiny organisms less than half the size of other small bacteria. (See Fig.2-6). They can only just be seen under a high power light microscope. They tend to live and multiply close to the surface of cells. They are respiratory spread and are mainly responsible for enzootic pneumonia (*Mycoplasma hyopneumoniae*), and mycoplasmal arthritis associated with joint infections (*Mycoplasma hyosynoviae*).

Mycoplasma can be grown on solid media; however, this is not easy and can only be done reliably in a few diagnostic laboratories. It is time consuming and often the identification of one strain is complicated by the presence of other strains. Few laboratories are able to identify them in smears under the microscope but PCRs are now becoming available.

Mycoplasma hyopneumoniae is found in the respiratory tract of pigs and survives for only a few hours outside the pig. New herds can be established free of this particular organism. Then the main method of reintroduction of the disease is through the purchased carrier pig or by windborne spread from a nearby herd or a vehicle carrying pigs. Two other less important mycoplasma are *Mycoplasma hyorhinis* and *Mycoplasma flocculare*. The former can affect the smooth membranes that cover the joints causing lameness, arthritis and pericarditis (inflammation of the heart sac). *Mycoplasma flocculare* causes small lesions that may be mistaken for enzootic pneumonia. It is often involved in pneumonia complexes.

OTHER BACTERIA

These can be readily seen under the microscope, particularly when they are stained. They are recognised by family group according to their shape, size, biochemical characteristics, antigenic characteristics and recently by identification of their DNA.

Most pathogenic bacteria can be grown easily in nutrient liquids and on solid media containing nutrients set in agar gel. Most grow profusely within 24 to 48 hours, although some such as the tuberculosis bacillus can take up to 3 weeks or more. They form little colonies consisting of billions of organisms and the shape and colour of these may be characteristic for a particular family or specific bacteria. A tiny smear from a colony spread on a glass slide and stained will give both the shape and the staining reaction of that particular bacteria. The stain commonly used is called a gram stain, and bacteria either stain positive (purple), or negative (red). This stain is of great help in carrying out primary observations. For example, the bacterium that causes meningitis in pigs, called *Streptococcus suis* type 2 is a small round organism in pairs or short chains that always stains positive or purple. Figs.2-7 and 2-8 show the different gram +ve and gram -ve bacteria and the diseases they cause.

Each bacterium has a number of specific characteristics that are peculiar to itself. Some, for example *An-*

RELATIVE SIZES OF THE INFECTIOUS AGENTS		
	Can be Seen	Approximate Size
Viruses	Electron microscope only	20-300 nm
Chlamydia	High power microscope	0.3 - 1 µ.m
Anaplasma	High power microscope	0.2 - 0.4 µ.m.
Mycoplasma	High power microscope	0.5 µ.m
Bacteria	High power microscope	0.5 - 30 µ.m
Fungi	Low power microscope	5 - 80 µ.m
Protozoa	Low power microscope	6 - 12 µ.m
Internal parasites	Low power microscope	5 - 350 mm
Mange	Low power microscope	0.5 mm
Lice	By eye	4 mm

1 metre = 100 cm = 1000mm
10^{-2} or $1/100$ metre = 1 centimetre (cm)
10^{-3} or $1/1000$ metre = 1 millimetre (mm)
10^{-6} or $1/1,000,000$ metre = 1 micrometre (µm or mcm)
10^{-9} or 1 billionth * metre = 1 nanometre (nm)
This gives you an idea of the actual size.
* Billion here - 1,000,000,000

(Fig.2-6)

GRAM NEGATIVE BACTERIA AND DISEASES	
Causal Bacterium	Pig Diseases
Actinobacillus pleuropneumoniae	Severe necrotic haemorrhagic pneumonia in growing pigs.
Actinobacillus suis and *equuli*	Focal pneumonia in piglets.
Bordetella bronchiseptica	Mild reversible atrophic rhinitis.
Brucella suis	Abortion Arthritis Boar infertility
Campylobacter coli, jejunum, hyointestinalis	Mild diarrhoea in piglets.
Escherichia coli (E. coli)	Piglet septicaemia and scour Post-weaning diarrhoea Oedema disease Mastitis and cystitis in sows
Haemophilus parasuis	Glässers disease
Klebsiella species	Mastitis
Lawsonia intracellularis	Porcine enteropathy (PIA, PHE, NE, RI)
Leptospira pomona	Infertility Stillbirths Weak piglets
Leptospira bratislava / muenchen	Infertility Vaginal discharge
Leptospira icterohaemorrhagiae	Haemorrhage Jaundice
Pasteurella multocida (toxigenic)	Atrophic rhinitis (progressive)
Pasteurella multocida (non-toxigenic)	Pneumonia (secondary, opportunist)
Salmonella choleraesuis	Generalised disease with pneumonia, diarrhoea and fever
Salmonella typhimurium, derby and others	Diarrhoea
Serpulina pilosicoli	Colitis
Serpulina hyodysenteriae	Swine dysentery
Serpulina (weak haemolytic sp)	Spirochaetal diarrhoea
Yersinia species	Diarrhoea

(Fig.2-7)

thrax bacillus, form spores which can survive outside the pig for many years. Organisms such as *E. coli* and salmonella can remain viable outside the pig for up to six months but *Mycoplasma hyopneumoniae*, the cause of enzootic pneumonia, probably for no longer than a few hours. Like viruses the survival of bacteria is also dependent upon the material surrounding them (faeces, soil, pus, urine, blood etc.), temperature, moisture and exposure to ultra-violet light. Again like viruses, they can survive indefinitely when frozen and for long periods in cold damp dark weather but only for a short time in very sunny weather. Such knowledge is important in controlling the spread of the disease.

Bacteria like viruses may attack specific parts of the anatomy or an individual system. For example, *Actinobacillus pleuropneumoniae* infects the pleura (smooth surface covering the lungs) and the lung tissue beneath. *E. coli* or salmonella invade the small intestine setting up an enteritis but *Salmonella choleraesuis*, the host adapted serotype of pig salmonellae, can affect the whole of the body including the lungs causing pneumonia.

Most bacterial diseases are characterised by specific clinical signs and these are shown in Fig.2-9. The common routes of bacterial spread are by direct contact, close respiratory droplet contact, infected faeces or mechanical transfer on shovels, boots, vehicles etc. You will see in Fig.2-17 some of the distances recorded in the field when disease did not transfer between one farm and another. They can be surprisingly small. For depopulation and re-population purposes however, those diseases with an airborne transmission of less than 230m should, in practice, be extended to at least 900m.

> ***Freezing prolongs the survival of infectious agents and sunlight and drying kills them.***

FUNGI

See chapter 13 for further information.

Fungi (moulds and yeasts) are found in damp conditions such as in badly stored cereals. In the process of multiplication some species produce poisons (mycotoxins) which when eaten, are capable of causing a variety of clinical signs. The more important mycotoxic diseases are shown in Fig.2-10.

The following factors are important on the farm to prevent fungi multiplying and producing toxins.
- Do not store moist corn or cereals
- Do not allow grain to ferment
- Examine feed hoppers daily.
- Treat grain bins regularly.
- Check holding bins for leakages and bridged feed

GRAM POSITIVE BACTERIA AND DISEASES	
Causal Bacteria	Pig Disease
Actinomyces (Corynebacterium) pyogenes	Abscesses and prevalent lesions.
Bacillus anthracis	Anthrax
Brucella suis	Brucellosis
Chlamydia psittaci	Abortion
Clostridium novyi	Acute hepatitis Sudden death
Clostridium perfringens	Piglet dysentery
Clostridium tetani	Tetanus
Corynebacterium (Eubacterium) suis	Cystitis/nephritis
Eperythrozoon suis	Anaemia Eperythrozoonosis Infertility Poor growth
Erysipelothrix rhusiopathiae	Erysipelas
Listeria monocytogenes	Abortions Encephalitis Septicaemia
Mycobacterium avium / intracellulare	Regressive tuberculosis
Mycoplasma hyopneumoniae	Enzootic pneumonia
Mycoplasma flocculare	Mild pneumonia (small lesions)
Mycoplasma hyorhinis	Secondary pneumonias
Mycoplasma hyosynoviae	Arthritis
Staphylococcus hyicus	Exudative epidermitis (greasy pig)
Other Staphylococci	Abscesses Mastitis
Streptococcus suis type 1	Arthritis and meningitis in piglets.
Streptococcus suis type 2, type 15	Meningitis in weaners and growers.
Streptococcus suis type 7	Arthritis Heart lesions
Streptococcus other types	Various

(Fig.2-8)

COMMON BACTERIAL DISEASES AND MAIN CLINICAL SIGNS					
Diseases	L	D	R	N	I	M
Actinobacillus pleuropneumonia			✓			
Anthrax		✓				✓
Atrophic rhinitis			✓			
Bordetellosis			✓			
Brucellosis	✓				✓	
Clostridial dysentery (piglets)		✓				✓
Cystitis / nephritis						✓
Eperythrozoonosis					✓	✓
Erysipelas (growing pigs)	✓				✓	✓
E. coli enteritis (piglets and weaners)		✓				
Enzootic pneumonia (mycoplasma)			✓			
Exudative epidermitis, greasy pig						✓
Glässers disease (polyserositis)	✓		✓	✓		
Leptospirosis					✓	
Mycoplasma arthritis (gilts)	✓					
Oedema disease (E. coli)				✓		
Pasteurellosis			✓			
Porcine enteropathy (PIA, PHE, NE, RI)		✓				
Salmonellosis		✓	✓	✓	✓	✓
Spirochaetal diarrhoea		✓				
Streptococcal infections	✓		✓	✓		
Sudden death in sows (clostridia)						✓
Swine dysentery		✓				
Tetanus				✓		
Tuberculosis						✓

L = Lameness   D = Diarrhoea   R = Respiratory   N = Nervous
I = Infertility   M = Miscellaneous (Urinary, Mastitis, Skin, Heart, Sudden death etc.)

(Fig.2-9)

monthly.
- Do not allow feed to waste and ferment in feed troughs.
- Always examine your basic feed ingredients.
- Visually check the final feed prior to feeding.

Several different species of fungi (called dermatophytes) infect the skin of the pig and cause ringworm. Ringworm is uncommon, although is a little more common in outdoor pigs than indoor pigs. It does no harm to pigs who seem unaware of it. It resolves spontaneously after a month or two and is unimportant. Occasionally fungi also cause abortion or mastitis in an individual pig but this is uncommon and no overall importance.

PARASITES
See chapter 11 for further information.

Parasites are organisms that either live in the body (internal parasites or endoparasites) or externally on or in the skin (ectoparasites). The smallest of the pathogenic parasites coccidia, are found in the intestine. They invade and live in the lining of the small intestine. The major parasites of the pig are listed in Fig.2-11.

Parasites unlike bacteria have a life cycle which is the process of development from the egg through larval stages and finally to the adult. Some parasites require an intermediate host, for example the earth worm is the intermediate host in the life cycle of the lung worm. This type of cycle is called an indirect one. A knowledge of the life cycle is important in preventing diseases. The most effective and cheapest way of controlling parasites is to break the cycle either by good hygiene or by removing the intermediate host if there is one.

Non Infectious Agents

TRAUMA

Trauma can be a major cause of disease on a pig farm and the common types of traumatic disease are shown in Fig.2-12. These are conditions that you will see constantly around pig farms. Most are preventable by good management and are dealt with in more detail in other chapters under the specific disease.

A GUIDE TO MYCOTOXIN LEVELS IN FEED: MILD TO ACUTE DISEASE				
Fungus	Toxins	No Clinical Effect	Toxic Level	Clinical Symptoms
Aspergillus sp	Aflatoxins	< 100ppb	300 - 2000ppb	Poor growth Liver damage Jaundice Immunosuppression
Aspergillus sp and Penicillium sp	Ochratoxin and Citrinin	< 100ppb	200 - 4000ppb	Reduced growth Thirst Kidney damage
Fusarium sp	T2 DAS DON (Vomitoxin)	< 2ppm	4 - 20ppm	Reduced feed intake Immuno-suppression Vomiting
Fusarium sp	Zearalenone (F2 toxin)	< 0.05ppm	1 - 30ppm	Infertility Anoestrus Rectal prolapse Pseudo pregnancy
			< 30ppm	Early embryo mortality Delayed repeat matings
Fusarium sp	Fumonisin	< 10ppm	20 - 175	Reduced feed intake Respiratory symptoms Fluid in lungs Abortion
Ergot	Ergotoxin	< 0.05%	0.1-1.0% Ergot bodies by weight (sclerotium)	Reduced feed intake. Gangrene of the extremities. Agalactia due to mammary gland failure.

ppm - parts per million **ppb** - parts per billion.
sp - species - each of these fungi have several species only some of which are toxic

(Fig.2-10)

THE COMMON PARASITES OF THE PIG AND SITES OF INFECTION		
Parasite	Site	Clinical Signs
Coccidia	Small intestine	10 day old scour
Demodectic mange	Skin	Rash Small nodules
Kidney worm (*Stephanurus dentatus*) (Southern USA and S. America. Not Europe)	Kidney	Wasting Blood in urine
Large roundworm (Ascaris)	Small intestine	Liver damage Reduced performance
Lice	Skin	Evident on the skin especially behind the ears but no lesions.
Flies - House fly, Black fly Stable fly, Blow fly Horse fly Screwworm fly		Skin lesions Small papules
Lung worm (*Metastrongylus*)	Lungs	Coughing Pneumonia
Nodular worm (*Oesophagostomum*)	Large intestine	Reduced performance
Red worm (*Hyostrongylus rubidius*)	Stomach	Emaciation Anaemia
Sarcoptic mange	Skin	Irritation; skin rash Thickened skin
Threadworm (*Strongyloides ransomi*)	Small intestine	Diarrhoea
Ticks	Skin	Evident but no lesions
Toxoplasma	Muscle	Abortion
Trichinella spiralis (uncommon)	Muscle	Very uncommon. Found at meat inspection
Whip worm (*Trichuris suis*)	Large intestine	Diarrhoea Dehydration

(Fig.2-11)

Good management reduces traumatic diseases.

HEREDITARY AND CONGENITAL DEFECTS
(DEVELOPMENTAL ABNORMALITIES)

Hereditary (genetic) and congenital diseases are quite common in swine and cover a range of conditions. The term "Hereditary" means that the condition was inherited by the piglet from the sow's or boar's genes. The term "Congenital" means "present at birth" but implies it is a development abnormality that occurred during the growth of the foetus while in the uterus, rather than an hereditary defect or abnormality. However some developmental abnormalities are not evident at birth, (for example, an inguinal hernia) and develop at a later stage. They are described as delayed developmental abnormalities. If a congenital defect occurs frequently and is related to a particular line or breed then it is likely to be hereditary.

> *Not all congenital defects are heritable.*

Most hereditary or congenital defects remain at a low incidence because breeding programmes cull affected animals. Sometimes however, a boar can be identified as being associated with a higher incidence of an abnormality than usual. A typical example would be umbilical hernia. (This condition can also be precipitated by abdominal pressure).

Embryo mortality varies considerably both between breeds and individuals and heredity plays an important but as yet ill-defined part. In most herds, records show that congenital malformations range from 0.5 to 2.5% with an average of approximately 1.5%. However, if all the defects were recorded then levels would approach 3%. Common developmental defects are described in Fig.2-13, the causes of which are often multifactorial in origin.

Another type of problem that occurs at birth is difficulty in farrowing associated with a small or abnormal development of the pelvis.

NUTRITIONAL DEFICIENCIES AND EXCESSES

See Chapter 14 for further information.

Current knowledge on the nutritional requirements of swine and the components of the different dietary ingredients have reduced significantly the problems associated with faulty nutrition. Deficiencies in the diet however do still occur from time to time and can be consid-

TRAUMATIC DISEASES

	Condition	Contact source
Piglets	Bush foot	Trauma by sows foot. Perforated metal slats.
	Face necrosis	Piglet teeth (fighting). Teeth clippers (poor technique).
	Fractured limbs	Sow trauma. Housing defects.
	Greasy pig disease	Faulty clippers or technique. Teeth damage (fighting).
	Joint infections	Floor pressure / De-tailing.
	Knee necrosis	Concrete - rough surfaces.
	Skin damage	From trauma by the sow.
	Tail necrosis	Concrete - rough surfaces.
	Teat necrosis	Any floor surface. Occurs within 48 hrs of birth. Oedema of teats.
Weaners	Greasy pig disease Pig pox	Infection triggered off by fighting and skin trauma.
Feeders	Bursitis	Floor surfaces.
	Bush foot	Poor concrete surfaces.
	Contact sores	Poor wet floor surfaces.
	Ear chewing	Other pigs.
	Flank suckling	Other pigs.
	Fractured limbs	Trauma by another pig. Housing defects.
	Greasy pig disease	Infection triggered off by fighting and skin trauma.
	Skin damage	Fighting.
	Tail biting	Other pigs.
Breeding stock	Bursitis	Floor trauma. Poor slat.
	Bush foot	Poor floor surfaces.
	Haematoma	Damage. Bruising.
	Leg weakness or Osteochondrosis	Sheer stresses on growth plates. Slippery floors.
	Long bone or pelvic fracture	Fighting. Trauma at service.
	Shoulder sores	Floor surface contact pressure.
	Skin abscess	Fighting.
	Vulval biting	Other sows.

(Fig.2-12)

COMMON DEVELOPMENTAL DEFECTS

Condition	Possible Cause	Comments
Bent legs	Unknown	Possibly exposure mid pregnancy to toxic agents.
	Heritable	Auto recessive gene.
	Poisons	Hemlock Black cherry
	Vitamin A	Excess dietary levels or by injection.
Congenital tremor	Swine fever virus	Type AI
	Unidentified virus (possibly circovirus)	Type AII
	Sex linked in male Landrace	Type AIII
	Recessive gene in the Saddleback	Type AIV
	Trichlorvon or Neguvon poisoning	Type AV
	Aujeszky's virus (pseudorabies)	Demonstration of virus to diagnose.
	Organophosphorus poisoning	Overdosing
Inguinal hernia	Heritable	Method unknown Environmental influences
Naval bleeding	Unknown	Associated with shavings
No rectum	Heritable	Environmental influences
Splay leg	Heritable	Common in the Landrace
	Fusarium toxin	Mouldy feeds
Umbilical hernia	Heritable	Environmental influences.

(Fig.2-13)

CHAPTER 2 - Understanding Disease

ered from four aspects: energy, protein, vitamins and minerals. Whereas most problems arise due to deficiencies, diseases can also occur due to excesses. The clinical signs of both are shown in Fig.2-14 and Fig.2-15. A consistent feature of vitamin deficiencies is poor growth but this can also be associated with many other factors.

If there is a problem in your herd I would refer you to the section in chapter 9 on the differential diagnosis of poor growth in weaner and feeder pigs under "Managing the Growing Pig....".

Mineral deficiencies are not uncommon today, particularly where the demands of lactation in the modern rapidly growing genotypes are difficult to satisfy

POISONS - TOXIC AGENTS
See chapter 13 for further information.

Poisoning by a variety of agents is still not uncommon in pigs today although less so than when herds were small and less intensive. Many substances if taken at excessive levels become toxic and cause disease.

Poisoning can occur in an individual pig or in a group or even affect a whole herd. In the latter two cases a number of animals will be affected at the same time all showing similar clinical signs. A study of the history may indicate a common exposure to the poison by contact or ingestion.

If fed to excess many dietary components including minerals and vitamins, can cause diseases. Many medicines are highly toxic if used above their therapeutic levels.

It is a common fault with stock people when treating animals to assume that twice the dose will act twice as well. This is a fallacy. Overdosing may well have the opposite effect.

Examples of common substances that may cause poisoning
- Antibacterial drugs - carbadox, furazolidone, monensin, sulphadimidine.
- Trace elements e.g. iron, copper, zinc, iodine, selenium, arsenic, mercury, lead, fluorine.

MINERALS. CLINICAL SIGNS OF DEFICIENCIES AND EXCESSES		
Mineral	Signs of Deficiency	Signs of Excess
Calcium	Agalactia Depressed milk yield * Fractures * Hypocalcaemia Osteomalacia * Osteoporosis * Posterior paralysis in sows * Rickets	Changes in bone formation If zinc is low (parakeratosis) more than 1% may cause problems. Reduced strength of bone
Copper	Leg weakness Loose faeces if suddenly withdrawn	* Jaundice 200 - 600g/tonne Haemorrhage Death
Iodine	Enlarged thyroid glands Reproductive failure Weak hairless pigs at birth	Rare > 800mg/kg
Iron	* Anaemia * Increased respiration More prone to piglet diseases Poor growth Pale skin	Death in piglets deficient in vitamin E Muscle degeneration > 5000 mg/kg
Magnesium	Infertility Rare Poor growth Weak joints	Loose faeces > 0.5% in diet.
Manganese	Infertility Rare Lameness Poor growth Weak piglets	Inappetance > 2000ppm
Phosphorus	Poor growth * Rickets See calcium also Soft bones	Changes in bone formation. Posterior paralysis in sows.
Potassium	Anorexia Rare Heart malfunction Incoordination Poor growth	Loose faeces > 1.2% in diet.
Salt (Sodium chloride)	Low water intake Poor growth and feed efficiency Unthriftiness	* Common Any level if water is short Death > 2 - 8% if water short Fits Incoordination Thirst
Selenium	* Mulberry heart disease Muscle changes Sudden mortality	Diarrhoea Feet deformity Lameness Respiratory distress Sudden death 5 - 10g/tonne
Water	* All systems affected Failure to thrive Predisposition to disease	Colic
Zinc	* Dry thick skin (parakeratosis) Poor appetite	Reduced feed intake > 3000g/tonne Up to 2500g/tonne in diet none.

* Likely to occur. Others uncommon or rare

(Fig.2-14)

- Coal tars.
- Gases - ammonia, carbon monoxide, hydrogen sulphide.
- Insecticides - organophosphorus, carbamates, lindane, dieldrin.
- Nutrients: essential minerals - copper, iodine, iron, manganese, selenium, zinc.
- Rat poison - warfarin
- Salt - if water is limited
- Toxic plants.

STRESS

Stress is a condition which occurs in all pigs when confronted with adverse management and environments. Better management of the environment has a beneficial effect on the health and the biological efficiency of the pig.

NUTRIENTS AND VITAMINS. CLINICAL SIGNS OF DEFICIENCIES AND EXCESSES		
Nutrient	**Signs of Deficiency**	**Signs of Excess**
Amino Acids	A predisposition to disease. Poor growth.	Digestive disturbances.
Biotin	Infertility. Anoestrus. Lameness *. Poor hoof quality *.	Unknown. Unlikely.
Choline	Poor litter size. Poor growth.	Unknown. Unlikely.
Cyanocobalamin (B_{12})	Poor growth. Infertility. Anaemia.	Unknown. Unlikely.
Energy *	Infertility *. Loss in weight. Poor fat deposition. Predisposition to: Cystitis pyelonephritis *. Post-weaning enteritis *. Respiratory disease *. Villus atrophy and malabsorption *. Thin sow syndrome *.	Deposition of excess fat.
Fat and fatty acids * (Linoleic)	Dry skin on sows and piglets. Loss of weight in lactation. Poor growth.	Colitis. Digestive disturbances. Loose faeces.
Folic Acid	Anaemia. Poor litter size. Poor growth.	Unknown. Unlikely.
Nicotinamide (Niacin)	Diarrhoea. Dermatitis. Poor growth. Paralysis.	Unknown. Unlikely.
Pantothenic Acid (B_5)	Poor appetite and growth. Goose-stepping gait. Diarrhoea.	Unknown. Unlikely.
Protein *	Lean tissue gain reduced. Poor growth. More prone to disease.	Diarrhoea.
Pyridoxine (B_6)	Poor growth.	Unknown.
Riboflavin (B2)	Infertility. Weak piglets.	Unknown. Unlikely.
Thiamine (B1)	Poor appetite and growth. Sudden death.	Unknown. Unlikely.
Vitamin A	Rare but reports of: Infertility. Incoordination. Poor bone growth. Poor sight. Congenital defects, born blind.	* Epiphyseal plate changes. * Increased incidence of OCD. * Increased requirements for vitamin E. Joint pain. * Leg weakness. * Mulberry heart disease.
Vitamin D_3	Fractures. Lameness. Rickets. Rubbery bones or osteomalacia. Swollen joints.	Calcification of soft tissues.
Vitamin E * (Mulberry Heart Disease)	Agalactia. Discoloration of fat. Gastric ulcers *. Liver, heart and muscle changes *. MMA syndrome. Oedema disease. Porcine stress syndrome. Predisposition to: App. E. coli diarrhoea. Respiratory disease. Swine dysentery. Reduced immune responses *. Sudden death. Udder oedema.	
Vitamin K	Enhances warfarin poisoning. Poor blood clotting.	Unknown. Unlikely.

* Likely to occur. Others uncommon or rare.

(Fig.2-15)

What does the pig do when stressed?

- It increases the leucocytes in the blood.
- It increases output of hormones (cortisol) from the adrenal gland and this depresses immunity.
- It becomes more susceptible to disease.
- It eats and drinks less.
- The growth rate and feed efficiency get worse for a period.
- It requires an increase in environmental temperature.

Major factors that may cause stress

- Shortage of water supply.
- Shortage of trough space.
- Excessive stocking density.
- Low, high or variable temperatures.
- Draughts.
- Movement, mixing, fighting.
- Verbal or physical abuse.
- Poor light.
- Low levels of selenium or vitamin E may increase the susceptibility to stress.
- High levels of vitamin A.
- Inadequate or poor nutrition.
- The act of farrowing or weaning.
- Transport.
- Changes in the environment e.g. changes in housing.
- Exposure to disease

How infectious agents are spread

To control infectious disease it is helpful to understand how organisms are disseminated and gain access to the pig. Each organism has individual properties that determine how long it will survive outside the pig, how infective it is, and how easily it is transmitted.
The methods by which disease spreads include the following:
- Direct contact with the infected pigs, including newly purchased pigs.
- Mechanical dissemination by vehicles, particularly pig transporters.
- Mechanically by on farm equipment, boots and clothing.
- Infection transmitted by people (e.g. influenza).
- Movement of birds, rats, mice, flies, dogs, cats and wildlife (e.g. wild boars).
- Environmental contamination on the pig farm (e.g. moving pigs into a contaminated pen, movement of contaminated faeces along defecating passages).
- Contaminated food and water.
- Airborne transmission in aerosal droplets or dirt.
- Biting insects (e.g. eperythrozoonosis).

Direct Contact Between Pigs

Infectious agents enter and leave the pig as shown in (Fig.2-16).

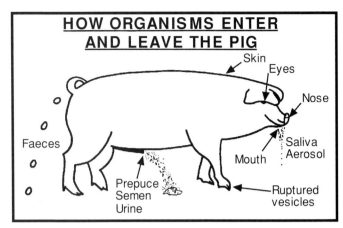

(Fig.2-16)

The common methods are by mouth (ingestion) or by inhalation. In general inhalation requires smaller doses of the organism than ingestion to set up an infection and produce disease because the acidity of the stomach and the normal bacterial flora of the intestines inhibit the multiplication of the organisms. Even smaller doses are required if infected material is splashed into the eyes. Some organisms, notably leptospira, can penetrate the mucous membrane lining the mouth and lips. Infections may enter the body through skin abrasions (e.g. erysipelothrix) and some may multiply in and on the skin (e.g. staphylococci causing greasy pig disease). Infections may also enter at mating either via the semen and seminal fluids or mechanically from the boar's prepucial sac, which is heavily infected with bacteria, or contamination. The penis may contaminate the vagina from the females dirty vulva and surrounding area.

Within the pig different infections multiply in different organs, enteric pathogens in the gut, respiratory pathogens in the respiratory tract, leptospira and some viruses in the kidneys, etc. and some become generalised and multiply throughout the body. The route by which the pathogen is spread will depend on the organs it has multiplied in.

Many live in faeces, some in the urine (e.g. leptospira) in vaginal discharges, semen, the skin. saliva, nasal discharges and expired air.

> *Bad management means increased mortality, more treatment costs, welfare problems for the pig, poor growth rate and poor food conversion.*
> *LESS PROFIT*

The main method of spread of respiratory diseases is by airborne droplet infection. The transmission of diseases by droplet spread in the air, is often restricted to as little as 10 metres but under the right climatic conditions can be many kilometres. Where pigs are in the same environment and particularly when in the same pen, or where the pens are separated by railings, organisms will

be transferred by direct body or nose to nose contact. Whether clinical disease develops or not is dependent upon a number of factors including:
- The resistance of the pig to the infection.
- The survival of the organism outside the pig.
- The virulence of the organism.
- The numbers of the organisms to which the pig is exposed.

Spread of infection may be within or between herds and between countries. The reader is unlikely to be involved in the third of these so this section will concentrate on the first two, particularly the second.

The ways in which infectious diseases spread within farms are similar to those by which they spread between farms except that the relative importance of each is different. In spread within farms, rodents, flies, equipment and airborne dust and aerosol are more important.

There are also additional modes of spread within farms that are unlikely between farms. Often slurry or solid manure is moved or drained between pens which have a common defecating alley, and there is direct contact between pigs within pens and often between pens. Even if there is not direct contact between pens, infections, including intestinal infections, can move in the dust-laden air. The respiratory tracts of the pigs act as vacuum cleaners, removing the dust from the air, sticking it against the mucus of the respiratory tract and moving it to the throat by the mucus elevator so that it can be swallowed. This commences from birth. Thus newborn piglets take their first breath, inhale *E. coli* and introduce the bacteria to their intestines.

Disease Dissemination by Vehicles

There is no doubt that vehicles which carry pigs, particularly those that carry slaughter pigs to the abattoir, pose a serious risk, so do vehicles picking up dead pigs for disposal. The risk from feed lorries is less but should not be ignored.

It is obvious that a truck driver unloading pigs at slaughter immediately after diseased pigs have been unloaded from a previous lorry, is likely to contaminate his boots and his lorry. Even if he washes the inside of his truck thoroughly and disinfects it he cannot be sure that he has eliminated all the contaminating disease organisms, including those in his driver's cab. When he calls at the next farm to collect pigs and helps to load them he may well contaminate the loading area and hence the herd. It is amazing how on many farms the water from the surface of the loading ramp drains directly back into the farm. Field experiences have documented two herd breakdowns with swine dysentery due to this. Cross-contamination between herds is also likely when trucks are picking up slaughter pigs or weaners from several different herds to make up a full load for delivery. It was shown in the UK that pig trucks were major factors in the spread of both TGE virus and swine vesicular disease (SVD) virus so it is likely to be true for other pathogens, particularly highly infectious ones.

Evidence for the spread of infectious disease by feed lorries is hard to find. In the USA it is thought that some farmers may carry grain to the local mill in farm vehicles that they have also used to carry pigs and that this is one source of contamination with TGE. It is the common practice of small mills to turn feed around quickly and therefore there is sufficient time for the virus to remain active. Storage would reduce this method of spread. The risk of a bulk feed lorry transmitting faeces-borne diseases on its wheels is very small but could occur over short distances. Diseases such as transmissible gastro-enteritis, porcine epidemic diarrhoea, swine dysentery, salmonellosis and swine vesicular disease might, in theory, be spread in this way. To maintain a vehicle dip to the required strength of a specific disinfectant is a costly procedure. The risks versus costs of this must be equated against the reduction in the amount of contamination on the lorry wheels as it travels along the roads together with the washing and the further diluting effect of a water dip. In general wheels are a negligible risk compared with other aspects of vehicular spread and wheel dips give a false sense of security. **Of greater risk however, is the feed pipe that attaches the lorry to the bin.** This is carried from farm to farm and often becomes heavily contaminated with faeces. Each farm therefore, should have its own connecting pipe particularly where the bins are not sited to the exterior of the farm. The siting of feed bins to the outside perimeter of the unit obviously reduces the risk.

The question is often asked "How long should a vehicle be left empty after the transportation of other pigs before the transportation of Defined High Health Status pigs (DHHS)?" This will depend on the diseases that the conventional pigs are thought to have, how thoroughly the vehicle is cleaned, the disinfectant used and the disease organisms that contaminated the vehicle.

As a guide:
- Remove all equipment and partitions from the vehicle.
- Completely remove all bedding and faeces.
- Soak the internal surfaces in water and detergent for at least $\frac{1}{2}$ hour.
- Pressure wash with hot water or use a steam cleaner.
- Pressure wash the exterior of the vehicle.
- Examine the efficiency of the above procedures. Repeat if there is visual contamination.
- Finally spray both internal and external surfaces with a non corrosive rapidly acting approved disinfectant such as Virkon S.
- Document the cleaning procedure. This is important from a legal point of view.
- If the vehicle is to transport DHHS pigs it must stand empty for 12 hours at least after disinfection provided the health status of the last occupying pigs was known. If not the period should be extended to at least 48 hours depending on the conditions of storage of the vehicle.

Problems can arise in countries during the winter when temperatures remain below freezing for long periods. Under such circumstances facilities must be made available to carry out efficient washing and disinfectant procedures and holding the vehicle in an equitable environment not subjected to freezing.

A loading bay should be provided at the exterior of the farm and it should have the following features:
- Facilities for the lorry driver to change boots and coveralls.
- A narrow passage for him to get around behind the pigs.
- Separate boots and coveralls for any farm personal working outside the unit.
- A pig passage way leading to it from the pig buildings or a system of one-way doors.
- It should be elevated to mid lorry height unless the lorry has hydraulic loading facilities.
- No bedding should be used on the ramp and water should be available for washing and disinfecting after loading.
- The loading ramp should drain away from the farm to a soak away or sealed tank.
- A specified approved disinfectant should be used that has rapid activity.
- There should be a holding area near the vehicle, gated off from the farm, so that pigs can be moved onto it without farm personnel entering.

Spread of Infection Between Different Ages of Pig Within a Farm

It was a commonly held belief, and still is in some places, that piglets pick up infectious disease from their dams. It is true for a number of potential pathogens such as *E. coli*, clostridia, fusiform bacteria, some streptococci and staphylococci but it is not true for many of the more serious enzootic pathogens. These are picked up after weaning from older pigs.

By the time a female pig has reached farrowing age, she has developed a powerful immunity to most of the serious pathogens enzootic in the herd and in most cases has thrown them off and is free from them. She passes the full spectrum of her humoral immunity on to her piglets, mostly in her colostrum and to some extent also in her milk. This makes the piglets immune to the same pathogens. Before weaning, the piglets are either not encountering the enzootic pathogens because the sow is not shedding them, or if they are encountering them, by say aerosol or from other parts of the farm on pig persons clothes etc. they are in low numbers. Their maternally derived immunity can prevent infection. See chapter 3 "Immunity".

After weaning, they are exposed to an increasing array and concentration of pathogens shed by older weaned and growing pigs. This is at the same time as they are suffering the extreme stress of weaning, when their maternally derived immunity is wearing off and their own active immunity has not had time to fully develop. As they grow older the total weight of the group and stocking density increases and the need for maximum ventilation grows. This is often inadequate, and enzootic infections particularly respiratory infections begin to cause clinical disease.

So the picture is one of enzootic infections moving down against a flow of piglets coming up.

Methods of disease control such as Medicated Early Weaning, Isowean, Segregated Weaning and Multi-site production make use of these facts to break the cycle of infection and they are discussed in chapter 3.

Environmental Contamination on the Farm

Organisms such as clostridia, erysipelas, salmonella and *E. coli* may contaminate the environment, soil or concrete surfaces (for example in the farrowing houses) and if attempts are not made to reduce or eliminate them they may overwhelm incoming pigs.

Most respiratory infections die out of the environment fairly quickly but faecal pathogens tend to be more persistent.

Diseases and organisms spread by pig faeces
- *Actinomyces (Corynebacterium) pyogenes*.
- Bacteroides.
- Campylobacters.
- Classical swine fever virus.
- Clostridia.
- *Corynebacterium (Eubacterium) suis*.
- *E. coli*.
- Enteroviruses.
- Porcine epidemic diarrhoea viruses.
- Erysipelothrix which cause erysipelas.
- Fusebacterium necrophorus.
- Klebsiella.
- *Lawsonia intracellularis* which causes porcine enteropathy (PE).
- Parasitic diseases (internal ones).
- Porcine parvovirus.
- Porcine reproductive respiratory syndrome (PRRS) virus.
- Rotavirus.
- Salmonellosis.
- The spirochetes which cause swine dysentery.
- Streptococci.
- Transmissible gastro-enteritis (TGE) virus.
- Yersinia.
- Foot-and-mouth disease.
- Swine vesicular disease virus.

Contamination by food and water

Water can become a major source of contamination in both outdoor and indoor pig producing systems. Outdoors the fouling of wallows by faeces and urine from sows provides a potential medium for the survival of some organisms. Leptospira from rats and other wildlife may contaminate streams and be drunk by pigs. Feed may be contaminated by salmonella from vermin and birds or its ingredients may have been contaminated at source. Diseases that can be spread by food and water include; *E. coli*, erysipelas, clostridia, salmonellosis and leptospirosis.

External parasites

Mange, lice and ticks can be carriers of some infectious agents and act as mechanical vectors or indirect hosts in diseases such as African swine fever, Japanese B. encephalitis and eperythrozoonosis. House flies may spread infections such as *Streptococcus suis*.

Inoculation

There are many diseases on the farm that result from contaminated skin damage. These include tail biting, ear nibbling, greasy pig disease, trauma to the gums following teeth removal, necrosis of knees in piglets, joint infections, eperythrozoonosis (needle contamination) and of course fighting.

Opportunist invaders

Opportunist invaders are those organisms that normally on their own would not cause disease but given the opportunity by additional factors will assume a pathogenic role. Typical examples include skin damage resulting in greasy pig disease, vulval discharges and endometritis.

Airborne transmission and Other Methods

If the organism is exhaled from the pig in large droplets, as is common with respiratory bacterial infections, then the actual spread of the organism is limited to probably no more than 50 metres and field studies suggest it is often less than 5 metres. Conversely, some viruses which are extremely small have been shown to be carried by wind for many kilometres under ideal conditions. For example foot-and-mouth disease virus was shown to have been windborne over land 20km (12 miles) and an incredible 300km (190 miles) over water. Aujeszky's virus has been carried 9km (6 miles) over land.

Diseases/organisms spread through the air by aerosol droplets

Short distances (i.e. a few metres)
- *Actinobacillus pleuropneumoniae* that causes severe haemorrhagic and necrotic pneumonia.
- Toxigenic *Pasteurella multocidia* that causes atrophic rhinitis.
- *Mycoplasma hyopneumoniae* that causes enzootic pneumonia. This can carry 2km.
- *Haemophilus parasuis* that causes glässers disease.
- *Mycoplasma hyosynoviae* that causes arthritis.
- Other pasteurella that are involved in pneumonia.
- *Streptococcus suis* that causes meningitis and other conditions.

Intermediate distances up to about 3km (2 miles)
- Enzootic pneumonia.
- Influenza, probably unproven.
- Porcine reproductive and respiratory syndrome (PRRS) virus.
- Porcine respiratory coronavirus (PRCV).

Relatively long distances >9km (6 miles)
- Aujeszky's disease.
- Foot-and-mouth disease.

Not all viruses become windborne. The viruses of TGE, porcine epidemic diarrhoea, porcine parvovirus, classical swine fever, African swine fever, encephalomyocarditis, or swine vesicular disease are not known to spread on the wind. Theoretically one would expect that viruses causing respiratory infections would be most likely to be spread on wind.

Bacterial infections are less likely to be carried so far on the wind because of the larger size of the droplets. Furthermore it has been shown that the great majority of airborne bacteria in pig farms are dead (although their endotoxins can still cause problems). Nevertheless there is strong evidence that *Mycoplasma hyopneumoniae* which causes enzootic pneumonia (EP) sometimes travels at least 3km (2 miles). Field experiences have shown that if another pig farm with EP is clearly visible from a newly repopulated pig farm which does not have EP, then sooner or later the healthy pig farm will break down with the disease. There is little firm evidence about the ability or frequency of the other bacterial infections being windborne.

The frustration about windborne infection is that you have no defence against it except in the choice of the location in which you build your pig farm. Keeping pigs in totally enclosed buildings is no defence. If the ventilation involves fans the air inlets act like vacuum cleaners. Filters fine enough to filter micro-organisms are possible but are impractical.

In hot dry summers the chance of aerosol spread between farms is low, but this does not always hold true for the same regions in winter, particularly at night. It is not surprising that epidemics of FMD occurred in winter.

Transmission by birds

The three porcine diseases that are definitely transmitted by birds are avian tuberculosis. transmissible gastroenteritis (TGE) and erysipelas, although it is likely that other infectious agents such as PRRS virus may be carried on birds' feet or pass through their alimentary tracts into their droppings.

Birds visit pig farms mainly in winter time, late fall or early spring, to eat pig feed. Pathogenic organisms on their feet could conceivably contaminate the feed. More important, their droppings contaminate the feed, the floors, and sometimes stored bedding, such as straw or shavings. In temperate and warm climates, pig buildings are often open on one or more sides. Bird proofing then involves extensive netting which is not often done in spite of the risk from birds. The opinion of farmers in England who have done this claim that it is cost effective in the savings made in feed alone. In extreme climates pig buildings are usually totally enclosed so the risk from birds is much reduced. Even then, there is still the possibility of birds defecating on stored or spilt food or stored bedding outside the buildings, the organisms in the faeces being carried in to the pigs on people's feet as well as on the bedding or feed.

In many countries the most dangerous birds are starlings. They tend to travel in large flocks, flying in a 30km (19 mile) radius and landing on numerous different pig farms in a day. In a study carried out it was estimated that about 30% of new outbreaks of TGE were due to starlings. When starlings ingest TGE virus, which is easily done when they are feeding on a pig farm during the acute stage of a TGE outbreak, they shed it in their droppings for up to 36 hours. There appears to be no evidence that porcine epidemic diarrhoea (PED) is spread by starlings but it would not be surprising if it were. Sea gulls have also been implicated in the spread of TGE in the UK. Porcine reproductive and respiratory syndrome (PRRS) virus has been shown to multiply in ducks but no work has been done to show whether it can multiply in other birds.

Birds with avian tuberculosis shed vast numbers of *Mycobacterium avium* in their droppings, which, when ingested by pigs cause typical tubercle lesions in the lymph nodes of the neck and mesentery, resulting in condemnation of the head and offal at slaughter. Sometimes individual herds suffer long periods with high condemnation rates. Bird-proofing the pig farm and removing all the stored bedding in some cases may not have the desired effect. It must be remembered that *Mycobacterium avium* is not a uniform species of bacterium but covers a wide spectrum of variants some of which multiply readily saprophytically (outside the pig). Some strains multiply, for example in peat used for bedding or in water tanks.

Birds are sometimes blamed for outbreaks of erysipelas in pigs. They can become infected by the causal organism, and may then shed it in their droppings. Most outbreaks however originate from the pigs themselves. The organism resides in the tonsils sub-clinically for long periods and becomes endemic in herds. For reasons that are not clear, probably related to stress, an individual carrier may develop clinical signs and then shed large numbers of virulent organism in the faeces.

Birds have been incriminated in the spread of diseases such as FMD and salmonella (and recently in the UK of PRRS) but it has rarely if ever been proved. Salmonellae can be carried and shed by birds in their droppings but often the serotypes are not those that would harm pigs. Highly infectious agents such as FMD could be carried for short periods mechanically on birds' feet but there is no firm evidence that this has played a significant role in spread. Sea gulls, may be involved in the carriage of materials contaminated by pig products, such as pig-meat wrappings from garbage dumps, into pig farms. (The wind may also blow such material into a pig farm if the garbage dump is nearby).

Transmission by flies
See chapter 11 for further information.

Flies are common on pig farms and have access to contaminated materials such as dead pigs, the secretions and excretions of diseased pigs and faeces. They frequently travel up to 2-3km (1-2 miles) between pig farms in breezy weather particularly in summer time and are attracted by smells that are slightly out of the line of the wind direction. Studies carried out in Cambridge showed that when the common house fly (*Musca domestica*) was fed on materials contaminated with *Streptococcus suis* type 2 the organism remained viable in the fly, probably in its crop, for up to five days and it would then contaminate whatever it fed on. Apparently, before feeding, the house fly tends to vomit its crop contents. Flies have also been shown to carry other infections, including *Serpulina hyodysenteriae*, the cause of swine dysentery. It seems reasonable to assume that they can carry many more infections than those that have been studied and reported. However, we should be wary about concluding that because they can carry an organism they necessarily play a role in its spread, The dose of organism that they carry may be extremely small and in some cases, such as *Serpulina hyodysenteriae*, may be below the infective dose required to establish the infection in a pig. Clinical observations suggest they play a role in disease in farrowing houses.

Transmission by rats and mice
What pig disease might they carry? It has been shown that *Serpulina hyodysenteriae*, the causal organism of swine dysentery, can infect mice and can be maintained in mouse colonies in pig farms. *S. hyodysenteriae*, isolated from mice on infected pig farms, has been shown to be pathogenic for pigs. Mice may provide one explanation why some pig farms break down with swine dysentery after they have been repopulated with clean stock or after attempts at eradication by blanket medication have been carried out. Although rats have been infected experimentally with *S. hyodysenteriae*, they are not thought to play any role in its spread in the field.

The rat is the natural host of the virus of encephalomyocarditis which is implicated in outbreaks of so called SMEDI (stillbirths, mummification, embryonic deaths and infertility) in the USA. It is thought that outbreaks occur in localised areas when rats are allowed to build up in numbers. In some countries the virus causes myocarditis and sudden death in pigs and other animals (e.g. zoo animals). In Cuba, this form of the disease is regarded as a major problem in pigs and has also caused deaths in apes, porcupines and cattle,

Rats and mice also carry and shed *Salmonella typhimurium* and other salmonella serotypes which affect pigs and dermatophytes, such as *Trichophytum menta-*

grophytes which cause ringworm in pigs but fortunately rarely. Rats seem to be resistant to infection with *Actinobacillus pleuropneumoniae* and *Streptococcus suis* type 2. Mice can be infected experimentally by large doses of *S. suis* type 2 but there is no evidence that they carry the organism under field conditions.

House-mice remain resident in piggeries and do not normally travel between them. Field mice may travel short distances but are not likely to be significant in the spread of pig disease. Rats are much more mobile. Individuals will frequently cover 1-2km ($^1/_2$-1 mile) in a night. However their movement between pig farms depends on a complex social relationship in the resident rat communities in farm buildings. Both rats and mice may be carried inadvertently between farms in vehicles such as feed trucks.

Other wildlife

The wild boar is a vector of pig disease, particularly in Germany at the time of writing, classical swine fever (hog cholera) has been found to be endemic in the wild boar population and contaminates domestic pig herds. The wild boar in Africa was, of course, the source of African swine fever to domestic pigs farms in Africa and subsequently to Portugal and Spain, (and to other countries).

Lawsonia intracellularis bacterium has been identified as the cause of porcine enteropathy and it has been transmitted experimentally to hamsters and mice. Porcine enteropathies in which the same antigen has been detected have also been seen in ferrets and rabbits. It seems likely therefore that this organism could be spread by a variety of other species and it is not surprising that the disease syndrome occurs sometimes in the most secure highest health herds.

A range of leptospira serovars are carried by wild animals but most are not normally pathogenic to pigs. Individual pigs may become ill with *Leptospira icterohaemorrhagiae* from rats. A main pig pathogenic serovar in North America and some other parts of the world (not the UK or Ireland) *L. pomona* is shed by hedgehogs and possibly mice and rats. Other serovars which affect pigs are present in wildlife in other countries however a serovar which is pathogenic in one country may not be pathogenic in other countries. The presence of *Brucella suis* in wild hares in Denmark and France has contaminated outdoor herds.

Domesticated / farm animals

What is the risk of keeping herds of high health status pigs near other farm livestock including poultry, or of keeping dogs and cats in such herds? In countries which do not have FMD, the risk in practice seems to be low. One can theorise about the contamination with salmonellae from calves, of toxigenic *Pasteurella multocidia* from cattle and sheep, of *Actinobacillus pleuropneumoniae* from cattle, sheep and deer, of *Erysipelothrix* from poultry and *Streptococcus suis* (various serotypes) from cattle, sheep, goats or horses. In practice, provided they are physically separated from each other, there is little risk. However, outbreaks of disease caused by some of these organisms sometimes occur without obvious explanation. The source might be other animals. Aujeszky's disease (pseudorabies) crosses species but the risk is mainly the other way around, (i.e. from the pigs to the cattle and dogs).

Dogs can shed the virus of TGE for up to 14 days after eating contaminated material such as dead piglets. This is clearly a risk when a nearby neighbour gets TGE but farm dogs do not usually wander great distances and there are so many other ways in which TGE can be spread between neighbouring herds that the importance of the dog as a common vector is probably small. Farm dogs have also been shown to carry *S. hyodysenteriae* but it is difficult to assess whether or not they play any role in the spread of swine dysentery. Recent studies have shown that *Leptospira bratislava* can be shed in dogs' urine. If the dog is a good watch dog then its benefits in keeping intruders and other animals at bay may outweigh its risk of introducing TGE, swine dysentery or leptospirosis. Pig farmers in regions where classical swine fever (hog cholera), African swine fever and FMD occur should be a little more careful about dogs because of the danger of carrying bones into the farm

Cats in pig farms are frowned upon in the UK. The reason is often the risk of atrophic rhinitis, but in the many SPF herds in Denmark, cats are kept routinely to control mice and rats. If they stray from the premises they are killed or not allowed to return. Atrophic rhinitis is not a common cause of breakdown in the large Danish SPF programme. The main cause of breakdowns is enzootic pneumonia with *Actinobacillus pleuropneumoniae* also a problem.

The two greatest risks of contamination to your herd are neighbouring infected pig herds and the introduction of disease through the purchased pig. It is always difficult to quantify the risk from neighbouring herds but Fig.2-17 shows the results of a field study looking at the minimum distances between herds when disease did not spread and the length of time observed. These results demonstrate minimum distances over which specific infections appear not to have travelled but they should not be used as a basis for a decision in practice. The recommended given distances should be used as a minimum for decision making purposes. If high health herds are being established a distance of at least 3.2km (2 miles) from other pigs is advised. However, the other factors must also be taken in to account.

Enzootic pneumonia, flu and PRRS are the three most difficult diseases to remain free from because they are windborne and are extremely common and widespread in the pig populations of most countries. The transfer of airborne mycoplasma is high within 800 metres of infected pigs but is reduced to almost negligible

CHAPTER 2 - Understanding Disease   **37**

proportions provided there are no other sources of infected pigs within a 3.2 km radius (2 miles). The respective sizes of the two farms and their distance apart must also be considered. A 50 sow herd producing weaners is much less likely to spread infection than a 1000 sow herd of feeder pigs because of the reduced numbers of infectious particles produced by the smaller weaner only population. Another factor is the type of terrain in which herds are located, flat treeless countryside is worst, trees break up aerosol plumes.

MINIMAL DISTANCES (FROM FIELD DATA) BETWEEN TWO PIG FARMS WHERE TRANSMISSION OF DISEASE HAS NOT OCCURRED

Disease	Actual Distance (m)	Observed Time Scale	Recommended Minimum Distance (m)
Actinobacillus pleuropneumonia (App)	500	5 years	500
Atrophic rhinitis (AR)	300	5 years	500
Aujeszky's disease (AD) (pseudorabies) (PR)	500	4 months. Then herd Infected	2000
Enzootic pneumonia (EP)	150	10 years	3200
Mange	100	5 years	500
Porcine reproductive and respiratory syndrome (PRSS)	800	3 years	2000
Streptococcal meningitis (SM)	300	12 years	3000
Swine dysentery (SD)	300	4 years	800
Transmissible gastro-enteritis (TGE)	400	4 months Then herd Infected	800

(Fig.2-17)

By People

The role of people as a mechanical means of transmitting disease has evoked considerable debate over the years. Indeed some of the severe restrictions such as seven days pig freedom prior to entry onto the farm, would perhaps suggest that the human is covered in pig pathogens. To try and clarify this the writer carried out a review on 122 pig farms, covering a 15 year period, to determine the changes in health status that had taken place since their establishment. (Figs.2-18 and 2-19). These changes were then related to the various entry precautions that were adopted on the different farms. It is interesting to note that in the 41 herds that required a period of pig freedom, there were 27 episodes of disease breakdown other than porcine corona virus and only one herd remained free of the latter. However, in 20 of these herds the breakdown was due to enzootic pneumonia which we now know is only transmitted by carrier pigs or through the air. The provision of boots and protective clothing are the important criteria for disease control.

THE APPEARANCE OF DISEASE IN HERDS RELATED TO HUMAN/PIG CONTACT AND TIME OF ENTRY INTO THE HERD.

	* 48 Hrs Pig Freedom	* 24 Hrs Pig Freedom or Same Day	* Boots Coveralls Only	No Precautions	Totals & % Breakdown	
No. farms	13	28	50	31	122	
Atrophic rhinitis (AR)	0 (13)	2 (24)	1 (48)	1 (21)	4/106	3%
Enzootic pneumonia (EP)	9 (13)	11 (22)	1 (2)	0 (0)	21/37	56%
Mange	0 (13)	1 (24)	0 (10)	0 (3)	1/50	2%
Porcine coronavirus (PRCV)	12 (12)	27 (28)	50 (50)	31 (31)	120/121	99%
Streptococcal meningitis (SM)	1 (13)	3 (26)	2 (50)	1 (31)	7/120	6%
Swine dysentery (SD)	0 (13)	0 (24)	1 (50)	3 (31)	4/118	3%

( ) = Number of herds susceptible   * On farm boots and coveralls used.

(Fig.2-18)

THE PERCENTAGE OF HERDS INFECTED WITH SPECIFIC DISEASES RELATED TO HUMAN / PIG CONTACT AND TIME OF ENTRY

	No Pig Contact on Day of Entry or Longer		No Time Limits	
Enzootic pneumonia (EP)	20 / 35	57%	1 / 2	50%
Streptococcal meningitis (SM)	4 / 39	10%	3 / 81	4%
Swine dysentery (SD)	0 / 37	0%	4 / 81	5%
Atrophic rhinitis (AR)	2 / 37	5%	2 / 69	3%
Mange	1 / 37	3%	0 / 13	0%

(Fig.2-19)

Recommendations for the control of people:

- No visitors should visit the farm at any time unless wearing boots and coveralls provided by the farmer.
- Visitors may be required to take a shower on entry, including a hair wash and to also ensure a complete change of clothes.
- A period of pig freedom(i.e. 1, 2, 3 nights away from other pigs) may be required when visiting DHHS (defined high health status) farms.
- No farm clothing should be used off the farm.
- Foot dips should be used for entry to the farm and be properly maintained with a rapid acting disinfectant.
- No equipment having had contact with other pigs should be allowed on the unit unless cleaned, disinfected and/or fumigated followed by a gap of at least seven days.
- Staff should not own other pigs nor visit other pig farms.
- Staff should not live on other pig farms.
- Staff should not visit markets or slaughter houses.
- No pig products should be brought onto the farm, or
- All pig products for consumption that are brought onto the farm must have been well cooked.
- All human food should be eaten in a designated area separated from the pig pens.
- Hands should always be washed after meals and after going to the toilet.

The minimum recommendation for a high health herd at a commercial level would be no pig contact on that day, a shower and the use of the unit's own protective clothing. The necessity for a shower is often questioned. It exercises a discipline, fosters an awareness and good attitude and forces the visitor to make a complete change of clothes. It also eliminates chance pig infections from contaminated dust. The showers must be kept clean and warm or they will not be used. The nucleus herd of a breeding pyramid should observe 24 to 48 hours of pig freedom. This is also often questioned. It is in fact difficult to argue a scientific case for it but there are several cases where veterinarians visiting successive herds have spread foot-and -mouth disease and there is at least one clear case of a pig manager bringing back TGE from another farm. The minimum of an overnight gap, showers and change of clothes is probably adequate. It is strongly recommended that all farms should provide boots and coveralls for every visitor. Provided these precautions are carried out, field experiences over many years shows that people are rarely implicated in the spread of disease.

The higher breakdown rates with EP and PRCV reflect their windborne spread which none of these precautions would prevent. Streptococcal meningitis may be spread by flies and the introduction of sub-carrier pigs

By Pigs

The health status of the herd

In an ideal world if the pig herd could be established and maintained completely free of all pathogenic organisms then from a disease view point there would be few limitations to maximising production. Unfortunately we do not live in such environments and because of factors often out of the control of the farm, there will always be a variety of pathogenic or potentially pathogenic organisms present.

The purchased pig is the most important potential source of new infections and whilst the donor herd may be well monitored to determine its health status, an infectious disease could be incubating at the time of purchase.

The situation is further complicated by the variety of terms that have been used to describe the perceived health status of a herd. They are imprecise and open to wide interpretation. There are four categories of health status.

- **Germ free (axenic)** - This is a pig which is thought to be totally free from infection with micro-organisms. Such pigs are produced by surgery (hysterotomy or hysterectomy) carried out on the pregnant sow near term. They are reared under completely sterile conditions usually in small containers enclosed in plastic balloons with filtered air and sterilised food and water. They can usually only be reared to a maximum of about six weeks because they get too big and unmanageable to maintain. They are for research purposes only. In fact, it is now realised that a germ free state is probably impossible to achieve. It is known that at least one retrovirus, which is inserted in the genetic DNA of every cell in the pigs' body, moves to the off spring from the parents. There are probably other as yet unknown viruses that behave similarly. Several viruses, for example, inclusion body rhinitis virus, although not inserted in the pigs' genes, also pass from mother to foetus before birth.
- **Gnotobiotic** - This term means "known life". It describes a pig which has been produced and reared initially as a germ free pig but while continuing to be barrier-maintained is then deliberately infected with known micro-organisms. Its micro flora is thus clearly known and defined. Again they can only be reared to about six weeks when retrovirus and other unknown viruses may be present.
- **Specific pathogen free (SPF)** - This term can be used to describe a pig or pigs, a herd or a disease control programme. It means that the herds are believed free from a short list of specified pathogens. Primary SPF piglets are usually produced in a similar way to germ free piglets and may be reared in isolators for about two weeks. During this time they may be given a probiotic flora (i.e. bacteria such as non pathogenic lactobacillus bacteria and streptococci which are meant to repress the growth of E. coli). They may also be given sterilised colostrum supplement. They are then removed from the isolator and placed in a very clean room under hygienic conditions. They become slowly contaminated with a simple bacterial flora derived from the attendants, dust in the air, and bacteria in their food and water but they remain free from specified pathogens (i.e. SPF). They can be used for research purposes or reared on to maturity and bred as the foundation stock of a new primary SPF herd.
- **Secondary SPF** pigs are piglets born to the primary SPF mothers and secondary SPF herds are herds set up with secondary SPF breeding stock. Such programmes are run by SPF associations of which the largest is in Denmark with somewhat smaller ones in Switzerland and the USA. The associations draw up strict disease control regulations for their members to follow and regularly carry out a series of laboratory tests (mainly serological) to test for the presence or absence of specified pathogens. These usually include toxigenic Pasteurella multocidia (atrophic rhinitis), *Mycoplasma hyopneumoniae* (enzootic pneumonia - EP), certain serotypes of *Actinobacillus pleuropneumoniae, Serpulina hyodysenteriae* (swine dysentery), *Sarcoptes scabiei* (mange) and lice. The herd breakdown rate with EP is usually high and there are also breakdowns with *Actinobacillus pleuropneumoniae* but at a lower rate. The other diseases are generally more consistently kept out.
- **Minimal disease (MD)** - This term was ill defined

and often became confused with SPF. There was an expectation by the pig farmer that there would be no more disease and the term also has negative connotations. This term was introduced in the early days of the development of multi-herd breeding companies to escape from the proscriptive rigidity of the SPF approach, which was found too inflexible for expanding international pyramids. It was realised in such pyramids that it was impossible to standardise health across all the herds using SPF and not necessary to do so. Furthermore it was realised that at a commercial level herds required compatibility of clinical freedom from disease rather than specified organisms per se. For example, *Actinobacillus pleuropneumoniae* comprises different strains varying in their virulence, some highly pathogenic and some non-pathogenic. It is an advantage for a commercial herd to contain non-pathogenic strains because they provide a level of immunity.

High health status (HHS)

Because of this and the problem with the term "minimal disease", the author proposed in the early 1970s a more positive term "High Health Status". This term has been widely taken up by pig breeders in the UK and North America and "Minimal Disease" has been largely discarded. It avoids some of the problems of minimal disease and gives a better indication of what the breeders are trying to achieve and what the commercial producer wants, but it is still imprecise and difficult to produce a specific definition and common understanding. The author therefore qualified it by adding "defined" i.e. "Defined High Health Status"(DHHS).

Defined high health status (DHHS)

This describes "a herd of recognised health status through the absence of the major infectious diseases". The diseases thought to be present or absent would be defined for that particular herd by the consulting veterinarian based upon clinical history and the results of pathological tests. The object of this approach is to ensure that each herd provides evidence of the absence of given diseases. It is important to emphasise that the term does not imply that animals are free of any infectious agent but that the observations and tests for the disease were all negative. This is important in legal terms since it is impossible to guarantee freedom from an organism or disease because at any one point in time the herd could unknowingly be incubating it. Furthermore an organism may be present, for example App that was non pathogenic i.e. the herd infected but no disease. It is also important that no antibacterial drugs are used routinely that would mask a virulent infection.

> *Remember in a DHHS herd you will always have some diseases. (See Fig.2-20).*

Using the term DHHS therefore, it becomes possible to describe the precise health profile of a particular herd with periodic veterinary documentation to that effect. It would be expected that most of the major infectious diseases would be absent under this definition and in Fig.2-20 an example of such a declaration for one farm is shown. This should be used for reference purposes and at **a veterinary level only,** where health compatibility can be discerned and assessed relative to the requirements of the recipient herd.

Such a declaration would be made by a veterinarian following clinical examination of the herd and receiving the results of any pathological tests. Examinations would be carried out every 2-3 months.

The history of the herd supported by other tests may allow some of the above to be declared absent and added to the defined health status. An example would be a long term herd history of freedom from piglet dysentery caused by *Clostridium perfringens* type C infection.

DEFINED HIGH HEALTH STATUS (DHHS) AN EXAMPLE		
Name Of Herd: Plantation Pigs	Declaration Date: 07-10-96	
Disease	Declared Health Status Results of Clinical Examination*	Possible Variations Could Include
Actinobacillus pleuropneumonia (App)	Negative	
Atrophic rhinitis (AR)	Negative	
Aujeszky's disease (AD)	Negative	
Brucellosis	Negative	
Enzootic pneumonia (EP)	No Evidence	Negative
Glässers disease	No Evidence	Negative
Influenza	Negative	No Evidence
Lice	Negative	
Porcine epidemic diarrhoea (PED)	No Evidence	
Porcine enteropathy (PE)	Negative	No Evidence
Porcine parvovirus (PPV)	No Evidence	
PRRS	No Evidence	Negative
Salmonellosis	Negative	
Sarcoptic mange	Negative	
Streptococcal meningitis (SM)	Negative	
Swine dysentery (SD)	Negative	
Swine pox	No Evidence	Negative
Transmissible gastro-enteritis (TGE)	Negative	
Tuberculosis	Negative	

Negative = Disease never diagnosed.
No Evidence = Infection has previously been diagnosed but it is not apparent at the time of declaration.
Present = Active disease.
* Based on long term history supported by pathological tests as necessary

(Fig.2-20)

Similarly, the absence of any clinical evidence of exudative epidermitis over a long period of time could allow a declaration based upon these observations. This however could not be based on specific bacteriology. It is emphasised that the assessment of DHHS must always be carried out by a competent pig veterinarian so that the information and criteria upon which a declaration is made accords with current accepted practices.

Purchase breeding stock from a DHHS herd or its equivalent.

Maintaining Freedom From Disease : Biosecurity

You can establish a high health status herd by building a new unit on a greenfield site or by depopulating your present farm, cleaning and disinfecting it thoroughly and repopulating it with pregnant gilts from a DHHS herd. Meanwhile you should consider carefully the location of the farm to be populated to decide what level of high health status would be appropriate. Then you should decide on the source of the new stock together with what measures you should adopt to prevent your new herd becoming contaminated.

Freedom from the main infectious diseases is a major contribution to the efficiency of production and to profitability. Thus the biosecurity measures that are taken to prevent new infections entering your herd, are of paramount importance.

The most important factor in biosecurity is the location. A secure location is one of very low pig density well away from any other pig herd, preferably in hilly or mountainous country and/or on the sea coast. If your farm is in such a location then the most important factor in biosecurity is a well designed and carefully operated loading bay particularly for loading slaughter pigs. You also need to control visiting people. If there are wild boar in the vicinity a stout perimeter fence is needed.

Of course, like most pig farmers, you may have no choice in your location because your farm is already up and running. With the help of your veterinarian, you should critically review the location your pig farm is in to assess what the risks are and what health status your herd can maintain. The worse your location the more important it is for you to take strict biosecurity measures.

The checklist in Fig.2-21 will help in determining

Infectious diseases that may be seen in a defined high health status herd
Avian TB.
Coccidiosis.
Coli septicaemia / diarrhoea.
Congenital tremor.
Cystitis / nephritis.
Erysipelas.
Exudative epidermitis. (Greasy pig disease).
Focal pneumonia (*Actinobacillus suis*).
Glässers disease.
Influenza.
Internal parasites.
Leptospira bratislava.
Mastitis.
Mycoplasmal arthritis (*Mycoplasma hyosynoviae*).
Oedema disease.
Piglet arthritis and meningitis (*Streptococci suis* Type 1).
Piglet dysentery (*Clostridia perfringens* type C).
Porcine enteropathy
Porcine epidemic diarrhoea.
Porcine parvovirus.
SMEDI
Tetanus.
Vomiting and wasting disease / ontario encephalomyelitis.
Vulval discharge

deficiencies. Fig.2-22 indicates the diseases that you should be able to maintain your herd free from and those diseases that are more difficult to keep out.

Selecting Your Source of Breeding Stock

The selection of the correct health status appropriate to your herd and location is vital before breeding stock are purchased. Your primary reason for purchase is to genetically upgrade your herd. Major requirements will be that they are available when you want them, in the numbers that are needed and at a price you can afford. But an overriding requirement is that they will not cause disease in your herd and lower your overall health status. At the onset therefore, consult with your veterinarian and ask him to determine at a veterinary level the information available about the proposed donor herd.

The investigations should include the disease history since its inception and those of any daughter herds that have been established from it. Also the health status and disease history of other herds it supplies. All veterinary reports should be requested and examined together with the results of tests for specific diseases and the frequency of such tests. The breeding history on the farm, should be checked together with any evidence of infectious reproductive disease. A detailed study of records of production parameters, growth and food conversion rates may be helpful. The biosecurity of the breeding pyramid

The minimum objective in establishing a high health status herd is to maintain the status quo for at least two years, reduce the days to slaughter (compared to the old herd) by 10 - 21 and improve the food conversion ratio by between 0.1 - 0.4. Ideally, a farrowing rate of 90% should be considered together with a grower mortality of less than 3.0%.
If you anticipate you can not maintain this for 2 years think again.

should be checked along with details of the health programme. The biosecurity of the donor herd itself must be assessed including the methods by which pigs or genetic material are brought into the herd. Finally a written veterinary statement should be obtained indicating that on both clinical and pathological grounds those selected diseases that you wish to keep out of your herd have not been diagnosed in the donor herd.

POSSIBLE SOURCES OF DISEASE ENTRY INTO YOUR FARM AND WHAT YOU SHOULD CONSIDER IN ORDER TO PREVENT IT	* Check your farm for disease risk
Before the farm is populated with new pigs:- Is your farm in a pig dense area?	☐
What is the position of your pig unit relative to other infected pig herds around it? - How far away is the nearest infected large infected herd? - Do you have an uninterrupted view of it? - Is the land around you flat or hilly, bare or wooded, on the coast or inland?	☐
Your foundation stock - is it of appropriate health status for your location? - Can you rely on a future continuous supply in adequate numbers of replacement stock of the same health status? - What precautions can you take against contamination?	☐
When the farm is being populated and afterwards:-	
Isolation - Do you have good isolation facilities for incoming stock? - How long are they to be kept in isolation? Is it long enough? - Do you check that there has been no disease outbreak in the herd of origin before you move them in?	☐
Transport - Are the trucks that bring your pigs clean? - Have they been to other farms? - Have they been careful not to drive behind or park beside other pig lorries? - Are the lorries that pick up your pigs for sale or slaughter empty when the arrive? - Are they clean? Have they been disinfected: - Does the driver wear clean boots and coveralls? - Do you have a safe loading area? - Does the water used to wash it run into or away from your pig buildings? - Are the loading procedures safe? Can the driver contaminate your herd?	☐
Visitors book - Do you make visitors sign a visitors book to affirm that they have not been near other pigs?	☐
Mechanical transmission - Are clean boots and coveralls provided at the entrance to your unit for all visitors and your staff? - Are there clean showers for visitors? Is there a proper changing area? - Do you make anyone who may have been near other pigs recently shower? - Do you make anyone who may have been near other pigs recently have a gap of say, 24 hours before they visit your unit. - Are toilets available for your staff and are they clean and hygienic? - Do you ever need to use equipment on your pig farm that has been in contact with other pigs? If so, how do you disinfect it?	☐
Bedding materials - Are they from a known clean source? - Are they contaminated by rats, mice or birds?	☐
Feed source - Are you satisfied with its quality?	☐
Feed lorries - Do they have to enter your pig compound? - Do you have your own bulk feed pipe?	☐
Water supply if not from the mains - Have you had it tested for bacteria? - Are your water storage tanks clean and rat proof? - Should you chlorinate it?	☐
Vectors - Flies - do you control them or are they a problem? - Rats and mice - do you have a regular efficient rodent control programme? - Birds - can they get to feed supplies and bedding stores? Should these be netted off? - Do you have a perimeter fence (including building walls) that would deter stray animals, including wild boar and human curiosity seekers?	☐
Human food - Do you allow it to be brought in to your pig buildings? - Do you allow pork meat products to be eaten on your farm? - Do you have a special area (canteen) where food must be eaten?	☐
Dead animal disposal - Do you have safe procedures? - Are they collected from your farm? - What do you do with casualty animals?	☐
You - If you are the unit owner or manager do you visit friends' pig herds?	☐

* Discuss these with your veterinarian and use the above as a check list.

(Fig.2-21)

Managing Pig Health and the Treatment of Disease

Buying breeding pigs - The ground rules

Step 1 Select the source based on:
- Availability.
- Genetics (including fecundity).
- Health.
- Market acceptability.
- Quality control.

Step 2 Determine with your veterinary advisor the health status of your own herd.

Step 3 Request veterinary liaison with the suppliers' veterinarian and get clarification of the health status of the donor herd.

Step 4 Assess the compatibility of health status.

Step 5 Determine the isolation requirements for incoming stock.

Step 6 Decide on vaccination and acclimatisation procedures.

DISEASES THAT YOU SHOULD BE ABLE TO KEEP OUT OF THE HERD		DISEASES DIFFICULT TO KEEP OUT
Reliably	Less Reliably	Difficult
Actinobacillus pleuropneumonia (App)	*	Arthritis (*Mycoplasma hyosynoviae*)
Atrophic rhinitis (AR)		Arthritis (*S. suis* type 1)
Aujeszky's disease (AD)	* *	Coccidiosis
Brucellosis		Congenital tremor
Enzootic pneumonia (EP)	*	Cystitis
Exotic diseases		Erysipelas
Leptospirosis (pomona)		Glässers disease
Lice		Influenza
Mange		Internal parasites
Porcine epidemic diarrhoea (PED)	* *	Piglet dysentery (*C. perfringens*)
Porcine reproductive and respiratory syndrome (PRRS)	* *	Porcine enteropathy (ileitis) PIA, PHE, NE, RI
Streptococcal meningitis (SM)	* *	Porcine parvovirus (PPV)
Swine dysentery (SD)		Rotavirus diarrhoea
Transmissible gastro-enteritis (TGE)	* *	Salmonellosis

* In pig dense areas   ** When a major disease out break is occurring

(Fig.2-22)

The donor herd

The suppliers may want to know the health status you require and offer you a choice of sources.
- Always purchase from a DHHS herd or equivalent if available.

What are the methods and risks of pig movement

Since incoming pigs are probably the greatest potential source of infection to your herd, the methods by which they are introduced or other methods by which you improve the genetic potential of your herd are vitally important.

Five methods are available:
- By introducing live pigs.
- By segregated early weaning SEW.
- By hysterectomy.
- By embryo transplants.
- By artificial insemination (AI).

Most diseases are kept out provided you don't bring them in via the pig.

Live pigs

a) Mature gilts and boars

Live pigs can be brought into your herd from a source herd of matching health status, or through SEW or hysterectomy and fostering if the source herd is of known but lower health status (depending on the disease to be eliminated).

If live pigs are brought into your herd with or without SEW it is advisable to hold them in isolation for a period before integrating them into your herd to check whether they develop disease and whether disease breaks out in the source herd. If the isolation premises are in a different site to your herd and not of the same biosecurity standards as your recipient herd, there could be a greater risk in holding them there rather than integrating them directly into your herd. The dangers of integrating them directly into your herd are obvious, namely, that if they are incubating an infectious disease sub-clinically then ultimately your herd will become infected. Perfect separate quarantine facilities are rarely available to commercial herds, particularly smaller enterprises but isolation that falls short of complete quarantine (e.g. on the same site) can be surprisingly effective. The incoming stock could be moved into a separate building on the same site preferably over 50 metres distant and this should be reasonably effective, provided separate boots and coveralls are used to tend the animals and provided the drainage from the building does not flow into your other pig buildings. If a separate building is not possible then a separate room sealed off from the main body of the herd is better than direct integration into the herd.

How long should the incubation period be? Here the importance of veterinarian liaison to match respective health status has already been highlighted.

If your herd is believed to be enzootic pneumonia (EP) free then it is advisable to place the incoming animals in isolation for a period of eight weeks. At the same time sentinel pigs (i.e. pigs from your herd due for slaughter) should be moved in and blood tested and / or slaughtered prior to the entry of the new pigs and their

Are you satisfied with your farm procedures.

lungs examined for EP freedom. If your herd is not free of EP, the length of isolation is debatable. Some veterinarians would advise six weeks but four is more practicable.

Should enteric or respiratory disease appear during the four week period either in the pigs in isolation or in the source herd the chances of preventing further damage by immediate slaughter would be reasonable.

b) Breeder weaners

Instead of buying in mature replacement gilts and boars you could buy in so-called breeder-weaners, say, 30kg live weight. This has the advantage of allowing them a long period of acclimatisation to your herd before you breed them. It also enables you to rear them yourself in the way you think best for future breeding gilts and allows you to carry out your own selection at slaughter weight. A disadvantage is that boars cannot be performance tested and therefore it is not feasible. Also, if you sell your pigs at 25-30kg or at weaning, you probably do not have the facilities to rear such pigs.

The advantages of buying in breeding stock at a commercial level, compared to the selection of the home produced gilt are its low cost, the availability of gilts when they are required, the genetic potential is constantly improved and if done carefully presents few problems. Some farms however prefer to breed their own breeding females and thereby only introduce into the herd, a small proportion of grand-parent females and boars. This policy often fails because of the difficulty of rearing the future female replacements within a commercial operation, the poorer reproductive performance and the fact that the gilts reared on the farm are often not available when required. This system is also a high cost one and often results in lower numbers of pigs reared. Extensive experiences have shown that provided there is good health liaison and sensible practical procedures then the herd health status can be maintained with the purchase of breeding stock.

c) Segregated early weaning (SEW) - Modified Medicated Early Weaning (MMEW)

The second method of bringing in live pigs from another herd is through a modification of the medicated early weaning (MEW) technique called by many segregated early weaning (SEW) and by one breeding company Isowean. This is based on the principle outlined earlier under "How infectious agents are spread". By the time females reach their first farrowing they have developed a strong immunity to the more serious enzootic pathogens in the herd and have eliminated most of them. Furthermore they pass such a strong maternal immunity to their offspring that the piglets are resistant to infection by most of these pathogens for varying periods depending on the pathogen. Thus if they are weaned immediately from the sow and moved to isolated premises at the appropriate age they

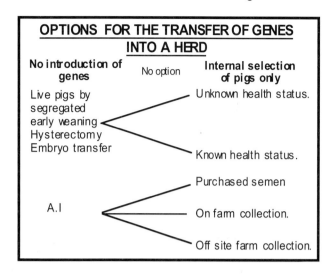

will be free of the pathogens you wish to eliminate.

Thus if you wished to obtain future breeding stock from a particular herd but your veterinarian thought that the general health of that herd was below that of your own you could obtain higher health status pigs free from the unwanted pathogen. If the pathogen you wished to avoid was *Mycoplasma hyopneumoniae*, (enzootic pneumonia), you could vaccinate the dams in the donor herd ahead of time to boost their immunity, put the sows and newborn piglets on an anti-mycoplasma drug such as tylosin or tiamulin and wean the pigs at ten days to the isolation facility on your farm. Isolation is necessary because if an unknown pathogen enters the donor herd it could go through the SEW system during the incubation period.

The SEW system is discussed in detail in chapter 3.

d) Hysterectomy and fostering

The fourth method of introduction of live pigs is through hysterectomy and fostering the piglets onto a newly farrowed sow in the recipient herd. This operation is carried out on day 113 of pregnancy when the sow is slaughtered. The womb containing the piglets is either removed 50 meters away to a pig-pathogen-free environment where the piglets are removed or it is passed through disinfectant trap into a sealed room. The litter is then immediately taken into the recipient herd and suckled onto a newly farrowed sow. If done properly the mortality rate is as low similar to that of your naturally

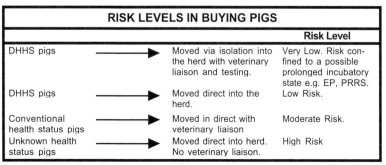

farrowed piglets.

The whole operation is synchronised using prostaglandins so that newly farrowed sows are available to act as foster mothers. (See chapter 15). Ideally the sow selected for the operation should be moved into isolation approximately eight weeks prior to the due date and monitored for evidence of disease. At the same time it should be blood sampled and tested for aujeszky's disease (AD) (pseudorabies), swine influenza, PRRS and other relevant diseases that could pass through the placental barrier including leptospirosis and brucellosis. The reason for blood testing for these diseases is that they are capable of passing from a recently infected mother to her piglets in the womb. This is most unlikely to happen with aujeszky's virus and PRRS if they are obviously immune, but it could happen with *Leptospira bratislava* and possibly *L. pomona*. If a sow is serologically positive for leptospira the risk can be diminished by treating her with either streptomycin or amoxycillin antibiotics prior to hysterectomy. If a sow is sero-positive for brucellosis it is better to discard her. It would appear also that porcine coronavirus does not cross the placenta and hysterectomy pigs from positive herds can be introduced into negative herds safely.

Hysterectomy is a safe procedure and in many hundreds of operations known to the authors there has been no evidence of transfer of disease.

e) Embryo transfer

Embryo transfer has been used successfully in several countries for the introduction of new genes but it has not been widely adopted probably because it requires two skilled teams, one to flush the fertilised eggs from the donor sow and one to insert them in the recipient sow. It has not been performed on anything like as big a scale as hysterectomy and fostering and therefore there is not the volume of field evidence to underline its safety, but in theory and on the limited evidence it is safe.

Its drawbacks are (1) that it needs two skilled teams, (2) it requires immaculate synchronisation and timing, (3) the embryos cannot be kept viable for more than a few hours and (4) unless done expertly results in a high failure rate and small litters. For practical purposes, SEW, hysterectomy and AI are much simpler.

f) Artificial insemination

The sixth method of introducing genes is by artificial insemination (AI). It is known that viruses of swine fever, aujeszky's disease, PRRS, parvovirus, and leptospira bacteria and *Brucella suis* could be introduced through AI mainly during the early stages of infection of the boar. If the boars first go thorough a true quarantine procedure and are screened for these infections then housed in an isolated AI stud (i.e. one in a secure location), with high standards of biosecurity and hygiene during the production of semen, then field experience indicates that the risks are very small. The advent of frozen semen, which hitherto has been largely unsatisfactory but which is now looking more promising, renders the use of AI much safer since the semen can be stored for a month or two, time enough to be sure that no new infection was incubating in the AI stud. AI does however, have the disadvantage that only half the genes are introduced into the herd.

Disinfection

Disinfectants are substances that kill both harmless and disease producing organisms. They act either as bacterial poisons, coagulate bacterial protein or act as oxidising or reducing agents. Antiseptics normally prevent bacterial multiplication and are used for cleaning skin or wounds. Some disinfectants in a more dilute form may act as antiseptics.

Common antiseptics used include:
- Chlorine based ones such as TCP.
- Quaternary ammonium compounds such as cetrimide
- Chloroxylenol (dettol).
- 1% crystal violet.
- Iodine.
- Alcohol
- 1% salt solutions.
- Hydrogen peroxide.

Disinfectants have two prime functions. First to prevent infectious agents gaining access to the farm and second equally important to control those organisms already on the farm and that persist in large numbers in the environment. The process of disinfection can be considered in three stages.
- The removal of the gross contamination within the building, that is the dried faeces, slurry and dust, by pressure washing preferably with hot water.
- The use of detergents to assist in the final removal of the organic material. Only after completion of these two should a disinfectant be applied.
- The use of the disinfectant.

Remember that the cheapest methods of disinfection are **the physical removal of contaminated material and final removal by water**.

> ***Water + detergent is >90% efficient in removing infections from a building.***

The effects of this are illustrated by a case of poor growth in finisher pigs. Two houses were involved, neither of which had been emptied or washed out for two and a half years. As an experiment groups of pigs were split into two on entry into the houses and weighed in and out again at point of slaughter. One of the houses was divided into sections and used on an all-in all-out basis. It was completely washed prior to the entry of each batch of pigs and the other house was used as a control with no changes. The growth curves of both groups were compared and by point of slaughter at 90kg there was approximately a nine days difference to the obvious advantage of the cleaned house. It is interesting in this case that only water and detergents were used without disinfectants. The all-in all-out procedures will also have contributed to the performance.

This phenomena of all-in all-out production associated with cleaning has been well known for a long time and yet on many farms it is still not practised. The reasons for the improved efficiencies are now better understood. In this study the pigs were no longer coming into an environment in which there was endemic disease. This was maintained by aerosol droplet infection from other pigs in the building and enteric organisms on floors and walls. The cleaned building was empty for periods of four days during and after the cleaning process and all the respiratory droplet organisms had time to be ventilated or precipitated from the air space. Whenever a pig enters an environment with older pigs already in the house, the large numbers of organisms present challenge the immune system of the incoming pigs and this process uses large amounts of protein and energy. This has effect of decreasing daily gain and food conversion efficiency whether serious specific diseases are present or not. This is a very important lesson to learn.

> **Pigs that are moved into houses that already have older pigs will always grow more slowly and be less efficient than those moved into an empty clean house.**

Colitis (inflammation of the large bowel) in growing pigs is now a common occurrence on pig farms. One of the major contributing factors is the continual use of pens, without washing and cleaning between batches.

Disciplines are almost invariably maintained in farrowing houses through all-in all-out procedures and by washing and disinfection. The same principles should apply equally across all pig buildings on the farm and in particular the mating area and the finishing houses. On many farms the mating pens have been in continual use for 25 years and we often wonder why reproductive performance has dropped gradually over intervening periods from farrowing rates of 90% to 80%. Other areas that require constant cleaning are foot dips and hands after handling diseased pigs. When a litter of young pigs have been treated for scour, the hands and clothing become heavily contaminated by as much as 15 to 20 billion organisms. ($^1/_2$ to 3 million will produce scour in the piglet).

> **Water + detergent is the cheapest disinfectant you have on the farm**

Facilities for washing and disinfecting hands to prevent the spread of infection should become an important part of environmental control.

A recommended routine for cleaning houses

1. Remove all muck and empty all slurry channels, tanks and gulleys.
2. Isolate the electricity supply.
3. Disconnect all moveable equipment, feeders, lamps etc. and open all inaccessible areas e.g. channels, fan boxes etc.
4. Brush down and sweep out the house.
5. Soak the complete building, roof to floor with a farm detergent or water, for 24 hours if possible.
6. Soak all moveable equipment and clean down.
7. Drain and flush out the water system, bowls, nipples, water tanks etc. and fill with a detergent steriliser. Leave for two hours drain and then refill with water.
8. Pressure wash the complete building using hot water or a steam cleaner.
9. Visually check the building.
10. Disinfect the complete house including all equipment and surrounds using a pressure washer or spray.
11. Follow this with fumigation using formalin gas where this is permitted with suitable precautions. Alternatively use a disinfectant such as Virkon S. (See Chapter 15)
12. Place a disinfectant foot bath outside the house and use prior to entry.
    Do not restock the house until dry. (A minimum of 48 hours).
    If you have to occupy the house before this then use a space heater to dry out the surfaces.

You will see from the above there are three chemicals required for the cleaning process.

First a detergent, which helps remove dirt and soiled material, second a detergent steriliser for cleaning and sterilising the water systems and finally a disinfectant to complete the cleaning process.

In houses where the floors are worn and in particularly farrowing pens it is good practice to brush the floor with lime wash (whitewash) after cleaning and disinfection. Carry out this procedure as follows:

- Wear goggles and gloves when handling this material since it is very irritant.
- Mix sufficient hydrated lime with water to produce a consistency of thin salad cream.
- Cover the farrowing house floor with the whitewash, using a soft household brush.
- Leave the surface for 48 hours to dry.
- Do not move the sow into the crate whilst the lime wash is wet. If you have to move the sow in before this do not brush the floor area where the sows udder will make contact.
- Lime wash can also be used on all concrete floors and can be of value in pens where, for example, greasy pig has become a problem. It is a very cheap disinfectant

and its value can be enhanced by adding 30g of phenolic disinfectant to 4.5 litres of lime wash.

Guidelines for fumigation

Using potassium permanganate and formalin

Formaldehyde is a noxious and highly toxic gas and exposure for only a short period can cause respiratory distress and with severe exposure ultimately coma. (Its use is forbidden in some countries).

Whenever fumigation is undertaken, there should be two people available. One in the house and one at the door to provide assistance if required.
- Wear protective goggles and a dampened face mask - these should be available to both persons.
- Use rubber gloves.
- Wet the house before fumigating and seal any openings.
- Always add formalin to the potassium permanganate. Have the exact quantities to be added ready in separate containers and add slowly.
Use high sided metal containers for mixing the compounds. Once the compounds are mixed vacate the house immediately.
- Ensure no livestock will be exposed to fumes that might escape.
- If the person in the house gets into difficulty, the person at the door should turn all fans on fully, open all doors and immediately pull the person out.
- Distribute the metal containers evenly through the house.
- Add 500mls formalin (40%) to 200grams of potassium permanganate per $28m^3$ of air space.
- Leave the building shut for 12 hours.
- Open up and ventilate eight hours before use.
- Place a notice on the door warning people "Fumigation in process".
- Oxygenating disinfectants such as Virkon S or Kwikstart sprayed as a fine mist, can be used as an alternate to fumigation with formalin. They are much safer and easier to handle.

Washing hands

Disinfection of hands should always take place after handling livestock, particularly where there has been faeces or urine contact. This is not least for personal hygiene reasons. (See chapter 17 Step 5 - Zoonoses....).

Hands should be washed following meals and after frozen or defrosted meat products have been handled because of the risk of transmission of such diseases as FMD, SVD and CSF.

The importance of washing hands after handling diseased pigs has already been highlighted in the case of scour in the farrowing houses. There is often a bewildering array of disinfectants available, each with attractive claims made as to their effectiveness. To make the best cost effective decision a number of questions should be asked.

Key points to consider when selecting a disinfectant (Fig.2-23)

- Always use a disinfectant that has been independently proven and has been shown to be effective against a wide range of infections but particularly those that are present on your farm. In many countries there are lists of approved disinfectants. Ask your veterinarian or supplier.
- Dilution rate - always read carefully the instructions as to use and in particular the amounts to be added to water for general disinfectant purposes. Check also the amounts required for the highly infectious diseases such as transmissible gastro-enteritis, aujeszky's disease and PRRS. From the cost of the concentrated disinfectant work out the cost of diluted chemical. A disinfectant costing £56 per 25 litres but with a dilution rate of 1:300 can be a much better buy than a disinfectant costing £56 per 25 litres and a dilution rate of 1:100.
- Time to act - there is always a minimum time before the disinfectant has killed micro organisms. Since most disinfectants are used at low temperatures always look at the killing time relative to this.
- Effectiveness in the presence of organic matter - this is important when using disinfectants on the farm, because invariably under such conditions they are going to come into contact with large amounts of organic matter. Some disinfectants such as chlorine are very quickly neutralised in the present of such materials. Footbaths contain high levels of organic matter due to continual contamination.
- Penetration - it is very important that the disinfectant has the ability to penetrate organic matter (detergency). In most cases however it is preferable to apply a detergent cleaner prior to the use of the disinfectant for more effective use.

Each group of disinfectants have their own special properties and an understanding of these will help you in your selection.

Detergents

These are cleansing agents which have good wetting powers and the properties of penetrating surfaces. Detergents can either be acid, alkaline or neutral. The neutral ones tend to be those such as soaps and liquids that are mainly used to remove soiled materials. They are often combined with the disinfectant to provide a dual action.

Disinfectants

The ideal disinfectant should be:
- Active quickly against a wide range of viruses, bacteria and fungi.
- Safe to handle.
- Active in the presence of dust or organic matter.
- Have a long period of activity.
- Non irritant, non staining, non toxic and non corro-

sive.
- Combined with a detergent or have such properties.
- Capable of use as an aerosol.
- Safe and effective when used in water systems.
- Capable of use through pressure washers.
- Coloured.

There are six classes of chemicals used for disinfection:
- Phenols.
- Chlorine based compounds.
- Iodine based compounds.
- Quaternary ammonia substances (QACs).
- Aldehydes.
- Peroxygen formulations.

Phenols

These are organic compounds that may or may not be combined with chlorine. They are usually effective in the present of organic matter but do not normally have a high detergent action. They are not however corrosive to metal but they can cause damage to plastic and rubber compounds. There action is moderately slow. Tar acids may be combined with other organic acids such as acetic and sulphuric acids to increase efficiency (e.g. Antec farm fluid S) to improve their effects against viruses.

Key facts about phenolic based disinfectants
- They are active in the present of organic matter.
- Their activity persists for a long period of time.
- They are ideal for vehicle dips and concrete floors.
- They have no detergent activity.
- Their rate of activity is slow two to twelve hours.
- They can be toxic and damage tissues.
- They are usually very effective against bacteria but not so good against viruses or spore producing bacteria.
- They are usually quite cheap.
- Some phenols such as chlorxylenols contain chlorine which adds properties of quick action.
- They taint milk and processed meat.

Chlorine based compounds

The chlorine based compounds can be considered in two groups. Those without organic compounds such as the hypochlorites which depend on the liberation of chlorine for their disinfection action and those that contain organic substances. Chlorine disinfectants have a very quick action but are very quickly neutralised in the presence of dirt or organic matter.

Key facts about the chlorine based disinfectants
- They can be very corrosive.
- They have a very quick action.
- They are inactivated by organic matter and hard waters.
- They do not persist for very long periods of time.
- They have no detergent activity.
- They are very active against viruses and bacteria.
- They may cause taint.
- They may be ozone unfriendly.
- They are very cheap.

Iodine based compounds

This group of disinfectants include substances called iodophors where the iodine is dissolved in a surface active agent and then phosphoric acid is added. Iodine substances are very safe, have low toxicity with almost no smell. When phosphoric acid however is added to the iodophors the disinfectant becomes a little more irritant and corrosive.

Key factors about iodine disinfectants (iodophors)
- Usually they have a high detergent activity.
- **They are ideal for foot baths.**
- They are brown in colour when very active becoming straw coloured when loosing their activity (used in footbaths for this reason).
- They are very quick in action.
- They are very effective against viruses and bacteria.
- They are moderately active in the present of organic matter.
- They tend to be more expensive.

Quaternary ammonia compounds (QACs)

These compounds may be used for cleaning and sterilising water systems and equipment and they are very efficient, particularly if the organic matter has been removed. They are not usually suitable for the disinfection of premises on their own because of the large amounts of organic materials present that immediately neutralise them. QACs are not compatible with soaps and they should not be mixed with other detergents. Some are used as antiseptics. They are more active against gram positive organisms.

Key factors about (QACs)
- They usually have little or no effect against fungi and bacterial spores.
- Inactive in the presence of organic matter.
- Inactivated by soaps and disinfectants.
- No activity against viruses.
- Suitable for cleaning water systems and smooth surfaces.

Aldehydes

These substances such as formaldehyde, are very toxic but are good disinfectants in aerosol form. There are now alternate products available that are equally effective and much safer to use (e.g. Virkon S).

Peroxygen compounds

These are the new broad spectrum disinfectants that are highly active against most micro-organisms. They are based on combinations of peroxyacetic acids or other derivatives, hydrogen peroxide, organic acids and anionic detergents. They are powerful oxygenating agents.

Managing Pig Health and the Treatment of Disease

THE CHARACTERISTICS OF THE DIFFERENT DISINFECTANT CHEMICALS						
	Chlorine Based	Peroxygen Compounds	Phenols Unchlorinated	Phenols Chlorinated	Iodophors	QAC Compounds
Can be used in aerosols	A Few	Yes	No	A Few	Yes	Yes
Corrosive to metal/rubber	No	No	Yes	Yes	No	No
Detergent action	No	Yes	No	Some	Yes	Yes
Effectiveness in presence of organic matter	Moderate	Yes	Yes	Yes	Moderate	No
Good action against bacteria	Moderate	Yes	Yes	Yes	Yes	Moderate
Good action against viruses	Yes	Yes	Poor	Poor	Yes	No
Persistent residues	No	No	Yes	No	Poor	Yes
Speed of action	Quick	Quick	Moderate	Moderate	Quick	Moderate
Staining	Some	No	Yes	Yes	Some	No
Suitable for foot baths	No	Yes	Yes	No	Yes	No
Toxic or irritant	Yes	No	Yes	Yes	Some	No

(Fig.2-23)

Precautions to be taken when using disinfectants

Always:
- Follow the manufacturers instructions carefully.
- Wear gloves and eye protectors when handling the concentrate.
- Wash concentrate off the skin immediately.
- Ensure the dilution is correct for the purpose being used.
- If there is contact with eyes wash immediately with copious amounts of water and seek medical help.
- Where foot baths are used ensure that these are cleaned and replenished regularly.
- Store in original container, tightly enclosed.
- Keep away from children.

What should you use on the farm

This would obviously depend on availability but the following should be considered:
- Foot baths - use an iodine based one.
- General disinfection of houses - use a phenol or organic acid based one.
- Water - use a QAC or chlorine based one.
- Concrete surfaces - use a phenol or organic acid based one.
- Broken floor surfaces not easily cleaned - use an oil based phenol type.
- Virus infections - use iodophors or peroxygen complexes (Virkon S). (Formalin fumigation is also effective).
- Bacterial problems - use iodophors or peroxygen complexes.
- Hands - use QAC compounds or soaps.
- Loading ramps - use a government approved disinfectant that is highly active against the major notifiable and transmissible diseases in your country.
- Aerosols - use formalin, chlorine, iodine or oxidising agents preferably the latter.

THE CONSEQUENCES AND SUBSEQUENT EFFECTS OF INTRODUCING A NEW DISEASE INTO THE HERD			
Disease	Time of Acute Disease (weeks)	Mortality Due to the Disease	
		During the Period of Acute Disease	During the Period of Chronic Disease.
Actinobacillus pleuropneumonia (App)	2 - 15	3 - 30 %	2 - 4 %
Atrophic rhinitis (AR)	8 - 26	1 - 5 % Weaners	1 %
Acute respiratory disease syndrome	2 - 15	3 - 10 % Weaners, Feeders	2 - 8% Weaners, Feeders
Enzootic pneumonia (EP)	4 - 18	2 - 14 % Sows	up to 3% Feeders
Parvovirus infertility	7 - 21	0.5 - 4 Pigs / Litter	0.5 - 1 Pigs / Litter
PRRS	8 - 16	5 - 30 % Piglets	0 - 1 Pigs a Litter
Streptococcal meningitis (SM)	4 - 12	4 - 12 % Weaners	1 - 5 %
Swine dysentery (SD)	3 - 12	1 - 4 % Post-weaning	1 - 1.5%
TGE	3 - 4	90 - 100% Piglets	1 - 4 %

(Fig.2-24)

The Costs of Disease

Economics and the high health herd

The most important reason for the establishment of a high health herd is to mitigate the severe effects of infectious disease. Most infectious diseases (excluding infections such as porcine parvovirus and leptospirosis) depress both the food conversion efficiency and daily live weight gain together with increases in mortality.

THE EFFECTS OF DISEASE ON GROWTH AND FOOD CONVERSION EFFICIENCY. (FCE)				
Disease	During Period Of Acute Disease		During Period of Chronic Disease	
	FCE	Days to 90kg	FCE	Days to 90kg
Actinobacillus pleuropneumonia (App)	0.1 - 0.4	7 - 30	0.1 - 0.3	4 - 15
Atrophic rhinitis (AR)	0.1 - 0.2	4 - 15	0.1 - 0.2	4 - 15
Chronic respiratory disease	0.1 - 0.4	7 - 30	0.1 - 0.3	7 - 28
Enzootic pneumonia (EP)	0.1 - 0.4	10 - 21	0.05 - 0.1	3 - 21
Mange	0.1	7 - 18	0.1	5 - 8
Streptococcal meningitis (SM)	0.05	1 - 3	0.05	0
Swine dysentery (SD)	0.1 - 0.3	5 - 20	0.3	4 - 5
TGE	0.1	4 - 10	0 - 0.15	0 - 3

(Fig.2-25)

CHAPTER 2 - Understanding Disease

The factors contributing to the cost of disease include

- Pig mortality - This results in increased production costs.
- Increased overhead costs.
- Increased feed costs.
- Loss of profit.
- Decreased feed efficiency.
- Increased stocking density.
- Slow growth - low daily liveweight gain.
- Less liveweight sold from the farm and a reduced throughput.
- An increased incidence of other diseases
- Increased labour costs.
- Increased veterinary costs and medicines.

Fig.2-24 shows the mortality associated with specific diseases, based on field data, both in the early acute phase when the organism first enters a non immune herd and after it has moved into an enzootic or chronic form.

Fig.2-25 shows the continuing effects on production once the acute episode has subsided.

Fig.2-26 shows the costs of outbreaks of disease (calculated and or actual) based upon specific mortalities, loss of production and/or reproduction and feed efficiency.

COSTS OF DISEASE FOR EACH 1% LOSS FROM TARGET PER 100 SOWS (FROM UK FIELD DATA)	
	£
Farrowing rate	800
Repeat matings	400
Abortion	900
Non pregnant sows	950
Non infectious infertility	700
Stillbirths	700
Piglet mortality	600
Crushed	600
Low viable	600
Scours	600
Losses post-weaning	800
Finishing pig losses	1300

(Fig.2-27)

Feed costs of £165 per tonne and a margin over feed of £24 per pig have been used in the calculations. Veterinary costs include in-feed medication. Clearly actual costs depend upon the price of feed and market prices in your country but the figures place relative values on the costs of disease.

These costs relate to the acute phase of the disease and subsequent effects over 12 months and obviously such costs depend upon the severity of the outbreak and

COSTS OF DISEASE OVER A 12 MONTH PERIOD PER 100 SOWS AND THE PROGENY OF 2000 PIGS TO 90KG (UK Field Data)						
Condition or Disease	Veterinary costs * (£)	Mortality and Culls	Performance Loss	Recorded Disease Level	Net Cost £ / Annum / 100 sows	Target Level
Foot-and-mouth disease	Slaughter policy	Slaughter policy	100%		50,000	
Swine vesicular disease	Slaughter policy	Slaughter policy	100%		50,000	
Swine fever	Slaughter policy	Slaughter policy	100%		50,000	
Atrophic rhinitis	300	2%	FCE, Dlwg	High	15,000	Zero
Aujeszky's (pseudorabies)	2250	375 pigs	FCE, Dlwg	High	16,800	Zero
Transmissible gastro-enteritis	540	315 pigs	10 - 14 days growth	High	12,400	Zero
Pneumonia complex	9000	2 - 6 %	FCE, Dlwg	Variable	10,000 - 16,000	Zero
Infertility viruses		402 piglets	Loss of margin over feed. Re-production	High	7, 500	Zero
Swine dysentery	14000	1%	FCE, Dlwg	Low	16,200	Zero
Farrowing rate		615 pigs	70%		15,000	89%
Repeat matings		106 piglets	17%		4,000	6 - 8%
Abortion		230 piglets	11%		9,200	1.0%
Non pregnant sows		92 pigs	6 %		3,800	2.0%
Non infectious infertility		410 pigs lost	Loss of margin over feed	72% farrowing rate	13,000	89
Piglet mortality	682		177 pigs	15 %	4,400	8 %
Stillbirths			84 pigs	8%	2,000	5 %
Crushed by sow		76 pigs	Loss of margin over feed	4%	1,900	1.0%
Poor viability		163 pigs	Loss of margin over feed	3.5%	1,500	1.0%
Piglet scours	555	50 pigs	Loss of margin over feed	2.5%	1,200	0.5%
Post-weaning losses	489	148	Loss of margin over feed + feed costs	8%	2,200	1.5%
Finishing losses	789	125	Loss of margin over feed + feed costs	7 %	7,400	1.5%

* Includes in-feed medication.
FCE = Food conversion efficiency.   **Dlwg** = Daily liveweight gain.

(Fig.2-26)

its period of continuation in that particular herd at that level of disease.

Based upon the figures in Fig-2-26 it is possible to produce guidelines of the costs of disease for a 1% adverse change from the target level as shown in 2-27.

Depopulation and Repopulation

The major costs of establishing a high health herd by depopulation and repopulation are related to the loss in cash flow and ongoing overhead costs between removing the old herd and its sale of pigs and the first pig sold at slaughter from the new one. In basic terms, the margin over feed per week represents the approximate costs of depopulation (building/maintenance costs need to be budgeted for). The farm must be emptied for a minimum of 4-6 weeks (8 weeks if swine dysentery exists in the farm) and further time lost will depend upon the date of commencement of the mating programme for the new incoming herd.

Depopulation can be carried out in one of two ways:

A. by complete removal of the herd at a fixed point in time, or
B. gradual removal towards a predetermined date.

Repopulation of the herd can be carried out with maiden or pregnant gilts that are up to two weeks from farrowing.

The most cost effective method is to remove the existing weaned and growing pigs to a totally separate well isolated site where their production can be completed. The donor herd should ideally have facilities to commence the new gilt mating programme and hold these to within two weeks of farrowing. Alternatively the pregnant gilts 21 days post-service could be moved to a holding site.

Fig.2-28 illustrates the actual programme used in the depopulation and repopulation of a 350 sow herd by method B. The breeding farm producing 30kg weaners was a separate site 5km away from the finishing farm. The new gilts were mated on the supply farm and then moved to a holding farm when they were 6 weeks in pig where they remained until 2 weeks prior to farrowing. The complete gilt herd of both maiden and pregnant animals was then moved into the depopulated farm over a period of 4-6 weeks.

The decision to use either method A or B is a complex one and it is dictated by such factors as the current economics of the pig industry, the levels and costs of disease, the availability of maiden or pregnant gilts, the type of herd and the availability of holding accommodation.

For the combined breeding and finishing farm planning will be different and the decisions will depend upon:

- The age / weight of the youngest pigs to be sold and the point of depopulation e.g. 30kg liveweight.
- The date of the last farrowing to produce 30kg pigs.
- The date on which the last disease sows are mated.
- The date when the new gilt mating programme commences. This will depend on whether the programme starts on the supply farm a holding farm or the repopulated farm.

From the above information it can be seen that method B as illustrated is by far the most cost effective (Fig.2-29) but equally the most complex. Method A can be improved further by selling diseased sows up to 6 weeks in pig and weaners at an earlier age.

Depopulation, repopulation costs

These represent 14 weeks of loss on a 350 sow herd - probably the very best that can be achieved. As a guide field experiences give approximate costs of £40,000 to £50,000 per 100 sows in a combined breeding finishing farm using the worst case scenario. To set against this however improvements of up to 0.4 in feed efficiency, 100g daily gain and significant reductions in mortality and medicinal costs should be achieved in the new herd. The repopulation would also allow the most updated genetics to be used to further obvious advantage.

If the finishing accommodation on a combined breeding finishing unit can be used for multi suckling then increasing the gilt mating programme and therefore the numbers of gilts farrowing is a very valuable procedure to consider. There are always a number of gilts which have to be culled after first weaning and this can also help reduce the herd to its proper size without the purchase of replacements in large batches. Farrowing a surplus number of gilts first time round costs more up front but gives a quicker return on cash flow.

Cleaning an existing pig farm is a no mean undertaking and you should be aware of the hard work that is involved. Furthermore, considerable expense will be involved in refurbishing the farm since many maintenance requirements are not evident until the buildings are empty. It is also an opportunity for major alterations.

In carrying out the cleaning and disinfection procedures efforts should be made to remove all faeces and manure from the farm. Slurry channels should be emptied and washed down and a visual and bacteriological check carried out once cleaning and disinfection has been completed.

It is vitally important that rats and mice are completely removed from the farm. Once all the houses have been cleaned then each in rotation should be sealed and fumigated with formaldehyde gas, or sprayed with a suitable disinfectant such as Virkon S. Dead pig pits should be covered with lime and finally buried.

Provided the farm is left empty for a period of 6-8 weeks few of the important disease organisms will survive except for SVD, CSF, ASF and salmonella.

Over the years clean herds have been established successfully by depopulation and repopulation for the following diseases.

- App.
- AR.
- Aujeszky's disease.
- EP.
- Foot-and-mouth disease.
- Mange.
- Salmonellosis.
- Swine fever.
- Streptococcal meningitis.
- Swine dysentery.
- Swine vesicular disease.
- TGE

Enzootic pneumonia and PRRS have however proved to be the most difficult diseases to keep out. The purchased pig has been the main cause of reinfection.

| METHOD B COSTS ||||
| In the illustrated herd these were calculated as follows ||||
	Breeding Farm £	Finishing Farm £	Total Costs £
Labour 15 weeks	9,400	2,350	11,750
Lost margin on 2025 pigs sold light	6,000		6,000
Cleaning	750	750	1,500
Maintenance	4,400	4,050	8,450
Other	3,750	1,900	5,650
Total costs	24,300	9,050	33,350

(Fig.2-29)

AN EXAMPLE OF A DEPOPULATION PLAN

Week number and action

Week	Action
1	Last diseased sows mated
2–17	Diseased sows sold after weaning. Breeding buildings cleaned and repaired as emptied
14	Last diseased sows farrow.
17	Last diseased sows weaned.
20	Last sows sold, weaners to holding farm.
21	Breeding farm empty, clean/disinfect.
22–27	—
27	First High Health gilts moved into cleaned farm.
28–32	—
30	First High Health gilts farrow.
33	First High Health gilts weaned.
34	Remaining diseased finishing pigs moved to holding farm.
35	Finishing farm empty, cleaning and disinfection programmed begins.
35–52	High Health gilts mated on supply farm
38	Last diseased fat pigs sold from holding farm.
41	—
42	First High Health weaners moved into cleaned finishing farm.
52	First sales of High Health finishing pigs.

TOTAL LOST INCOME 14 WEEKS.... (weeks 38–52)

(Fig. 2-28)

3 Managing Health and Disease

Management components of health control..55
Immunity - how the pig responds to infection 56
    Innate (i.e. Inherited) and non-specific resistance....................................58
    Acquired specific immunity..60
    The role of passive immunity in the development of actively
    acquired immunity 62
    Serological tests..62
    Vaccination...63
    Immunosuppression..65
Medicinal control of disease 66
Eradicating disease..66
Recognising disease on the farm 66
    The use of sight..66
    Observation of the group..67
    Changes in behaviour...67
    The use of smell 67
    The use of touch 67
    The use of sound..67
Clinical examination of the herd 67
    Assessing health, management and disease in outdoor production 70
The management and treatment of the sick pig 74
    The design of the hospital pen..75
Disposal of dead pigs..76
The consultant or specialist veterinarian..76
Staff training and education...77
    An example of management failures and disease 81
The use of records..82
    Recording objectives..82
Planning for efficient production and disease control 88
    Management procedures for maximising the mating programme...............88
Management of the environment 89
    Environmental factors affecting dry sows..90
    Environmental factors affecting lactating sows and sucking pigs 90
    Environmental factors affecting growing pigs 91
    Air quality..91
    Environmental temperatures 92
    Stocking densities..93
    Segregated weaning and disease control procedures................................94
Nutrition and feeding... 101
Water 102

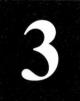

Managing Health and Disease

There are many factors that affect the economic viability of modern day pig production. For a business to be successful it must take account of all of them. Disease is one that plays a significant role. The important factors that you might be able to control and improve are highlighted here. You should find it of value to consider each and assess them in relation to your own pig farm.

There are other factors, such as government regulations which are completely out of your control and so are omitted from this check list. Likewise, money available to the consumer is a national problem, rather than one at farm level. The important criteria on the farm, however, are the price of feed and the efficiency with which this is converted into liveweight gain and ultimately lean meat. The interaction between people, management, the environment and disease, dictates the efficiency of these conversions.

Manipulate any of these and improve your profitability.

Management Components of Health Control

Chapter 2 discussed the various organisms that can produce disease. In many cases the causes are multifactorial involving an interaction between the pig, the environment the management and the organism. The components of this interaction are listed below. If the biological efficiency of your pigs is to be maximised it is necessary to give detailed attention to these eleven points.
- Immunity of the pig. How the pig responds to infection.
- Medicinal control of disease.
- Eradicating disease.
- Recognising and monitoring disease at a clinical level.
- Treatment of sick and casualty pigs.
- The use of a veterinary consultant.
- Staff training and education.
- Understanding how to use records.
- Planning for efficient production.
- Management manipulation of the system and the environment.
- Good nutrition.

These factors are placed into perspective in Fig.3-1,

FACTORS THAT AFFECT THE ECONOMIC VIABILITY OF MODERN DAY PIG PRODUCTION
- Application of new technology.
- Continuing education / training.
- Control of pollution.
- Daily liveweight gain.
- Disease control and treatment.
- Efficiency of feed conversion to lean meat.
- Efficiency of pen utilisation.
- Environmental restrictions.
- Equipment cost and quality.
- Genetic potential of the pigs.
- Its control and treatment.
- Labour cost.
- Management and motivation of people.
- Management decisions.
- Market outlets.
- Methods of feeding.
- Number of pigs sold per year.
- Nutrition and quality of the feed.
- Planning.
- Price of feed.
- Reproductive performance.
- Size of the herd.
- Slaughter price.
- Stocking densities.
- The control of pollution.
- Transport cost.
- Use of records.
- Weight and grade of pigs sold at slaughter.
- Welfare requirements.

which also highlights how they should be adopted towards maximising pig health. Pig health is interpreted as maximum biological efficiency.

Maintaining an efficient healthy pig farm starts with good planning. To achieve this it is necessary to have an efficient recording system. This can be a simple manual or a computer programme that identifies both production details and health levels and measures results against predetermined levels of efficiency. It is also necessary to identify those diseases that are present in the herd and take measures to prevent new diseases entering. The risks of disease being introduced by purchased pigs have been dealt with in chapter 2 but the management and integration of the gilt and the boar when they first enter the herd also needs to be addressed. Finally the services of an experienced veterinarian can have a major impact not only on the profitability of the farm but also improving on the status quo.

The infectious organisms that cause disease in pigs are viruses, bacteria, fungi and parasites. At a clinical level they can be divided into three groups.
1. Primary (non-indigenous) pathogens.
2. Enzootic opportunist pathogens.

Managing Pig Health and the Treatment of Disease

3. Harmless commensals.

Primary pathogens are not present in all herds but when they enter a susceptible herd they usually cause disease. They are responsible for major infectious diseases such as swine fever, foot and mouth disease, transmissible-gastro-enteritis, aujeszky's disease (pseudorabies), enzootic pneumonia, atrophic rhinitis, swine dysentery. Such diseases occur at varying levels depending upon the pathogenicity (virulence) of the strain (i.e. its capacity to produce disease) the numbers of organisms that are presented to the pig and the degree of immunity that exists in the herd to the infectious agent.

Enzootic opportunist pathogens are those that are always present in all herds and yet do not cause disease unless there are deficiencies in the environment. Such organisms include streptococci responsible for joint infections, coliform bacteria causing piglet diarrhoea, virulent staphylococci that cause greasy pig disease, and klebsiella associated with mastitis to mention but a few.

Harmless commensals are found on the skin, in the respiratory and alimentary tract, vagina and prepuce. They are mostly bacteria, of which there are hundreds of species in the large intestine alone, but some are fungi and protozoa. Very few viruses can be regarded as harmless commensals.

Immunity - How the Pig Responds to Infection

Infection is considered to have taken place when a virus, bacterium or parasite enters a pig and starts to multiply. If it is a potentially pathogenic organism it may change the normal structure and function of the pig. A study of these changes is called pathology and organisms causing disease are described as pathogens. Fig.3-2 shows the sequence of events that may take place when an infectious pathogen infects the pig.

Infection creates two scenarios; the first is when there is no disease. The immune mechanism of the pig responds to challenge and the infectious agent is either eliminated or remains within the body in a carrier state. The carrier pig may or may not shed the organism or may shed it intermittently. The second scenario is that of disease which is followed by an immune response and complete recovery and elimination of the pathogen or recovery with a carrier state, or death. Whether the organism causes disease or not is dependent on how viru-

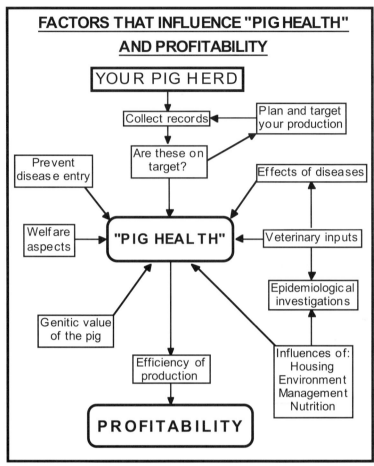
(Fig.3-1)

lent (the capability of the organism to produce disease) it is, how many organisms are present, what other concurrent infections are present, what protective mechanisms are available in the pig to prevent disease and what environmental or other factors are present that will lower the pigs immunity. For example, certain strains of *Actinobacillus pleuropneumoniae* are only mildly pathogenic and do not normally produce disease. However if they are in combination with PRRS virus the presence of both could produce severe pneumonia. A non pregnant gilt exposed to parvovirus infection only develops an immune response but no signs of disease because disease only occurs in the developing foetus. Nevertheless the gilt would become serologically positive in laboratory tests.

> **Bad management allows opportunist pathogens to produce disease.**

A successful and healthy pig farm is one in balance and harmony with the organisms that are present both in the environment and the pig. It is the manipulation of this balance that is so important to health and disease and ultimately to productivity and profitability.

> **Group 1 - Primary pathogens produce disease in a susceptible herd. You are better off without them.**

CHAPTER 3 - Managing Health and Disease

Disease is a numbers game :
- *A minimum number of infectious particles is required.*
- *The numbers required depends on the virulence of the organism*
- *The number required depends on the level of immunity.*

It follows that if the numbers of organisms in the environment can be maintained at a minimum then the threshold level of organisms necessary to produce disease is unlikely to be reached. Examples here would be the excellent growth rates that can be achieved with all-in all-out systems in nurseries or flat decks, when pigs are housed on weld mesh or slatted floors and they are divorced from their faeces and potential enteric organisms. Likewise in respiratory diseases, the more pigs there are in a common air space, and the smaller the cubic capacity of that air space relative to the numbers of pigs, then the greater will be the numbers of aerosol organisms and the more severe disease.

To be a successful pig producer you should have some idea of how pigs resist infectious disease. Unfortunately, it is a complex subject and although here an attempt has been made to simplify it, it will probably still seem a little complicated.

The technical terms used in immunology (i.e. the study of immunity) are a major part of the problem. If you have not had a good grounding in biology they may be like a foreign language. If that is the case, or even if it is not, start by reading through the terminology below.

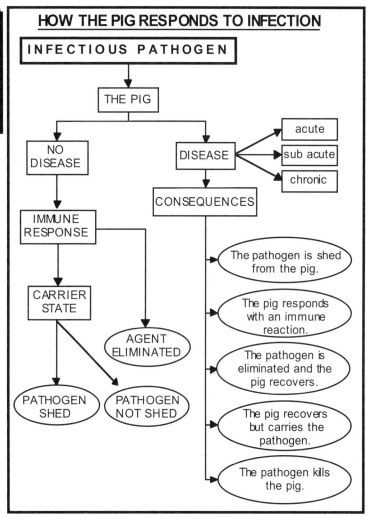

(Fig.3-2)

Terminology

Adjuvant - A substance added to an inactivated vaccine to make it more effective.
Antibodies - Complex large proteins (called gamma-globulins) which are produced by specialised cells in response to invading antigens and which stick specifically to the invading antigen neutralising it or triggering off a destructive reaction.
Antigen - Foreign invading substance (i.e. a substance which is not normally part of the pig's body), usually consisting of protein or part of a protein, which stimulates the body to produce antibodies. Antigens exist on the surfaces of bacteria, viruses and parasites.
Antiserum - Serum with high antibody levels against a specific infection. It has usually been produced experimentally in laboratory animals by injecting the infection into them.
Blood sample - Whole blood sample taken hygienically with a syringe into a bottle or by a pin prick through the skin absorbing the droplet of blood with blotting paper.

Commensal bacteria - Bacteria that live permanently in or on the body without causing disease.
Epithelium - Cellular membrane (e.g. mucous membranes) containing epithelial and other cells.
Humoral immunity - Blood-borne immunity.
Hyperimmune antiserum - The same as antiserum above but emphasising its high titre.
Lymphocytes - Specialised defence cells in lymph nodes, other lymphatic tissue and the blood which produce antibodies or take part in cellular immunity.
Mucous membranes - Cellular membranes (e.g. those lining the gut) which secrete a sticky substance called

Remember:
Expose your pigs to too many pathogenic organisms and you have sick pigs - poor performers.
Lower the level of pathogens in the environment and you have healthy pigs - high performers.

mucus on to their surfaces.
Mucus - A clear sticky semi-liquid secreted by cells in mucous membranes.
Pathogenic infection - An infectious organism which has the potential to cause disease. This is in contrast to the many organisms that live normally in or on the body which never cause disease and are called commensals.

> **Resistance to infectious disease is a key to herd health.**

Phagocytes - Cells of the body whose special task is to engulf bacteria, viruses, or parasites in an attempt to destroy them. They are also called macrophages.
Phagocytosis - The process whereby the specialised cells of the body engulf bacteria, viruses or parasites in an attempt to destroy them.
Plasma sample - A whole blood sample taken hygienically with a syringe and mixed with an anti-clotting agent so that it remains liquid. The sample is spun fast in a centrifuge and the red and white blood cells sediment to a firm pellet at the bottom leaving a clear liquid - the plasma.
Serology - Tests done in the laboratory to detect the level of specific antibodies in serum samples ("ology" means study of - so literally serology means "study of serum").
Serum sample - A whole blood sample taken hygienically with a syringe and allowed to clot. The serum is the clear straw-coloured liquid which can be drawn of with a pipette. It contains the antibodies.
Titre - The concentration of a specific antibody in a serum sample. It is expressed as the amount by which the serum has to be diluted before a serological test goes negative.
Virulence - How pathogenic an organism is. Organisms with a high capability of causing disease are called highly virulent.

The main components that make up the resistance of a pig to infection may also seem complicated but if you refer to Fig.3-3 as you read it should also help you to understand the text better. You do not need to understand all the components but take note of the following:.
- What antibodies are.
- What stimulates them to be produced.
- The importance of colostrum and milk in providing immunity.
- Why blood tests are done and how they are interpreted.
- How vaccines work.

Innate (i.e. inherited) and Non-Specific Resistance

Innate and non-specific resistance is that which all pigs are born with or, in the case of some forms of non-specific resistance, that which develops as the pigs grow regardless of what infections they are exposed to. They consist of:
Physical barriers - These are the external and internal body surfaces of the respiratory, alimentary and urogenital tracts, namely skin, horn and hair externally; and internally, the membranes that line the nose, sinuses, throat and the tracheal and bronchial air tubes, the mouth, stomach and intestines; the vagina, uterus, bladder and urinary tubes. Other internal barriers include joint capsules and the blood-brain barrier.
Chemical barriers - The mucous on the surface of mucous membranes and some other body fluids such as saliva and tears contain antibacterial and anti-viral substances such as lysozyme and interferon. The acid in the stomach also inactivates bacteria and viruses to some degree.
Complement system - This is a series of at least 20 proteins (enzymes) in the blood that attack foreign cellular material in a sequential cascading manner, the first one or two acting and stimulating the next to act and so on. "Foreign" means non-self, i.e. material that is not part of the pig's normal body. Although complement acts non-specifically its action may be enhanced by some specific antibodies.

You may wonder how complement distinguishes between "self" and "non-self". It does so because the pig's own cells have a coating of special pig-protective protein that acts like Teflon in a non-stick saucepan. It specifically stops the pig's own complement from sticking to surfaces of its own cells to ensure they are not destroyed. If it can not stick, it can not destroy. Viruses, bacteria and parasites do not possess this special pig protein so they are not protected.

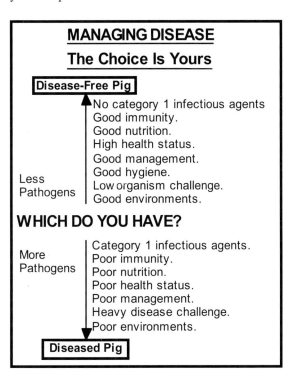

Phagocytosis - Certain defence cells, called phagocytes, can engulf foreign material such as an invading bacterium in an attempt to destroy it within the body's tissue or to carry it away (e.g. to the gut) in order to eliminate it from the body. Phagocytes fall into two groups, polymorphs and monocytes.

The first group, the polymorphs, are part of the blood white cell population. They circulate in the blood but respond quickly when pathogenic infection occurs. They rapidly migrate out of the blood stream to attack the infection. Some virulent bacteria are covered with a slippery capsule which inhibits the polymorphs from engulfing them. A specific antibody (called an opsonin) is then required to stick to the capsule enabling the polymorph to engulf it. One type of polymorph (eosinophil) tends to attack parasites.

The second group of phagocytes; monocytes, also start initially as part of the blood white cell population. They circulate in the blood to start with but then migrate into the tissues and onto inner body surfaces to become local tissue macrophages or they wander through the tissues as wandering macrophages. These macrophages are usually capable of engulfing viruses and bacteria non-specifically, i.e. without the aid of specific antibodies.

Bacteria, viruses, parasites and toxins contain antigens. Antigens stimulate antibody production.

Macrophages engulf bacteria and viruses in order to destroy them or remove them from the body but they are not always successful. Some virulent bacteria and viruses can survive and multiply inside macrophages often destroying the macrophages. For example, the virus of PRRS (porcine reproductive and respiratory syndrome) multiplies in the macrophages of the lungs and destroys them thus compromising the lung immunity.

Virulent strains of the bacterium *Streptococcus suis* type 2 and some other bacteria that cause meningitis, behave like the Greek legend of the Trojan horse. To get through the blood-brain barrier, which is normally resistant to penetration by bacteria, they hide in migrating monocytes. The monocytes then migrate through the blood-brain barrier to become brain macrophages where the bacteria break out to cause meningitis.

Probiotic flora - The skin, mouth, stomach, intestines, vagina and prepuce have a complex mixture of non disease producing organisms, mostly bacteria, that have evolved over thousands of years to live in intimate relationship with each other. They are usually limited to one part of the host. Some of them are antagonistic to invading pathogenic bacteria and inhibit their growth. Examples in the gut are the inhibitory activities of bacteroides organisms against *E. coli* or lactobacillus

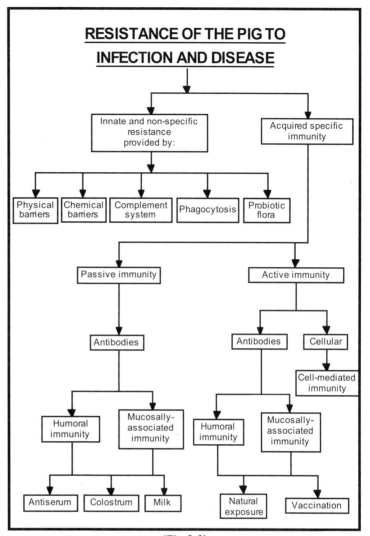

(Fig.3-3)

against salmonella. This 'indigenous flora' is not inherited, i.e. piglets are not born with it. However it is related to the pig's individual characteristics because it differs from the indigenous flora of other species. It is always the same mixture in any individual pig throughout life. As the pigs grow this indigenous flora becomes increasingly complex.

Lactobacillus bacteria inhibit the multiplication of other pathogenic bacteria by secreting lactic acid. Lactic acid is available commercially to put in water or feed in order to reduce bacterial multiplication.

Various combinations of probiotic bacteria, (usually streptococci and/or lactobacilli) are also available commercially for feeding to newborn pigs or to restore the flora of pigs which have been lost through treatment with oral antibiotics. Experimentally probiotics have been shown to be effective but they are sometimes disappointing when applied on the farm. See chapter 14.

Acquired Specific Immunity

This is the immunity that the pig acquires as it goes through life. It may be obtained actively or passively.

Actively produced specific antibodies

When a foreign protein or part of a protein (called an antigen) enters the body, the body responds by producing antibodies in the lymphocytes of its lymphatic tissues. This is known as antigenic stimulation.

Antigens stimulate the production of antibodies which circulate in the blood and body fluids. They are secreted onto epithelial surfaces and specifically adhere to the antigen. The surface of the antibody fits snugly on to the complex corrugated surface of the antigen. The adherent antibodies may then have one of several effects. They may:
- neutralise the antigen (common with some viruses), or
- enable white blood cells to phagocytose it (such antibodies are called opsonins), or
- in conjunction with complement, disable and possibly destroy it.

In some infections they may have little or no effect.

Active antibody production in pigs is mostly brought about by natural exposure of the lymphocytes to the surface proteins on viruses, bacteria and parasites or by exposure to toxins.

It can also be induced artificially by the inoculation of vaccines or toxoids (denatured toxins which have lost their potency but retain their ability to stimulate antibodies).

Or it can be stimulated by the deliberate feeding of substances such as faeces (i.e. so-called 'feed back').

Delayed production

When a new pathogen invades a pig the antibody response takes about 10 to 14 days to reach maximum levels. This delay is important in relation to natural infection and also to vaccination, since protection is not immediate. Pigs keep meeting new infections throughout their lives, particularly when they are young. If a new infection is pathogenic it may be 5 to 7 days before specific antibodies against the pathogen start to appear, during which time the pig could succumb to disease.

Furthermore if it occurs at a time when the pig is disadvantaged, e.g. having just been moved and mixed in a different pen or during a change of feed, the antibody response may be partly suppressed.

When a pathogen which has infected the pig previously invades the pig again the antibody response is much quicker because the lymphocytes which were primed by the first infection are still present. This is also true in a pig which has not been previously infected but has been vaccinated.

Antibodies are large proteins called immunoglobulins (Ig) of which there are three main types, IgG, IgM and IgA. They can be humoral (i.e. circulating in the blood and body fluids) and thus getting into all the body organs and tissues, or they can be local on the surface of mucous membranes such as those lining the respiratory and alimentary tract. These are called mucosal associated antibodies.

Humoral antibodies

Over 80% of the humoral immunoglobulin circulating in the blood of the mature pig is IgG, about 10% is IgM and most of the rest is IgA.

If a pig is vaccinated by intramuscular or subcutaneous injection against an infectious pathogen that invades the body (e.g. against diseases such as erysipelas or swine fever) the humoral antibodies produced are effective in blocking the invasion.

> **To produce maximum immunity in the intestine the intestines themselves have to be antigenically stimulated.**

Mucosal associated antibodies

If a pig is vaccinated (e.g. into the muscle or under the skin) against an intestinal infection such as TGE virus or enterotoxigenic *E. coli* which multiply and do their damage in the gut, the humoral antibody response induced is unlikely to prevent the organism multiplying in the gut or to greatly reduce the diarrhoea that results.

To be fully effective in the gut, the immunising antigen must stimulate a local immunity mainly by acting on the lymphatic tissues of the intestines ("Peyer's patches"). This results in the production of IgA just below the surface layer of the gut. The IgA passes through the cells of the mucous membrane and attaches

> **Stress depresses the pig's immune response.**

to another molecule called the secretory component. It is then called secretory IgA and consists of two IgA antibody molecules joined together by the secretory component. This combination increases their potency, makes them resistant to digestion by gut enzymes, and more readily absorbed by mucus. Since the mucus coats the whole lining of the intestines and the respiratory tract, the secretory IgA acts as a shield against potentially pathogenic infections.

In contrast to humoral antibodies, therefore, mucosal associated antibodies in the pig are principally IgA, in the form of secretory IgA.

> **High colostrum intake soon after birth is vital to the survival of the piglet.**

Cell-mediated immunity

There are two broad categories of immune reaction to infection:
1. Humoral immunity in which a major component is antibodies in the blood.
2. Cell-mediated immunity which need not involve antibodies.

Although they can occur independently, they usually both occur at the same time with greatly enhanced benefit. Cell-mediated immunity is initiated by lymphocytes originating from the thymus gland (T lymphocytes), whereas humoral immunity involves lymphocytes that are derived originally from the bone marrow (B lymphocytes). Cell-mediated immunity also involves other types of cell such as macrophages and natural killer cells.

Whereas it's important for you as a pig farmer to have some understanding of humoral immunity because of its association with blood testing, maternal immunity (colostrum and milk) and vaccination, it is much less important for you to understand cell-mediated immunity except to be aware that it exists.

Passively acquired immunity

So far we have been considering active immune reactions that result from stimulation of the pig's immune system by invading antigens but immunity can be passive without the pig's immune system being stimulated. Passively acquired immunity, usually termed "passive immunity", is acquired naturally by the newborn piglet through the ingestion of colostrum and milk or artificially by the injection of antiserum or oral dosing of colostrum substitutes.

Colostrum

Unlike human babies and puppies, no antibodies are transferred through the placenta from the sow to her piglets before birth. Normally, piglets are born in a vulnerable state without any humoral or mucosal associated antibodies and no acquired cell-mediated immunity. Fortunately, towards the end of gestation when the sow's mammary glands develop, the first secretion they produce, colostrum, is rich in antibodies representing the whole spectrum of the sow's own circulating antibodies. A first instinct of the newborn piglet is to find and suck a teat. Normally, a sow has voluntary control over milk let down, but during farrowing this control is weak. The piglets nuzzle the teat and surrounding gland and then suck the teat. This results in a rapid let-down of colostrum. In the first twelve to twenty four hours of life the piglet's intestines are able to absorb whole antibodies before the enzymes in the intestines digest them. Consequently, within a short period after a good first suck, the piglet's blood contains the full spectrum of its dam's antibodies often at about the same level as that of the sow.

Four points must be emphasised.
1. Without maternal antibodies the piglet is highly susceptible to infection. It is essential for the piglet's survival that it drinks colostrum soon after birth before pathogenic micro-organisms have had time to multiply and invade. It is also essential that it ingests enough colostrum to provide adequate protection until it has actively produced its own humoral antibodies.

> **Good hygiene in the farrowing house is essential for survival even if levels of colostral antibodies in the piglet's blood are high.**

2. The ability of the piglet's intestine to absorb colostral antibody is short-lived, but is shortened still further when the piglet has drunk. Thus, if a piglet that has had no colostrum, is to be cross-fostered onto another sow, or given substitute colostrum orally, it should be done in the first few hours of life and no other nutrients should be given in advance. The fostering sow must also still have colostrum available.

> **Piglets with low levels of maternal antibody in their blood stream are likely to die.**

3. Being passively acquired the amount of antibody in the blood stream is finite and can be exhausted by exposure to excessive antigen. Put another way, there is a maximum amount of colostral antibody that a pig can absorb into its blood stream. Overwhelming doses of bacteria will use it all up.

> **Maternal antibodies against different pathogens decline at different rates. Most have gone by 8-12 weeks of age.**

4. The passively acquired colostral antibodies in the blood gradually waste away to about half the initial level by about ten to fourteen days, although they may persist at a reasonably protective level against most pathogenic antigens for six to twelve weeks. (See Fig.3-4). The time taken to decline to ineffective levels varies depending upon the amount of colostral antibody taken in by the piglet and on the type of infection or toxin against which the antibody acts. In some exceptional cases (e.g. against *Mycoplasma hyopneumoniae*, parvovirus and *Leptospira bratislava* they may persist much longer, sometimes up to four and a half months.

> **To achieve maximum survival rates piglets must receive colostrum as soon as possible after birth.**

Milk

Mucosally-associated antibodies are present as IgA and secretory IgA in colostrum but at low levels relative to the other types of antibody (IgG and IgM). However, the normal milk which follows colostrum contains sufficient secretory IgA to get absorbed in the surface mucus and protect the piglets intestines provided the piglet sucks the sow every one to two hours. This is sometimes called lactogenic immunity.

Feed-back

It is not surprising that mature sows provide a better maternal protection to their piglets than first litter gilts. They are older and have had greater exposure to infections. The protection provided by gilts is frequently inadequate, for example, to cope with the challenge of virulent *E. coli*. Thus gilt litters tend to suffer from diarrhoea more often than sow litters. To boost the protection of their piglets it is good practice to expose gilts to farrowing or weaner house faeces for about four weeks prior to their anticipated farrowing. High dose levels however are required to be effective in the case of *E. coli*.

In severe intractable outbreaks of *E. coli* diarrhoea, TGE or PED, diarrhoeic piglet faeces may be mopped up from the floor with paper towels and put through a grinder along with the intestines of dead piglets. These should be untreated piglets in the case of *E. coli* diarrhoea because the antibiotics will neutralise the effect. The resultant emulsion is suspended in an equal quantity of water and a cupful poured on to the feed of sows and gilts which are in late pregnancy. This is done twice or three times per week from about four weeks until one week before farrowing. Some people grind up bits of afterbirth with the faeces because they think that it makes the feed-back more effective. This procedure is not recommended because organisms such as *Eperythrozoon suis*, leptospira, toxoplasma and PRRS virus may be spread. Furthermore it may predispose gilts to cannibalism and savaging.

Feedback is usually an effective method of stopping an outbreak of neonatal scour in piglets caused by viruses. There is of course a delay before the effect comes about because the pregnant sows and gilts need at least ten days to respond fully. There is much less effect on scouring which occurs at 10-14 days of age compared to that which occurs within 5 days of birth.

There are other dangers in using feed-back. It is not effective against piglet dysentery caused by *Clostridium perfringens* type C and may make the situation worse. Also it should not be used in herds with endemic swine dysentery, or if it is used, it should be done on a modest scale with care (e.g. anti-dysentery drugs may have to be included in the soup). Nor should it be used when there are clinical cases of other diseases (e.g. erysipelas) occurring in the herd because it will spread them. An additional problem is that many people find feed-back aesthetically displeasing and are reluctant to do it. On balance it is not recommend except for TGE.

> **Regular suckling coats the lining of the piglet's intestines with lactogenic (milk) antibody and protects against diarrhoea.**

An effective alternative for *E. coli* diarrhoea originally used in the USA was to grow the *E. coli* from the diarrhoeic piglets in milk and feed the milk to pregnant females. This method has been largely superseded by the introduction of commercial vaccines which are very efficient to stimulating an immunity.

> **Feed-back can be risky.**

It is common practice to expose gilts to faeces from the floors of service pens 4 to 5 weeks before mating. This is done to ensure that the maiden gilts have been exposed to both parvovirus and other potentially damaging organisms well before they become pregnant. There are now however, efficient vaccines against parvovirus.

Antiserum

Antibodies can also be acquired passively by injecting antisera. They will protect the pig for 7 to 10 days against the specific infection that the antiserum was prepared against. This used to be a common practice in pig medicine before antibacterial drugs and effective vaccines were widely available. This is rarely done now.

The Role of Passive Immunity in the Development of Actively Acquired Immunity

The newborn piglet is exposed to a vast array of antigens from the moment it is born. Its immune system is naive and immature but competent to respond and produce an active immunity. The maternally derived immunity has to provide sufficient protection long enough while the piglet gradually develops its own active immunity. This is illustrated in Fig.3-4. In the wild a sow continues to suckle her offspring for several months. Weaning is gradual with plenty of time and opportunity for a wide range of antigenic stimulation. However, in modern pig production weaning is abrupt and at an unnaturally young age (e.g. 3 to 4 weeks). After weaning, the circulating humoral antibodies persist and continues to provide an effective protection against invasion of the pig's body. However at weaning, milk, the source of mucosal-associated antibodies is suddenly cut off. The antibodies that are present in the mucous decline within a day or so.

Serological Tests

Humoral antibodies that have been stimulated by infection can be used in blood tests in the diagnostic laboratory to diagnose what the infection is or to screen a

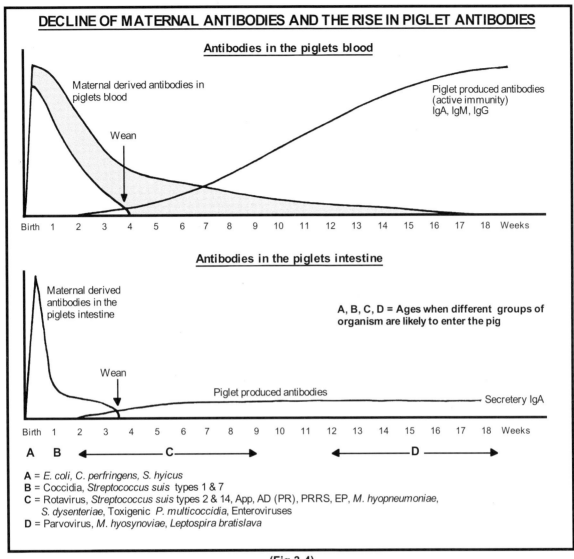

(Fig.3-4)

herd for the presence or absence of an infection.

Numerous serological tests are available e.g. agglutination tests, conglutination tests, complement fixation tests, fluorescent antibody tests, ELISAs etc. Different tests are useful for different infections. The laboratory has to decide which one is best in each case.

When carrying out such tests, either the laboratory can use commercially available antiserum to test against organisms that have been isolated, or they can use double serum samples (two samples taken over a period of time) from the sick pigs to test for specific antibodies using known antigens. Why double serum samples? Because if just one sample is taken and it is positive you do not know whether the antibodies are carried over from an old infection, which has long since gone, or whether it is associated with your current disease problem. The first sample is called "Acute" the second called "Convalescent" which is taken 7 to 14 days later. If the antibodies are due to the current infection, they will be rising from zero or very low to high. If they remain level or fall it is probably a past infection. When antibody levels rise it is called a rising titre, a titre being the term used to express the concentration of specific antibody in a given serum sample. This is measured by the amount the serum has to be diluted before the test becomes negative (i.e. the antibodies have been diluted to a non-detectable level). So if the titre rises from, say, 1:10 to 1:100, it means that the laboratory had to dilute the second serum sample by 10 times indicating infection. Most tests have a bottom threshold titre below which the test is deemed negative. They may also have a narrow middle band which is deemed to be suspicious and a higher titre above which the test is deemed positive.

Vaccination

Vaccines contain antigens from viruses, bacteria, bacterial toxins, or parasites. They are given to pigs, usually by injection, to stimulate an immune response which will protect the pigs against later natural infection with the organism from which the vaccine was derived. Most stimulate both a humoral response and a cell-mediated response.

Vaccines can be live, containing living organisms which will multiply in the pig, or inactivated, containing only killed organisms which will not multiply in the pig.

In live vaccines the organism has usually been attenuated (i.e. its virulence has been reduced) so that although it will multiply in the pig it will not normally cause any disease. Examples are the PRRS vaccine (although some may cause mild reactions), aujeszky's disease (pseudorabies) vaccines and classical swine fever vaccines. Live attenuated vaccines have the advantage that because they multiply in the pig they give a bigger antigenic stimulus resulting in stronger longer-lasting immunity. They have the disadvantage that they may die in wrong storage conditions (e.g. heat) or during dosing (e.g. by exposure to antiseptics or disinfectants) and are then useless. It is also important that they are stable and not able to return to full virulence.

Inactivated (dead) vaccines may contain whole organisms, antigenic parts of organisms or antigens which have been synthesised chemically. An example of a commonly used whole organism vaccine is the erysipelas vaccine. (In North America such vaccines are often called Bacterins).
For example : -
Erysipelas vaccine
This is made by growing the erysipelas bacteria in a liquid nutrient broth (several strains may be used).

The bacteria are then killed.
↓
A liquid or adjuvant is added to the bacterial suspension.
↓
This produces the vaccine.
↓
A predetermined number of bacteria are injected into the pig. The first dose (usually 2ml).
↓
A second dose is required to complete the immune response. Usually given 14 to 24 days after the first.
↓
7 days after the second dose the pig is protected.

Synthesised antigen vaccines are still largely in the experimental stage.

The immunity produced by inactivated vaccines can be enhanced by adding substances or adjuvants such as aluminium hydroxide or certain types of oil. You should take care, however, if you use vaccines with oily adjuvants because they can cause serious local reactions if you accidentally inject yourself, e.g. your hand.

Inactivated vaccines may also contain toxins which have been modified so that they still stimulate an immune response but are no longer toxic to the animal. Toxins which have been modified in this way are called toxoids. The classic vaccine of this type is the tetanus toxoid which is used commonly in horses but rarely in pigs. In pigs, some of the *E. coli* vaccines against piglet diarrhoea and the clostridial vaccines against piglet dysentery also contain toxoids.

> **Remember however, vaccination is never 100%.**

Autogenous vaccines

Autogenous vaccines are bacterial vaccines that are manufactured from the specific pathogenic bacteria isolated from the diseased pig. They are usually made under a licence for use only on that farm. You should consult with your veterinarian. These are available from Salus (QP) Ltd. They can be useful when serious disease outbreaks occur and standard commercial vaccines are not available.

Such vaccines could be made from most bacteria including :-
- *Actinobacillus pleuropneumoniae*
- *E. coli*
- *Haemophilus parasuis*
- Pasteurella
- Salmonella
- *Streptococcus suis*
- *Staphylococcus hyicus* (Greasy pig disease)

One drawback to vaccinating a herd is that you cannot then use blood tests to check whether the organism is present in the herd or not. All the pigs will test positive which has obvious implications for an eradication programme based on blood tests, for example the eradication of swine fever or aujeszky's disease (pseudorabies). To get over this, gene-deleted vaccines have been developed. A part of the organism's gene which codes for an antigen has been removed so that when the organism multiplies in the pig it does not stimulate antibodies against that antigen. Special blood tests can then distinguish between the array of disease antibodies and those stimulated by the vaccine. A new generation of such gene manipulated vaccines, and possibly also synthetic polypeptide vaccines, can be anticipated.

Autogenous vaccines are those prepared with infectious pathogens from the herd which is to be vaccinated. The causal organisms has to be isolated, grown up, killed, and made into a safe vaccine form. Autogenous vaccines may be useful when serious disease outbreaks occur and standard commercial vaccines are not available.

Vaccine usage

Fig.3-5 lists the pig diseases for which vaccines are available. This list is not exhaustive and some vaccines will be available in some countries and not in others. However they are used in most countries both to protect against disease and to assist in eradication programmes. Some examples of commercial vaccines available are shown in chapter 4 these are but a few of the many available.

Vaccines commonly used on pig farms throughout the world include erysipelas, parvovirus infection (SMEDI syndrome), *E. coli* diarrhoea, clostridial dysentery of piglets, enzootic pneumonia caused by *Mycoplasma hyopneumoniae*, necrotic pleuropneumonia caused by *Actinobacillus pleuropneumoniae* and atrophic rhinitis caused by toxigenic *Pasteurella multocida*. In many countries, vaccines against disease, such as, salmonellosis, PRRS and TGE are also used depending on commercial availability.

In the European Union vaccination against classical swine fever has been stopped in a programme aimed at stamping the disease out. Vaccination against foot-and-mouth disease has also been stopped for a similar reason. Aujeszky's disease (pseudorabies) virus is widespread everywhere in the EU except in the UK and Denmark. With the exception of these two countries vaccination is widely practised. A blanket vaccination regime for all herds is being applied in some countries such as the Netherlands in an attempt to build up a national herd immunity resulting in the eradication of the virus.

North America is free from FMD and CSF so vaccination is not practised but PR vaccines are widely used in conjunction with eradication programmes. Elsewhere in the world, the situation regarding these three diseases varies, so vaccination policies also vary.

The effectiveness of vaccines

This varies, because of the need to stimulate mucosal immunity locally. As mentioned earlier, vaccines given by injection against respiratory and intestinal disease are generally not as effective as those against systemic or generalised diseases. An exception to this is the vaccine for enzootic pneumonia (*M. hyopneumoniae*) because it stimulates cell-mediated immunity. If, however, they are fed or sprayed into the upper respiratory tract they may produce a stronger local immunity. The vaccine against piglet dysentery is a toxoid and if given routinely to sows in adequate doses is usually reasonably effective in providing passive protection via the colostrum.

Sometimes vaccines do not work particularly well on

MAJOR VIRUS DISEASES THAT MAY BE CONTROLLED BY VACCINATION [+]
Aujeszky's disease
Foot-and-mouth disease
Porcine parvovirus
PRRS
Swine fever
Swine influenza
TGE

BACTERIAL DISEASES THAT MAY BE CONTROLLED BY VACCINATION [+]
Any bacterial disease by autogenous vaccines, e.g. greasy pig disease
Actinobacillus pleuropneumonia
Atrophic rhinitis
Clostridial diseases
E. coli diarrhoea
Enzootic pneumonia
Erysipelas
Glässers disease (*Haemophilus parasuis*)
Leptospirosis
Pasteurellosis
Streptococcal meningitis

[+] The availability of vaccines varies from country to country.

(Fig.3-5)

a farm and in such cases the following possibilities need to be considered:
- The vaccine was contaminated.
- The vaccine was not capable of producing the required immunity.
- The pig was already incubating the disease when it was vaccinated.
- The vaccine had been incorrectly stored. High temperatures reduce the effectiveness. (Always keep vaccines in a refrigerator but do not freeze).
- The vaccine had been exposed to sunlight.
- The vaccine had gone out of date.
- The needle and syringe were dirty or faulty.
- Chemical sterilisation destroyed the vaccine.
- The animal had inadvertently missed being vaccinated. This is particularly common with parvovirus vaccination in the gilt.
- Vaccine response was poor because there was maternal antibody present.
- The vaccine was deposited in fat and was not absorbed. Faulty injection techniques

Immunosuppression

There are many factors that suppress both innate and acquired immunity levels but in pigs infectious agents are the most common ones. These include:
- *Mycoplasma hyopneumoniae* the cause of enzootic pneumonia.
- *Pasteurella multocida*.
- Aujeszky's disease virus.
- Swine influenza virus.
- African swine fever virus.
- PRRS virus.

These agents may destroy the macrophages or lymphocytes, or delay or reduce the efficiency of the immune response, or damage the innate defences.

Weaning time is also a period of immuno-suppression by withdrawal of the sows milk that contains the protective mechanisms of IgA. When pigs are mixed, moved or stressed the plasma cortisol levels rise with a similar effect and the demand for vitamin E rises.

Medicinal Control of Disease
See chapter 4 for further information.

Prevention
Specific details of this are discussed elsewhere under the relevant diseases. Diseases can be prevented or controlled effectively if treatment is applied during the incubation period, that is the period from the time of exposure to the organism to the onset of clinical disease. This is sometimes called prophylactic (i.e. preventative) or strategic medication. This medication must be given at the correct time which is determined by the pattern of the disease on the farm and by trial and error.

Eradicating Disease
Some diseases can be eradicated by a combination of medication, vaccination and management or even by management procedures alone. Fig.3-6 illustrates those that have been successfully removed from combined breeding feeding herds.

The methods by which these are carried out are described under the specific diseases.

Recognising Disease on the Farm
Early recognition is the first priority for managing disease. It is carried out by the stockperson using the senses of sight, sound, touch and smell to detect the abnormal animal and to differentiate it from the normal animals. Every day, a clinical examination of all pigs should be carried out. On a 100 sow farm, this could take up to half an hour per day and on a large farm, it becomes a major daily task but can be split between department levels. How many managers in organising their farms allow such a time period for this function?

The Use of Sight
- Inappetance is obvious where an animal is housed and fed as an individual, such as a sow in confinement, but in group housed animals this is not easy to detect. The failure to eat, or a drop in feed intake in a pen of apparently normal pigs, must immediately arouse suspicions and the initial check should be for lack of water which is usually the most important sudden cause of inappetance involving all pigs in a group. If the water supply is normal look for signs of disease.
- Listlessness or a dull appearance of the pig will be quickly detected by the good stockperson as early signs of illness.
- Shivering and raising of hair over the body is an important feature of disease and is one of the very early sign of streptococcal meningitis or joint infections in the sucking pig. Look for this sign next time you examine each individual in the litter. A pig laid on its belly and shivering with its hair on end compared to the rest of the group, is either scoured or lame from a generalised septicaemia (bacteria in the blood stream).
- Loss of body weight is a first indication of inappetance or dehydration due to diarrhoea or pneumonia.

DISEASES THAT CAN BE ERADICATED BY MEDICATION, VACCINATION AND OR MANAGEMENT PROCEDURES
Atrophic rhinitis
Aujeszky's disease (pseudorabies)
Enzootic pneumonia
Lice
Mange
PRRS
Salmonella choleraesuis
Swine dysentery
TGE

(Fig.3-6)

- Discharges from the nose or eyes indicate an upper respiratory infection. Excess salivation from the mouth indicates an exotic disease such as vesicular disease. In sows, a discharge from the vulva could indicate vaginitis, cystitis, pyelonephritis or endometritis.
- Faecal changes can indicate a wide range of diseases but sloppy faeces can also be quite normal. Look for signs of mucous or blood indicative of swine dysentery, salmonella infections gastric ulceration or proliferative haemorrhagic enteropathy. Constipation may be important in the development of udder oedema and agalactia at farrowing.

Examine all pigs carefully everyday.

- Vomiting can be a sign of diseases such as transmissible gastro-enteritis, or in individual pigs it may indicate gastric ulceration. In the sucking pig, gastroenteritis associated with *E. coli* infections is often seen. Injections with long-acting penicillin may also cause pigs to vomit.
- Skin changes help in identifying diseases, typified by acute or chronic lesions of mange and lice although the latter are now uncommon. Erysipelas may not be evident by sight but running the flat of the hand over the skin will indicate tell-tale lesions of raised areas. A blueing of the extremities could indicate acute viral infections, acute bacterial septicaemia or a toxic state, as seen in flu, PRRS infections or acute mastitis and metritis. Acute pneumonia or pneumonia associated with heart sac infection can give a similar picture.
- Respiration rates. If any of the above changes have been identified cast your eye across the pen of pigs and compare the respiratory rates of both the normal and the suspect animals. Assess, whether the breathing is

a deep chest movement, due to consolidation of the lungs and a shortage of oxygen, or very shallow abdominal breathing indicative of pleurisy and pain. Finally the circumstances surrounding the death of a pig is an important observation, especially when backed up by post-mortem examination. The timing and place where pigs die in a herd relative to clinical observations can often help in identifying and understanding a problem

Observation of the Group

Daily, regular time should be set aside for the examination of all pigs. Allow at least 5-10 seconds to observe each pen of pigs. The environment of the house must also be assessed by noting the following:
- Temperature.
- Humidity.
- Ventilation.
- Smell.
- Pig behaviour.
- Appetite.
- Human reaction.
- Ammonia levels as experienced through breathing and the effect on eyes.
- Abnormal changes in slurry and bedding.

> *Always examine the environment in a house at pig level.*

Changes in Behaviour

The pig is a social animal and in a healthy condition remains part of a group, In disease however it tends to rest on its own or often be rejected by the other pigs even to the extent of being attacked. Altered lying patterns in a pen must always be regarded with suspicion. Conversely where a number of pigs are ill or the environment is inadequate huddling is common. The reluctance of pigs to rise or show an interest in the observer must always warrant a more detailed examination.

The Use of Smell

The odour of a dead pig is one that we have all experienced from time to time. However, odours also occur with scour, bad feed or infected tissues. The smell of piglet scour on outdoor sows can help detect affected litters. The quality of the air through the sense of smell will highlight poor ventilation rates, high levels of gases, or high or low humidity. What is uncomfortable for ourselves is also likely to be the same to the pig.

The Use of Touch

It is essential to handle a sick pig, to detect changes in skin temperatures, the significance of abnormal fluids or lumps on the skin. The limbs should always be palpated in cases of lameness, for possible fractures or swellings in the joints. In the newly farrowed sow, always palpate the udder to detect any early changes of agalactia or mastitis.

The Use of Sound

Be extremely wary if there are no pig noises when you enter a building. A disaster could have occurred due to electrocution, suffocation, or high levels of toxic gases such as carbon monoxide or hydrogen sulphide.

> *Remember a happy healthy pig will usually approach and make contact with you.*

> *Manage your farm by walking around it not by staying in the office.*

Clinical Examination of the Herd

The daily clinical appraisal of the various sections of the herd should be carried using a series of checklists held on a clipboard. The observations should combine all the senses described. Suggested checklists are outlined below as examples.

Managing Pig Health and the Treatment of Disease

A CHECKLIST FOR THE FARROWING AREA - INDOORS	
	Comments
Water availability.	
Sows' body condition at entry.	
Sow condition at weaning.	
Feed intakes.	
Are any sows not in pig?	
Late or early farrowings.	
Farrowing problems.	
Mastitis or metritis.	
Quality of piglets at birth.	
Sow mortality, prolapses etc.	
Sow health problems.	
Litter sizes, still-births, mummified piglets.	
Congenital conditions.	
Scour levels. Treatments.	
Quality of the environment, hygiene, dry floors, temperature.	
Creep temperatures.	
Health of piglets, evenness of growth.	
Respiratory disease, rhinitis, pneumonia.	
Parasites. Fly control.	
Are medication procedures being carried out properly e.g. mange, worming, vaccination?	
Are other procedures being done properly?	
All-in all-out procedures.	
Use of footbaths.	
Building maintenance.	
Your additions.	

A CHECKLIST FOR THE SERVICE/MATING AREA - INDOORS	
	Comments
Condition of sows at weaning.	
Hair growth.	
Feed levels from weaning to service.	
Boar sow ratio.	
Boar usage.	
Service procedure. Supervision.	
Fertility levels.	
Assess the litter size relative to service procedures.	
The environment at weaning, floors, drainage, temperature.	
Weaning to service intervals.	
Discharges, mastitis, diseases.	
Trauma, stress.	
Lameness.	
Boar condition, health, service performance.	
Your additions.	

Chapter 3

CHAPTER 3 - Managing Health and Disease

A CHECK LIST FOR THE DRY SOW AREA - INDOORS	
	Comments
Assess the environment - temperatures, humidity.	
Housing problems, tethers, stalls.	
Welfare problems.	
General sow contentment or restlessness.	
Body condition. Feed levels, inappetance.	
Chronic mastitis.	
Vulval discharges.	
Sows not in pig.	
Sows repeating.	
Abortions.	
Oestrus abnormalities.	
Condition of the faeces.	
Culls. Reasons for and causes.	
Mortality levels and causes.	
Prolapses.	
Vaccination programmes.	
Your additions.	

A CHECKLIST FOR THE PIGLET WEANING AREA - INDOORS	
	Comments
Age and weight at weaning.	
Evenness of growth.	
Water availability.	
Feed, access, type and quality.	
Stocking density.	
Lying patterns of the pigs.	
Environmental temperature.	
Growth of the pig in the first ten days post-weaning.	
Respiratory diseases, rhinitis, pneumonia.	
Enteric diseases.	
Condition of faeces.	
Environment - ventilation, humidity.	
Insulation.	
Vermin control.	
Fly control.	
Skin conditions, mange, greasy pig disease.	
Lameness.	
Welfare aspects.	
Building maintenance.	
Your additions.	

Managing Pig Health and the Treatment of Disease

A CHECKLIST FOR THE GROWING AND FINISHING AREAS - INDOORS	
	Comments
Assess weight for age.	
Stocking densities.	
Evenness of growth.	
Nutrition and growth in different houses.	
Application of feed and types.	
Effect of movement of pigs.	
Environment in different houses.	
Quality of environment, insulation, temperatures, humidity, draughts.	
Temperature fluctuations.	
Lying patterns of the pigs.	
Feed conversion efficiency.	
Daily liveweight gain.	
Appearance of the pigs skin - mange, hair growth.	
Appearance of faeces.	
Respiratory diseases.	
Enteric diseases.	
Diseases, mortality, prolapses.	
Culls	
Parasites.	

Assessing Health, Management and Disease in Outdoor Production

Successful outdoor production is dependant upon the interaction between breed, the variables of the climate, soil type and management. Routine clinical examinations need to include the following.

DISEASES AND CONDITIONS THAT MAY BE EXPERIENCED IN OUTDOOR PRODUCTION	
	Comments
Clostridial infections, necrotic enteritis.	
Coccidiosis.	
Endometritis - vulval discharges.	
Internal parasites.	
Lameness:	
Bush foot.	
Erysipelas.	
Mycoplasma arthritis.	
OCD.	
Physical damage.	
Leptospirosis.	
Lice.	
Mange.	
Mastitis.	
Parvovirus.	
PRRS.	
Summer infertility, abortions, embryo reabsorption.	
Sunburn / heat stroke.	
TGE.	
Variable litter size.	

Refer to relevant chapters for information relating to specific diseases.

CHAPTER 3 - Managing Health and Disease

A CHECKLIST FOR THE FARROWING AREA - OUTDOOR PRODUCTION	
	Comments
Huts or arks	
Air flow, draughts, condensation.	
Bedding type quality amount - dryness.	
Door flaps.	
Environment	
Fenders	
Insulation	
Level ground.	
Nose ring to prevent digging.	
Provision of solid floors.	
Siting against prevailing wind.	
Size for breed of sow.	
Soil type / nesting.	
Wallows / shade.	
Feeding / nutrition	
Ad lib / hoppers.	
Amount fed sow / year.	
Feed levels.	
Only dry feed.	
Ration composition.	
Wastage.	
Water availability.	
Sows	
Accuracy of recording.	
Behavioural problems.	
Body condition, body score.	
Born alive, dead, reared.	
Efficiency of breeding female.	
Gilt mothering qualities.	
Lactator ration used.	
Management efficiency.	
Mastitis, agalactia.	
Numbers born alive.	
Treatment required.	
Variability of body condition.	
Piglets	
Born dead.	
Effects of bedding on viability.	
Losses due to foxes, crows.	
Iron injections.	
Management at farrowing.	
Mortality %.	
Quality of piglets at weaning.	
Savaging.	
Scour.	
Stolen piglets.	
Teeth clipping.	
Treatments required.	

Managing Pig Health and the Treatment of Disease

A CHECKLIST FOR THE DRY SOW AND WEANING AREAS - OUTDOOR PRODUCTION	
	Comments
Huts or Kennels.	
Effects of weather.	
Environment	
Ground conditions / bedding.	
Lying patterns.	
Siting - position, draughts.	
Soil type.	
Stocking density.	
Feeding / nutrition	
Feed intake - Service to 21 days.	
- Last 3 weeks of pregnancy.	
Feed used / sow / year.	
Type of ration - composition.	
Wastage.	
Water availability.	
Sows	
Barren returns.	
Body condition.	
Diseases evident.	
Efficiency of identification tags etc.	
Fertility records.	
Grass types / mycotoxins.	
Lameness / mastitis.	
Management quality.	
Parity spread.	
Sunburn / heat stroke.	
Wallows / shades.	
Boars. Service paddocks	
Age.	
Boar usage.	
Boars condition.	
Efficiency of boar type.	
Feeding / nutrition.	
Group sizes.	
Lameness - disease.	
Libido.	
Management and mating.	
Penis problems.	
Use of AI.	
Wallows / shades.	
Gilts	
Acclimatisation.	
Age, weight, oestrus.	
Anoestrus.	
Fertility.	
Flushing.	
Introduction to cobs.	
Lameness.	
Litter size.	
Management quality.	
Nutrition / back fat measurements.	
Vaccination.	
Weaners	
Bedding, dryness, ventilation, draughts.	
Environment in huts.	
Growth, daily liveweight gain.	
Health and disease at weaning.	
Management quality.	
Medication.	
Mortality.	
Nutrition and feeding.	
Respiratory, enteric diseases.	
Spacing of huts.	
Use one area per week.	
Water supply.	
Weaning weight body condition.	

CHAPTER 3 - Managing Health and Disease

PREVENTIVE MEDICATIONS - OUTDOOR PRODUCTION	
	Comments
Vaccinations to consider	
Atrophic rhinitis.	
Clostridia.	
E. coli.	
Enzootic pneumonia, mycoplasma.	
Erysipelas.	
Leptospira.	
Parvovirus.	
TGE.	
Other medications to consider	
In-feed medication.	
Iron injections.	
Water medication	
Anthelmintics.	

BIOSECURITY AND MANAGEMENT AUDIT - INDOOR AND OUTDOOR PRODUCTION	
	Comments
Bedding source, quality.	
Bird contamination.	
Boots, coveralls.	
Casualty pens.	
Casualty stock disposal.	
Control of substances hazardous to health.	
Dead stock disposal.	
Destruction of pigs.	
Feed storage.	
First aid box.	
Fly control.	
Foot dips.	
Health and safety.	
Loading ramp - Disinfectant used.	
Medications:	
Cleanliness of equipment.	
Medication in feed bins.	
Records of use.	
Refrigerator.	
Storage.	
Use of syringes, needles.	
Withdrawal periods.	
Movement records.	
Perimeter fence.	
Pig freedom times.	
Rodent control.	
Shower facilities.	
Signing in book.	
Siting of feed bins.	
Stocking rates.	
Transport and pig movement.	

If these lists are used daily, regular disciplines will be established in each area of the farm that will raise efficiency and awareness and identify sick pigs early.

The Management and Treatment of the Sick Pig

Once a sick pig has been recognised the following sequence of events is suggested:
- Identify the animal by spray or tag.
- Carefully examine the pig and its environment.
- What do you think is wrong with it? (If in doubt seek veterinary advice).
- Take the rectal temperature.
- Is it necessary to treat the condition?
- What drug has been recommended for treatment by the veterinarian?
- What nursing/welfare provisions are there?
- Should the pig be left in the pen?
- What method of drug administration should be used?
- What dose level should be given and how often should the drug be given?
- Determine method of administration the site of injection, syringe and needle type.
- Assess the response daily
- Normal temperature 38.6°C to 39.5°C (101.5 to 102.5°F)
- Respiratory rate at 20°C (70°F) 25-30 per minute.

Having recognised the sick pig and the cause of the problem, a decision must be made whether to treat it in the pen or move it to a specialised "hospital pen". Treatment consists of three very important aspects, good nursing, good nutrition and necessary medicines. It is in the first of these that there is often a lack of awareness. Any pig that is so disadvantaged, either through lameness or sickness, that it cannot fend for itself, should immediately be moved into a hospital pen.

Sick pigs should only be left in the pen if they are still able to move around freely, have an uninhibited access to the drinker and are only inappetent for a maximum of 24 hours.

On every pig farm there should be 6 to 8 separate hospital pens per hundred sows. At least two pens should be available for weaners, two for growers, two for feeder pigs and two pens for lame or disadvantaged sows. Each pen should satisfy the following criteria:
- The floor should be solid and well drained.
- It should be deep bedded on straw, shavings or other suitable material.
- It should be well lit so that examinations are easily carried out.
- There should be easy access to food and water, preferably by a water bowl and ad lib feeder.
- One person on the farm should be appointed responsible for all sick pigs.
- There should be a maximum of six pigs per pen with a floor area of up to $1m^2$ per pig for pigs up to 100kg and $3m^2$ per sow.

> **Your farm should have hospital pens.**

- Adequate temperatures must be maintained in these pens and invariably this will involve either the provision of extra heating or the siting of the pens in a very warm building. To achieve this in weaners and the young growing pigs, it is necessary to provide an insulated micro-environment within the building, consisting of an insulated floor sides and roof with an infra-red bulb or alternative heat source controlled by a thermostat. Pigs will respond much more quickly if they are in a warm, well bedded environment. On one farm regularly visited by the author all ill pigs, no matter how mild, are always moved into a series of 30 small hospital pens. The owner often relates how many of these pigs reach slaughter weight days ahead of their healthy contemporaries. There is a lesson here.

The disadvantaged pig can be managed in one of four ways: (Fig.3-7 and 3-8).

1. Sell to a slaughter outlet

This assumes that the pig is destined for sale through normal outlets and would include a pig that has been in a sick pen and has recovered, or one that is fit to travel, has no condition likely to render the carcase unfit for human consumption and no drug residues.

> **Sick pigs should be moved to a hospital pen.**

2. Treat the pig

Treatment would be given on the assumption that the pig will respond and ultimately be fit for normal slaughter. Having made this decision, a careful review should be made of the progress on a day by day basis and if the pig is not responding, either the treatment should be changed, further advice sought, or it should be destroyed.

3. Casualty slaughter

The animal should be capable of being transported to the nearest available slaughter house without compromising its welfare. A veterinary slaughter certificate or owner declaration may be required, depending on the welfare rules and regulations. Such animals might be lame or with fresh rectal or vaginal prolapses, or maybe slow growing pigs. On farm slaughter of the pig may be necessary for welfare reasons, for example a broken leg or acute severe lameness. This should only be carried out if the carcase is likely to be fit for human consumption.

4. Destroy the pig

There should be facilities on the farm for humane destruction of all ages of pigs. (See chapter 15 Slaughter).

> **Hospital pens should be warm and comfortable.**

The Design of the Hospital Pen

The hospital pen should be the most comfortable warm area on the farm with easy access to feed and water because the environmental requirements of the sick pig are exacting. For example the newly weaned pig affected with malabsorption will have lost most of its body fat and could require an effective temperature of 30°C (95°F). Hospital pens should cater for three groups of pigs, those in the immediate post-weaned period, those in the growing and finishing period and sows. In the weaning and the growing period there should be two types, one to handle the acutely ill pigs and the second to hold the recovered pigs.

This is similar to the straw based weaner accommodation shown in Fig.3-46 only smaller. It consists of an inner well heated chamber with strip curtains separated from a cooler outer section. In some designs the floor is heated as well and this provides an excellent environment. The complete pen is deep bedded in at least 300mm of straw or other bedding so that the disadvantaged pig can select its required environment. This is vital for the recovery of those pigs who have lost body fat. The walls and roof of the accommodation should be insulated with 100-150mm of foam or fibre glass depending on the temperature of the external environment. Provision should be made for a separate water tank leading to a water bowl so that medication can be applied as necessary. Feed should be readily accessible by open dishes in the case of weaners and well sited hoppers in the case of growing pigs. The sow accommodation should provide a good grip for the feet on the floor particularly for those sows that are lame (e.g. leg weakness). The stocking densities should range from $0.2m^2$ per pig for weaners through to $3m^2$ for the sow.

Management features of the sick pen

- For the acutely ill pigs it should contain no more than 5 or 6 pigs.

MANAGING SICK GROWING AND FINISHING PIGS	
Condition	Action
Lameness:	
Totally off the back legs	Destroy
Acutely lame with swollen infected joints. Severe.	Treat and assess Destroy
Lame with no obvious cause, no open wounds and no temperature	Casualty slaughter or treat
Severely damaged claw	Casualty slaughter or treat
Recently broken legs.	Destroy or casualty slaughter on the farm.
Severe sprains and dislocations	Treat and assess.
Injuries:	
Tail - bitten	Treat
Tail swollen, abscessed	Destroy
Tail treated / recovered	Sell
Swelling without open wound.	Treat
Severe traumatic injuries e.g. recent open wound	Destroy or casualty slaughter if fit to travel or treat.
Ear - bitten, flank bitten other recent wounds	Treat move to hospital pen. It is essential that these cases are isolated immediately and during treatment.
Rectal prolapse	Replace and suture then sell for normal slaughter ASAP.
Severe rectal prolapse	Replace then immediately slaughter or destroy
Ruptures:	
Small	Sell for normal slaughter
Large	Sell for normal slaughter at lowest possible weight. Casualty transport conditions should apply.
Large with ulcerated skin.	Destroy - unfit to travel move to straw pen. Sell as normal pig when recovered or casualty slaughter if skin lesions still present at slaughter weight.
Runts and ailing pigs	
Mild	Treat
Severe	Destroy

MANAGING THE SICK SOW	
Conditions	Action
Prolapse of the uterus	Destroy.
Prolapse of the vagina	Replace and retain by suture.
Prolapse of the rectum	Replace suture and casualty slaughter.
Rectal stricture	Destroy as soon as noticed.
Open wounds	Treat.
Cuts and wounds Mild	Treat sell when healed.
Severe	Destroy.
Shoulder sores and ulcerated hocks	Treat and move to a bedded area. Then sell when healed.
Lameness:	
Off back legs	Destroy.
Acutely lame	Treat and assess.
Severely swollen infected joints.	Treat and assess or destroy.
Not severe	Treat and assess.
Lame, no obvious cause but weight on all legs.	Casualty slaughter or treat.
No obvious wounds and no temperature	Treat.
Emaciated condition	Destroy.
Dystocia. (Difficult farrowing)	Treat then review and retain only if sow expels pigs and recovers. N.B. If live pigs are present consider on-farm hysterectomy. or Destroy. N.B. Never send a sow with retained piglets for slaughter; in almost all countries it will be condemned.

(Fig.3-7)

(Fig.3-8)

- Pigs should be examined twice daily and assessed.
- The pen should be well lit and bedded.
- There should be no draughts and it should be warm.
- One person should be appointed responsible for these pens.
- Medication and electrolytes should be administered daily and recorded.
- There should be easy access to the pens for observation.
- Water should be available in a bowl at an accessible height for the smallest pig.

Disposal of Dead Pigs

Dead pigs can be a source of continuing problems. They attract birds, rats and mice and are a breeding ground for flies. Vehicles collecting them pose a serious threat of disease to your herd.

There are five options for the disposal of dead pigs:
1. A self digestion pit dug into the ground and lined with concrete rings. This will cope with pigs up to 50kg. This is only of use in ground with a low water table and in temperate climates.
2. Composting in a deep straw manure heap or using other materials. Pigs will decompose totally within three weeks provided they are placed into the centre of the manure heap and buried at a minimum depth of 1.2m. This is only of value in temperate climates. Make sure there is no access for foxes and other animals. This method can be used for pigs up to 150kg weight.
3. Burial. This will depend on the water table and local restrictions
4. Incineration on the farm.
5. Removal by a licensed person for incineration or disposal elsewhere. (N.B. This is the only option allowed in some countries).

Care needs to be taken for disease security at the collection site of dead animals. It should be out of the vicinity of the farm and at least 200m away; 400m if live pigs are involved. There should be an entry to the collecting area on the farm side and an exit on the opposite side for collection by the disposing lorry. An example of a reception area is shown in Fig.3-9. There are many variations of design. In some countries the design is stipulated by the authorities.

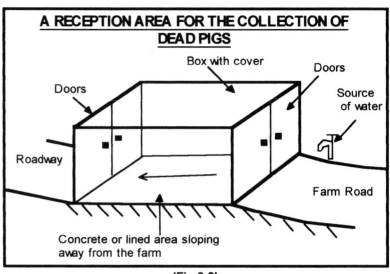
(Fig.3-9)

> **Poor pig disposal leads to the spread of disease.**

> **Vehicles collecting dead or sick pigs pose a disease risk to your herd.**

> **Give serious consideration to the disposal of dead pigs.**

The Consultant or Specialist Veterinarian

Traditionally veterinary services have consisted of attending sick animals and the diagnosis of disease and treatment. This fire brigade type of work has usually been carried out by the general practitioner dealing with other species as well, in a multi-species mixed practice. As pig units during the past ten to twenty years have become larger and their techniques of production more sophisticated, the level of knowledge and expertise required from the veterinarian has increased substantially. As a result more-specialised comprehensive veterinary services have developed. They differ in different countries in the way they have become organised but the basic requirements are similar. In the UK a second service has developed, that of the independent pig specialist, who spends the majority of his or her time working amongst pigs on his clients farm within the frame-work of the general practice to which he belongs. A third even more specialised role is that of the person who is totally dealing with pig health, management and production and who could be classified as a consultant. He or she not only attends herds within the practice but also is invited to advise on herds in other practices often at considerable distances away. There is a fourth role within the industry, that of the specialist veterinarian fully employed by large pig organisations or ancillary industries, but his job perspective can often (but not always) become more of an administrative and decision making one rather than "hands on" on the pig farm.

A somewhat similar development of veterinary services has developed in North America except that here a number of very large pig producing organisations have emerged each comprising of 100k to 200k sows and their progeny. These employ full-time veterinarians with highly specialised roles. Similar developments have occurred in some countries of South America and Australasia.

Nevertheless, the actual resources required in different countries have some comparisons even if the organisations are different. The three different types of service shown in Fig.3-10 are those most commonly found in the UK.

Veterinary services should be used to:-
- Increase efficiency.
- Further educate and help understanding.
- Contribute to management.
- Control disease.
- Prevent disease.

SWINE PRACTITIONER SERVICES			
Service Provided	General Practitioner (G.P.)	Specialist Working at least 3/4 time with pigs	Specialist Working Full Time Amongst Pigs (Consultant)
Emergency services	✓	≈	-
Diagnosis of disease	✓	✓	✓
Treatment of disease	✓	✓	≈
Disease control	≈	✓	✓
Production control	-	✓	✓
Management control	-	✓	✓
Epidemiology	-	✓	✓
Diagnostic services	-	≈	✓
Statutory work	✓	≈	-
Computer technology	-	≈	✓
Information technology	-	≈	✓
Education	-	≈	✓
Nutritional advice	-	≈	✓
Environmental control	-	✓	✓
Waste control	-	≈	≈
Corporate decisions	-	✓	✓
Profitability	-	≈	✓
R & D	-	≈	✓

Key: ✓ Yes — No ≈ Variable

(Fig.3-10)

The fundamental needs of the modern pig unit are to maximise production and efficiency and thus the return on the investment. The achievement of maximum profitability however must be carried out within the economic constraints and accepted practices of animal welfare. Part of the service must include a routine visit to the farm every two to three months, or in the case of the large farm a shorter period, so that studies of the inter relationships between management, the pig, the environment and organisms can be carried out, relative to the problems. The most successful farms are those which achieve high productivity and give attention to detail. They invariably have good team work, disease control and understand how to maximise biological efficiency. A major role of the veterinarian at his periodic visit must be to help in this understanding and awareness of the problems on the farm and identify the procedures to correct them. Fig.3-11 shows a format that could be used at the veterinary visit. It starts with a discussion and an examination of records followed by a clinical examination of the herd or vice versa. At each visit a special topic for discussion and education should be pre-planned, that relates to a problem area on the farm. During the clinical examination of the herd the personnel responsible for each area of the farm should accompany the veterinarian to give their observations and discuss weaknesses and strengths. This also provides an opportunity for education and motivation.

A written report of the observations and advice should be provided so that it can be used and acted upon pending the next visit. It is also a reminder of the dis-

A PROCEDURE FOR THE ROUTINE VETERINARY VISIT
- Pre-visit preparation
- Assess previous recommendations.
- The clinical examination of the herd.
- The discussion and examination of records.
- An educational topic.
- A review of general problems.
- Actions to be taken.
- Preparation for the next visit.
- The report.

(Fig.3-11)

cussions that took place and it can highlight agreed recommendations not acted upon.

The veterinarian can influence the relationships between people, management and pig and this communication and the dissemination of knowledge associated with it, can be one of the main attractions for the purchase of veterinary services, particularly when the results are increased profitability.

Fig.3-12 shows some of these inter relationships that occur, starting with the bank, the spouse or partner, the owner, the pig and finally profit. Within each group of people there must be constant interactions and dialogues with the ultimate aim of improving profitability.

Fig.3-13 outlines detailed interactions by the specialist or consultant on the farm and some guidelines. The frequency and time necessary for the veterinary visits relative to herd sizes, is shown in Fig.3-14. It should be noted that a new emerging role involves participation in quality assurance schemes and auditing the farm against required standards.

What services do you require from your veterinarian?

Staff Training and Education

Farms that have been highly successful for long periods of time invariably have a good management structure and rapport between pig people and pigs. In other words people management in all aspects is probably the most crucial part of successful pig farming. If there is a problem of production or disease, it usually arises from bad management decisions, their implications, or its complete failure.

> **It costs nothing to say "well done"**

In order to achieve good management on the farm it is necessary to understand and satisfy the fundamental needs of the people at work. These needs, in a sequential order, can be listed as follows:

To satisfy basic biological needs

These in essence are the provision of an acceptable standard of living both at work and at home through an adequate wage and the availability of affordable medical services.

To be in a secure position

Satisfaction of the biological needs leads to the second requirement, that of security in the position of good employment. People at this level are constantly seeking reassurance about their job, are very conservative, do not take risks and motivation can be very poor. It is in this group that education and training can have the greatest impact and allow development into the next levels of needs.

To belong to the business

Through education, training and friendships teamwork develops, where people ask questions and at the same time listen and are developing and becoming motivated in their job. At this point the managers or people in control play an important part by providing good relationships with the workers. From friendship and sense of belonging comes achievement. A sense of achievement on the pig farm involves recognition by senior management and in the process builds self esteem. Furthermore it starts the process of motivation.

Motivation is created on the pig farm by the feed back of information and the employee being recognised for his contributions. When people are given the responsibility for a job not only does that give them recognition but enables them to develop their own initiatives and thereby move into more challenging roles. From this a highly motivated team work develops, with staff helping to solve problems.

To become confident

Through the development of a sense of achievement people will then develop confidence in their jobs and direct and help others. This is the point at which efficiency across the farm improves considerably.

To develop new skills

The final and ultimate part of the process is where the confidence reaches a level such that through further education and application, new skills can take place. A typi-

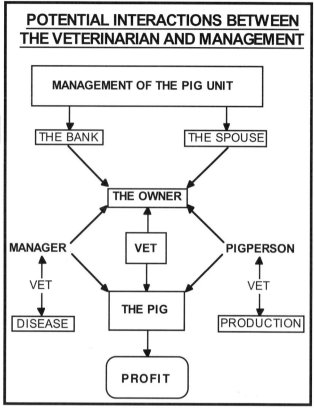

(Fig.3-12)

cal example of this is when the farrowing house manager is promoted to under manager or the under manager is promoted to full manager. This must be the ultimate goal of the education process throughout the farm, though of course the pathways upwards will be limited by the capabilities of each individual and the size of the farm.

The objectives of training and education

These essentially can be grouped into five areas:
1. Education per se.
2. To provide a better understanding of the job.
3. To provide a better working relationship both with pig people and managers.
4. To provide a better environment for the pig and improve its welfare.
5. Finally to increase efficiency of not only production and health but also the economic viability of the farm.

What is important to the employees in their work?

A number of surveys have been carried out in different occupations and the results in order of preference generally are very much the same. These include:
- An interesting job.
- Appreciation for the work that is done.
- Being involved in the job - This is important because

CHAPTER 3 - Managing Health and Disease 79

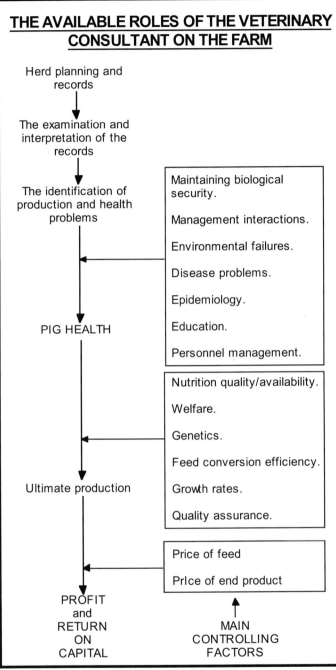

(Fig.3-13)

nel achievement and gratification from the boss.
- A good environment in which to work.
- Good office facilities.

All the above are provided by education.

Are you providing your employees with the above? Why not ask them?

If as an employer or manager you provide education then it is quite pertinent to ask the question "How do I benefit"? Such benefits would include:
- More consistent standards of work.
- You have more confidence in the staff.
- The system of pig farming becomes more efficient.
- The system is much better maintained.
- There are fewer disasters or mistakes.
- There is a great deal more staff motivation and therefore work practices become more efficient.
- The staff become aware of their responsibilities when working with people and they are much more flexible.
- There is a much lower staff turn over.

The same question must then be asked "How does the employee benefit from education"?:
- There is more involvement in the job.
- There is better understanding of objectives and goals and greater achievement.
- There is a great deal more job satisfaction and more motivation.
- Confidence in abilities develops.
- There is a status of being skilled.
- Skills can be documented and thereby recognised.
- The prospects of achievement become apparent and through this, enhancement of the job position.
- There are less accidents at work.

Are you a successful employer or a manager?

This is a very important question to ask yourself. It can be answered by the difficulties you have in obtaining employees or the time which they remain in your employment. It is interesting to look at the characteristics of the good manager. Check yourself against this list and pick out the areas which you consider are weaknesses then develop them into strengths.

Characteristics of a good owner/manager
- Manages people well with skill and understanding.
- Has as much interest in people as in the work.
- Demonstrates technical competence.
- Has good business and financial skills.
- Is able to motivate people and provide education.

it does provide people with considerable motivation particularly if owners and managers are prepared to listen and take note.
- A good salary or wage for the job which in it self provides a considerable amount of the basic security need.
- Confidence and trust - this further promotes motivation and in particular self esteem.
- Incentives - these range from increased rewards financially, through bonus schemes to the sense of person-

Chapter 3

- Is a good communicator and aware of peoples needs.
- Has good organisational competence.
- Is a clear decision maker having listened to the various relevant thoughts from people.
- Provides a good work experience.
- Gives employees an opportunity to contribute to the debate.
- Always gives a perception of responsibility.
- Provides a challenge and encouragement.
- Rewards people through personal achievement, recognition, authority, status and pay.
- Provides a constant and enthusiastic environment within which the employees can work.
- Makes every effort to ensure that the employees are involved in all planning and decision making and in particular has the quality to go and ask questions and listen.
- Involves people in their job. This is one of the highest priorities in most employees.
- Always creates an atmosphere of constant good relationships where employees are not frightened to communicate their ideas or indeed their feelings about their job.
- Provides a clear avenue for the expressions of frustrations and any on going problems.
- Expects and receives excellent performance from the staff and conveys a belief that they are capable of carrying this out.
- Should say "thank you - well done", often.
- It is interesting to note that the successful managers are those that have a sense of personal fulfilment. This also creates an excellent environment for employees.

Finally there is a strong relationship between motivation and the belief that improved performance will lead to financial rewards. However, the methods by which the reward is determined needs careful thought and clarification. If you develop a bonus system always assess it first on a wide range of theoretical scenarios before you commit yourself to it.

How should you improve education on the farm?

There are four or five clearly identified areas of job specification where programmes of education need to be developed. These areas can be categorised as follows:

The Trainee Stockperson
↓
The Stockperson
↓
The Training Manager or Under Manager
↓
The Manager
↓
The Owner

At a farm level, training can be provide by both the manager and or owner, the veterinarian and other people introduced to the farm for that purpose. The manager should play a pivotal role in this by his constant daily instruction, the assessment of various techniques, by staff meetings and by using his records.

At a stockperson level each farm should have a simple manual of the different daily tasks so that when instructions and training have been given and competency assessed they can then be documented.

This type of training programme would be considered as basic and be undertaken over a one to two year period. It would be suitable for the new recruit or school-leaver.

The veterinarian would have a part to play in the basic training through promoting understanding and the development of short seminars on the farm as part of his visit contribution.

Topics that should be considered in the basic training programme

- Technical pig production terms and their understanding.
- Aspects of safety on the pig farm.
- Management of:
  - Boars
  - Dry sows
  - Farrowing houses.

HERD SIZE Suggested Visit Frequency and Veterinary Time on the Farm		
No. of Sows	Visit Frequency in weeks	Hours per Annum
50 - 100	8 - 12	16
150 - 250	8 - 12	27
300 - 400	6 - 8	36
450 - 600	4 - 6	48
600+	4 - 6	90

(Fig.3-14)

Always make it clear that any bonus system is a reward and not a right.

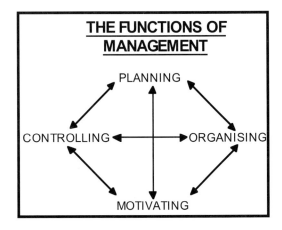

THE FUNCTIONS OF MANAGEMENT

- Weaner production.
- Feeder pig production.
- The hospital pen.
- Understanding reproduction.
- Artificial insemination techniques.
- Pregnancy testing.
- Recording and the use of records.
- Understanding genetics and breeding.
- Recognising the healthy and diseased pig.
- The disposal of dead stock.
- The role of disinfectants in disease.
- The management of drugs on the farm.
- The administration of drugs on the farm.
- Nutrition and the application of feed.
- Slurry disposal.
- The use of pressure washers, electricity.
- Managing the gilt.
- Welding and maintenance.
- Understanding simple pig production economics.

Within each of these topics there will be further individual areas of education. For example in the farrowing house a list should be made of all the various tasks that are carried out including:
- Preparing the house for occupancy.
- Recording farrowing details.
- Preparing the sow for farrowing.
- The signs of farrowing.
- How to assist at farrowing.
- Removing teeth and tails.
- Injecting with iron.
- Managing the litter.
- Recognising disease.
- Recognising piglet diseases.
- Assessing the healthy and diseased udder.
- Castration, tattooing.
- Feeding the sow.
- Controlling the environment.
- Moving the sow
- Catching the litter in preparation for tasks.

Each of these would provide a short course of instruction followed by "doing", followed by assessment.

Intermediate training

This area of training is aimed at the experienced stockperson or the person responsible for a section of the farm or a trainee manager. It should involve attending day courses that included personnel management and more advanced training of the basic topics. Veterinary seminars on the understanding of diseases should be an important part of this. This can be carried out either on the farm at the veterinary visit, if there are sufficient people to justify this, or alternatively by the development of seminars at the veterinary practice or at the agriculture schools. The following topics should form part of the veterinary training programme:
- Understanding infectious agents.

> *Use this book for training on your farm. It is written for that purpose.*

- Anatomy of the pig.
- The use and misuse of drugs.
- How diseases are spread.
- The healthy and the diseased pig.
- The collection, understanding and use of records.
- The relevance of disease control to profitable pig farming.
- Understanding reproduction in the male.
- Understanding reproduction in the female.
- Non- infectious infertility.
- Infectious infertility.
- The process of farrowing.
- Approaching farm problems.
- Aspects of vaccination.
- Welfare of the pig.
- Notifiable diseases.
- Respiratory diseases.
- Problems of the dry sow.
- Nutrition, production and disease.
- Controlling parasites.
- Skin diseases.

> *Have a copy of this book accessible to all staff at all times. Do not lock it away.*

Advanced training

This should be aimed at the under manger, the manager and the group farm manager. Instruction courses here would involve attending specific educational seminars. At a veterinary level these would include the topics already mentioned for intermediates but they would now be dealt with in a more detailed and scientific way and include a greater understanding, particularly of the epidemiology and the control of disease. Instruction techniques and the ability to teach people should be a major part of this training programme together with people management, business management and communication skills. Training in the areas of business management and the use of computers form a essential part of modern day pig production. The greatest complaint of people working on pig farms is style of management and lack of appreciation. The education of the manager in this respect is important.

An Example of Management Failures and Disease

The following sequence of events highlights how bad

> *If you want a good farm, have a good manager.*

management and decisions can result in disasters.

The farm was a 500 sow herd where the management made the decision to expand from 500 to 600 sows through the purchase of gilts. Unfortunately the health status of the purchased gilts was not checked out and they infected the herd with atrophic rhinitis. To coincide with the herd expansion a decision was also made to develop a building programme which was not completed in time. The number of breeding females increased and so did the stocking densities in the service area resulting in poor hygiene and stress with increases in services and boar usage. The increased number of services resulted in high numbers of animals farrowing with no increase in farrowing accommodation. Finally the resulting shortened lactation length, due to shortage of farrowing accommodation, caused ascending vaginal infection and endometritis post-service. This together with the increased boar usage and poor hygiene resulted in a major infertility problem. The increased throughput of sows through the farrowing houses resulted in major scour problems which together with the poor hygiene increased the severity of the rhinitis. The shortened lactation length together with the scour precipitated post-weaning problems, increased stocking density and further increased problems with rhinitis. The final insult was the fact that the shortened lactation length resulted in poor litter size. The end result therefore of the original management decisions resulted in a herd with severe rhinitis, low litter size, increased pre-weaning mortality, heavy discharges and an infertility problem. The farm went out of business.

The Use of Records

The previous sections have illustrated some of the consequences of management failure, particularly in planning, that can lead not only to production problems but also to major disease breakdowns. The collection of records and their use are vital components necessary to develop management strategies. Whilst there are many computer programmes available for recording pig herds and many of these are highly efficient, nevertheless it is important to understand the basic principles of using records for production and disease control.

Recording Objectives

Before spending a considerable amount of money on a computer programme, a lot of time entering data and producing a great deal of paper it is important to answer a simple question. "What are we trying to do?" There are five reasons for producing information:
1. To improve overall efficiency.
2. To maximise profitability.
3. To produce end data that defines:
   - Production levels.
   - Reproduction levels.
   - Management achievements.
   - Economics.
   - The use of feeds.
   - Growth performance.
   - The levels of disease.
   - The levels of medicinal treatment.
4. For epidemiological studies to understand problems.
5. Finally as aids for daily use by management.

Fig.3-15 shows the pathways for using data so that management control, production and disease can be monitored and better understood.

There are 3 major areas crucial to management decisions, namely economics, production and feed. The total liveweight of pigs leaving the farm is fundamental to profitability. Every extra kilogram of liveweight sold increases the margin over feed with few extra overheads. Likewise matching the type of pig to the best market is another important management decision.

Production is monitored from individual records of the sow, sucking pig, weaner and grower-finisher and in each of these disease, treatment and mortality levels are recorded.

Feed usage, the third recording area, is also the largest cost centre, and the monitoring of costs per tonne, costs of liveweight gain and efficiency of use are vital. It is here that the greatest use of records and computer technology can be made but it is also the area where there is often the least input.

Fig.3-16 shows data from national information in the UK to illustrate the costs as a percentage of sales. It can be seen that the veterinary medicines costs were 2.12% of the net sales. These might at first sight appear small but it does not take into account the costs of any disease, poor production and poor feed efficiency which on some farms could be a further 8-10%. Veterinary services in this respect can be highly cost effective.

Recorded information can be classified into four main categories for practical use:
- **Action information** - This is used on a weekly basis by the manager and staff. It should provide data relating to animals that are due for service, pregnancy testing, vaccination, and farrowing. Most computers forecast what is likely to happen in the weeks ahead.
- **End data** - This is summary information produced as rolling averages of the previous month, several months or years. It indicates on a cumulative basis what has been happening during any defined period. This helps to monitor the efficiency of the production and the effects of disease and it is used against target figures to identify problem areas. End data does not however provide information for epidemiological analysis and problem solving.
- **Epidemiological information** - This is the detail that produces the end data and consists of a number of individual pieces of information. Unfortunately many computerised systems do not retain this, or if they do its presentation is in such a vast amount or in an illogical format that it can be extremely difficult for the

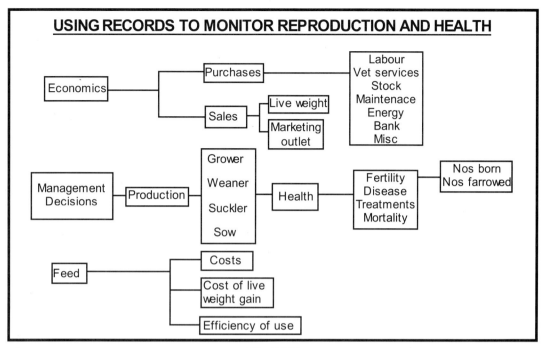
(Fig.3-15)

pig farmer or the veterinarian to use and assimilate. A much more simple procedure is to identify the specific points of information that are required relative to the problem and analyse these manually. Using this method we can then utilise the observations and clinical examinations of the stock people, identify the animals which form the core group of the problem and then study them to identify any common features.
- **Forecasting information** - This is used for planning and targeting and there are a number of useful computer programmes that respond to changing productions and disease information and allow more reliable decisions to be made.

What ever system of record keeping is used or proposed to be used on the farm, consider the following questions:
- What are you trying to do?
- Is it possible to do it?
- How do you record it?
- Is the effort going to be worthwhile?
- Is the method of collection and presentation simple and straightforward?
- Is the information to be collected accurate and reliable?
- How do you intend to use the information?

The consultant veterinarian has an important role to play in the analysis of recorded information and in its epidemiological use.

The following simple formats and examples have proved of value in both monitoring and investigating problems on the farm. Fig.3-17 to Fig.3-27.

These records could be documented weekly and the format is valuable as a monitor to achieving efficient production. It allows remedial action to be taken.

BREEDING AND FEEDING HERDS
Extracted Data from National Information UK September 1996 *

Pigs Sold Per Sow Per Annum - 20.6
Sale Weight - 85 - 100kg
Price - Average cost feed / tonne £145
      Feed cost / pig produced £44
      Sale price per pig £73.00

	Percentage of Net Output (Pig sales less breeding purchases)
Feed costs (total)	59
Margin over feed	41
Variable costs	
Vet / med.	2.12
Transport	1.15
Electric / heat	1.33
Water	0.64
Bedding	0.5
Miscellaneous	0.97
Total	**6.71**
Fixed costs	
Labour	7.7
Buildings, machinery, other	4.65

* Meat and Livestock Commission 1996

(Fig 3-16)

Managing Pig Health and the Treatment of Disease

HERD TARGETS FOR PRODUCTION AND DISEASE												
	Jan	Feb	Mar	Apr	May	Jun	Jul	Aug	Sep	Oct	Nov	Dec
No. of breeding females	*216*	*218*	*221*									
Target:	**220**	**220**	**220**	**220**	**220**	**220**	**220**	**220**	**220**	**220**	**220**	**220**
Total matings (+ gilts)	*46*	*88*	*131*									
Cumulative targets:	**47**	**94**	**141**	**188**	**235**	**282**	**329**	**376**	**423**	**470**	**517**	**564**
Gilt matings	*7*	*12*	*18*									
Cumulative target:	**7**	**14**	**21**	**28**	**35**	**42**	**49**	**56**	**63**	**70**	**77**	**84**
Repeat matings	*3*	*5*	*11*									
Cumulative target:	**4**	**8**	**12**	**16**	**20**	**24**	**28**	**32**	**36**	**40**	**44**	**48**
Nos. farrowed	*41*	*84*	*123*									
Cumulative target:	**42**	**84**	**126**	**168**	**210**	**252**	**294**	**336**	**378**	**420**	**462**	**504**
Nos. born alive	*476*	*899*	*1339*									
Cumulative target:	**474**	**948**	**1422**	**1896**	**2370**	**2844**	**3318**	**3792**	**4266**	**4740**	**5214**	**5688**
Pre-weaning mortality	*32*	*72*	*108*									
Cumulative target:	**40**	**80**	**120**	**160**	**200**	**240**	**280**	**320**	**360**	**400**	**440**	**480**
Nos. weaned	*440*	*863*	*1253*									
Cumulative target:	**434**	**868**	**1302**	**1736**	**2170**	**2604**	**3038**	**3472**	**3906**	**4340**	**4774**	**5208**
Weaner mortality	*5*	*12*	*19*									
Cumulative target:	**7**	**14**	**21**	**28**	**35**	**42**	**49**	**56**	**63**	**70**	**77**	**84**
Grower / finisher mortality	*3*	*10*	*16*									
Cumulative target:	**7**	**14**	**21**	**28**	**35**	**42**	**49**	**56**	**63**	**70**	**77**	**84**
Weaners sold												
Cumulative target:	-	-	-	-	-	-	-	-	-	-	-	-
Finishers sold	*401*	*816*	*1246*									
Cumulative target:	**420**	**840**	**1260**	**1680**	**2100**	**2520**	**2940**	**3360**	**3780**	**4200**	**4620**	**5040**
Sows sold	*4*	*9*	*14*									
Cumulative target:	**6**	**12**	**18**	**24**	**30**	**36**	**42**	**48**	**54**	**60**	**66**	**72**

An Example of targets set for a 220 sow herd selling finished pigs.

(Fig.3-17)

CHAPTER 3 - Managing Health and Disease

RECORDING SOW PROBLEMS										
Unit: *Poplar Farm*				Total number of sows: *400*						
Month / Week				Jan	Feb	Mar	Apr	May	etc.	Target % *	Target Nos. per Month
Matings Sow First time				71	62	50					64
Repeats				6	4	4				< 8	5
Gilt First time				10	16	12				< 5	15
Repeats				2	3	1				< 2	1
PD% Doubtful negative				2	3	2				< 2	1
No. treated - hormones				-	-	-				< 1	0
Anoestrus sows			C	-	-	-				< 3	0.5
Anoestrus gilts			C	1	-	1				< 5	0.5
Repeats / infertility			C	2	1	1				< 2	< 2
Not in Pig			C	2	1	1				< 1	< 1
Abortions			D/C	-	-	-				< 1	< 0.5
Discharge from vulva			T	2	1	-				< 1	< 1
			D/C	1	-	-				< 1	< 1
Mastitis			T	-	-	-				< 5	1
			D/C	-	-	-				< 2	2
No milk			T/C	2	-	-					2 - 4
Lame			T	3	4	2				< 20 p.a.	1
			D/C	1	-	1				< 12 p.a.	1
Miscellaneous problems			T	-	-	1				2 p.m.	
			D/C	-	-	-				1 p.m.	
No of farrowings				70	64	67				73	73
Assisted farrowings				-	2	1					< 3
Prolapse			T/D/C	1	-	-				< 8 p.a.	
Fever			T	1	-	-				1 p.m.	
			D/C	-	-	-				-	
Haemorrhage			T	-	-	-				< 1 p.m.	
			D/C	-	-	-				< 3 p.a.	
Litters savaged			T/C	1	-	-				< 2	
Low Nos. born / reared			C	2	-	-				< 8	
Total normal sow sales				4	8	12				15 p.m.	
Total sow deaths										< 20 p.a.	< 2
Sows destroyed on the farm			D							< 4 p.a.	
Problem sows shipped or culled			C							< 4 p.a.	

T= Numbers treated   **D/C** = Numbers died or culled.
* As a percentage of sows mated or farrowed in your defined period.   Per month (**p.m.**)   Per annum (**p.a.**)

(Fig.3-18)

RECORDING MATING

Week / Month....... *January.*

Sow No.	Date Weaned	Date First Mated	First or Repeat Matings	No. Services	Boar Used	Lost Days	Date Due to Farrow	Comments
317	1-1-97	6-1-97	1	3	27/27/26	5	30-4-97	-
27	1-1-97	28-1-97	1	2	3B	27	25-4-97	Mastitis
64	Gilt	2-2-97	2	3	8/4/4	29	27-5-97	Bled

(Fig.3-19)

RECORDING FAILURES TO FARROW

MONTH: April   **TOTAL SERVED:** 104
CATEGORY: (See below)

Sow No.	Parity	Date First Mated	1st or Repeat Mating	Boar used	Cause of Failure	Date of Failure	Days Interval	Result/history/ Stockperson/ comments
75	7	10-12-96	1	16	Dis	24-2-97	76	Discharge
161	5	12-12-96	2	4	-	2-2-97	52	Poor service
67	8	3-1-97	1	60	D/C	27-3-97	83	Fighting
724	1	2-3-97	1	24	Ab	4-5-97	63	Lame

Cause of failure: **(Rp)** = Repeats   **(Ab)** = Abortion   **(NIP)** = Not In Pig   **(Dis)** = Disease   **(D/C)** = Death/Culled

(Fig.3-20)

RECORDING BOAR MATINGS AND SOWS THAT FARROW FROM THEM

Boar	Matings	Repeats	Non Return Rate	Farrowed From the Matings	FR %	Average Born Alive	Pigs / 100 Matings / Farrowed
4	23	6	74%	16	70%	10.1	707
5	19	1	95%	18	95%	10.4	988
7	12	0	100%	11	92%	11.4	1048
9	16	3	81%	13	81%	12.1	980
10	24	1	96%	22	92%	11.9	1094

(Fig.3-21)

RECORDING SOW DEATHS

Sow No.	Date Served	Boar Used	Date of Death	State Pregnancy	Parity	Condition	Illness / Treatment	PM Findings or Cause of Death	History
126	7-9-96	60	17-9-96	Unknown	6	Poor	Ill fever	Peritonitis	Bled at service

(Fig.3-22)

CHAPTER 3 - Managing Health and Disease

RECORDING VULVAL DISCHARGES				
Identification of sow	420	16		
Date of farrowing	4-7-96	6-8-96		
Date weaned	25-7-96	20-8-96		
Date mated	30-7-96	29-8-96		
Parity	7	2		
Boar used	20/20	14/147		
Date of discharge	28-8-96	30-9-96		
No. days from mating	24	32		
Description of discharge	Mucus	white/pus		
Results of first pregnancy diagnosis	-ve	+ve		
Results of second pregnancy diagnosis	-ve	-ve		
Date of farrowing or otherwise	Culled	Culled		

(Fig.3-23)

RECORDING LITTER SIZE DETAILS BY PARITY
Month / Week:..

Sow No.	Litter No.	Date Farrowed	Boar Used	No. Alive	No. Dead	No. Mummified	No. Weaned	Days Suckled
604	7	24-8-96	23/23	14	3	1	13	19
906	1	29-10-96	29/29	3	3	3	9 (6 fostered)	-

(Fig.3-24)

RECORDING PIGLET DIARRHOEA FOR INVESTIGATION

Date Scour Noted	Sow No.	Parity	Date Farrowed	No. Pigs in Litter	No. Affected	No. Deaths	Comments: Vaccine Used, Treatment Given
23-4-96	52	2	22-4-96	11	All	2	Not vaccinated Neomycin
27-4-96	604	1	26-4-96	9	All	6	Not vaccinated Trimethoprim
28-4-96	606	1	26-4-96	10	All	0	Enrofloxacin. Responded

(Fig.3-25)

RECORDING OF WEANING / FINISHING PIG DISEASES

Period		Jan	Feb	Mar	Apr	May	Jun	etc.	Total	Target % *
Lameness	T	12	2	1					15	< 1
	D/C	1	-	-					1	< 0.5
Haemorrhage	T	-	-	1					1	< 1
(Pale pig)	D/C	1	-	-					1	< 0.5
Pneumonia	T	24	36	52					112	1
	D/C	1	4	6					11	< 0.5
Scour	T	2	3	2					7	< 2
	D/C	-	-	-					-	< 0.5
Prolapse	T	16	14	14					44	< 1.5
	D/C	-	-	-					-	< 1
Blown-up	T	4	3	1					8	< 1
(Rectal stricture)	D/C	2	1	1					4	All
Fever	T	-	-	-					-	< 1
	D/C	-	-	-					-	0
Stress	T	2	-	-					2	1
(Fighting)	D/C	-	-	1					1	0.5
Runt	T	8	7	9					24	< 1.5
Poor pigs	D/C	1	1	1					3	< 1
Meningitis	T	-	-	-					-	< 2
	D/C	-	-	-					-	< 2
Miscellaneous	T	-	1	-					1	< 2
(Middle ear)	D/C	-	1	-					1	< 1
Total deaths	D/C								22	< 4
Total treated									214	< 5
Total to cull pen										< 1.5
Pigs at risk		2100	2010	2221						

T = Number treated   D/C = number died or culled.
* As a percentage of the population at risk in your defined period.

(Fig.3-26)

RECORDING WEANER OR FINISHER MORTALITY

Week:..................   Month.......Feb 1996

Date	Weight of Pig	Age of Pig	Name of House & Time In	Feed Being Used	Condition Good/Moderate/Poor	Cause	Comment / Observation
3-2	60kg	16 wks	G1	346	G	Blown up	Sudden
8-2	85kg	20 wks	73	1-64	G	?	Pale

(Fig.3-27)

Planning for Efficient Production and Disease Control

One of the most difficult management tasks is to control the numbers of sows and gilts mated in any given period of time. If for example the programme requires 20 matings per week and only 10 are carried out followed by 30 in the next week major problems may arise in managing these animals through the housing system. The effects of these are shown in Fig.3-28. Problems first arise through the overuse of boars leading to infertility problems and variable litter size. As stocking densities increase more animals enter the housing system than it is designed for. In the farrowing houses there is a failure of the all-in all-out system resulting in early weaning and more fostering. There is an increased number of pigs to be transferred into the weaner and growers accommodation at any one time with increased stocking densities, permanently populated houses and the movement of pigs from one house to another thus disturbing the status quo. The end result of all these various changes is disease or poor growth depending on the severity of the mating control failure and pathogenic organisms present on the farm.

Management Procedures for Maximising the Mating Programme

Managing the mating program for maximum throughput without creating pig flow problems requires good forward planning to achieve consistency.

Calculate the entry to exit time per crate in days e.g.
    21 days mean lactation length
    3 days cleaning time
    4 days entry to farrowing
Total = 28 days

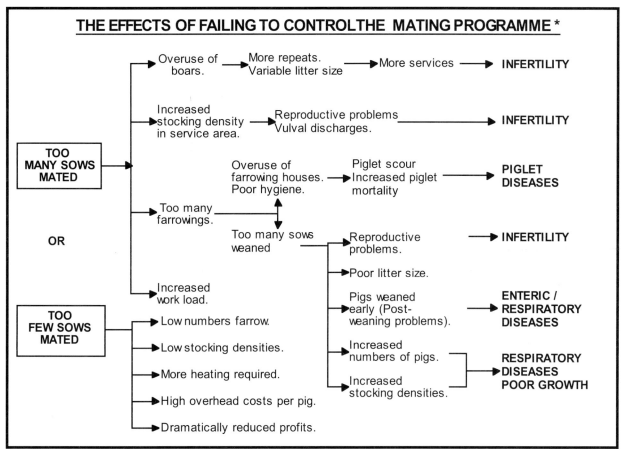
(Fig.3-28)

* The term mating and service are often considered the same. Mating here means the complete process i.e. includes 1, 2 or 3 services etc.

In theory therefore each crate could be used 365 ÷ 28 = 13 times per annum. Calculate the actual number. This will indicate the efficiency of use.

Maintaining regular batch farrowings each week, or each farrowing period, is dependant upon the following:
- Sows coming into oestrus regularly after weaning.
- A good conception and consistent farrowing rate.
- A knowledge of the farrowing rates weekly or monthly.
- A planned input of gilts to replace culled sows.
- Anticipation of oestrus in the gilts.
- Planning at least 8 weeks ahead to determine the breeding females that will be weaned and due for mating.
- The effects of disease.

There are a number of management tools that can be used:-

1. Modern computer programmes will list out sows that fail to maintain a pregnancy on a week by week basis. (Fig.3-29). This format can also be carried out manually from the weekly mating sheets. When sows reach their twelfth week of pregnancy (forecast week) those animals still pregnant, viable or those due to be culled for age or disease can be identified. This will indicate those available for mating in 7 weeks time. The anticipated matings can be brought to target by planned gilt matings for that week.
2. Fig.3-30 shows a farm example on a weekly basis whereby production is monitored against the cumulative targets. Such a method gives an opportunity to manipulate the system if there is a major loss and compensate for it.
3. For small herds up to 350 sows a circular calendar can provide an excellent and simple visual method. (Fig.3-31). Sows due for culling can be identified by a colour code. In this particular herd summer infertility is a regular phenomenon with increased matings carried out to compensate and disadvantages sows culled.
4. Another option to maintaining the programme is to serve all sows weaned each week and cull some sows $3^{1}/_{2}$ weeks later to adjust the number of pregnancies to those required.

Management of the Environment

When faced with a problem it is always an interesting proposition to ask the question,

How might I make this problem worse?

Such an approach invariably highlights areas for corrective action.

A FARM EXAMPLE

Week	Target Matings+	Sows Mated	Week No. 1	2	3	4	5	6	7	8	9	10	11	12	13	14	15	16	FR%	Suckling 17	18	19	M 20
								Sows Still in Pig															
1	10	10	10	10	10	**9**	9	9	9	9	9	9	9	9	9	9	9	9	90	9	9	9	9
2	10	11	11	11	11	11	**9**	9	9	9	9	9	9	9	9	9	9		81				
3	10	9	9	9	9	9	9	9	9	9	9	**8**	8	8	8	8			88				
4	10	12	12	12	12	12	12	**11**	11	11	11	11	11	11					91				
5	10	10	10	10	10	10	10	10	10	10	10	10	10						100				
6	10	11	11	11	11	11	11	11	11	11	**10**	10							90				
7	10	9	9	9	9	9	9	9	**7**	7	7	6							66				
8	10	11	11	11	11	11	11	11	11	11									100				
9	10	10	10	10	10	**9**	9	9	9	9									99				
10	10	10	10	10	10	**9**	9	9	9										90				
	etc.													Planning Week									

The numbers in bold indicate sows dropping out.   M No. sows mated   + Females available for mating.   FR% Farrowing rate

(Fig.3-29)

There are a number of common environmental failures that are associated with problems and loss of performance in the dry sows, lactating sows, sucking pigs and the growing pigs. These call for management actions.

Environmental Factors Affecting Dry Sows
- Catabolic state from weaning to 21 days post-service.
- Grouping sows at weaning. Fighting
- Poor light intensity.
- Fluctuating lighting patterns.
- Fluctuating temperatures day and night.
- High air flow, draughts.
- House temperatures above the upper critical temperature.
- House temperatures below the lower critical temperature.
- Low mating house temperatures.
- Poor water availability.
- Small badly designed tethers or stalls.
- Faulty floor surfaces.
- Wet poorly drained floors.

Environmental Factors Affecting Lactating Sows and Sucking Pigs
- Cross-fostering different age groups of piglets.
- Mechanical transfer of infections between litters.
- High feed levels pre and immediately post farrowing.
- Fluctuating farrowing house temperatures.
- Failure to determine the best farrowing house temperature.
- Draughty creep areas, low creep temperatures.
- Draughts on the sow.
- Continuous throughput. No all-in all-out system.
- Failure to wash, disinfect and dry between batches.
- Poor crate design.
- Wet poorly drained floors.

AN ACTUAL EXAMPLE OF HERD TARGETS CUMULATIVE BY WEEK

Week No. Date	1 06-4	2 13-4	3 20-4	4 27-4	5 04-5	6 11-5	7 18-5	8 25-5	9 01-6	10 8-6	11 15-6	12 22-6
Total matings	14	30	43	56	64	75	83	91	103	111	127	134
Cumulative targets: (11.1)	11	22	33	44	55	66	77	88	99	111	122	133
Gilt Matings	6	8	8	10	10	11	14	14	14	14	16	16
Cumulative targets: (1.9)	2	3	5	7	9	11	13	15	17	19	20	22
Repeats	0	2	4	6	6	8	8	8	8	8	10	10
Cumulative targets: (0.9)	1	2	2	3	4	5	6	7	8	9	10	11
No. Farrowed	9	22	25	36	47	56	65	72	84	95	105	116
Cumulative targets: (9.9)	9.9	19	29	39	49	59	69	79	89	99	108	118
Born Alive	100	242	280	413	541	640	743	820	945	1078	1195	1325
Cumulative targets: (118)	118	236	354	472	590	708	826	944	1062	1180	1290	1416
Weaned	110	218	328	415	522	588	689	748	895	999	1100	1224
Cumulative targets: (104)	104	208	312	416	520	624	728	832	936	1040	1140	1248

Target ( ) actual weekly target
220 sows
2.35 litters / sow / year
Piglets born alive 11.9
Piglets weaned per litter 10.5
24.7 pigs reared

(Fig.3-30)

- Leaking feed troughs.
- Poor water supply.
- Poor lighting.
- Delayed faeces removal from behind the sow.
- Fly problems.

Environmental Factors Affecting Growing Pigs

- Incorrect house temperatures, particularly fluctuations.
- Pigs held below their lower critical temperature.
- High ventilation rates, air flow and draughts.
- Low or fluctuating humidity together with low temperatures.
- Poor insulation.
- Worn out environmental controllers and sensors.
- Floor types, poor drainage, wet floors, slats with draughts.
- Constant mixing and movement of pigs.
- Moving pigs too soon from one house to another.
- High stocking density.
- Large group sizes and small cubic air space.
- Continually populated houses with endemic disease.
- Feed changes when pigs are moved from one house to another together with lower levels of nutrition.
- Inadequate trough spaces or water availability.
- Poor or inadequate nutrition.
- Continual exposure to faeces.
- High levels of toxic gases.

The first requirement of good management is to prevent the build up of infection through the cleaning and disinfection of buildings, maintaining low stocking densities and good environments. Reducing stress through the effects of fluctuating temperatures and the influences of humidity and ventilation on organisms in the air is the second part. The third part is the provision of good nutrition and in particular, adequate levels of energy, protein and lysine.

Air Quality

The quality of the air in the pig building depends on a number of factors including the stocking density, the cubic capacity of the building, the lower critical and upper critical temperatures, concentrations of gases and levels of dust.

As the number of infectious organisms and the pigs' exposure to them increases, there is an increasing risk of disease. Control of the environment therefore must constantly aim to reduce these levels.

Bacteria and viruses spread from pig to pig by direct contact, indirect contact (e.g. on walls or floors), on equipment and people, and by airborne dust and droplets. The latter mode of spread is obviously associated with air quality.

In dry airborne dust most of the infectious organism die quickly but their toxins (e.g. endotoxins) can still be harmful to the pig when inhaled. Aerosol droplets con-

A CIRCULAR CALENDAR USED ON A FARM FOR MONITORING THE MATING PROGRAMME

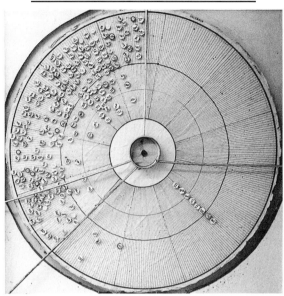

Sows start at the top move to the left to farrow and are then weaned. Weaned sows are on the right awaiting mating to start the cycle again.

(Fig.3-31)

taining organisms dry out rapidly at low humidity and the organisms die. At the middle range of humidities the droplets do not dry and the organisms remain viable and infective. At very high humidities (>90%) droplets and dust pick up water, increase in size, and are precipitated out of the air.

Size of the dust particles or aerosol droplets has a bearing on the pigs' defences. When very small particles or droplets are inhaled they are sucked deep into the lungs, sometimes as far as the terminal air sacs (alveoli). Larger particles and droplets tend to be filtered out in the nose and throat or in the upper airways of the lungs.

> *If you have a problem check through the relevant list.*

Using systems that do not operate on an all-in all-out basis the incoming pigs meet with heavy doses of respiratory and enteric organisms which are being shed by the older pigs already there. The most harmful time for this to happen is in first stage and second stage weaner accommodation at a time when the antibodies from the sows colostrum and milk are waning and before the pig has had time to fully develop its own. Overwhelming aerosal build-up of organisms also tend to occupy finishing rooms that contain heavier pigs.

The constant high challenge to the respiratory system results in major mobilisation of the pigs immune systems which is costly in energy and lowers the pigs growth rate.

The situation may be worsened by suppression of the

pigs' immune system caused by mixing, moving, stress, overcrowding, inadequate nutrition, and high levels of irritant slurry gases. Increased ventilation helps in reducing gases but does not have much effect on airborne dust and droplets. Infact it may make airborne dust levels worse. It also may create evaporative cooling over the pigs which will not help their resistance. Chilling tends to trigger disease.

Reducing stocking density and avoiding overcrowding have the biggest effect on improving air quality and reducing airborne organisms with a resultant boost to growth rate and efficiency of feed conversion to meat. This increased growth also serves to decrease the stocking density by faster throughput. Changing from dry feeding to liquid feeding also reduces dust levels and respiratory disease.

A checklist for maintaining air quality

- Assess the quality at the daily inspection.
- Humidity.
- Condensation.
- Smell. Levels of ammonia.
- Dust levels.
- Assess the lying patterns of the pigs. Are there draughts?
- Check temperature fluctuations.
- Check that fans and inlets are functioning.
- Strip and clean the inlets and outlets between batches of pigs.
- Test that controller systems are functioning correctly each week.
- Test the fail safe mechanism twice weekly.
- Assess levels of disease.
- Check the stocking density of the pigs relative to the cubic capacity of the house.
- Check that stocking densities are not above recommended levels.

Environmental Temperatures

It is important to maintain the pig within an equitable temperature range and this is called the thermo-neutral zone. It is dependent upon the type of floor, its insulation properties, the air speed and temperature and the insulation of the building.

> **Overcrowding leads to respiratory disease and poor growth rate which slows throughput further increasing the overcrowding.**

This is particularly so if the pig is at a critical time in relation to disease challenge, or when under environmental stress. For example if it coincides with a move from solid concrete or straw bedded floors to concrete slats. The temperature requirement for the pig might have been 20°C (68°F) before the move but could well be 25°C (77°F) for the first days in the new accommodation.

> **Failure to keep the pig within its temperature comfort zone contributes to the development of disease.**

Pigs that are within their comfort zone will lie on their sides barely touching their neighbours.

The point at which pigs must increase heat production to keep warm is called the lower critical temperature (LCT). Many factors affect this including body weight, feed intake, age, insulation of the building and in particular the floor type. There is an upper critical temperature (UCT) and the range between the upper and lower ones is called the thermo-neutral zone as shown in Fig.3-32.

> **Lowering stocking density improves air quality and growth rate which decreases stocking density further.**

Fig.3-33 gives guidelines to the temperature requirements necessary at different phases in the production cycle. Adverse temperatures have effects at the following critical times:

- From birth to 48 hours.
- From 8-14 days of age.
- From weaning to 7 days post-weaning.
- On movement from first to second stage weaner accommodation.
- A change in the type of flooring e.g. solid to slats, bedded to non-bedded.
- A change of housing or nutrition.
- A change in stocking density.
- A move from dry to wet feeding.
- A move to poorly insulated houses.
- Movement into a wet house.
- Fluctuations in external temperatures due to ventilation and air speed.
- Faulty environmental controllers.
- Low energy diets or unpalatable feed.
- Restricted feeding.
- Failure to eat sufficient feed.
- Thin pigs.
- Disease.
- The sow during lactation.
- From weaning to 21 days post-mating.
- In the last six weeks of pregnancy.

Because there are so many variables it is difficult to be categorical about specific temperatures for different weights of pig. Approximate guidelines for different floor types are shown in Fig.3-34 but the ultimate determinant is the pig itself, by its behaviour, lying patterns and

> **Adjust the temperature of the building by the lying habits of the pig. Then when the pig is comfortable note the temperature required.**

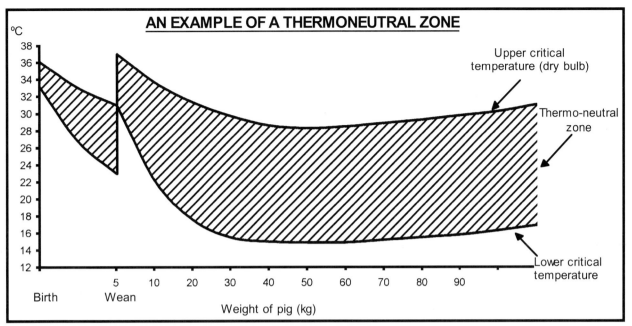

(Fig.3-32)

performance.

For every degree below the LCT (lower critical temperature) a growing pig looses approximately 10-12g of liveweight gain per day. A level of 1°C below the LCT during the growing period could cost £1.00 in extra feed per pig. Fig.3-35.

Draughts at any age can result in the pig experiencing significantly lower temperatures than might be registered by an air temperature thermometer. This is the wind chill factor.

Stocking Densities

Disease levels, growth rates, feed efficiency and mortality are closely correlated to stocking densities but the threshold level will vary with age and weight of pig, its health status, the cubic capacity of the building and from farm to farm.

For example a farm that is free of EP, PRRS and APP would accommodate a much higher stocking density than an infected farm because the latter would be prone to pneumonia, due to the presence of the infectious agents.

A guide to stocking density that would be considered acceptable from a welfare view point is shown in Fig.3-36.

Let the pig tell you if it has the correct environmental temperature.

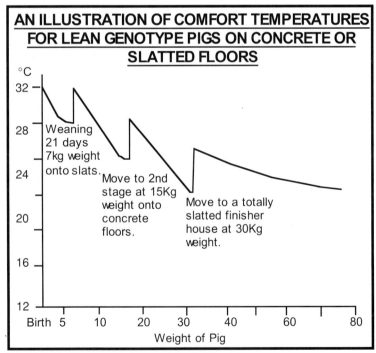

(Fig.3-33)

Factors to consider in assessing stocking densities

- Type of flooring and drainage.
- Age of pig and type of housing.
- Quality of insulation in the floor.
- Quality of insulation of the building.
- Type of feeding system.

- Availability of feed.
- Temperature requirements of the pig.
- Can the pigs produce sufficient heat?
- Are the pigs huddled?
- Air flow and draughts.
- Welfare requirements.
- Are mortality levels higher than the target?
- Is there disease?
- Is tail biting or vice a problem?
- Measure the daily liveweight gain and weight for age.
- Is there variation in growth within the pen?
- Levels of respiratory or enteric disease.

Draughts in pig houses are expensive.

What are the best stocking densities for maximum efficiency of output?

The guidelines in Fig.3-36 could be used but in order to measure true economic output in the most efficient terms it is necessary to measure lbs or kg of liveweight sold per unit of space per 12 months. To determine this the following information is needed:
- The total occupied floor area of the unit.
- The opening and closing period liveweights.
- The weight the pigs entering the pens.
- The weight of pigs sold.

The weight sold per unit of space is then calculated as follows:

$$\frac{(\text{wt sold} + \text{closing period wt}) - (\text{wt entered} + \text{opening period wt})}{\text{Total pen space (square ft. or metres)}}$$

Powel and Brunn in Canada showed responses at varying mean stocking densities Fig.3-37. It can be seen that whilst daily gain, feed intake and feed conversion were better at the lower level stocking density level of $0.81m^2$ the economic benefits in terms of meat sold were better at $0.49m^2$. Fig.3-38 shows predicted space for the best ADG and FCE.

Segregated Weaning and Disease Control Procedures

The sow during her lifetime becomes strongly immune to most of the infectious diseases present in the herd in which she is kept. She passes on this immunity in the form of colostral antibodies to her piglets in the first few hours of life and later also in the form of milk antibodies.

In addition because she has developed such a strong immunity the sow has thrown off many of the infections that commonly affect younger growing pigs, such as *My-*

A GUIDE (ONLY) TO AIR TEMPERATURE ACCORDING TO FLOOR TYPE

Weight Pig kg (lbs)	Straw °C (°F)	Concrete °C (°F)	Perforated Metal °C (°F)	Slatted °C (°F)
5 (11)	27-30 (81-86)	28-31 (82-88)	29-32 (84-90)	30-32 (86-90)
10 (22)	20-24 (68-75)	22-26 (72-79)	24-28 (75-82)	25-28 (77-82)
20 (44)	15-23 (59-73)	16-24 (61-75)	19-26 (66-79)	19-25 (66-77)
30 (66)	13-23 (55-73)	14-24 (57-75)	18-25 (64-77)	17-25 (63-77)
90 (198)	11-22 (52-72)	12-23 (54-73)	17-25 (63-77)	15-24 (59-75)

To convert to °F double the °C and add 30. This will give a simple approximation
(Fig.3-34)

THE EFFECT OF TEMPERATURES ON GROWTH
Bacon Pig 18 - 90 kg

		°C Below LCT 1°C	5°C
Growth g/day	600g	588	540
Days to slaughter	120	122	133
Extra feed		5.75 kg	31.0
Cost / pig at a feed cost (£170/tonne)		£1.00	£5.00

(Fig.3-35)

A GUIDE TO STOCKING DENSITIES. SLATTED SYSTEMS

Weight of Pig		Area		Pig weight	
kg	lbs	sq.m	sq.ft	kg/sq.m	lbs/sq.ft
5	11	0.09	1	55	11
10	22	0.15	1.5	66	15
20	44	0.2	2.5	100	17
30	66	0.3	3.0	100	22
40	88	0.34	3.6	115	24
50	110	0.4	4.3	125	25
60	132	0.45	5.0	133	26
70	154	0.5	5.6	140	27
80	176	0.55	6.0	145	29
90	198	0.6	6.6	150	30
100	220	0.65	7.0	153	30
200(sow)	441	2.8	30	74	15
Boar mating pen		9.3	100		
Boar housing only		7.5	80		
Sow loose-housed		2.8	30		
Sow confined		1.5	16		
Gilt housing during oestrus		2.8	30		
Farrowing crate		4.6	50		

As a guide 0.1sq.m / 10kg liveweight or 1sq.ft / 10kg liveweight
For straw based grower systems add 30%
(Fig.3-36)

Av. Pen Space Per Pig		ADG		ADF		FCE	Weight Meat Sold
m^2	ft^2	g	lbs	kg	lbs		Tonnes
0.49	5.3	640	1.41	2.23	4.92	3.49	125
0.57	6.2	663	1.46	2.28	5.02	3.42	109
0.66	7.1	681	1.50	2.31	5.10	3.38	98
0.73	7.9	704	1.55	2.32	5.18	3.36	90
0.81	8.8	731	1.61	2.39	5.27	3.31	82

ADG = average daily gain.
ADF = average daily feed intake.
FCE = feed conversion efficiency.

(Fig.3-37)

WEIGHT SPACE AND BEST PERFORMANCE			
Weight Of Pig		Space	
kg.	lbs.	m²	ft²
23 - 55	50 - 120	0.65	7
55 - 114	120 - 250	0.93	10

(Fig.3-38)

coplasma hyopneumoniae (causing enzootic pneumonia) and *Actinobacillus pleuropneumoniae* (causing necrotic pleuropneumonia). Two major factors are involved:
1. The sow is not shedding many infectious pathogens, and
2. The piglet is strongly protected against infection.

In the majority of cases piglets start becoming infected after they are weaned, when the milk antibodies have stopped and the colostrum antibodies are wearing off. They become infected from the older pigs in the first and second stage weaner accommodation and further infected when they enter the grower accommodation. Thus in herds in which respiratory infections are endemic the pigs only start to show clinical signs when they are 7-10 weeks old.

This important principal is now used to control or eliminate disease.

Terminology

As so often happens when new procedures are developed a variety of different ill-defined terms are invented to describe them. So lets first list and then define the terms used for the procedures related to segregated weaning. (Fig.3-39).

What do these terms mean?
Medicated Early Weaning (MEW)
See chapter 4 for further information.

Pregnant sows are removed from the herd in small groups at about 110 days of pregnancy. (Fig.3-40). They are washed and medicated against whatever infections are to be eliminated. Farrowing is induced with prostaglandins at 113-114 days of age. The piglets are medicated from birth and weaned away to a separate clean site at 5-6 days of age. The sows may also be vaccinated against one or more infections in the herd before being moved to the farrowing accommodation.
Aim: To produce high health status breeding stock free from the infectious pathogens present in the herd of origin.

Original Terms	Alternative Terms
Medicate Early Weaning (MEW)	Classical MEW.
Modified Medicated Early Weaning (MMEW). Isowean. Segregated Weaning (SW).	Segregated Early Weaning (SEW).
Partial depopulation (Partial depop.)	Segregated Disease Control (SDC).
Two-site production.	Two-site segregated weaning.
Multi-site production.	Multiple-farm segregated weaning.

(Fig.3-39)

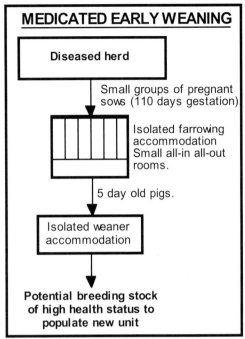

(Fig.3-40)

Piglets whilst suckling the sow catch very few of the infections present in the herd.

Weaned pigs catch infectious disease from older growing pigs.

Effectiveness: This has been used successfully by breeding organisations on a large scale. It is comparable to primary SPF repopulation.

It is not a practicable procedure for commercial operations. It will only be effective if the source herd does not have active disease.

Modified Medicated Early Weaning (MMEW)

This is the same as MEW except that the sows are not removed to isolated farrowing accommodation but are allowed to farrow in the herd of origin the pigs being weaned away to a separate site at 5-10 days. (Fig.3-41). The age of weaning depends on the infectious pathogens that are to be eliminated.

Aim: The same as MEW but less all-embracing. The range of infectious pathogens to be eliminated is not quite so comprehensive. MMEW can also be used to move pigs from a diseased herd to a healthy herd.

Effectiveness: A well known veterinarian in the USA, Hank Harris studied the effectiveness of this procedure and produced pigs free from different infections, from herds in which they were endemic. (Fig.3-42 and 3-43). He found that different infections required different weaning ages and some need medication and / or vaccination of the sows and / or piglets. The development of three site and multi-site production systems were then developed by him.

These were developed for breeding organisations but have now been applied widely to commercial operations. Also the source herd must not have new infections. If it becomes infected with a new pathogen during the procedure the pathogen is likely to break through the system. Because of this, if it is used for moving pigs from a diseased herd to a healthy one, strict 4-8 week quarantine and testing has to be incorporated into the procedure.

Segregated early weaning (SEW)

This is the same as MEW but may be done without the use of medications.
Aim and Effectiveness: The same as MMEW.

Segregated weaning (SW)

This is the same as SEW except that the piglets are weaned away from the farm at a more conventional weaning age, say, 18-23 days.

Aim: When used routinely its purpose is to produce healthy slaughter pigs.
Effectiveness: Obviously this is not as comprehensively effective as MEW, MMEW or SEW but it is more practicable for commercial production and is the basis of three-site production and where combined with all-in all-out systems is highly effective in producing healthy high-performance weaners, growers and finishers.

Isowean

This term (short for Isolated weaning) has become much broader in its meaning and is now used to cover MMEW, SEW, SW and even sometimes three-site and multi-site production.

Partial depopulation or segregated disease control

This method applies the principles of SW but in the combined breeding/finishing herd. To start the system pigs are weaned for a period of 6-10 weeks into separate naturally ventilated straw based accommodation or outside farrowing arks. They should be far enough away from the endemically infected pigs to prevent droplet spread (>15m). The growing finishing herd of endemically infected pigs is either then totally depopulated or each house is emptied sequentially. The segregated pigs are returned in to the hous-

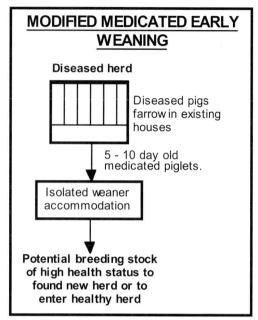

(Fig.3-41)

ing system without contact with the infected pigs if these are still on the farm.

This method can be applied to the breeding/finishing farm which cannot adopt a true SW system. If the farm has a problem with endemic respiratory disease it is first necessary to break the cycle. This is carried out by rearing the pig's into separate accommodation for a period of six to eight weeks or so, whilst the remainder of the pigs are sold off the farm. (Fig.3-44). Such pigs are weaned either within the farm perimeter or its surrounds depending on facilities, into either straw based kennels or outdoor arcs. They are not allowed droplet contact with endemically infected pigs in the existing houses and as

SEGREGATED EARLY WEANING		
The Oldest Age at Which Pigs can be Weaned to a Segregated Site and be Reliably Free From Contamination by Pathogenic Organisms Endemic in the Herd		
Infection / Disease	Age (Days)	Medication / Vaccination * for added safety
Actinobacillus pleuropneumoniae (App)	< 28	Medication + Vaccination
Aujeszky's virus	21	Vaccination
Bordetella bronchiseptica (AR)	5	Medication + Vaccination
Influenza virus	16	None
Mycoplasma hyopneumoniae (EP)	10	Medication + Vaccination
Pasteurella multocida (toxigenic) (AR)	8 - 10	Medication + Vaccination
PRCV	? < 14	None
PRRS virus	< 16 (NR)	None
Salmonella cholerae-suis	16	Medication
Other salmonella spp.	? < 21	Medication

Some of these data suggested by D.L.Harris (1996 - personal communication)
* Vaccination of the sow >2 weeks before farrowing
    Medication of the sow and/or piglets with an appropriate drug against the organism.
    Medication and vaccination are not always necessary but increase the reliability.
? Not known or guesswork
(NR) on present evidence not reliable.

(Fig.3-42)

far as possible are separated on a weekly basis. In practice the distance under natural ventilation need be as little as 15m and under fan assisted ventilation 35m

A Dutch straw barn can make ideal temporary accommodation for housing the weaners. Each weeks weaners should be separated by walls made of straw bales (or outdoor arcs 15m apart). During the next 6 to 9 weeks as the endemically infected pigs are sold from the farm each house is depopulated washed and disinfected. Once the weaner to finisher accommodation has been emptied and cleaned (Fig.3-44 method 1) the segregated weaners re-enter the buildings.

Each building however must be split into sections, each to hold one weeks worth of pigs (or part) so that an all in, all-out management operation is established. This is important to its continuing success. The design and layout of temporary (or permanent) accommodation that can be used is shown in Fig.3-45 and Fig.3-46 and some farms with the availability of straw have continued to use this method very successfully.

Most combined breeding and finishing farms, even if established as high health herds, ultimately become infected with one or more pathogens. These become endemic due to the continual use and management of pig houses (Fig.3-47) with worsening feed efficiency, reduced daily liveweight gain and poor profitability. Furthermore when a pig is moved into a house already occupied with other pigs it is exposed for the first time to a new range of organisms, both pathogenic and non pathogenic. It is now recognised that this exposure, even though there may be no clinical disease, stimulates the immune system, with increased demands for energy and lysine and the result is poor growth. Segregated weaning systems break the cycle and production and health can be maintained by continuing SDC principles on the farm.

Infections of the respiratory tract seem to have the

ENTERIC DISEASES

The Oldest Age at Which Pigs can be Weaned to a Segregated Site and be Free From Contamination by Pathogenic Organisms Endemic in the Herd

Enteric Diseases	Age (Days)	Medication / Vaccination * of the sow for added safety
Coccidia	—	Not possible
E. coli	—	Not possible
Internal parasites	< 14	Medication
Parvovirus	< 28	Vaccination
Salmonella	? < 21	Medication
Swine dysentery	< 21	Medication
TGE	? 21	None

* Vaccination of the sow > two weeks before farrowing.
? not known or guess work

(Fig.3-43)

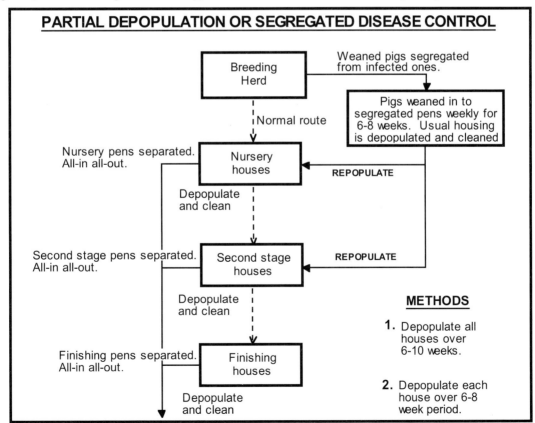

(Fig.3-44)

biggest adverse effect on efficiency of lean meat growth. This is probably because a disproportionately large portion of the body's immune cells are in or associated with the respiratory tract. Every time the pig breathes in air it inhales bacteria and viruses along with dust and toxic gases. The effect of this on a respiratory tract that is already chronically infected and diseased is to repeatedly stimulate the immune system to fight off the insult. The energy required for this is very high. It has to be derived from the pig's food to the deprivation of growth.

The respiratory tract is the main antigen sampler and immune stimulator of the pig's body.

To illustrate this a trial experiment was carried out on a breeding finishing farm where respiratory disease was endemic. 128 pigs were weaned at an average of 27 days of age and immediately moved off site to a clean straw yard with no other pig contact. 143 pigs were left on the farm as controls. See Fig.3-48. The growth rate differences were spectacular, a 16% improvement in feed conversion efficiency and a 74% improvement in daily liveweight gain (dlwg) at the end of 49 days. Half the healthy pigs were then returned to the farm where FCE became worse by 21% and dlwg by 40% over the next 48 days.

It is significant to note that the off site weaned pigs were still infected with enzootic pneumonia and PRRS.

SDC can also be carried out by building, instead of total weaner/finisher depopulation but the decision would depend upon the siting and distances apart of the buildings. Systems using SDC in pig dense areas would wean between 21 and 24 days of age. At these ages EP and PRRS will be maintained but other pathogens eliminated or controlled.

Factors to consider when adopting partial depopulation - SDC

- Discuss with your veterinarian the disease profile on the farm. It should be possible to eliminate from the breeding herd the following diseases if they exist.
  Mange - by medication. (See chapter 11).
  Atrophic rhinitis - by sow vaccination after a six month period.
  Severe pleuropneumonia - by preventing droplet spread, and vaccinating and medicating the sow herd.
  Swine dysentery - by medication. (See chapter 9).
- EP - will not be eliminated but it can be controlled effectively by vaccinating piglets at one

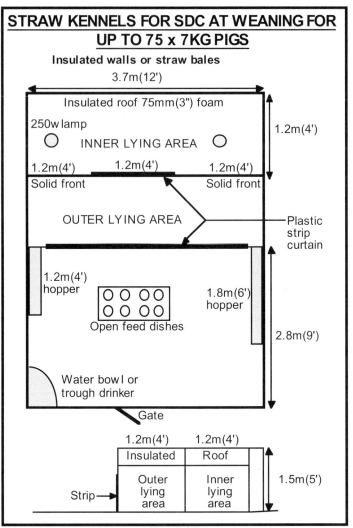

(Fig.3-45)

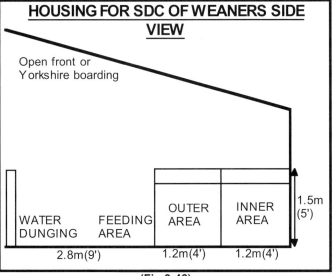

(Fig.3-46)

and three weeks of age.
- PRRS - may remain but its effects will be minimal with endemic diseases removed and a segregated all-in all-out system.
- The weaning age could vary between 16-26 days depending upon the level of disease control required.
- The SDC programme is best carried out during warmer months of the year.
- All houses or sections of houses must be adapted for all-in all-out use.
- All weaner and finishing pigs should be sold from the farm before the segregated weaners re-enter the building again. Pigs may enter the houses after they have been cleaned and empty for 14 days.
- A study of the pig flow should be made to see if by better use of houses, greater control of the system can be achieved.
- Allow a two week period between depopulation and repopulation of each house.
- If a swine dysentery eradication programme is being carried out allow at least 4 weeks depending on disinfection procedures. (See chapter 9).
- Consider batch farrowing to give better use of buildings.

Field experiences and the advantages of SDC

- There is no loss in pig production and minimal loss in sale weight of pigs and cash flow.
- Respiratory and enteric diseases can be controlled effectively.
- Post-weaning mortalities have been reduced from 12 to 4% and maintained.
- Continuous in-feed medication can be removed and only occasional strategic medication may be required.
- Increases in daily liveweight gains of up to 22% have been achieved.
- Buildings can be altered and maintenance carried out.
- Significant improvements in health status can be maintained.
- Mange, atrophic rhinitis, pleuropneumonia and swine dysentery may be successfully eradicated.

Successful systems have been maintained for at least 3 years. (At the time of writing).

SDC is an effective method of upgrading health status without total depopulation of the herd, which might not be advisable in a pig dense area.

Two site production

Traditionally, weaners have been reared to about 30kg on the same site as the dry sows and farrowing accommodation. However, the term "Two Site" in the present context implies that the piglets are weaned at three weeks of age to a second separate site where they are housed to slaughter weight. (Fig.3-49)

Aim: To produce healthy growers and finishers.

Here the breeding farm produces only piglets to weaning and moves these to a separate combined nursery and finishing farm.

The finishing farm would ideally have separate houses but more likely separate sections for each weeks supply of weaned pigs. To reduce droplet spread infections each house should be separated by at least 15m.

In this system it would be advisable to vaccinate pigs

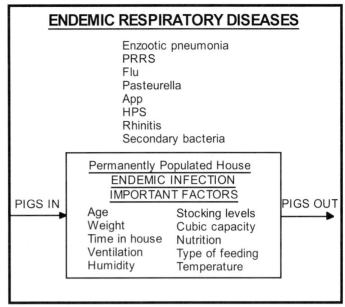

(Fig.3-47)

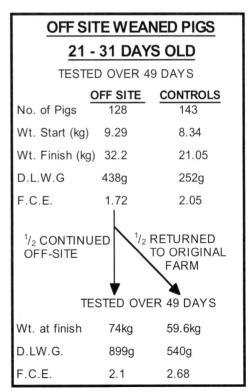

(Fig.3-48)

against mycoplasma pneumonia and wean between 16-24 days of age depending upon the disease status to be achieved. In the European Union routine weaning under 21 days is not allowed unless for health reasons.

Three site production

The sows and boars are on the first site where the piglets are born and suckled. They are then weaned to a second site and at 25-30kgs are moved to the third site for growing and finishing. (Fig.3-50)

Aim: To break the cycle of infection.

Here as the name implies the system is separated into breeding, nursery and finishing sites. The latter site can be further adapted by housing separation as in two site SEW to allow all-in all-out on a weekly basis.

Co-operative production

Groups of producers can combine to take advantage of 3-site or multi-site production in many different ways including changing some farms to breeding only, some to nursery production and others to finishing.

Batch farrowing

Instead of farrowing weekly the mating programme is adjusted to farrow larger groups less frequently and thus wean larger populations of similar aged pigs. The segregated weaning principle then becomes easier to apply. Other advantages include better use of buildings, all-in all-out, greater attention to detail at farrowing and the more efficient use of AI. Furthermore pigs in the growing finishing periods can be fed more specialised diets along their growth curve.

Multi-site production

The sows are all on one or more sites where they farrow. On the same day of the week the piglets are all weaned away to an all-in all-out nursery where they are reared for seven weeks. In each successive week all the suckled piglets are weaned to different all-in all-out nursery sites. After 7 weeks the first nursery is emptied, cleaned and disinfected and refilled with young weaners again. There are thus 8 separate nursery sites. Each successive week when a nursery is emptied the 30kg weaners are moved to separate all-in all-out grower/finisher sites. There are 16 of these filled and emptied in rotation

Aim: To break the cycle of infection and maximise growth and feed conversion.

Effectiveness: This is very effective on a commercial basis for large scale commercial production. The all-in all-out system mitigates against the occasional leak of single pathogens coming through, however they will only affect one nursery site and one finisher site. Producers have made the mistake of mixing up SEW and SW weaning too young.

Using this system a number of breeding farms may co-operate and supply piglets all of similar ages together on a week by week basis to the separate weaning units. See Fig.3-51. For it to be successful however the age at weaning needs to be tightly controlled and pigs of older age must under no circumstances be fostered backwards. They should be removed from the system. Furthermore if there is a disease outbreak such as TGE on one of the breeding farms the result can be disastrous.

The distances between breeding farm, nurseries, growing buildings and finishing houses should ideally be at least 3km (2 miles) apart to take full advantage of SEW. The closer to each other they are the greater the risk of windborne spread of diseases such as enzootic pneumonia, PRRS,

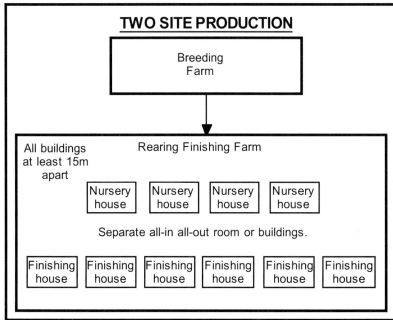

(Fig.3-49)

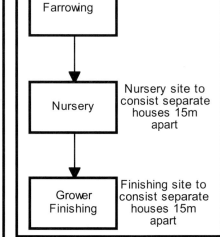

(Fig.3-50)

flu and aujeszky's disease. However for droplet spread disease such as rhinitis, meningitis, pleuropneumonia and dysentery 500m is adequate but clearly the risk is slightly increased.

Single sow herd multi-site production

This principle is illustrated in Fig.3-52. There are eight separate nurseries holding pigs until 10 weeks of age. They are then moved to separate finisher accommodation each week, again all-in all-out. For this to operate in practice, the sow herd has to have at least 1500-2000 sows.

Multi-sites, and variations of it, have been applied successfully and on a large scale in the USA, Mexico and Chile and it is now catching on in the UK and Spain. It has the huge advantages of combining all-in all-out production by site with those of segregated weaning. Ideally it requires 45,000 sows in the combined first site if the sows are treated separately or 24,000 if they are not but effective systems can be achieved with fewer numbers. The development of outdoor sow herds provides an ideal base for multi-site production.

The SW principle can be adopted with advantages to disease control in many different ways and that method best suited for the farming system must be identified.

It should be pointed out that SW is not a fool proof system and it can create considerable problems if there are a few piglets carrying disease amongst a naive population. Typical examples would be mycoplasma pneumonia, actinobacillus pleuropneumonia or TGE. Streptococcal meningitis is not controlled by SW and serious outbreaks have occurred.

Nutrition and Feeding

(See chapter 14 for further information).

Nutrition and feeding provide an important tool for management manipulation in the control of disease. The quality of the feed, its methods of presentation and the amounts of feed provided are part of the disease prevention process.

More detailed discussion is given in chapter 14, but it is relevant at this point to highlight the periods in the production cycle when feed levels and quality of nutrition should be carefully considered and monitored.

The gilt (See chapters 7 and 8)

- Selection to the onset of puberty.
- Puberty to point of mating.
- Mating to 21 days post-mating.

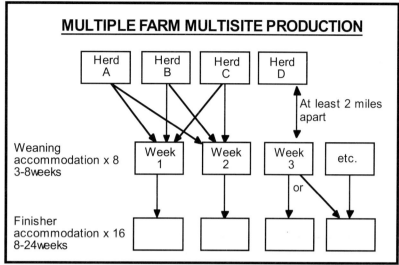

(Fig.3-51)

- During the last month of pregnancy.
- Farrowing to 3 days post-mating.
- During lactation.

The sow (See chapters 7 and 8)

- Weaning to service.
- Service to 2 days.
- 2 to 21 days post-mating.
- 7 days before farrowing.
- During lactation.

The piglet

- 7 to 21 days of age.
- During disease outbreaks.

The weaner (See chapter 9)

- Weaning to day 14.
- Dietary change unsuitable for weight and age of the pig.
- Whenever a housing change is made.
- During disease outbreaks.

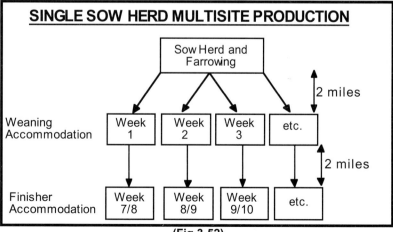

(Fig.3-52)

Grower and finisher pigs

- Any dietary changes.
- A change from dry to wet feeding.
- Changes in house temperature.
- Changes in the feeding system.
- After pigs are mixed.
- Environmental changes.
- When new cereals or corn are introduced.

Water

The ready availability of clean fresh water is essential. Insufficient attention is given to this on many farms. It is useful to consider the role that water plays in the normal metabolic functions of the pig.

- It helps to maintain and control body temperature, through both the intake and during exhalation when the heat is dissipated from the pig. It is lost in three ways, either by respiration, in the urine or in the faeces.
- An imbalance between water intake and loss results in dehydration and increased concentration of urine. Clinical signs include very dry faeces, hollow eyes and a dehydrated skin.
- It is responsible for transporting food and waste products throughout the body. Waste products are eliminated via water through the kidneys.
- Hormones are transported around the body through the blood stream.
- Water regulates the acid alkali balance in the body through the controls exerted by the kidney.
- Water is used in protein synthesis. The digestive process will not function without it. Any restriction of water therefore will affect the above vital functions.

The piglet

Within 6 hours of birth water should be made available in a shallow dish or a trough because fluid intake is so vital at an early age. An efficient dish used for both creep and water in the farrowing pen is shown in Fig.3-53. It is interesting to note how many piglets within 24 hours will drink small amounts of water when given the opportunity. Nipple drinkers are not a very attractive method of presenting the water to the piglet. Water consumption of piglets during lactation is also influenced by the farrowing house temperature and at 28°C (82°F) in a warm creep area water requirements will increase dramatically. The provision of water to the piglet in the first week causes no harm and is more likely of benefit. For pigs from one to three weeks of age clean water is best presented in an open type drinker rather than a nipple drinker. The water in dishes and drinkers must be clean and fresh.

The weaned pig

The pig experiences dramatic changes at weaning by the sudden move from a liquid to a solid diet. The con-

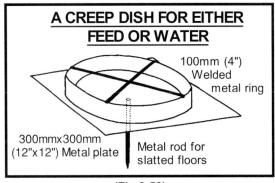

(Fig.3-53)

ditioned reflex, calling the pigs to suckle regularly is also lost. Dehydration associated with poor water intake and marked villus atrophy is a common occurrence within the first 7 days of weaning. Ensure the flow rate is at least 0.6 litres per minute from nipple drinkers. It is advisable to offer water in small open drinkers or water bowls daily for the first 5 to 7 days post-weaning. The loss of milk at weaning time and villus atrophy reduce the availability of liquid to the pig for the first 48 hours.

The sow

The changes in water intake from pregnancy to lactation are considerable. Sows that have a lower water intake during lactation generally rear poorer litters and it is important therefore to encourage the sow to drink the moment she enters the farrowing quarters. This is best carried out by giving 4.5 litres of water twice daily into the feed trough until 2-3 days post farrowing. The water flow through a nipple drinker for the lactating sow should approximate 1.5 to 2 litres per minute. Water intake in the dry sow varies from 9-18 litres per day and in lactation from 18 to 36 litres.

Guidelines for water requirements, water flow rates and drinker to pig ratios are given in Figures 3-54, 3-55 and 3-56.

Water quality

The variables in water quality include organisms, the physical characteristics and the mineral content. Water can become contaminated with pathogenic and non pathogenic bacteria and viruses. The presence of coliform bacteria (i.e. *E. coli* and related bacteria) is an indication of faecal contamination and a potential source of disease. (Fig.3-57).

The chemical quality of water can be assessed by determining the total dissolved solids, the pH (the alkalinity or the acidity), the iron content and the presence of nitrates or nitrites. Further testing would include levels of sulphates, magnesium, chloride, potassium, calcium, sodium and manganese. The total solids in water represent the amount of matter that is actually dissolved. If this level is less than 1000ppm it is of no significance but once it reaches over 6000ppm it becomes unfit for

CHAPTER 3 - Managing Health and Disease

WATER REQUIREMENTS

Guidelines For the Use of Nipple Drinkers		Water Consumption		
Weight of Pig (kg)	Height from Floor to Drinker (mm)	Age (Weeks)	Weight (kg)	Litres Per Day
5 - 10	100 - 250	8	20	1
10 - 30	300 - 400	9	25	2.5
30 - 50	400 - 600	10	28	3.3
50 - 100	600 - 750	12	39	4.2
100 +	750 - 900	14	50	5
	750 - 900	17	70	7
	750 - 900	21	90	8.9

(Fig.3-54)

GUIDELINES FOR WATER FLOW FROM NIPPLE DRINKERS

Pigs / Weight (kg)	Litres / minute
Piglet	0.3
Weaner 7 - 25 kg	1.0
Grower 25 - 50kg	1.4
Finisher 50 - 110kg	1.7
Dry sow	2.0
Lactating sow	2.0

(Fig.3-55)

DRINKER TO PIG RATIOS *

Type	Ratio
Nipple	1 : 15 to 1 : 10 Weaner to finisher
Bite	1 : 15 to 1 : 10 Weaner to finisher
Bowl	1: 17 finishers
Trough	300mm per 20 finishers 300mm per 15 sows

* UK welfare guidelines

(Fig.3-56)

pigs. Generally if the total solid content is low it is usually of good quality and the water is safe to drink. The pH level of good water varies between 6.5 and 8.

Hardness of water is dependent on the levels of calcium and magnesium present but these have no effect on animal health. Hardness does however result in the accumulation of scale causing pipes to gradually block and the flow rate drops unnoticed. This is a common problem on farms that have metal pipes of at least four years standing.

Iron can cause problems in water, with brown coloured staining. Certain types of bacteria can grow and cause blockage of pipes.

High levels of nitrates and nitrites can interfere with the use of vitamin A by the pig and they may be responsible for high still-birth rates.

A Summary of the effects of high nutrient levels in water

Sodium and chloride
- If this is above 250-500ppm then a brackish taste may develop.
- High levels of sodium chloride (salt) affect palatability and can adversely affect pig productivity and performance.
- Sodium sulphate is a laxative and mildly irritant.

Calcium and magnesium
- There are no effects on animal health unless their are high levels of the sulphates which result in the accumulation of scale (as $Mg(OH)_2$ and $CaCO_3$) and over a period of time the diameter of pipes is reduced with the poor flow rates.

Iron and copper
- High levels of copper have a catalytic effect on the oxidation of iron and if the iron levels are high precipitation of iron occurs when water is pumped, resulting in problems with the delivery system.
- Iron also supports the growth of certain types of bacteria causing foul odours and blocked water systems.

Sulphate
- High levels of sulphate in association with magnesium and sodium can cause diarrhoea.

Manganese
- High levels promote oxidation leading to a reddish

GUIDELINES TO WATER QUALITY SUITABLE FOR PIGS

	ppm (parts per million) Less than
Calcium	1000
Chloride	400
Copper	5
Fluoride	2-3
Hardness calcium carbonate	< 60 Soft > 200 Hard
Iron	0.5
Lead	0.1
Magnesium	400
Manganese	0.1
Mercury	0.003
Nitrites	10
Nitrates	50
Phosphorus	7.8
Potassium	3
Sodium	150
Selenium	0.05
Solids dissolved	1000
Sulphate	1000
Zinc	40
Total viable bacterial counts (TVC) per ml 37°C (99°F) 22°C (72°F)	Low but more important no fluctuation between samples. Target $< 2 \times 10^2$ $> 1 \times 10^4$ poor
Coliforms/100ml	Zero

(Fig.3-57)

tinge in the water.

Nitrates / nitrites
- Nitrites can change the structure of the haemoglobin in blood rendering it incapable of transporting oxygen. If levels are high the blood is a dark colour due to lowered levels of oxygen.
- Extremely high levels of nitrates / nitrites in water, impair the utilisation of vitamin A in pigs and a reduc-

tion in performance - such levels however are very rarely found under practical conditions but levels can be sufficiently high to increase stillbirths.

4 Treating Disease

Understanding medicines... 107
    Legal requirements 107
    How medicines are prescribed... 107
Understanding dosage levels 108
    In-feed medications... 108
    Injectable medicines.. 108
    Water medication 108
Controlling and storing medicines 109
    Disposing of medicines 109
Types of medicine and their application 110
Anti bacterial drugs and their uses.. 111
    Types of antibacterial drug.. 111
    Aminoglycosides 111
    Cephalosporins.. 111
    Macrolides... 111
    Penicillins 112
    Quinalones... 112
    Sulphonamides.. 112
    Tetracyclines... 112
    Other antibacterial drugs 112
    Antibacterial sensitivity tests... 112
Administrating medicines by injection... 112
    Using the syringe and needle 113
    Self inoculation... 113
    Sites of injection... 113
Administrating medicines topically 114
Administrating medicines in water... 115
    Group treatment.. 115
    Individual pig treatment 116
Administrating medicines in-feed... 117
    Factors to consider when using in-feed medication................ 117
    Strategic medication 118
    Pulse medication... 120
    Continuous medication 120
Medicated early weaning (MEW)... 120
    Trade name of antibacterial drugs 120
Anaesthetics, sedatives, analgesics 121
    Products available 121
Parasecticides.. 122
Vaccines.. 124
Hormones.. 125
    Hormones used to control the oestrus cycle........................... 126
Growth promoters 126
    Probiotics.. 127
Electrolytes... 127
    Rehydration by mouth 128
Examples of some pig vaccines available in the EU and elsewhere 1997 129

Chapter 4

Treating Disease

Understanding Medicines

You are advised to consult your veterinarian when assessing information given in this chapter.

The treatment of disease in the modern pig unit is complex, with a wide range of medicines available for a variety of conditions. This chapter looks at some of the complexities and interactions involved in the use of medicines so that treatments can be carried out efficiently and without risk.

Specific treatments for diseases are discussed later in their relevant chapters.

Legal Requirements

Based on EU directives.

Medicines must be used safely and correctly in food producing animals to ensure there are no residues. Most countries across the world have strict controls over both the methods of prescribing and the uses of medicines. In the EU for example medicines may be considered in five groups, which are adapted in the UK as follows:.

1. **GSL**: This describes the **G**eneral **S**ales **L**ist and includes a variety of medicines that are available to the general public over the counter.
2. **P**: This describes those medicines that are available over the counter only from a qualified **P**harmacist where his expert advice and guidance can be given or supplied by a veterinarian for animals under his care.
3. **PML**: Into this category are designated over the counter **P**harmacy **M**erchant **L**ists. Included in this group are recognised and certified merchants who are able to sell from a prescribed list of drugs direct to the farming community.
4. **POM**: These are **P**rescription **O**nly **M**edicines that are only available on the direction of a veterinarian.
5. **Controlled Drugs:** This category covers the addictive drugs such as morphine, heroin and pethidine.

The major categories concerning the pig farmer are the P, PML and POMs.

When a medicine is supplied to the farm the following information should be available:-
- A description of the medicine.
- The date of manufacture.
- The date of dispensing.
- The date of expiry.
- The client's name and address.
- The species to be treated.
- The date of withdrawal.
- The dose rate and instructions for use.
- Name and address of the supplier.
- Manufacturer's batch No.
- The name and address of the veterinarian prescribing.
- A typical bottle label would appear as shown.

> *List the generic names of the drugs on your farm. You will then recognise their use in the chapter. The information will be on the bottle label.*

How Medicines are Prescribed

Most medicines have two names, one which describes the chemical which is the active principle, often referred to as the **generic name**, and the second, the manufacturer's own **trade name**. For example, oxytetracycline hydrochloride (OTC) is the generic name

AN EXAMPLE OF A MEDICINE LABEL		
FOR ANIMAL TREATMENT ONLY	Duphacycline * LA Oxytetracycline 20%	Store at room temperature not exceeding 25ºC. Protect from light.
100 ml. Each ml contains: Oxytetracycline Dehydrate BP equivalent to 200 mg Oxytetracycline base as the magnesium complex in an aqueous solution. Duphacycline LA is indicated for the treatment and control of conditions caused by or associated with organisms susceptible to the action of oxytetracycline. By deep intramuscular injection to cattle, pigs and sheep.	Mr Jones, Horse Farm Date .... The Grower Pigs Pneumonia	Do not dilute. Keep out of the reach of children. Once a vial has been broken open the contents should be used within 4 weeks. Discard unused material. Wash hands after use. Avoid contact with eyes. For use: see leaflet:
Dosage: 1ml per 10 kg body weight.	Give 1ml/10 kg twice. 2 days apart.	PL: 1596/4160
Warnings: Not recommended for cats, dogs and horses. Milk for human consumption must not be taken during treatment. Milk for human consumption may only be taken after 7 days from the last treatment. Animals for human consumption should not be slaughtered within 14 days of injection. Not for use in animals suffering from renal or hepatic damage. Do not use in ewes producing milk for human consumption.	The Willow Vet Group Frankstone	SOLVAY DUPHAR VETERINARY * SOUTHAMPTON SO30 4QH A division of Solvay Veterinary Ltd. Duphacycline is a trademark of SOLVAY DUPHAR B.V., WEESP, HOLLAND. Lot: 5511-03 Exp: Dec 98 * Now Fort Dodge.

for a broad spectrum antibiotic. Terramycin is the trade given to it by Pfizer Ltd. Other trade names for the same drug include, tetramin, duphacycline, engemycin and so on. These vary from country to country. Throughout this book the generic names are used with references to some commonly used trade names.

You will be familiar with the trade names of medicines used on your farm but also try to remember the generic names, because this will help you to understand how they function and how to identify them irrespective of a trade name.

Understanding Dosage Levels

All medicines have a recommended therapeutic range, expressed in milligrams per kilogram (mg/kg) of live body weight. This range is used by the veterinarian so that he can decide whether a higher or lower dose level is required. Dose levels may also change with varying body weights.

In-feed Medications

These are prescribed by grams (g) of active or generic substance per tonne of feed. For example, 500g per tonne (1000kg) of oxytetracycline (OTC) means that there are 500g of active drug mixed in a tonne of feed. However, the manufacturer's product is normally available as a supplement - a mixture of the generic substance and usually a cereal base. Terramycin (OTC) 10% feed supplement means that OTC is present at a 10% level. Thus 1kg would contain 10% or 100g of oxytetracycline. To mix 500g of active ingredient per tonne in this case would therefore, require 5kg of the feed supplement.

Examples of in-feed medication are shown in (Fig.4-1). Feed can be analysed for the levels of antibiotic added. For technical and analytical reasons, do not expect 100% recovery rate. It can often be as little as 40-60%.

Injectable Medicines

Injectable medicines contain the active principle suspended or dissolved in a liquid. The label on the bottle indicates the actual amount of drug usually as mg per ml. Each drug has a recommended dose level expressed in mg/kg or mg/lb of live weight and instructions as to its administration, frequency and any side effects or contraindications.

For information:

1000ng (nanograms)	= 1ug (microgram) also mcg
1000ug	= 1mg (milligram)
1000mg	= 1g (gram)
1000g	= 1kg (kilogram)
1000kg	= 1T (tonne)
mg / kg = g / tonne	= ppm (parts per million)
mg / kg x 0.0001	= %
ppm x 0.0001	= %
1000ul (microlitres)	= 1cc (cubic centimetre) or 1ml (millilitre)
1000ml	= 1 litre

For conversions to imperial measurements see appendix.

Example: Terramycin Q100 injectable solution contains 100 mg/ml of OTC.

The therapeutic level is 10mg per kg live weight daily and thus the daily dose level becomes 1ml/10kg of body weight.

In practice, instead of referring to mg /kg, it is normal for the veterinarian to prescribe on the basis of 1ml/kg of live weight, but guidelines are also usually printed on the label.

Water Medication

Treating pigs via the drinking water involves the

A GUIDE TO IN-FEED ANTIBIOTICS AND THEIR USE IN RESPIRATORY DISEASE AND MENINGITIS

Drug Active Principle (dose level in g/tonne)	EP	App	CRD	AR	SM	Some Trade Names * of Premixes
Amoxycillin (300-500)		✓	✓	✓	✓	Stabox
Chlortetracycline (CTC) (400-800)	✓	✓	✓	✓	✓	Aureosup, Aurofac, Auromix, CTC 50
CTC (165) with sulphadimidine (164) and procaine penicillin (83)	✓	✓	✓	✓	✓	Microfac, Cyfac, ASP 250
Lincomycin (110-220)	✓		✓			Lincomix
Lincomycin (44) Spectinomycin (44)	✓		✓			Linco-spectin
Oxytetracycline (OTC) (400-800)	✓	✓	✓	✓	✓	Terramycin, Tetramin, Oxytet
Phenoxymethyl penicillin (200-300)		✓			✓	Potencil
Tiamulin (100)	✓		✓			Tiamutin, Denagard
Tilmicosin	✓	✓	✓	✓		Pulmotil
Trimethoprim/sulpha (250/750)		✓	✓	✓	✓	Duphatrim, Trimediazine,
Tylosin (100)	✓					Tylan

EP Enzootic pneumonia App Actinobacillus pleuropneumonia
CRD Chronic respiratory disease AR Atrophic rhinitis
SM Streptococcal meningitis caused by *Streptococcus suis* type 2.
* Compare the trade names in your country against the active principle
(Combinations of the above drugs may be used, particularly with CRD)

(Fig.4-1)

A FORMAT FOR RECORDING TREATMENTS

Date Commenced	Animal	Identification	Condition / Disease	Drug Used / Bottle Number	Dose Per Day (ml) Day	Withdrawal Period (Days)	Date of Clearance	Administered By.
1-1-97	Sow	163	Mastitis	OTC		14	17-1-97	JD
2-2-97	60kg	1246	Lame	Pen Strep		21	23-2-97	JD

same principles, a daily intake of the active principle based on mg/kg of live weight. In practice however, it is better to consider this by the active drug required per day per tonne of live weight of pig. For example, if the water soluble preparation consists of 100% pure active drug, (in other words no carrier added to it), then for most antibiotics, this level would range from approximately 15-25g/tonne of live weight per day. If, however, the powder contains only 50% of active principle (the other 50% would be a carrier, usually a sugar or citric acid base), then the dose would be 30-50g/tonne of live weight or twice the amount. The initial calculation, however, would be based upon mg/kg live weight. As a guide pigs drink 100 litres of water per tonne of liveweight per day. For example a treatment level of 10mg/kg of active drug and using a 50% powder, 20g/tonne would be required. In practice if the administration is by nipple drinkers the level is increased by up to 20% to allow for wastage.

Controlling and Storing Medicines

To achieve the maximum response to medicines and prevent any abuses, discipline should be maintained in their control, administration and storage. Consider all drugs to be dangerous. Many become potentially toxic if the recommended levels of treatment are exceeded or if they are given in the wrong way.

Some drugs have a very narrow range between treatment levels and poisoning. A good example is monensin, 100g/tonne is the therapeutic level and 300g is toxic.

Light and heat destroy drugs and freezing also has an adverse effect, particularly on vaccines.

Check list for medicines

- Provide a locked room or cupboard for all your drugs.
- Provide a refrigerator for vaccines and other drugs as required. Use a maximum minimum thermometer and record temperatures daily.
- Allow only certain designated people to have direct access to the main drug store.
- Document all drugs in and out of the drug store.
- Insist on empty bottles being returned before a second bottle is taken out. This prevents black market trade.
- Agree with your veterinarian the minimum amounts that are required for a given period of time and follow his advice on usage.
- Make sure that all bottles are labelled for the correct use, that withdrawal periods are displayed and personnel are aware of them.

> *Follow the instructions precisely.*

- Keep a daily record of all medicines used on the farm.
- Make sure you have safety data sheets to hand in case of accidents.
- Ask your veterinarian to check your storage and usage of medicines regularly to ensure that the recommendations are being carried out

> *Always be aware of the withdrawal period before slaughter.*

- Check regularly that medicines are in date.
- Make sure that all drugs, syringes and needles are kept well away from children and people not on the staff.
- Dispose of empty bottles, needles and syringes safely.

Disposing of Medicines

This must be carried out with care to prevent environmental contamination and accidental human or animal contamination.

There are three ways of safe disposal.

Empty bottles

These should be placed into a plastic bag and disposed of within the local authority guidelines or rules.

Syringes

Needles <u>must always</u> be removed from the syringe, and the syringes placed in polythene bags, marked "Syringes only" and incinerated.

DRUGS THAT SHOULD BE STORED IN THE REFRIGERATOR 2-8°C (36-46°F)	DRUGS THAT SHOULD BE STORED IN A DARK, COOL PLACE 18-22°C (64-71°F)
Iron injections. All vaccines including part opened bottles. Hormone injections, e.g. pituitary extract or milk letdown. Any bottles that have been opened and are in use. Any other medicines where the label indicates this temperature requirement.	Sedatives, vitamins and minerals. Stimulants. Antibiotics. In-feed and water soluble preparations. Disinfectants.

Needles and needle holders

These should be placed into a Sharps box, to be taken away for incineration. A Sharps box is a very strong polythene box, with an automatically closing lid where the needles can be dropped through and retained safely. (See Fig.4-2). It is good practice to cut the tip off the needles so that they cannot be misused. Simple used - needle guillotines are available for this.

> *Always check and follow the manufacturers recommendations.*

Types of Medicine and Their Application

Medicines used in the swine industry can be grouped into eight broad areas:-
- Antibiotics and antibacterial substances.
- Minerals, for example iron, vitamins and electrolytes.
- Sedatives and analgesics (painkillers).
- Parasecticides to treat mange, lice and worms.
- Vaccines and sera (and miscellaneous drugs).
- Hormones.
- Growth promoters and probiotics.
- Colostrum supplements.

> *Always consult the label for withdrawal times.*

For each individual medicament a manufacturers data sheet will be available, which gives guidelines as to its use, specific precautions and any contra-indications.

Medicines can be administered to individual pigs or groups of pigs for treatment or to prevent disease.

Individual treatments are usually given by mouth in the case of piglets, by injection in older pigs and occasionally onto the skin or per vagina. In outbreaks of disease, group treatments are carried out by in-feed medication, injections or in the water. Treatment for mange or lice may involve the use of sprays. Where medicines are used to prevent disease, they can be used in a number of ways as illustrated in Fig.4-3. The most efficient and cost-effective method of treatment is to administer drugs, either by injection or by mouth, to the individual pig. Sick animals do not eat much, and contrary to popular opinion, they do not drink much either. In outbreaks of disease therefore the treatment of sick pigs in the feed or water is not medically efficient. Furthermore in a group of pigs affected with pneumonia for example, it is unlikely that more than 20% of such animals have sufficient lesions to require treatment and 80% of the group would therefore be treated unnecessarily. This cost must be added to that of the sick 20%. However group medication can be of value in preventing more disease developing. There can be practical problems with treating large numbers of individual pigs. Nevertheless, the response

SHARPS CONTAINER

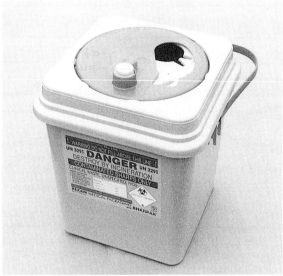

A container for holding needles and syringes. When full it is sealed and disposed of by incineration

(Fig.4-2)

A DATA SHEET EXAMPLE *

DUPHAPEN
Presentation Procaine Penicillin Injection BP. A sterile white aqueous suspension containing Procaine Penicillin BP 300,000 iu./ml.

Uses Duphapen Injection is indicated in the treatment of systemic infections caused by or associated with organisms sensitive to penicillin. When administered by intramuscular injection it will provide an effective therapeutic blood level for approximately 24 hours.

Dosage and administration Shake well before use.
By intramuscular injection only.

Routine daily dosage
Horses and cattle:	10 - 20ml
Calves, foals, sheep, pigs and goats	3 - 10ml
Dogs	0.5 - 5ml
Cats	0.5 - 1ml

Contra-indications, warnings etc. Do not use in known cases of hypersensitivity to penicillin's.
Do not inject intravenously.
Occasionally in suckling and fattening pigs administration of products containing procaine penicillin may cause a transient pyrexia, vomiting, shivering, listlessness and incoordination. Additionally in pregnant sows and gilts a vulval discharge which could be associated with abortion has been reported.
Milk taken from cows during treatment and for 48 hours (4 milkings) after treatment must not be used for human consumption. Meat for 18 days.

Pharmaceutical precautions Store at room temperature not exceeding 25ºC. Protect from light.

Legal category POM

Package quantities Multi dose vials of 40 ml and 100 ml.

Further information Nil.
Duphar Ltd
Product licence number 1596 /4011
(* Courtesy of Fort Dodge)

is much better.

Medicines are administered in a variety of ways depending on the type of drug and its availability. Some drugs are toxic by injection and may only be available by mouth, whereas others may be applied and absorbed through the skin. It takes a period of time for any drug to be absorbed into the system to reach levels sufficient to have a therapeutic effect and then be excreted from the body. The frequency of treatment is determined using this knowledge.

The following methods of administration are used in the pig :-

- **By injection** - Intravenous, subcutaneous, intradermal and intramuscular.
- **Topical** - The medicine is applied to the surface of the body. An example would be the use of pour-on organophosphorus preparations or sprays for the control of mange.
- **Oral** - Most injectable antibiotics are also available for oral administration.
- **Via the Uterus** - Pessaries (small slow-melting tablets) can be placed into the uterus following interference at farrowing. Likewise, antibiotics can be deposited into the anterior vagina in cases of infection.
- **Via the Rectum** - This is not a normal method for administrations in the pig, although in cases of meningitis associated with salt poisoning and water deprivation, water can be dripped into the rectum to correct the imbalance. (See chapter 15 Flutter valve)

The method of administration will be indicated on the label of the bottle, and this should always be followed. For example, intravenous injections are used for anaesthesia, intradermal injections to test animals for tuberculosis, and subcutaneous injections for certain types of antibiotics or some vaccines. The most common route of injection however is intramuscular for antibiotics, iron injections, and oil-based vaccines. Occasionally, injections might be given into the joint for arthritis or into the mammary glands for mastitis.

Remember antibiotics will not kill viruses, only bacteria.

Anti Bacterial Drugs and Their Uses

Antibacterial drugs are either produced from the fermentation of moulds (antibiotics) or they are synthesised chemically.

They act in one of two ways, by either killing bacteria, in which case they are called BACTERICIDAL, or by inhibiting bacterial multiplication, in which case they are called BACTERIOSTATIC.

Bactericidal antibiotics generally act quicker than bacteriostatic ones.

Bacteria however often multiply after a primary virus infection and antibiotics are used to control these secondary infections.

THE USE OF MEDICINES	
Methods of Treatment	Methods of Prevention
The Individual Pig	**Strategic medication**
By injection	In-feed
Topical application	In the water
Oral	By injection
Per vagina	**Continuous medication**
Per rectum	In feed
Groups of Pigs	**Intermittent medication**
In-feed	In-feed or in the water
By injection	**Pulse medication**
In the water	In-feed or in the water
By topical application	Medication and early weaning

(Fig.4-3)

Antibiotics act in one of three ways.
- They destroy the bacterial cell wall - e.g. penicillins, cephalosporins.
- They interfere with the protein metabolism inside the cell e.g. oxytetracycline, chlortetracycline, streptomycin.
- They interfere with the protein synthesis of the cell nucleus - e.g. sulphonamides.

Remember sick pigs do not usually eat or drink much

Types of Antibacterial Drug

AMINOGLYCOSIDES

These antibiotics contain sugars and include:
Apramycin   (Apralan)
Framycetin   (Framomycin)
Gentamycin   (Pangram)
Neomycin   (Neobiotic)
Spectinomycin   (Spectam)
Streptomycin   (Devomycin)
(Examples of trade names)

They are very active against gram-negative bacteria such as *E. coli* and are used to treat piglet scours and to control bacteria in the digestive tract. They are bactericidal and are poorly absorbed from the intestinal tract. The use of streptomycin is banned in some countries.

CEPHALOSPORINS

Most of these drugs are poorly absorbed from the intestine and are therefore given by injection. They include:
Cephalexin   (Ceporex)
Ceftiofur   (Excenel)

Ceftiofur has a wide range of activity and is an excellent drug for the treatment of respiratory disease.

MACROLIDES

This group includes:
Erythromycin   (Erythrocin)

Tiamulin   (Tiamutin)
Tilmicosin (Pulmotil)
Tylosin   (Tylan)
Lincomycin (Lincocin)

They are mainly active against gram-positive bacteria and specifically act against mycoplasma such as *M. hyopneumoniae* the cause of enzootic pneumonia and most are also active against *Serpulina hyodysenteriae* the cause of swine dysentery. Chloramphenicol is also a member of this group but its use in food producing animals has been banned in some countries. They are all bactericidal.

PENICILLINS

There are three types:
1. Penicillin G. benzathine - This is not used orally because it is destroyed in the stomach. It is used only by injection and is very active against gram-positive bacteria including staphylococci, streptococci, erysipelothrix and clostridia and some activity against actinobacillus spp, pasteurella haemophilus and leptospira. It has a prolonged action.
   Penicillin G. procaine - This is slowly released giving a prolonged action.
2. Acid Resistant.
   Phenoxymethyl penicillin - This is the oral form, it is absorbed from the digestive system and not destroyed by gastric juices.
3. Semi-synthetic.
   Ampicillin, amoxycillin, cloxacillin - All these have a wide range of activity against gram-positive and gram-negative bacteria

All the penicillins are bactericidal.

QUINALONES

These drugs are new to veterinary medicine. Enrofloxacin (Baytril) is used in pigs. They are very active against gram-positive and negative organisms and thus of value in both respiratory and enteric disease.

SULPHONAMIDES

There are approximately thirty different ones available but the common ones used in pigs are sulphadimidine (also called sulphamezathene) and sulphadiazine. The former recycles in the environment via faeces and can be responsible for tissue residue failures at slaughter particularly in the kidneys. Sulphonamides are often combined with synthetic substances called trimethoprim and baquiloprim. They are then termed potentiated sulphonamides and have a wider spectrum of activity. Sulphonamides are bacteriostatic but have a wide range of activity against both gram-positive and gram-negative organisms and they are also active against chlamydia, toxoplasma and coccidia spp.

TETRACYCLINES

These antibiotics are produced from streptomyces fungi and are widely used in pig medicine. Tetracyclines include oxytetracycline (OTC) and chlortetracyline (CTC). They have a wide range of activity against gram-positive and gram-negative bacteria. They are bacteriostatic at low levels but may become bactericidal at high doses and are used in respiratory diseases and secondary bacterial infections. The common ones are OTC (terramycin) and CTC (aureomycin).

OTHER ANTIBACTERIAL DRUGS

Dimetridazole (Emtryl) - This may be used either in feed or water. It acts mainly on anaerobic bacteria and it used specifically in swine dysentery and colitis.
Nitrofurans - These are mainly active against gram-negative organisms found in the intestinal tract and are available for feed medication.
   Furazolidone (Neftin) - Available for in-feed medication or oral use
   Furaltadone - Another nitrofuran used against salmonella and *E. coli* infections by water medication.
   Nifulidone - This is only available for water medication.
They all may be bactericidal or bacteriostatic.

Antibacterial Sensitivity Tests

Some antibacterial drugs are more active against gram-positive than gram-negative bacteria and others are the reverse. This gives a guide to the choice of drug to be used. Drug sensitivity tests carried out in laboratories give a better guide against specific infections, but this is not a perfect one. Some bacteria which are sensitive in laboratory tests are not sensitive in diseased animals. They may be multiplying in sites where the drug cannot reach them, or the antibiotic is not reaching them in high enough concentrations.

In its simplest and commonest form the test is carried out by growing the bacteria in a growth medium and then suspending them in a saline solution. A thin film of this is spread over the surface of a culture plate and left to dry. Discs of cardboard impregnated with different antibiotics are placed on the surface and the plate is then incubated. The drug diffuses out into the growth medium radially. If the organism is killed by the antibiotic there is a clear zone of no growth around the disc. If the organism is resistant to the drug it grows right up to the disc. Such tests usually take 12 - 24 hrs. Some bacteria however take weeks to grow.

Administrating Medicines by Injection

An understanding of the basic anatomy of the skin

and its underlying structures is helpful if medicines are to be injected efficiently. The outer layer of the skin consists of the epidermis or surface, beneath which is the thicker dermis consisting of living cells which are multiplying (Fig.4-4). The skin is attached to the underlying muscle by a combination of subcutaneous fat and fibrous "connective" tissue. An injection directly into the skin or the dermis (intradermal) requires a tiny needle less than 5mm long. This is used when testing for tuberculosis. Fat itself has a poor blood supply and an injection into fat is poorly absorbed. Abscesses are also more likely to develop. Subcutaneous injections must only be given where there is a minimal amount of fat.

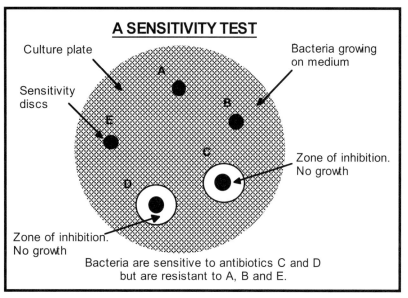

A SENSITIVITY TEST

Bacteria are sensitive to antibiotics C and D but are resistant to A, B and E.

Using the Syringe and Needle

- On most pig farms 2ml, 10ml and 20ml syringes are required.
- Always use disposable ones, they are sterile and easy to manage.
- Use syringes with a side rather than a centre nozzle because they break less easily.
- Use only one drug in one syringe. Some drugs are incompatible when mixed.
- Use one syringe for one injecting session and then dispose of it.
- Always wipe the bottle top clean with cotton wool and surgical spirit before use.
- Multi dose syringes must be kept in the refrigerator when not in use and cleaned and sterilised by boiling (10 minutes at 100°C(212°F)) between injecting sessions.
- Always keep part-used bottles in a refrigerator.
- Always use disposable needles that have a protective cap. This will keep the needle clean and prevent self inoculation.
- Change the needle frequently and determine the frequency by the ease of penetration into the tissues.
- Always change the needle <u>immediately</u> if:
  - The end becomes burred.
  - You drop it on the floor.
  - It makes contact with the external environment.
- NEVER clean it with your fingers or wipe it with your clothing. Use fresh cotton wool and surgical spirit to clean the needle after 2 to 3 inoculations.
- Always use a separate needle for each individual animal when injecting breeding stock to prevent spread of *Eperythrozoon suis* by blood inoculation.
- The practical procedures for using a syringe and needle to administer iron are described in chapter 15.

Self Inoculation

If you inoculate yourself accidentally you should take the following actions.

1. Report immediately to the person to whom you are responsible on the farm.
2. Look at the label on the bottle. Does it give any emergency procedures?
3. Read the leaflet or data sheets held on the farm for example, in the UK, Control of Substances Hazardous to health (COSHH) Safety Regulations. If not available ring your veterinarian, or your medical doctor.
4. If you are using an oil based vaccine (see the bottle label) go to the casualty department of a hospital immediately with the bottle. Such vaccines can cause blood vessels to go into spasm with potential loss of blood supply and consequent loss of tissue (e.g. a finger). The tissues usually require opening up and the injection flushing out.

Sites of Injection

- **Subcutaneous** - The ideal site for the small pig is inside the thigh beneath the fold of the skin or, beneath the skin behind the shoulder. In the growing and mature animals, the best site is approximately 25-75mm behind and on the level of the base of the ear, using a

MEDICATION BY INJECTION
Advantages
It is the best and most effective method.
It is most cost effective.
The dose rate is accurately given.
Treatment commences immediately the injection is given.
Medication is not dependant on water or feed intake.
Sick pigs can be identified early and treated.
The stockperson observes the pigs more efficiently.
There is a better assessment of the response.
Withdrawal periods can be accurately determined.
Disadvantages
Stress involved in handling the pigs.
Extra labour costs.
Practical difficulties for the staff.
It is more expensive.

25mm needle at a 45° angle.
- **Intravenous** - There are three sites for injecting drugs directly into the blood stream, the ear veins, the jugular vein and the anterior vena cava or large vein that leaves the heart. The ear vein is the most common method particularly for anaesthetics and occasionally calcium injections. The skin over the outer part of the ear is cleaned with cotton wool and surgical spirit which also demarcates the veins. They are then raised by applying pressure to the base of the ear. The pig should be restrained by a wire noose or rope around the upper jaw and or by sedation using azaperone (stresnil). For techniques see chapter 15.
- **Intramuscular** - The common preferred site in weaners, growers, finishers and adults is up to 70mm behind the base of the ear. Small piglets are often injected into the ham of the hind leg because there is not much muscle on the neck. This is not recommended in growers/finishers because of the possibility of abscesses.

Fig.4-5 lists some of the common antibiotics that are administered by injection. The first column gives the mg/ml of active drug and the second the mg/kg of live weight to achieve therapeutic levels. How much body weight 1ml will treat is then calculated and the number of ml required to treat the pig is then calculated. This varies with the concentration or mg/ml of the antibiotic.

Withdrawal period - This is the time between the last dose of drug administered and the time when the level of residue in the muscle, liver, kidney, fat or skin is equal or less than the maximum residue limit (MRL) allowed in carcasses. The MRL in the EU is the legally permitted maximum concentration allowed. Fig.4-5 gives guidelines of the periods for the different antibiotics but for the exact period it is necessary to refer to the current relevant data sheet.

Where a withdrawal period for pig meat is not specified a standard period of 28 days is recommended.

A guideline to the use of antibiotics in specific diseases is shown in Fig.4-6 but you are advised to discuss these with your veterinarian.

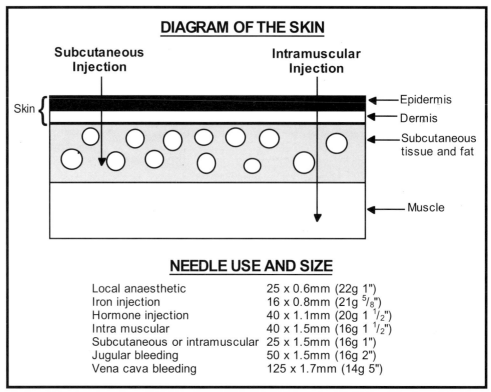

(Fig.4-4)

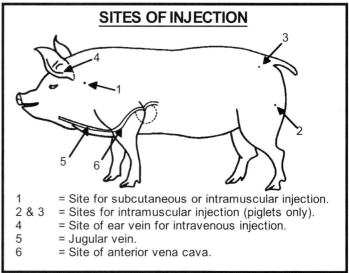

Administrating Medicines Topically

These can be applied to the nose, mouth, ears, eyes, skin and feet. Treatments to the skin are either applied by spray, liquid or immersion of the pig, and used against skin parasites, such as mange or lice or greasy pig disease. Some drugs are poured onto the skin from which they may be absorbed and distributed throughout the body. Mange is treated this way using 20% phosmet (Porect). Topical administration of medicines is simple cheap and causes the pig least stress. As techniques develop it could be come an increasingly used procedure.

Administrating Medicines in Water

Group Treatment

The practical problems of giving medication in water can be considerable. On many farms, the water pipes are old, and if the antibiotic powder contains sugars or acids there is a tendency for mineral deposits to form and block the pipe, or yeasts multiply, producing a jelly which does likewise. It then becomes a major problem to clean them out. Water soluble antibiotics should be used in a pure form where possible or with a minimum carrier base. Water tanks can be quite small, and it is therefore necessary to introduce the antibiotic to the water four or five times a day. If water is taken direct from the mains supply, water medication is impossible unless a proportioner is used. Some water authorities prohibit the use of water direct from the mains supply. Up to 40% of the antibiotic may be wasted through inefficient nipple drinkers. Small groups of pigs are best medicated using a 180 litre barrel with a water bowl attached to the bottom. This is a very efficient method of administration but impractical on a large scale.

Fig.4-7 shows a range of antibiotics available for water use and dose levels per tonne of liveweight. For example amoxycillin powder 50% contains 50% of the active drug amoxycillin, and 50% of a carrier, either citric acid or a sugar such as dextrose. A dose level of 15mg/kg liveweight of amoxycillin requires a dose of 30g/tonne of liveweight per day of total powder but in practice this level would be raised to approximately 40g/tonne to allow for the losses in the water through the nipple drinker.

How to apply antibiotic powder to water in header tanks

1. Calculate the total kg of liveweight to be medicated in tonnes.

INJECTABLE DRUGS AVAILABLE FOR BACTERIAL INFECTIONS					
	Strength	Dose			
Antibiotic (Check availability in your country)	mg/ml	mg/kg	kg wt treated by 1ml	Some Trade Names	* Days Withdrawal
Amoxycillin	150	10 - 20	8 - 15	Amoxinsol Amphipen Amoxi Betamox Amfipen	18
Ampicillin	150	2 - 7	20 - 75	Penbritin Polyflex	28
Ceftiofur	50	3	16	Excenel Naxcel	12 hours
Cephalexin	18%	7-10	18	Ceporex	2
Clavulanic acid plus amoxycillin	35/140	8.75	20	Synulox	14
Enrofloxacin	100	2.5	40	Baytril	10
Framycetin	150	5	30	Framomycin	49
Lincomycin	100	5 - 10	20	Lincocin Linco	2
Oxytetracycline	100	10 - 20	20	Duphacycline Terramycin Embacycline Oxytet	15
Procaine pen plus dihydrostreptomycin	150/250	15 - 25 25	20	Depomycin Streptopen	21
Procaine penicillin	300	15 - 25	20	Depocillin	5
Spectinomycin	100	20	5	Spectam	5
Streptomycin sulphate	150	10 - 25	6 - 15	Streptomycin sulphate	21
Sulphadimidine	333	100	3	Vesadin	7
Tiamulin	200	10	20 - 30	Tiamutin Denagard	10
Trimethoprim/sulpha	40/200	18 - 20	16	Delvoprim Trivetrin Duphatrim	5
Tylosin	200	2 - 10	10	Tylan Tyluvet	7

* Refer to current data sheets.

(Fig.4-5)

MEDICATION IN WATER
Advantages
It is easy to administer. It can be effective in a short period of time and can be given in the early stages of disease. It can be introduced very quickly. Large numbers of pigs can be treated at low cost. It can be used strategically.
Disadvantages
Healthy pigs are treated. Sick pigs often don't drink. There is considerable wastage if used via nipple drinkers. Water pipes tend to block up. The design of the pipe system may not be suitable.

2. Calculate the g of powder required for the 24 hour period. Add 10-20% extra if nipple drinkers are used.
3. **The water intake per tonne of liveweight per 24 hours will be approximately 100 litres.**
4. Calculate the total water used in 24 hours.
5. Divide the header tank capacity into the total water used which gives the times that the tank is emptied in 24 hours.
6. Divide the powder and add pro rata to the tank. Stir each time.

Example

Medication with Amoxycillin - 50% at 15mg/kg. Water bowls used.
4 tonnes of live weight at 30g powder per tonne = 120g.
400 litres of water consumed
If a 200 litre tank is available then 400/200 = the tank will empty twice in 24 hours
Place 60g or half the powder in the tank early in the morning and the other half at the end of the day.

Individual Pig Treatment

This is most commonly used in sucking piglets for scours and other bacterial infections. Fig.4-8 lists drugs available.

When you decide to treat pigs orally (or by injection) ask yourself the following questions:

- Should I consult my veterinarian?
- Have I identified every individual affected piglet?.
- Is this condition one that has been reliably diagnosed before or is it a new one?
- Is it necessary to treat it?
- Do I have drugs to treat this condition or are they readily available?
- Are there any welfare or nursing implications?
- Should the affected pig(s) be moved to a hospital pen?
- Is oral dosing the best or should I use a different method of administration?
- What dose should be given? Have I the right information on this?
- How often should the drug to be given and for how long?
- Are any adverse effects likely?

Then you should:

- Record when the treatment started and its progression.
- Assess the response on a day-by-day basis.
- If there is no response within 24 hours consult your veterinarian.

ANTIBACTERIAL DRUGS WHICH MAY BE USED FOR SPECIFIC DISEASES

Antibiotics	Amoxicillin	Ampicillin	Ceftiofur (Excenel)	Cephalexin	Synulox	Enrofloxacin (Baytril)	Framycetin (Framomycin)	Lincomycin (Lincocin)	Penicillin / Streptomycin	Procain Penicillin	Speclinomycin (Spectan)	Sulphonomide	Tetracycline	Tiamulin (Tiamutin)	Trimethoprim/Sulpha	Tylosin
Actinobacillosis pleuropneumonia	✓	✓	✓	✓	✓	✓			✓	✓		✓	✓		✓	
Atrophic rhinitis	✓	✓	✓	✓	✓	✓			✓	✓		✓	✓		✓	✓
E. coli diarrhoea	✓	✓	✓	✓	✓	✓	✓				✓	✓			✓	
Colitis						✓	✓	✓			✓	✓	✓	✓	✓	✓
Chronic respiratory disease	✓	✓	✓		✓			✓					✓		✓	
Cystitis	✓			✓		✓			✓	✓			✓		✓	
Enzootic pneumonia						✓		✓					✓	✓	✓	✓
Erysipelas	✓	✓		✓					✓	✓			✓			
Greasy pig disease	✓	✓	✓	✓	✓			✓			✓		✓		✓	
Generalised bacterial infections	✓	✓		✓	✓											
Joint infections	✓	✓		✓				✓					✓		✓	✓
Leptospirosis	✓	✓											✓			
Mastitis metritis	✓	✓		✓	✓	✓		✓	✓				✓		✓	✓
Meningitis		✓		✓					✓	✓		✓			✓	
Mycoplasmal arthritis						✓		✓					✓	✓	✓	
Pasteurellosis	✓	✓		✓		✓			✓	✓		✓	✓	✓	✓	✓
Porcine enteropathy						✓	✓				•		✓	✓	✓	
Salmonellosis	✓	✓	✓	✓	✓						✓				✓	
Swine dysentery								✓						✓	✓	✓

Remember: bacterial drug sensitivities can vary

(Fig.4-6)

DOSE LEVELS OF WATER SOLUBLE DRUGS

	% Active Drug	Dose mg/kg	g/Tonne Live Weight *	Some Trade Names	Days Withdrawal*
Amoxycillin P	50	10 - 15	20 - 30	Amoxinsol	1
Apramycin P	30	7-12	23 - 39	Apralan	14
Chlortetracycline P	100	10 - 20	10 - 20	Aureomycin	10
Dimetridazole P	40	18 - 25	45 - 62	Emtryl	7
Lincomycin P	40	4.5 - 11	11 - 27	Lincocin	1
Neomycin P	70	11	16	Neobiotic	14
Oxytetracycline P	80	10 - 30	12 - 37	Terramycin	5
Tiamulin P	45	8.8	20	Tiamutin	1
Tilmicosin L	250mg/ml	12 - 20	50-80 ml/tonne	Pulmotil	*
Trimethoprim/sulpha P	2 / 10	24	240	Cosumix	3
Tylosin P	100	15	15	Tylan	0

* For guidance only. Refer to relevant data sheet .   P = Powder   L = Liquid

(Fig.4-7)

ORAL DRUGS AVAILABLE TO TREAT PIGLET SCOUR

	mg/ml	mg/kg wt	1 to 5 kg wt treated (ml)	Some Trade Names
Amoxicillin	40	7 - 15	1	Clamoxyl
Apramycin	18	10 - 20	1	Apralan
Enrofloxacin	5	1.5	1 - 2	Baytril
Furazolidone	50	50	1	Neftin
Neomycin	50	35	1	Neobiotic pump
Spectinomycin	50	50	2 - 4	Spectam scour halt
Toltrazuril	25	6.25	see page 264	Baycox
Trimethoprim/sulpha	10/50		1 - 2	Duphatrim Noradine Tribrissen

(Fig.4-8)

CHAPTER 4 - Treating Disease

Administrating Medicines In-Feed

The inclusion of antibiotics, in-feed is the most common method of controlling and preventing diseases. (Fig.4-9).

In-feed medication can be an effective means of control when used over several weeks.

In-feed medication is wasteful in that it is inevitably given to healthy pigs that do not need it as well as to the diseased pigs that do need it. In-feed supplements can also be used as top dressings, that is, sprinkling small amounts over the feed to administer the antibiotic. Top dressing is a very suitable method for small groups of pigs and individually fed animals, such as sows and boars.

Factors to consider when using In-Feed Medication

- At the time of the disease outbreak, there may be no bin capacity available to hold the medicated feed and

THERAPEUTIC DRUGS THAT MAY BE AVAILABLE FOR IN-FEED USE.
Doses and some Disease Indications

Active Drug	g/Tonne in-Feed * (Dose in mg/kg liveweight)	Common uses	
Amoxycillin	300 - 600 (15)	Greasy pig disease Streptococcal meningitis Pasteurellosis	Respiratory bacterial infections Secondary bacterial infections
Amprolium	125	Coccidiosis	
Apramycin	100 - 150 (10)	E. coli Post-weaning diarrhoea	Salmonellosis
Arsanilic acid or sodium arsanilate	250 - 400	Swine dysentery Eperythrozoonosis	
Bacitracin	275	Bacterial enteritis Clostridial enteritis	
Carbadox	55	Colitis	Swine dysentery
Chlortetracycline	300 - 800 (20)	Greasy pig disease	Respiratory disease
Chlortetracycline Penicillin Sulphadimidine	165 82 165	Enteric disease Greasy pig disease	Respiratory disease
Dichlorvos	380 - 550 (10 - 21)	Internal parasite control	
Dimetridazole	200 - 500	Colitis	Swine dysentery
Fenbendazole	14 - 53 (5)	Internal parasites	
Flubendazole	30	Round worms	
Furazolidone	200 - 400	Post-weaning enteritis	
Hygromycin	14	Control of ascaris, nodular and whip worms	
Intagen	1.5 - 5kg premix per tonne	Oral E. coli vaccine	Prevent scour in piglets
Ivermectin	2 (100mcg)	Internal parasites lice and mange	
Levamisole	800	Internal parasites	
Lincomycin	44 - 220 (5 - 10)	Greasy pig disease Mycoplasmal pneumonia & arthritis	Respiratory disease
Lincomycin Spectinomycin	44 44	E. coli infections Mastitis Mycoplasma pneumonia	Salmonella infection Swine dysentery
Monensin	100	Colitis	Swine dysentery
Neomycin	163 (11)	Colitis E. coli infections	Enteritis Salmonella
Oxibendazole	40 - 100 (1.6)	Internal parasites.	
Oxytetracycline	200 - 800 (20)	Greasy pig disease Respiratory disease	Secondary infection
Phenoxy methyl penicillin	200 - 400	Actinobacillus pneumonia Streptococcal meningitis	Clostridial infections Necrotic enteritis
Pyrantel tartrate	100 - 880	Internal parasites	
Salinomycin	30 - 60	Colitis	Non specific enteritis
Sulphadimidine	100 - 300	Enteric disease Greasy pig disease	Respiratory disease
Thiabendazole	50 - 100	Internal parasites	
Thiophanate	168 - 500 (6 - 7)	Internal parasites	
Tiamulin	30 - 100 (1.5 - 2)	Mycoplasma pneumonia & arthritis	Swine dysentery
Tilmicosin	200 - 400	Mycoplasma pneumonia Pasteurella	Actinobacillus pneumonia
Trimethoprim/sulphas	Varies See data sheets (15 - 30)	Atrophic rhinitis Colitis Enteric disease	Post-weaning diarrhoea Respiratory disease
Tylosin	100	Mycoplasma pneumonia	Swine dysentery
Zinc oxide	2500g zinc	Post-weaning enteritis	

* To convert g/ton (2000lbs) reduce the in-feed levels by 10%

(Fig.4-9)

- bagged food is sometimes required.
- If strategic medication is used, hold one bin for medicated feed only.
- If medicated feed is placed in a bin containing non medicated feed, the time of the feed reaching the pigs and the withdrawal will be unknown.
- Bagged food is more expensive.
- There can be a delay in manufacturing and delivering the medicated feed.
- Sick pigs often do not eat or have reduced feed intake and therefore won't receive sufficient antibiotic.
- If the appetite is poor the drug inclusion rate may need to be increased by up to 30%, provided it is safe to do so.
- In-feed drugs may require a product licence for use in food producing animals and therefore the availability of drugs is narrow.
- Each particular drug has its own withdrawal period and this may mean it is impracticable to use in pigs near the point of slaughter.
- Automatic feed lines make the application of in-feed medication to selective groups difficult.
- The bin containing the medicated feed should be marked with the date it entered and the date when empty. Withdrawal times can then be calculated.

Strategic Medication

This method applies treatment at the anticipated beginning of the disease or during the incubation period. To carry this out, there are a number of essential components:-

- The specific organism associated with the disease should be identified.
- The drug sensitivity of the organism should be identified.
- The incubation period (the time from exposure to the organism to clinical symptoms) should be known.
- Last, and most important, the point at which the disease process starts and when it becomes clinically apparent should be determined. Medication can then commence prior to this point.

Strategic medication (Fig.4-10) is usually carried out in the feed but it can also be applied in the drinking water or by injection using long-acting preparations. It can also be applied to eliminate disease from a group of pigs. A good example would be to prevent possible swine dysentery in purchased pigs on entering a finishing herd. In this case the feed could be medicated with either lincomycin (110g/tonne) or tiamulin (100g/tonne) for the first 14 days during isolation on the farm. If strategic medication is carried out routinely, medicated feed must be held continuously in a designated bin.

A typical example would be the use of high levels of oxytetracycline, (500-800g to the tonne), in growing pigs to control severe outbreaks of enzootic pneumonia. The procedure would be to medicate all the pigs for seven days, one week after entry into the houses or approximately ten days prior to the commencement of clinical symptoms.

STRATEGIC MEDICATION. SOME DRUGS THAT COULD BE USED		
	Respiratory Diseases	Enteric Diseases
Injections	Long-acting OTC Long-acting amoxycillin Long-acting penicillin Lincomycin Tiamulin Tylosin Ceftiofur (Excenel)	Trimethoprim/sulpha Lincomycin Tiamulin Amoxycillin Dimetridazole
Water soluble antibiotics	Amoxycillin CTC Lincomycin Tiamulin Tilmicosin OTC	Neomycin Trimethoprim/sulpha Framycetin Apramycin
In-feed inclusions	800g/tonne OTC or CTC 220g/tonne lincomycin 100g/tonne tiamulin 200 - 400g/tonne tilmicosin	100g/tonne tiamulin 110g/tonne lincomycin 100g/tonne apramycin

(Fig.4-10)

Thus each week a selected group of pigs would commence treatment to prevent the development of extensive lesions in the lungs and yet allow immunity to develop. An alternative strategy would be an injection of long-acting OTC given at a predetermined point. This method is of course more labour intensive. Strategic medication by injection is easier to apply in younger pigs. Fig.4-11 indicates some of the diseases where it can be used and the times of application.

The following on-farm case histories illustrate some of the uses for strategic medication:-

Enzootic pneumonia

Farm A was a 200 sow herd producing pigs for sale at 90kg. Its buildings were poorly insulated and due to the bad economic state of the industry at the time, no capital was available to improve the environment other than by managerial means. Severe bouts of coughing developed on this farm approximately three weeks after pigs moved from the first stage rearing accommodation into the finishing houses. Post mortem and lung examinations showed extensive lesions of enzootic pneumonia associated with secondary pasteurella infections, the latter shown to be sensitive to chlortetracycline (CTC). The first cases of clinical pneumonia became evident starting 10 days after the pigs moved into the finishing house. Commencing on day eight after entry, pigs were medicated with 600gm/tonne CTC for a period of seven days. This had a dramatic effect on reducing the incidence of disease and in particular, the numbers of pigs requiring individual treatment. The variability in growth was reduced. Initially, this was a herd with young breeding but as they matured, the time of onset of disease changed to appear five weeks after moving in to the finishing houses. The strategic medication was therefore given two weeks later.

Atrophic rhinitis (AR)

Herd B was a 1200 sow unit showing clinical atrophic rhinitis at a visual level of 15%. Toxigenic pasteurella and bordetella bacteria were isolated and were found to be sensitive to trimethoprim and amoxycillin. All piglets were injected with a long-acting preparation of the latter drug at day seven, and again at weaning at 21 days. Pigs were further medicated with oxytetracycline in-feed for 14 days post-weaning. For a period of six months following this, the incidence of atrophic rhinitis at a visual level dropped to 2%. It then, however, started to rise again to a 7% level. Apparently the stockperson had decided to inject the pigs at 10-14 days of age because this was more convenient. This allowed early establishment of pasteurella organisms in the nose and a considerable amount of damage. When the injections were moved back to the seven day point the problem again returned to low levels. This example illustrates the importance of determining by trial and error, the critical point at which strategic drug therapy should be given. At the time of this disease problem vaccines to prevent atrophic rhinitis were not available

Actinobacillus (Haemophilus) pleuropneumonia (App)

This disease can be a very difficult one to control especially in its severe form. Herd C was a 250 sow herd producing pigs for slaughter at around 70kg liveweight. At nine weeks of age pigs were moved from the nurseries (flat decks) into a second stage rearing accommodation and within seven days of entry, severe outbreaks of pleuropneumoniae occurred. In view of the very short incubation period of this disease (12-48 hours) strategic medication can be difficult to apply. In this particular case, medication was applied immediately the first clinical case became apparent. To obtain a very rapid response, chlortetracycline was placed in the header tanks in the drinking water for a period of 72 hours. The response on this farm was quite dramatic, but perhaps even more importantly, the trigger factors associated with a drop in energy intake and variable temperatures in the house were then corrected. This reduced the strategic medication requirements which illustrates the importance of management.

Streptococcal meningitis (SM)

Farm D was a 350 sow herd previously free of streptococcal meningitis. It became infected with a virulent strain of *Streptococcus suis* type 2 through the purchase of a group of gilts which were carrying the infection. The introduction of disease caused severe problems in the nurseries (flat decks) where it regularly appeared approximately 16 days after entry into the house. All pigs were medicated through the drinking water with potassium penicillin V commencing on day 10 through to day 17. High numbers of pigs become carriers of the organism in their tonsils within 2 weeks of occupying nurseries and a variable number of such animals then develop the disease. The object of applying water medication at this stage was to reduce the level of infection. The disease reached its peak with some 15% of each batch of pigs moved into the house requiring individual treatment. Strategic medication reduced this down to less than 1%.

Swine dysentery (SD)

Farm E was a finishing farm purchasing approximately 10,000 pigs per annum. It had previously been infected with swine dysentery and an eradication programme was successfully carried out. It was however, periodically committed to buying pigs from unknown sources, in response to market forces. In order therefore, to protect the herd all incoming pigs were strategically medicated in groups of 200 when they entered the farm whilst in isolation premises. These premises were completely emptied and disinfected between batches. On arrival the pigs were medicated in the water with ronidazol for a period of five days, together with in-feed medication at 60gm/tonne for a further seven days. These procedures prevented the appearance of disease.

THE TIMING OF STRATEGIC MEDICATION USING EITHER LONG-ACTING INJECTIONS OR IN-FEED MEDICATION

Age Weeks		EP	App	AR	SM	HPS
Birth	1			←		
	2			←		←
	3		←			
	4			←		
Weaning						
	1			←	←	←
	2			←	←	
	3					
8	4		←	←	←	←
Feeding						
	1		←			
	2					
	3					
	4					
	5					
14	6	←				
Feeding						
	1					
	2	←				
	3					
	4					
	5					
	6					
	7				←	
22	8					

← = Age when medication may be started.
EP = Enzootic pneumonia
App = Actinobacillus pleuropneumonia
AR = Atrophic rhinitis
SM = Meningitis caused by *Streptococcus suis* type 2
HPS = *Haemophilus parasuis* causing glässers disease

(Fig.4-11)

These on farm situations illustrate some of the methods by which strategic medication can be used to good effect to control disease and at the same time be cost effective. There are a variety of drugs available and Fig.4-10 lists some of these, together with in-feed dose rates. However, if you are thinking of adopting strategic medication discuss it with your veterinarian first so that he can advise you on the best type of drug, the dose level and its timing. Fig.4-11 shows possible time applications for strategic medication.

Pulse Medication

Pulse medication is an alternative programme to continuous medication for the control of disease. The medication is given either in water or feed for short periods of only 48-72 hours.

Only drugs with short withdrawal periods can be used if pigs are near market weight. Treatment costs are reduced compared to continuous medication. It does need careful control to ensure that withdrawal periods are observed and is difficult to carry out where automated feeding systems are used. It is more ideal for use in wet feeding systems.

Pulse medication has been used successfully in the control of pneumonia, using a combination of 300g/tonne of CTC and 30g/tonne of tiamulin. Such medication could be used for two days followed by four days off. Results on farms have shown an improvement in food conversion of 0.2, daily liveweight gain of 6.7%, and considerable reductions in lung scores at slaughter.

Continuous Medication

Pigs are medicated continuously for periods of up to 12 weeks during the critical periods of exposure to disease. Dose levels are usually lower than those used for treatment. Fig.4-1 lists the in-feed levels that can be used for the various respiratory diseases.

Continuous medication can be expensive but in permanently populated houses with mixed ages of pigs it can work well with considerable growth enhancement which helps offset the cost.

There is continual suppression of organisms. In severe endemic disease the system can break down. There may also be problems with withdrawal periods in finishing pigs. Continuous medication should therefore be regarded as a last resort. Always ask three questions if continuous medication is necessary:
1. Why is there a problem?
2. What has gone wrong with the management?
3. CAN THIS BE CORRECTED?

Medicated Early Weaning (MEW)

See chapter 3 for further information

This is a specialised technique for producing high health status breeding stock from a disease herd. It is used mainly by breeding (seed stock) companies rather than commercial producers although systems such as three-site and multi-site production which have evolved from it, are highly applicable to commercial production.

Basically, MEW breaks the cycle of infection by farrowing groups of sows in isolation and weaning their piglets to clean premises at about 5-7 days of age. Medication of the sow and piglets, and sometimes vaccination of the sow, are added safeguards depending upon what particular infections are to be eliminated.

This method produces excellent results in removing most bacterial infections. However, it is possible to produce a pig that is so devoid of pig organisms, that it cannot be acclimatised into conventional herds. Also if a new herd is established by this method it can be very susceptible to even low pathogenic organisms. The technique is used mainly to establish new high health herds.

Procedures

- Sows are moved into isolated farrowing houses at least 5 days before farrowing, 800m from the nearest pig.
- An all in - all out system is used. Each batch of sows is washed prior to entry.
- Farrowing is induced with prostaglandin injections at day 113.
- Sows are medicated from entry into the farrowing house until the piglets are weaned.
- The piglets are weaned at 5 days and reared in groups in isolated housing.
- The piglets are medicated from birth to 10 days of age.

A possible medication regime

Sows: Injected with potentiated sulphonamide containing 40mg trimethoprim, 200mg sulphonamide/ml (TMS), on entry into the farrowing accommodation at the recommended treatment level.
From entry to weaning the feed is medicated with TMS at therapeutic doses, and water soluble tiamulin is given twice daily.

Piglets: Injected daily with TMS until weaning.
Post weaned pigs - Injected with TMS and dosed orally daily with tiamulin for 5 days.

Bacterial diseases that can be eradicated by MEW:
- Actinobacillus pleuropneumonia
- Atrophic rhinitis
- Enzootic pneumonia
- Glässers disease (*Haemophilus parasuis*)
- Mange (Treatment of the sow with ivermectins is required).
- Streptococcal meningitis
- Swine dysentery

Trade Names of Antibacterial Drugs

Finally, to give a better understanding of antibacterial substances and trade names, Fig.4-12 illustrates some of the commercial products available for the different generic antibiotics in the UK, EU and elsewhere.

ANTIBACTERIAL DRUGS AND SOME TRADE NAMES

Active Principle	Trade Names in the UK and the EU *	List Trade Names in Your Country for Reference if Different
Amoxycillin	Amfipen, Amoxi, Amoxinsol, Amoxypen, Betomax, Bimoxyl, Clamoxyl, Duphamox, Micromox, Qualamox, Trioxyl.	
Ampicillin	Duphacillin, Embacillin, Intacillin, Norbritten, Penbritin, Polyflex, Vidocillin.	
Apramycin	Apralan.	
Baquiloprim sulpha	Zaquilan.	
Clavulanic acid and amoxycillin	Synulox.	
Cephalexin	Ceporex.	
Ceftiofur	Excenel.	
Chlortetracycline	ASP250, Aureomycin, Aurofac, CTC250.	
Chlortetracycline + pen + sulpha	Cyfac, Microfac, ASP 250	
Enrofloxacin	Baytril.	
Erythromycin	Eryterocin, Erythromycin, Erythro200.	
Framycetin	Framycetin.	
Furazolidone	Furoxone, Furazolidone, Microdone, Neftin.	
Gentamycin	Gentamycin, Pangram	
Lincomycin	Lincocin, Lincospectam.	
Neomycin	Neobiotic.	
Oxytetracycline	Alamycin, Duphacycline, Embacycline, Engemycin, Intacycline, Neoterramycin, Oxytet, Oxytetrin, Terramycin, Tetramin, Tectin, Tetroxy, Tetsol.	
Penicillin	Crystapen, Duphapen, Duplicillin, Ethacillin, Norocillin, Penicillin, Potencil, Propen.	
Penicillin / streptomycin	Depomycin, Duphapen strep, Milimycin, Pen strep, Penicillin PS, Streptopen.	
Spectinomycin	Spectam.	
Sulphadimidine	Bimadine, Intradine, Sulphoxine.	
Tiamulin	Tiamutin, Denagard.	
Tilmicosin	Pulmotil	
Trimethoprim/sulpha	Bimotrim, Cosumix, Delvoprim, Duphatrim, Letrox, Norodine, Porsyn, Scorprin, Strinacin, Sulphatrim, Tribrissen, Trivetrin, Trimediazine, Trimidoxine, Uniprim	
Tylosin	Bilosin, Tylan, Tylamix, Tylasul, Tylosin, Tyluvet.	

* Check with your veterinarian to determine the trade names in your country.

(Fig.4-12)

By producing a list of products available in your country you can compare the costs of the active drugs made by different manufacturers. These lists will alter with time with new additions and deletions. Discuss aspects of this with your veterinarian.

Antibiotics and antibacterial medicines are the most widely used drugs on a day to day basis in the control of pig diseases but other products must also be considered. These include:
- Anaesthetics, sedatives and analgesics.
- Parasecticides. Wormers.
- Vaccines.
- Hormones.
- Growth promoters and probiotics.
- Electrolytes.

Anaesthetics, Sedatives, Analgesics

The indications for anaesthesia in the pig are limited but include caesarean section, vasectomy and ovum transplants, operations that are carried out by a veterinarian. Most other surgical procedures can be carried out by the use of tranquillisers and local anaesthetics. Anaesthesia is carried out by intravenous injection, inhalation, spinal anaesthesia or local infiltration of tissues. The first three are only used by a veterinarian but local anaesthesia is frequently necessary to suture small skin wounds or replace rectal prolapses. Sedatives are frequently used by non veterinary pig people.

Products Available
Drugs used for general anaesthesia
Halothane - Inhalation POM
Pentobarbitone - Intravenous injection POM
Tanopestone - Intravenous injection POM
POM = Prescription Only Medicine for veterinary use only.

A sow may also be killed for an emergency hysterectomy by shooting and bleeding by cutting the jugular veins, or destroying the spinal cord using a pithing rod. Only after pithing or bleeding is complete anaesthesia achieved to allow removal of the piglets. Details of this procedure are given in chapter 15.

Drugs used for local anaesthesia
Procaine
Lignocaine
Amethocaine
Some Trade Names (all injections)

Corneocaine	POM
Dunlop local	PML
Lignovet	PML
Lignocaine adrenalin	POM
Lignocaine A	POM
Lignol	PML
Nopain plus	PML

PML = Pharmacy Merchant List.

Check with your veterinarian for trade names in your country.

Sedatives

There are three drugs available for sedating pigs, acetylpromazine (ACP), azaperone (stresnil) and primidone (mysoline).

ACP (10mg/ml injection POM)

This drug is used in animals to prevent travel sickness and occasionally in pigs as a general sedative at a dose level of 0.1mg/kg liveweight. It is also useful for treating abdominal pain in cases of colic or to provide sedation together with local anaesthesia.

Azaperone (40mg/ml injection POM) Trade name Stresnil

This is a sedative and analgesic widely used in pigs and very effective.

Indications for use:
- To prevent fighting.
- Sedation prior to anaesthesia.
- To examine pigs feet.
- To prevent a gilt savaging her newborn piglets.
- To calm an excitable animal.
- Prior to mixing or transportation.
- To facilitate any manipulative procedure.

The dose level is 0.5 to 2ml/20kg body weight. The effects of the drug are dose dependent. When used at 2ml/20kg the pig is completely sedated after 20 minutes and lies on its side. The lower level of 0.5ml/20kg will prevent fighting when pigs are mixed.

Some guidelines to dose levels:
- Prevention of fighting in adult and growing pigs 1ml/50 kg
- To prevent savaging 2ml/20kg
- Sedation prior to anaesthesia 2ml/20kg
- Sedation prior to manipulation 1ml/20kg

It is important not to disturb the pig for 15 minutes after injection. Distractions will reduce the effectiveness of the drug.

Primidone (Mysoline POM 250mg tablets)

This is an excellent yet little used drug for preventing the savaging of piglets particularly by gilts. One tablet per 12kg body weight per 24 hours divided into two doses given am and late pm is advised. Treatment should commence at least 24 hours before farrowing and continue for at least 24 hours after farrowing. The tablets should be crushed onto the food.

Analgesics

Phenylbutazone
Some trade names:
- Tomanol POM injection
- Equipalazone POM injection
- Equipalazone POM powder

This drug is very useful in treating painful conditions such as acute lameness and torn muscles, bush foot infections or acute mastitis. It can be given by injection, by powder or by mouth and its use will be advised by your veterinarian.

Parasecticides

See chapter 11 Parasites for further information.

Drugs to control parasite infections act variously on the adult worm, the egg or the larva.

Fig.4-13 shows the drugs available and the methods of application. Medicaments can be given by mouth in the water or feed, by injection or on the skin.

The treatment and control of specific parasites is discussed fully in chapter 11.

SOME DRUGS AVAILABLE * TO TREAT PARASITES OF THE SKIN (ECTOPARASITES) AND INTERNAL PARASITES (ENDOPARASITES)

Active Drug	Some trade Names	Presentation / Dose Levels *	Large white worm	Eggs	Red stomach worm	Larvae	Lice	Lung worms	Mange mites	Nodular worms	Kidney worms	Thread worms	Ticks	Muscle worms	Stomach worms	Whip worms	Withdrawal period Days*	Cost comparison / spectrum of activity
Amitraz 12.4%	Taktic	Topical liquid concentrate 40ml to 10l water					✓										7	2.5
Amitraz 2%	Topline	Pour on to skin					✓										7	3.6
Doramectin	Dectomax	Injection. 1ml/33kg liveweight. (300mcg doramectin/kg liveweight)	✓		✓		✓	✓	✓	✓		✓			✓		28	15
Febantel	Bayverm	In feed pellets	✓	✓	✓	✓		✓		✓					✓	✓	35	3.6
Fenbendazole	Panacur	Pellets for top dressing. In feed for 1 day	✓	✓	✓	✓		✓		✓	✓	✓			✓	✓	5	1.0
Flubendazole 5%	Flubenol	Powder. Top dress or in feed for 10 days	✓	✓	✓	✓		✓		✓		✓			✓	✓	7	1.6
Ivermectin 1%	Ivomec injection	1ml/33kg. (300mcg ivermectin/kg liveweight)	✓	✓	✓	✓	✓	✓	✓	✓	✓	✓			✓	✓	28	15
Ivermectin 0.6%	Ivomec premix	Powder in feed 330g to 1kg premix/tonne	✓	✓	✓	✓	✓	✓	✓	✓	✓	✓			✓	✓	5	10
Levamisole 7.5%	Levacide/Levadin	Injection	✓	✓	✓	✓		✓		✓	✓	✓			✓	✓	28	3
Oxibendazole 2-20%	Loditac	In feed for 10 days or pellets for top dressing	✓	✓	✓	✓				✓	✓				✓	✓	14	3.6
Phosmet 20%	Porect	Topical liquid pour onto skin 1ml/10kg liveweight					✓		✓				✓				35	4.8
Thiophanate 22.5%	Nemafax 14	Powder in feed for 14 days	✓	✓	✓	✓				✓		✓			✓	✓	7	2.8

* See manufacturers data sheets for further details.   Some bendazole compounds may have activity against muscle worm.

(Fig.4-13)

Vaccines

So far most of the chapter has dealt with the treatment of disease but therapeutics also includes the use of products to prevent disease and the most common of these are vaccines which stimulate the immune system. Vaccination involves exposing the pig to the protein components (called the antigen) of the infectious agent. Some vaccines contain living organisms that have been altered so that they cannot produce disease but still produce an immunity. Most contain killed or inactivated organisms.

The immune system responds by producing antibodies that destroy the infectious agents, usually in co-operation with specialised body cells or by neutralising the toxins that are responsible for the disease. This process of stimulating immunity is called vaccination.

Vaccines contain antigens from viruses, bacteria, bacterial toxins, or parasites. They are given to pigs, usually by injection, to stimulate an immune response which will protect the pigs against later natural infection with the organism from which the vaccine was derived. Most stimulate both a humoral response and a cell-mediated response.

Vaccines can either contain viable organisms that will multiply in the pig, or inactivated ones that will not multiply in the pig.

In live vaccines the organism has usually been attenuated (i.e. its virulence has been reduced) so that although it multiples in the pig it does not normally cause disease. Examples are the PRRS vaccine, aujeszky's disease (pseudorabies) vaccines and classical swine fever vaccines. Live attenuated vaccines have the advantage that because they multiply in the pig they give a bigger antigenic stimulus resulting in stronger longer-lasting immunity. They have the disadvantage that they may become inactivated in wrong storage conditions (e.g. heat) or during dosing, by exposure to antiseptics or disinfectants, and are then useless. It is also important that they are stable and not able to return to full virulence.

Inactivated (dead) vaccines may contain whole organisms, antigenic parts of organisms or antigens which have been synthesised chemically. Synthesised antigen vaccines are still largely in the experimental stage.

The immunity produced by inactivated vaccines can be enhanced by substances called adjuvants such as aluminium hydroxide of certain types of oil. You should take care, however, if you use vaccines with oily adjuvants because they can cause serious local reactions if you accidentally inject them into yourself, e.g. your hand.

Inactivated vaccines may also contain toxins which have been modified so that they still stimulate an immune response but are no longer toxic to the animal. Toxins which have been modified in this way are called toxoids. The classic vaccine of this type is the tetanus toxoid which is used commonly in horses but rarely in pigs. In pigs, some of the *E. coli* vaccines against piglet diarrhoea and the clostridial vaccines against piglet dysentery contain toxoids.

> *Remember, vaccination is never 100%*

Autogenous Vaccines

Autogenous vaccines are bacterial vaccines that are manufactured from the specific pathogenic bacteria isolated from the diseased pig. They are usually made under a licence for use only on that farm. You should consult with your veterinarian. These are available from Salus (QP) Ltd. They can be useful when serious disease outbreaks occur and standard commercial vaccines are not available.

Such vaccines could be made from most bacteria including :-
- *Actinobacillus pleuropneumoniae*
- *E. coli*
- *Haemophilus parasuis*
- *Pasteurella*
- *Salmonella*
- *Streptococcus suis*
- *Staphylococcus hyicus* (Greasy pig disease)

One drawback to vaccinating a herd is that you cannot then use blood tests to check whether the organism is present in the herd or not. All the pigs will test positive which has obvious implications for an eradication programme based on blood tests, for example the eradication of swine fever or aujeszky's disease (pseudorabies). To get over this, gene-deleted vaccines have been developed. A part of the organism's gene which codes for an antigen has been removed so that when the organism multiplies in the pig it does not stimulate antibodies against that antigen. Special blood tests can then distinguish between the array of disease antibodies and those stimulated by the vaccine. A new generation of such gene manipulated vaccines, and possibly also synthetic polypeptide vaccines, can be anticipated.

Autogenous vaccines are those prepared with infectious pathogens from the herd which is to be vaccinated. The causal organisms has to be isolated, grown up, killed, and made into a safe vaccine form. Autogenous vaccines may be useful when serious disease outbreaks occur and standard commercial vaccines are not available.

Vaccine usage

Fig.4-14 lists the pig diseases for which vaccines are available. This list is not exhaustive and some vaccines will be available in some countries and not in others. However they are used in most countries both to protect against disease and to assist in eradication programmes. Some examples of commercial vaccines available are shown in chapter 4 these are but a few of the many available.

Vaccines commonly used on pig farms throughout the world include erysipelas, parvovirus infection (SMEDI syndrome), *E. coli* diarrhoea, clostridial dysentery of piglets, enzootic pneumonia caused by *Mycoplasma hyopneumoniae*, necrotic pleuropneumonia caused by *Actinobacillus pleuropneumoniae* and atrophic rhinitis caused by toxigenic *Pasteurella multocida*. In many countries, vaccines against disease, such as, salmonellosis, PRRS and TGE are also used depending on commercial availability.

In the European Union vaccination against classical swine fever has been stopped in a programme aimed at stamping the disease out. Vaccination against foot-and-mouth disease has also been stopped for a similar reason. Aujeszky's disease (pseudorabies) virus is widespread everywhere in the EU except in the UK and Denmark. With the exception of these two countries vaccination is widely practised. A blanket vaccination regime for all herds is being applied in some countries such as the Netherlands in an attempt to build up a national herd immunity resulting in the eradication of the virus.

North America is free from FMD and CSF so vaccination is not practised but PR vaccines are widely used in conjunction with eradication programmes. Elsewhere in the world, the situation regarding these three diseases varies, so vaccination policies also vary.

The effectiveness of vaccines

This varies, because of the need to stimulate mucosal immunity locally. As mentioned earlier, vaccines given by injection against respiratory and intestinal disease are generally not as effective as those against systemic or generalised diseases. An exception to this is the vaccine for enzootic pneumonia (*M. hyopneumoniae*) because it stimulates cell-mediated immunity. If, however, they are fed or sprayed into the upper respiratory tract they may produce a stronger local immunity. The vaccine against piglet dysentery is a toxoid and if given routinely to sows in adequate doses is usually reasonably effective in providing passive protection via the colostrum.

Sometimes vaccines do not work particularly well on a farm and in such cases the following possibilities need to be considered:
- The vaccine was contaminated.
- The vaccine was not capable of producing the required immunity.
- The pig was already incubating the disease when it was vaccinated.
- The vaccine had been incorrectly stored. High temperatures reduce the effectiveness. (Always keep vaccines in a refrigerator but do not freeze).
- The vaccine had been exposed to sunlight.
- The vaccine had gone out of date.
- The needle and syringe were dirty or faulty.
- Chemical sterilisation destroyed the vaccine.
- The animal had inadvertently missed being vaccinated.

MAJOR VIRUS DISEASES THAT MAY BE CONTROLLED BY VACCINATION +
Aujeszky's disease
Foot-and-mouth disease
Porcine parvovirus
PRRS
Swine fever
Swine influenza
TGE

BACTERIAL DISEASES THAT MAY BE CONTROLLED BY VACCINATION +
Any bacterial disease by autogenous vaccines, e.g. greasy pig disease
Actinobacillus pleuropneumonia
Atrophic rhinitis
Clostridial diseases
E. coli diarrhoea
Enzootic pneumonia
Erysipelas
Glässers disease (*Haemophilus parasuis*)
Leptospirosis
Pasteurellosis
Streptococcal meningitis

+ The availability of vaccines varies from country to country.

(Fig.4-14)

This is particularly common with parvovirus vaccination in the gilt.
- Vaccine response was poor because there was maternal antibody present.
- The vaccine was deposited in fat and was not absorbed. Faulty injection techniques.

Hormones

These products are usually under the direct control of your veterinarian i.e. POM (prescription only medicines) products. As a general statement the use of hormones that act on the ovaries to stimulate oestrus should be avoided because the stage of the oestrus cycle cannot be accurately determined. However at specific times their use can be advantageous. Hormones used in the pig include the following:-

Prostaglandins

See chapter 8; Controlled farrowings.

These are substances that following injection, cause the corpus luteum to regress. The corpus luteum is present in the ovaries during the middle period of the oestrus cycle and during pregnancy. Its removal may either initiate oestrus, abortion or farrowing depending on the stage of the reproductive cycle.

There are three uses:
1. Given within 36 hours post-farrowing to improve subsequent fertility and litter size.
2. To resolve endometritis or womb infection.
3. To synchronise farrowing by injecting the sow from day 113 of pregnancy. Farrowing usually commences within 24 hours.

Prostaglandins are potentially hazardous to women and should never be handled by them. Fig 4-16 shows a format recommended for their control and use on the farm

Milk let down products

These are hormones produced by the anterior pituitary gland at the base of the brain. Their action is to release milk from the mammary gland and cause contractions of the uterus. They may be given to promote the farrowing process provided there are no mechanical obstructions. They are also useful in promoting milk flow when the udder is congested. Specific uses are discussed in chapter 7.

> *If a gilt has not cycled by 240 days of age cull it. It is infertile or subfertile. (Assuming it is not pregnant!!)*

Hormones Used to Control the Oestrus Cycle

These can be used to synchronise oestrus in groups of gilts or in sows after weaning.

Regumate Porcine (POM)

This is an oil based product containing the active principle altrenogest - a progesterone substance. Progesterone is produced by the ovary when the sow is in the middle of the oestrus cycle or pregnant. It suppresses oestrus in the non pregnant female if it is given daily and when it is removed the sow or gilt will come into heat.

Its main use is to synchronise oestrus by medicating batches of gilts daily for 18 days, (5mls per day per gilt is placed on the feed). At the end of this period following its withdrawal most gilts will be in heat within 5-7 days.

It can also be used in sows at weaning time to synchronise oestrus but this should not be necessary at a commercial level. Regumate should only be used in gilts that have shown oestrus. Some trials have shown an increase in litter size following its use.

PG600 (POM)

This product contains hormones that stimulate the production and release of follicles from the ovary. They are called gonadotrophins. PG600 is used to stimulate gilts that have failed to show oestrus but in such cases it is not uncommon for only 50% to respond, and come into heat. Furthermore some gilts will be mated only to become pseudo pregnant and not farrow. It is better to cull anoestrus gilts - they are telling you they are infertile.

Gilts treated with PG600 should be served towards the end of the heat period.

PG600 can be used where there are anoestrus problems in first litter gilts. Litter size is often improved.

A Suggested Format for the Safe Use of Prostaglandin Products

1. I .... understand and will carry out the following procedures for the safe use and administration of Prostaglandin (trade name ....), for the induction of farrowing in sows.
2. I have read and understand the packing leaflet / data sheet.
3. The handling of this product is restricted to myself and .... who shall be bound by these rules.
4. At ALL TIMES the product will be stored in a nominated locked place.
5. No other person shall have access to the product or handle it.
6. It will only be administered to sows which are my property and on my farm / farms for the induction of farrowing as directed.
7. I will record the date of administration of each dose with records of the number of sows and dose volume given. These records will be available for inspection on request.
8. Supplies of the product will only be issued to me personally by a qualified veterinarian. I will sign for each consignment.
9. Empty containers will be placed in a sealed polythene bag, and returned to the issuing veterinary practice at which time a new supply may be issued.
10. I agree to receiving instruction as to the handling, storage, administration and recording of the use of this product.
11. A new sterile syringe and needle will be used each time the product is administered. After these injections have been given the syringes and needles will be rinsed out and either returned to the veterinary practice or safely destroyed on the farm as agreed.
12. Waterproof gloves will be worn by the operator handling the product. Accidental spillage will be washed off the skin immediately and in event of accidental injection, medical advice will be promptly sought.
13. I understand that contact with prostaglandin products by women of child bearing age or by asthmatics is to be avoided.
14. These rules will be displayed where the product is to be stored.
15. I understand that failure to comply with these instructions at any time would result in withdrawal of stocks and no further issue of the product.

Signed .... Name and Address ....
....
....

Site of storage of prostaglandin if different to above:
....
....

Date ....
Countersignature of veterinarian
....
Date ....

(Fig.4-16)

SOME MILK LET DOWN PRODUCTS AVAILABLE

Commercial Name	Active Principle	Dose
Hyposton POM	Oxytocin (10 units / ml)	0.5 - 1ml
Oxytocin POM	Oxytocin (10 units / ml)	0.5 - 1ml

Gilts are injected on the day of weaning and a normal oestrus follows. However if this is necessary, your management and or nutrition in lactation is probably wrong and you should read chapter 5.

Growth Promoters

The aim of efficient pig production is to maximise growth. This can be aided by the inclusion of specific growth promoting substances to the feed. It is worth remembering that growth is also maximised by:

- The correct levels of vitamins in the diet.
- The correct levels of minerals, protein and energy.
- Metallic compounds such as copper.
- Some sedatives.
- Anabolic steroids.
- The effects of management, the environment, disease, genetics and housing.

The inclusion of anti microbial substances in the feed is the most common and cost effective method of promoting growth. Such growth promoters at very low levels have the effect of reducing the activity of the organisms in the gut which increases the efficiency of the absorption of food from the intestine and suppresses any harmful products of bacterial metabolism.

How cost effective are growth promoters.?

A summary of data over the past 15 years shows the following:
- Improvements in average daily gain of up to 4 %.
- Improvements in average daily feed intake by 0.2 - 1.4 %.
- Improvements in food conversion rate by 2.5 - 3.9 %.

However the more healthy the herd and the fewer the diseases, the less will be the effect.

The question is often asked "Are these substances harmful to the health of either animals or man?". To date there is no evidence to suggest they have any adverse effect whatsoever.

Licensed growth promoters usually have a nil withdrawal period, and most are antibiotics that have little or no therapeutic action in the pig. (There are a few exceptions to this, for example tylosin).

The characteristics required for a growth promoter:
- They must be non toxic.
- Performance must be improved with economic benefit.
- There must be no adverse effects in relation to other antibiotics.
- They must not alter the normal bacteria in the gut, or allow one organism to predominate over another, for example salmonella.
- They must not pollute the environment.
- They must not increase drug resistance or be involved in the transfer of drug resistance between one bacterial species and another.

Growth promoters available in pig feeds are shown in Fig.4-17.

Probiotics

See chapter 14 for further information.

These are harmless naturally occurring bacteria. When given by mouth they help to maintain a balanced micro environment in the gut and inhibit the multiplication of pathogens such as *E. coli*. They include acid producing strains of lactobacilli, streptococci and yeasts.

In some cases they are claimed to improve feed efficiency, daily live weight gain and health but evidence for this in most cases is not convincing.

GROWTH PROMOTERS THAT MAY BE AVAILABLE *			
Active Drug	Dose Active Drug (g /Tonne)	Some Trade Names	Comments g/tonne
Alivamycin	10 - 40	Maxus	20-40g up to 4 months old. 10 - 20g up to 4 - 6 months old.
Bambermycin	10 - 20	Flavomycin	Up to 6 months of age.
Carbadox	15 - 30	Carbadox	Not permitted in some countries.
Chlortetracycline	10 - 55	Aureomycin	Not permitted in some countries.
Copper carbonate	100 - 175 (Copper)	Ukasta Ltd	100g max. to finishers 175g up to 17 wks old
Copper sulphate	100 - 175 (Copper)	Ukasta Ltd	100g max. to finishers 175g up to 17 wks old
Cupric oxide	100 - 175 (Copper)	Ukasta Ltd	100g max. to finishers 175g up to 17 wks old
Lincomycin	20	Lincomix	Not permitted in some countries.
Olaqunidox	15 - 100	Enterodox	Use up to 4 months of age.
Oxytetracycline	10 - 55	Terramycin	Not permitted in some countries.
Procaine penicillin	10 - 50		Not permitted in some countries.
Salinomycin	15 - 60	Salocin	Pigs up to 40kg 30 - 60g. Pigs to slaughter 15 - 30g.
Spiramycin	5 - 80	Spira	Max. age to 3 months only.
Tiamulin	10	Tiamutin	Not permitted in some countries.
Tylosin	10 - 40	Tylan	Up to 4 months old 40g. Up to 6 months old 20g.
Virginiamycin	5 - 50	Stafac	Up to 4 months old 50g. 4 - 6 months old 20g.
Zinc bacitracin	5 - 50	Albac	5 - 50g. Up to 6 months old.

* Consult data sheet of your country or your veterinarian

(Fig.4-17)

SOME AVAILABLE PROSTAGLANDINS		
Commercial Name	Active Principle	Route
Alphacept POM	Alfaprostol	Intramuscular
Iliren POM	Tiaprost	Intramuscular
Lutalyse POM	Dinoprost	Intramuscular
Planate POM	Cloprostenol	Intramuscular
Prosolvin POM	Luprostiol	Intramuscular

Electrolytes

Approximately 55% of a pigs body weight is made up of water. In young lean animals it is much higher (70%) and in fat ones lower because fat contains little water.

The fluid balance in the body is regulated by the kidney and in particular the concentrations of sodium (Na), chloride (Cl), potassium (P), hydrogen ions, bicarbonate, protein, calcium and magnesium in the tissues. These substances are called electrolytes.

A pig could loose 5% of its body weight in fluid losses with little clinical effect but at 15% it would die.

Such losses equate to 40-160ml/kg of body weight. If the pig cannot maintain its fluid balance by intake relative to normal or abnormal losses dehydration will result.

Diarrhoea and vomiting are by far the most important causes in the young pig particularly during sucking and in the immediate post-weaning period.

Certain types of *E. coli* and salmonella produce toxins which cause fluids to be excreted into the small intestine. This is called secretory diarrhoea.

Conversely viral infections such as TGE virus, PED virus and rotavirus destroy the villi in the intestine causing a marked reduction in the absorptive capacity of the digestive system and dehydration. This is called malabsorption or osmotic diarrhoea. It is also common in a milder form in pigs that have been weaned 2 days or more. It may then occur with or without diarrhoea.

Rehydration by Mouth

This is the most practical method for use in sucking pigs and weaners. Glucose water and electrolytes when combined with the amino acid glycine are well absorbed from the small intestine.

A typical electrolyte formulation would comprise %

Glucose	67.5
Sodium chloride	14.3
Glycine	10.4
Potassium dihydrogen phosphate	6.8
Citric acid	0.8
Potassium citrate	0.2

It is mixed with water at a rate of 30g per litre for the first 24 hours and followed by 15g per litre until the pig has recovered. The solution should be provided fresh daily in easily accessible drinkers.

A number of commercial electrolyte solutions are available but all should contain glycine.

THE COMMON CAUSES OF DEHYDRATION IN THE PIG

Condition	Common Causes
Diarrhoea	**Viruses**: 　Epidemic diarrhoea 　Rotavirus 　Swine fever 　Transmissible gastro-enteritis (TGE) **Bacteria**: 　Campylobacter 　Clostridia 　Coccidia 　E. coli 　Salmonella 　Serpulina causing swine dysentery
Vomiting	E. coli Haemagglutinating encephalitis virus TGE
Fever	Many virus and bacterial diseases Pleuropneumonia Pneumonia
Water shortage	Blocked water pipes Meningitis
Toxic conditions	Greasy pig disease Mastitis
Kidney failure	Cystitis Pyelonephritis
Haemorrhage	Bloody gut Haemorrhagic enteritis Trauma

EXAMPLES OF SOME PIG VACCINES AVAILABLE IN THE EU AND ELSEWHERE 1997 *

Vaccines	Company	Organism/Type	Initial Dose	Booster	Comments
Respiratory disease					
Carovax (Pneumonia)	Mallinckrodt	*Pasteurella haemolytica* and *P. multocida*	2ml and second dose 4 wks later.	2ml pre-farrowing.	Sows and Pigs.
Ingelvac	Boehringer	PRRS Live modified virus	Single dose 2ml Intramuscular.	None	Pigs 3 - 18 weeks old only.
Pastacidin (Pneumonia)	Hoechst	*Pasteurella haemolytica* and *P. multocida*	1ml and second dose 2-3 wks later	4 wks before farrowing.	Sows and growing pigs.
Porcilis AR-T (Rhinitis)	Intervet	Pasteurella toxin Bordetella	2ml and second dose 6 wks. Can give at any age in sows.	2-6 wks before farrowing.	Deep intramuscular injection. Sows only.
Nobi porvac (Aujeszky's)	Intervet	Aujeszky's virus. Live attenuated	2ml to pigs 10 weeks plus sows 2 x 2 ml 4 weeks apart.	2 - 3 times yearly.	Differential test available. All pigs.
PR vac killed	Smith Kline Beecham	Aujeszky's virus inactivated.	2ml at weaning	Twice yearly to sows.	Differential SN test available. Sows and growers.
Stellamune	Pfizer	*Mycoplasma hyopneumoniae*	2ml and second dose 2 - 4 weeks later	-	Pigs from 1 - 10 weeks of age.
Suvaxyn M. Hyo	Fort Dodge	*Mycoplasma hyopneumoniae*	2ml and second dose 2 - 4 weeks later	-	Pigs from 1 - 10 weeks of age.
Suvaxyn HPP	Fort Dodge	*Actinobacillus pleuropneumoniae*	2ml and second dose 2 wks later.		Pigs 6 weeks onwards
Suvaxyn rhinitis	Fort Dodge	*Bordetella bronchiseptica*	1ml and second dose 2-3 wks later. Sows 4 wks pre-farrowing.	4 wks before farrowing.	Sows and Pigs.
***E. coli* scour**					
Ecopig	Smith Kline Beecham	LT Enterotoxin	5ml 3wks pre-farrowing	1-4 days post-farrowing	Sows
Gletvax	Mallinckrodt	*E. coli* & clostridia	5ml 4 and 2 wks pre-farrowing.	2 wks pre-farrowing.	Sows
Intagen premix	Roche PML	*E. coli* antigens	In feed		Sows and Pigs
Porcilis porcol 5	Intervet POM	LT Toxin K88 K99 987P antigens	2ml twice 3 wks pre-farrowing. 5 wks apart	Every 6 months	Sows Boost at weaning
Porcovac plus	Hoechst	*E. coli* antigens	5ml 6 and 3 wks pre-farrowing.	3 wks pre-farrowing.	Piglets 2mls at 10 and 24 days old.
Porcovac plus	Hoechst PML	*E. coli* antigens	2ml 6 and 3 wks pre-farrowing.	3 wks pre-farrowing.	Sows
Suvaxyn *E. coli* P4	Fort Dodge	K88 99 987P F-41 antigens	2ml 4 and 2 wks pre-farrowing.	2 wks pre-farrowing.	Sows
Erysipelas					
Colisorb	Hoechst	Erysipelas, *E. coli*	6 and 3 wks pre-farrowing.	3 wks pre-farrowing.	Sows
Erysorb plus	Hoechst	Erysipelas	6 and 3 wks pre-farrowing.	3 wks pre-farrowing.	The boost can be given at weaning. Gilts injected 12-16 wks of age.
Suvaxyn erysipelas	Fort Dodge	Erysipelas	2ml 6 and 3 wks pre-farrowing.	3 wks pre-farrowing.	Boost sows at weaning time. Gilts injected 12-16 wks of age.
Parvovirus					
Nobi-vac parvo	Intervet	Parvovirus oil based.	2ml	See data sheet.	Gilts over 6 months of age.
Parvovax	Rhone Merieux	Parvovirus oil based.	2ml pre-service boost after farrowing.	Annually. See data sheet.	Gilts over 6 months of age.
Porculin parvo	Mallinckrodt	Parvovirus oil based.	2ml. See data sheet.	See data sheet	Gilts over 6 months of age.
Suvaxyn gestafend 6	Fort Dodge	Inactivated leptospira parvovirus	See data sheets.	To sows and gilts.	
Suvaxyn parvo	Fort Dodge	Parvovirus	2ml pre-service.	After farrowing. See data sheet.	Gilts over 6 months of age.
Suvaxyn parvo 2	Fort Dodge	Parvovirus oil based	2ml repeat 3wks later.	See data sheet.	Gilts over 6 months of age.
Virus diarrhoea					
TGE vaccine	Smith Kline Beecham	Modified live TGE virus	See data sheets	See data sheets	See data sheets
Scourmune	Schering-Plough	Modified live virus. Inactivated. TGE and Rotavirus	See data sheets	See data sheets	See data sheets
Autogenous					
All types bacterial.	Salus QP Ltd	Made from farm bacteria	2 doses required 2 - 3 weeks apart.	Variable	Contact Salus QP Ltd

* This table should only be used as a guide Refer to current data sheets

Chapter 4

5 Reproduction: Non Infectious Infertility

The breeding female 133
The use and interpretation of records.. 135
Understanding farrowing rates and production losses......................... 136
Embryo and foetal losses 137
    Group 1 losses - anoestrus 137
    Acclimatisation of gilts 140
    Light 142
    Group 2 losses - ovulation and egg production 143
    Group 3 losses - fertilisation.. 144
    Group 4 losses - implantation.. 145
    Group 5 losses - foetal death and the mummified pig 147
Detecting pregnancy 148
    Methods of pregnancy diagnosis (PD) 148
    A practical format for diagnosing pregnancy on the farm........... 149
Abortion and seasonal infertility 149
    Non infectious causes 150
    Infectious causes.. 151
Group 6 losses - stillborn pigs 153
Low litter size 153
The boar 154
    Anatomy and physiology... 154
    Facts about semen 155
    Fertilisation 156
    Libido... 157
Mating procedures.. 157
    Single service (supervised) 157
    Skip services 158
    Multiple services.. 159
    Key points to a successful mating.. 159
    Artificial insemination (AI) 160
    Fungal poisoning - mycotoxicosis... 160

Chapter 5

5 Reproduction: Non Infectious Infertility

The Breeding Female

Problems associated with reproductive failure are often complex. In trying to resolve such problems it is essential to understand the important factors that maximise biological efficiency.

Key points to maximising reproductive performance

- Use the breed of female that is suitable for your system.
- Ensure that the breeding female exhibits good hybrid vigour.
- Monitor the age of the sow and her continuing performance.
- Collect the required records and use them to understand the problem.
- Ensure an even parity spread across the herd. Litters 3-5 are most productive.
- Use high levels of feed energy, protein and lysine in lactation and maximise feed intake.
- Provide an equitable environment with even temperatures. Cleanliness is essential.
- Compare the reproductive performance to the lactation length.
- Maintain good body condition throughout pregnancy.
- Have a sufficient number of boars available so that they need only be used once every 24 hours at most.
- Maintain sow health and immunity to disease.
- Assess the age of the gilt at first service, relative to life time performance in the herd.
- Assess the effectiveness of sow management from weaning to 21 days post-service.
- Make sure that the right type of stockperson is in charge of mating. The ability of the stockperson has a direct effect on reproductive performance

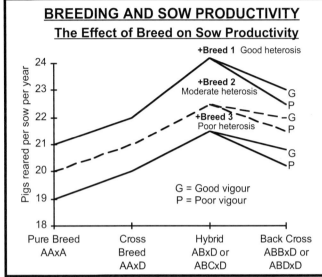

AAxA: Pure-bred female mated with a boar of the same breed on-line.
AAxD: Pure-bred female mated with boar of a different breed or sire line. This does not necessarily increase the numbers of piglets born but the improved vigour of the piglets mean that more survive to weaning.
ABx D or ABCxD: Two way or three way crossbred females mated to a different breed or boar line, A, B and C. Should be prolific dam lines.
ABBxD: Back cross female mated with a different breed or boar line. Both A and B are prolific breeds or dam lines.
ABDxD: Back-cross female mated with the same breed or boar line used in the back-cross. The back-cross has 50% non prolific boar line.

(Fig.5-1)

Do not be tempted to breed from an F2 female if her sire was a boar line.

Most of the major breeding (seedstock) companies now develop lines rather than standard breeds. The lines are generally based on breeds but have been developed differently. Thus one line "A" may be based predominantly on the Large White breed but has been developed as a dam line by selecting for prolificacy (No. of piglets born alive per litter and No. of litters born per year) and mothering ability (No. of piglets weaned per sow per year). Line "D" may also be based on the Large White breed but has been developed as a sire line by selecting primarily for growth rate, feed conversion efficiency and lean meat. This sire line development is often done at the expense of prolificacy and so if you are a commercial producer you should never select female back-crosses sired by such boars for breeding.

Efficient reproduction starts with females of high genetic potential for prolificacy and this includes good hybrid vigour (heterosis). The hybrid female is the progeny of the male of one breed or dam line (A), crossed with the female of another breed or dam line (B) to produce the commercial F1 gilt (AB). This animal is usually highly prolific in terms of pigs produced per sow per year. Some breeding companies cross the F1 with a third breed or dam line (C) to produce their commercial hybrid or three way cross. Such pigs are designated by a variety of numbers and names and Fig.5-1, illustrates the differences that may occur between (ABxC) crosses de-

CROSS BREEDING
More pigs.
Heavier and more even piglets at birth.
Better mothering ability.
Better production of milk.
More pigs reared.
Better fertility.
More libido in the boar.
Better conformation of teats and legs.
Increased longevity.

(Fig.5-2)

pending on the level of hybrid vigour. Pure breeding produces the worst scenario, hence the reason why, at a commercial level no farmers should use pure bred females and boars of the same breed. In the past it has been common practice, commercially, to breed back from the F1 by using a boar of the same breed to produce a further breeding female that is $\tfrac{3}{4}$ pure breed (A), $\tfrac{1}{4}$ alternate breed (B). However, there is invariably loss of hybrid vigour and even in farms that are efficient, performance is usually less efficient than the F1.

Fig.5-2 lists the essential features of different breeding combinations and it is important when selecting the source of your gilts to remember that there can be a considerable difference in the prolificacy of the dam lines and in the expression of hybrid vigour between one breeding company and another.

The age of the sow also plays an important part in reproductive efficiency. In Fig.5-3 you will see that the best reproductive performance is in litters 3, 4 and 5. Although by litter 8 the total number of pigs born may be greater there is often wide variation in the size of individual pigs at birth, an increasing number being too small or runts. There is also an increase in the numbers of stillborn with a reduction in live births. Furthermore, with age sows tend to be more clumsy and lazy, with higher levels of pigs laid on and an increased mortality, often 3% or more above those of the efficient parities. Sows in litters 3 to 5 should rear at least 24 pigs per annum but by the 8th litter and above this often drops below 21. Levels of reproductive efficiency should also be compared to those being achieved by the incoming gilts. Culling decisions should be made in light of the performance of your first litter gilts, the maintenance of the mating programme and the availability of older sows as foster mothers.

The parity distribution in the herd necessary to maximise production is shown in Fig.5-4.

Sow management from the day of weaning to 21 days post-service influences reproductive efficiency. If you have a problem, this is the first area that should be assessed.

Consider the overall plan in Fig.5-5 which defines the critical parameters necessary to maximise reproductive efficiency.

The maintenance of gilt and sow numbers is the

AN EXAMPLE OF THE EFFECTS OF AGE ON REPRODUCTIVE EFFICIENCY *				
		Litter Number		
	Gilt	2	3 - 5	8+
Pigs Born	10.7	11.3	11.7	12.2
Alive	10.2	10.6	11.0	10.4
Dead %	5	5.5	6	15
Fostered (essential ones) %	3	4	8	10
Mortality				
Laid on %	3	3	3	5
Starvation %	1	1	1	2
Other	5	5	4	6
Total mortality %	9	9	8	13
No. weaned	9.3	9.5	10.1	9.1
Farrowing rate %	85	87	90	83
Litters/sow/year	2.3	2.28	2.4	2.25
Pigs reared/ sow/year	21.4	21.6	24.3	20.5

* Based on studies of field records

(Fig.5-3)

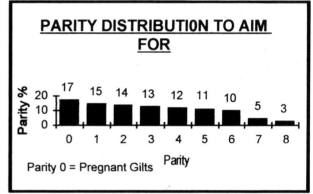

(Fig.5-4)

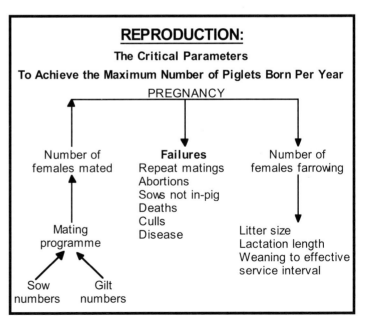

(Fig.5-5)

first critical factor. There must always be sufficient females available to maintain a mating programme.

A shortfall in numbers available is the most common failure on most pig farms.

From point of mating to point of farrowing there can be a variety of pregnancy failures which are dealt with later in this chapter. For every 100 sows served in a given period of time less than 100 will farrow. This in percentage terms is described as the farrowing rate. Failures of animals to farrow are associated with repeat matings, abortions, sows not in-pig, deaths, culls and/or disease.

Farrowing Rate =
$$\frac{\text{Nos. of sows farrowed}}{\text{Nos. of sows served}} \times 100$$

How to approach a problem on the farm

Of all the problems on the pig farm, understanding and resolving a reproductive problem can be the most challenging. However, if a logical approach is taken, the causes of the reproductive failures can usually be worked out and corrective actions taken. The approach outlined in Fig.5-6 relates the performance of the herd to accepted levels of efficiency, this then defines the area of failure and finally the problem is identified. Further investigations are then necessary to understand what has precipitated the problem and these are carried out by examining the management procedures, records and performing appropriate pathological tests. An important objective here is to determine if the problem is of infectious or non infectious origin or a combination of both. The end results are either farrowing rate loss, a reduced litter size, anoestrus or any combination.

The Use and Interpretation of Records

The causes of infertility cannot be determined and corrective action taken without collecting reliable information and using it in a meaningful way. Records required for each breeding female to understand reproductive failure:-
- The sow number.
- The number of litters or parity.
- The dates of mating, farrowing and weaning.
- The number of services at each mating.
- The service quality. (Rate each service as 1, 2 or 3 - good, moderate or poor).
- The boar used or AI.
- The lactation length.
- Mummified piglets and their size.
- The numbers born alive/dead.
- The weaning to service interval.

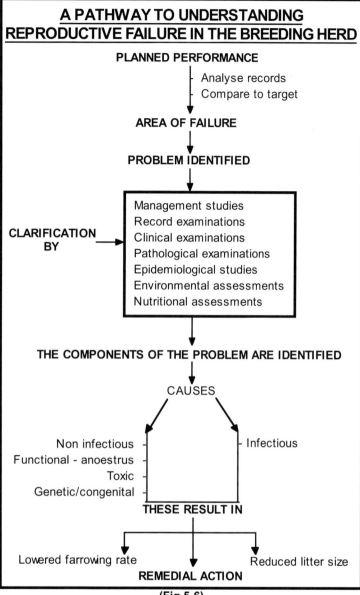
(Fig.5-6)

Remember: Failure to maintain the optimum mating programme is the most common and most costly failure on many pig farms today. See chapter 3.

Records required for the breeding herd
- Litter size variation * (scatter).
- Repeat matings - and their intervals in days.
- Abortions - and the age of foetuses
- Females found not in pig.
- Discharges - The time when they occur post-service, observations and the outcome.

- Parity distribution.
* Percentage of litters with total born (alive/dead/mummified) less than 9.

Whilst the above information looks rather daunting it is normally recorded in the mating book and on the sow and litter card on most farms. If a problem arises it is a simple procedure to identify the sows involved, collect the individual data and look for common features.

Fig.5-7 provides data against which your own farm performance can be related.

These suggested targets and action levels for the various parameters are not absolute but rather broad guidelines.

> *Monitor reproduction by farrowing rate loss. Record abnormalities in both the boar and the sow.*

Understanding Farrowing Rates and Production Losses

In Fig.5-8 the components of farrowing rate loss are defined at the best levels of biological efficiency. A 7% failure of repeat matings made up of 5% at a normal interval of 18-22 days and a further 2% outside this would be a good target to achieve. A continuing farrowing rate of 89% for a minimum period of 12 months would be considered excellent and this would give approximately 10 non productive days per sow from the first day of mating to the mating for the next pregnancy. Depending on the lactation length 2.3 to 2.4 litters per sow per year would result. It should be noted however that these figures do not take into account the period from the day of entry of the gilt into the herd to its first mating. Non productive days in this respect often go unrecognised and can be significant.

Analysing the farrowing rate losses

Pregnancy losses from mating should be documented on a daily basis as they occur. Fig.5-9 shows a simple recording sheet that you could adopt. This type of approach is usually of more value than using computerised information, because the precise detail required is often not recorded in the programme.

This is particularly so in the column "Results/History/Comments", where the stockpersons' observations

REFERENCE DATA FOR REPRODUCTIVE EFFICIENCY IN A BREEDING HERD (28 day weaning)		
A 100 Sow Module	Suggested Targets	Action Level
No. of gilts available for service at any time	6	4
Age at first service (days)	220 +/- 10	240
No. of productive sows	100	95
Average days from weaning to first mating	6	7
Repeat matings		
- Regular returns (18-22 days) %	5	6
- Irregular returns (23 days +) %	2	5
Non productive days per sow.	12	14
Abortions %	< 1	> 2
Sows not in pig %	1	> 2
Sows culled pregnant %	< 1	> 2
Deaths during pregnancy	1	> 2
Farrowing rate %	89	85
Vaginal discharge - more than >5 days post-service	1	> 2
Sows culled per year %	36	42
Sow parity at culling	6	8
Pigs born alive	11.2	10.9
Pigs born dead %	5	7
Piglets mummified % < 100mm	< 0.5	1
Piglets mummified % > 100mm	1	1.5
Number of boars	5	4
Mean age (months) boars	21	24
Age at culling (years) boars	3	> 3

(Fig.5-7)

FARROWING RATE LOSSES No Infertility Problems		
	Loss/100 Services	Lost Days
Normal repeats	5	105
Abnormal repeats	2	60
Abortions	< 1	40
Endometritis	< 1	21
Sows not in pig	1	90
Culls disease	1	30
Deaths	1	40
TOTAL LOSS	11%	386

Farrowing rate 89%
Empty days from service to service = 10
4 week weaning 2.38 litters per sow per annum
3 week weaning 2.50 litters per sow per annum

(Fig.5-8)

RECORD OF FAILURES TO FARROW								
MONTH: April					TOTAL SERVED:		104	
CATEGORY: (See below)								
Sow No.	Parity	Date First Mated	1st or Repeat Mating	Boar used	Cause of Failure	Date of Failure	Days Interval	Result/history/ Stockperson/ comments
161	5	12-12-96	2	4	-	2-2-97	52	Poor service
75	7	10-12-96	1	16	Dis	24-2-97	76	Discharge
67	8	3-1-97	1	60	D	27-3-97	83	Fighting
724	1	2-3-97	1	24	Ab	4-5-97	63	Lame

Cause of failure: **(Rp)** = Repeats   **(Ab)** = Abortion   **(NIP)** = Not In Pig   **(Dis)** = Disease   **(D/C)** = Death/Culled

(Fig.5-9)

CHAPTER 5 - Reproduction: Non Infectious Infertility **137**

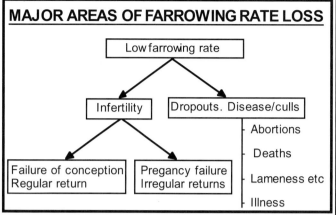

(Fig.5-10)

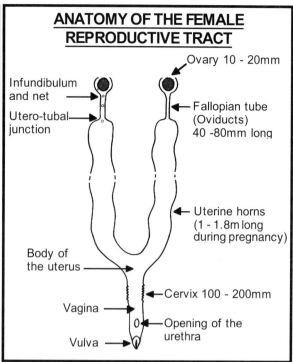

(Fig.5-11)

can be very helpful in understanding the problem. For example, farrowing rate problems may not be associated with reproductive efficiency but due to lameness and subsequent abortion or embryo absorption. Lame boars or lame sows can be associated with farrowing rate loss and if such information is not collected the core of the problem may be missed. Fig.5-10 shows the overall picture if you have a low farrowing rate.

Embryo and Foetal Losses

To help you understand the processes of fertilisation and pregnancy Figs.5-11 and 5-12 show the anatomy of the reproductive tract of the female.

Note in Fig.5-12 that the opening of the urethra (tube from the bladder) lies on the floor of the vagina, approximately 70mm inside. If a boar has very long back legs the penis enters the vagina in a downward movement and the tip of the penis sometimes enters the urethra. In such cases the sow shows pain and there is the potential for damage which can result in cystitis or infection of the bladder. Two uterine arteries branch off the main aorta and supply blood to the womb. In the pregnant state the changes in blood flow in these arteries are used to diagnose early pregnancy. See chapter 15.

By studying records and carrying out clinical observations and pathological tests it is usually possible to determine precisely where reproductive failure has occurred. Such failures can be conveniently grouped into six categories related to stages in the reproductive cycle. In most cases failure can be narrowed down to one or two of these. (Fig.5-13). However, to determine the causes of the loss it is first necessary to understand reproductive physiology, both in the sow and in the boar. The stages of development from fertilisation to farrowing and the consequences of each group failing are shown in Fig.5-14. You should spend time studying this to appreciate the procedures that are available for corrective action on the farm.

Group 1 Losses - Anoestrus

Anoestrus is common both in the maiden gilt and in

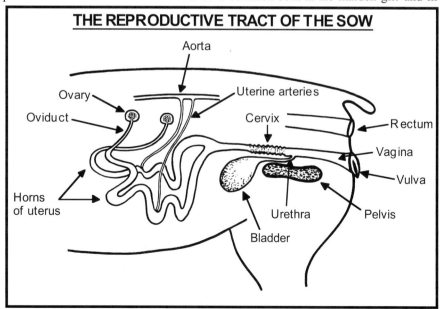

(Fig.5-12)

Chapter 5

Approximately £2.50 is lost for every day of pregnancy failure.

the sow post-weaning. Puberty is initiated in the gilt by complex hormonal mechanisms that are associated with growth and age. The hybrid gilt commences oestrus from around 160 days of age onwards but some exotic breeds such as the meishan come into heat much earlier.

Factors in the external environment stimulate the higher centres of the brain which activates the pituitary gland (Fig.5-15). This tiny gland at the base of the brain produces the hormones which start the oestrus cycle (the hormone surge). There are primarily two hormones involved; the follicle stimulating hormone (FSH), which as the name implies causes the ovaries to be stimulated and to produce follicles containing eggs. The second is the luteinising hormone (LH) which at the point of oestrus is excreted into the bloodstream to act on the follicles and cause the eggs to be released. The developing follicle at the time of oestrus is about the size of a small cherry. There may be up to 15 to 18 of them in each ovary. After the egg has been released from the follicle and ovary the remaining tissues develop into a body called the corpus luteum. This produces the hormone progesterone and the levels in the blood rise as oestrus subsides. The hormone changes are depicted in

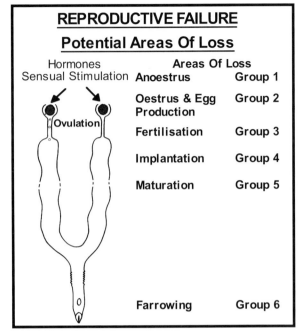

(Fig.5-13)

Fig.5-16.

Oestrus is initiated by the ovary which produces the other female hormone, oestrogen and it is this that is

EMBRYO AND FOETAL DEATH AND THE CONSEQUENCES

The Age and Position of Embryos	The Failure	The Result
Day 0 - Ovulation	No Ovulation	Anoestrus
Day 0 - Fertilisation	No Fertilisation	Normal 21 day return
Day 2 - Fertilised ova descend	Total embryo mortality prior to day 10	Normal 21 day return
Day 3 - Embryo size :0.2mm - 0.5mm	Only 5 or less embryos present at day 10	Delayed return to oestrus at 24 - 38 days.
Day 4 to 12 - Embryos move between horns	Implantation occurs but all embryos die before day 35 and are absorbed	Sow not in pig, pseudo pregnancy. Return between 40 - 70 days
	1 - 2 embryos survive after day 35	Litter size 1 - 2 pigs born Delayed farrowing
Day 12 to 14 - Implantation (pregnancy) 5mm - 10mm	All embryos die after day 35 mummified A foetus dies after day 35	Sow pregnant but does not farrow Mummified

(Fig.5-14)

SIGNS OF OESTRUS	REASONS FOR FAILURE TO DETECT OESTRUS
Swelling of the vulva, redness and small amounts of mucous. Changes in vocal sounds. Standing immobile next to the boar. Standing when back pressure is applied with ears pricked. Standing when mounted by other females. Seeking contact with a boar Nosing the flank of other females or boars. Smelling the prepuce. Permitting the boars to mount and mate.	Lack of understanding and appreciation by the stockperson. Lack of experience. Overwork. Insufficient time to observe animals. Lack of light. Dark environment. Poor lighting resulting in poor observation. Cold or excessively hot summer weather. Too many gilts in the group and poor observation. No boar stimulation. Apprehension from either pig persons or other animals. Pain, particularly in joints and muscles. Lack of libido in the boar. Boar too heavy. Illness in the boar. Female not expected in heat.

responsible for the outward signs of heat. After ovulation oestrogen levels drop as the progesterone rises. Females with high levels of progesterone in the first three days after mating are more likely to create an improved environment for the survival of the fertilised egg. High levels of feed intake in the first two to three days may lower progesterone levels and thereby result in an increase in embryo mortality.

Key factors that stop the hormone surge and produce anoestrus in the gilt
- Age - immaturity.
- Bad external environment
- Bullying. Stress.
- Disease.
- High stocking density.
- Lameness. Pain.
- No contact with the boar and his pheromones.
- Poor light.
- Poor nutrition.
- Poor management.
- Sunburn. Skin damage.

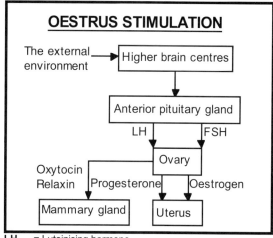
(Fig.5-15)

Anoestrus problems in gilts or sows can be a major cause of economic loss, the significance of which is often unrecognised.

The most common problem is failure of the stockperson to recognise oestrus. Field experience shows that approximately one third of anoestrus gilts examined at slaughter have been cycling, one third are pregnant and only one third are actually in anoestrus.

If there is an oestrus problem in your gilts then consider the following five areas and identify the potential failures in the system.

Key points to stimulating oestrus in the gilt
- Develop a successful management system
- Create good health
- Acclimatisation of new gilts - create a low stress environment
- Provide good nutrition
- Satisfy the gilt's physiological needs

Develop a successful management system

It is important to develop a predictable method of management, an example of which is shown in Fig.5-17.

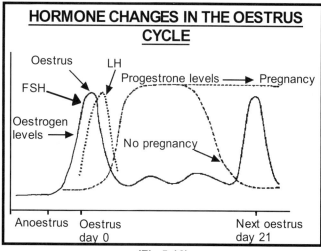
(Fig.5-16)

Note this starts with a large group of gilts, fed on a good grower diet ad lib to 90kg weight and given mature boar or V-boar (vasectomised) contact. In some herds however, particularly those with a very lean genotype, it may be better to feed a dry sow diet with a lower lysine level (0.7%) to increase fat deposition. The rate of growth and nutrition also needs to be considered if leg weakness is a problem. The type of nutritional intake becomes an important variable. Does the gilt respond to the existing system of feeding and management? If she does not then make a change. A P2 fat measurement of at least 18mm should be achieved by point of mating. Heat is observed during the initial period in the holding pool and once gilts have been identified at their first oestrus they should be ear tagged and moved into the service area in small groups of no more than six. The stocking density should provide for approximately 2.7m^2 per animal.

> *The most common "cause" of anoestrus is either:*
> *Failure to detect heat - or the gilt is already pregnant!*

The stages of the oestrus cycle
DAY 0 - 1 **Proestrus** - This is the period just prior to standing for mating. The vulva reddens and the gilt becomes sexually active.
DAYS 1 - 3 **Oestrus** - The gilt stands firmly to the boar.
DAYS 3 - 6 **Metoestrus** - The corpus luteum develops and produces progesterone and the period of sexual activity disappears.
DAYS 6 - 18 **Proestrus** - The quiet period prior to the next oestrus.
DAYS 18 - 22 **Oestrus again.**

Key points to a good gilt management system :
- Ear tag all gilts and record them as they come into heat.
- Vaccinate gilts against porcine parvovirus in the holding pool at around 90kg as you tag them.
- Move cull sows at weaning into this pool because as they come into heat urine containing oestrogen acts as a stimulus. An alternative technique is to spray urine from sows in heat onto the noses of anoestrus gilts.
- Preferably use an old vasectomised boar in the holding pool for intermittent periods of 10 days. If you use an entire boar - be sure he cannot mate gilts
- Change the boar in the holding pool of gilts regularly every 7-10 days.
- Alternatively expose the gilts to the boar for 20 minutes daily under observation. Only use mature boars.
- A high stocking density of less than 1.4m^2 per animal will have a marked depressant effect on oestrus.
- Provide a minimum of 10-14 hours of light per day, that is adequate to read a newspaper at floor level and 10-14 hours of darkness.
- Make sure pens are clean, dry and draught free and not in heavy shadows.
- Make sure there are no disease problems e.g. worms, mange, enteric or respiratory diseases.
- Determine the most responsive feeding programme and ad lib feed 2-3 weeks prior to expected matings.
- Acclimatise the gilts to your farm.

A GILT MANAGEMENT SYSTEM TO PRODUCE OESTRUS

Mature boar contact or V boar. → Holding pool. 6-30 gilts for 6-8 weeks. — Gilts enter at 75-90kg live weight.

Observe heat, eartag and record. — Acclimatise to organisms on the farm with old boars and/or young, growing pigs.

M O V E

Mature boar contact. — Service pool 3-6 gilts. — Sight of the boar. Smell of the boar. Provide light for 14 hours a day.

Ad libitum feed/exercise. — Allow 2.7m^2 per gilt

V = vasectomised — Oestrus

(Fig.5-17)

Create good health

The health status and nutrition of the gilt is very important in deciding whether she will come into oestrus or not. Look at the group of gilts. Are they a good weight for age or is growth variable or poor? If this is the case is there any clinical evidence of disease, mange for example, which may be responsible for anoestrus. Active respiratory diseases, or previous pneumonia, heart sac infection or pleurisy can inhibit puberty and the onset of oestrus. Atrophic rhinitis can destroy the sensitivity of the nose and therefore the response to pheromones (male hormones). If gilts are regularly moved into continually populated pens, heavy parasite burdens and coccidia can build up that can interfere with the digestive process. Anoestrus problems have been associated with these.

> *Remember a happy comfortable gilt is a fertile one.*

Acclimatisation of Gilts

Gilts that you introduce to your herd from elsewhere must be "acclimatised" over a period of up to 6 to 8 weeks prior to mating. This acclimatisation allows the gilts to adjust to your feed, housing and management system but above all to those pathogenic organisms enzootic in your herd that they may have no immunity to. Major problems arise when gilts from high health status herds (e.g. a herd free from EP, App, PRRS, AD/PR, AR) are put straight into a herd in which these infections are present and active. The gilts become ill and fail to

> *Never serve on first oestrus unless you want a poor litter.*

come in heat or fail to conceive. They may be made permanently infertile. In such cases vaccination of the gilts on arrival against, for e.g. EP, AD/PR, App and even in extreme cases *H. parasuis*, help the acclimatisation and possibly allow it to be shortened. A period of medicated feed - at half to three quarters therapeutic level may also help, say, for the first three weeks. Even when the incoming gilts are from a herd thought to be of similar status to your own, a minimum of three weeks acclimatisation is necessary.

If possible (and its not possible on many weaner producer farms) the incoming gilts should be segregated from the main herd for at least the first three weeks of acclimatisation. Some seedstock suppliers insist on this. It gives time to remove the gilts off your farm if disease breaks out in the source herd. The process of acclimatisation involves exposing the group of gilts to likely sources of virus or bacterial contamination. The exact procedures depend upon the diseases present in your herd compared with the herd of origin.
The following should be considered:

- Identify the diseases the gilt has been exposed to in the donor herd and those present in your herd.
- Decide whether the gilts move into isolation or direct into the herd. If the latter place them in a pen with separate drainage and air space for 4 to 6 weeks and use separate boots and protective clothing.
- Parvovirus - Vaccinate the gilts 2-3 weeks prior to mating additionally expose them to grower faeces (8-16 weeks of age). Place 3.3kg into the pen three times a week.
- Aujeszky's disease - Vaccinate on arrival.
- TGE - If gilts are naive vaccinate in isolation if your herd carries the virus or if no vaccine is available expose them to weaner faeces soon after arrival.
- Congenital tremor - Expose the gilts to faeces from the farrowing house three times a week. Wipe the vulva of recently served sows with tissues to collect semen secretions and place these in the pen three times a week.
- Rotavirus - Expose the gilts to weaner faeces three times a week.
- Atrophic rhinitis - Vaccinate on arrival.
- Erysipelas - Vaccinate on arrival.
- *E. coli* - Expose gilts three times a week to weaner and/or farrowing house faeces. Vaccinate during pregnancy.
- Leptospirosis - Vaccinate on arrival.
- Enzootic pneumonia - If the incoming pigs come from a herd free from EP vaccinate prior to arrival or well before if possible.
- Porcine reproductive respiratory syndrome - Where possible buy in sero-positive gilts into a sero-positive herd. If gilts are naive either vaccinate whilst in isolation on arrival or expose to an infected environment on the farm for one to two hours. A building containing pigs 6 to 12 weeks of age is ideal. Expose naive gilts to PRRS at six weeks prior to mating. An alternate is to house a small number of pigs in the isolation premises.
- Judge the result of acclimatisation by the response. Avoid using placenta for feed-back it can spread disease and may increase the risk of cannibalism a farrowing.

Checklists for the health of your gilts
Assess health and disease. Do you have:
- Variable growth
- Coughing
- Evidence of rhinitis
- Mange
- Pneumonia
- Lameness and stiffness on movement
- Failure of the gilt to stand to the boar - Osteochondrosis or leg weakness
- Poor feed intake or an incorrect diet.

> *By 210 days of age good fertile gilts should have come into oestrus.*

> *If a gilt has not come into oestrus by 240 days consider culling her. She is telling you she is infertile.*

Provide good nutrition

The methods of feeding the gilt and the composition of the diet will depend on the genotype. They will also depend on the environmental needs of the gilt relative to housing, temperature and insulation of the buildings. To determine the best system requires a degree of trial and error on the farm - the objective being to produce the second or third oestrus cycle within a predetermined time span so that the service programme can be accomplished satisfactorily.

Key points to success:
- Gilts should arrive on the farm at approximately 85kg and be fed a dry sow diet until 100kg. This will also allow time for acclimatisation.
- It is necessary to increase backfat in the modern genotype to 18-20mm at the P2 measurement. This is best carried out feeding a low lysine ration, such as that contained in a sow breeder ration (13.4MJ DE/kg and 0.8% lysine). Feed to appetite.
- Approximately 2-3 weeks prior to moving into the service area for mating ad lib feeding should take place. This is to maximise ovulation rate. Use a good lactator or grower diet containing 14MJ DE/kg and 1% lysine.
- Low protein, low energy, or poor quality diets in the period leading up to puberty will often produce a deep state of anoestrus that in some cases is permanent. Assess the response to the diet used.
- Do not leave gilts in a finisher house to point of service, many will never cycle and nutritional requirements may not be satisfied.

Satisfy the gilt's physiological needs

Oestrus should commence from approximately 165-200 days of age. Movement from one pen to another with close boar contact provides the greatest stimulus.

Key Points to Success:
- Age at puberty is dependant on breed. Pure breeds are often slower coming into oestrus.
- House a vasectomised boar in the group.
- The major chemical substances that stimulate oestrus are pheromones found in boar's saliva and in preputial secretions. These are more powerful in old boars, however make sure they cannot mate.
- Provide direct pheromone contact.
- Rotate boars to give a different contact every 7-10 days.
- Provide a dry, warm well lit environment. Would you be comfortable in your gilt housing? If so, then it will satisfy the gilt.
- Provide 14 hours of good light (you should be able to read a newspaper in the darkest corner).
- Wherever possible always move gilts to the boar for contact.

A SUMMARY OF THE CAUSES OF ANOESTRUS

Cause	Relative Importance	
	Gilts	Sows
Large groups / Badly matched groups / High stocking densities	+++	++
Confinement stalls	+++	+
No boar contact	+++	+
Genetic	+	-
Poor photo stimulation	+++	+
Catabolic state	+++	+++
High temperatures	+	+++

- not very important   +++ very important

Parasites, Poor diet, Food spoilage, Illness → Predispose to → Dietary deficiencies or catabolism → Anoestrus

Poor Environment ← Damp floor, Draughts, Poor bedding, Low air temp

Light

To maintain a viable pregnancy requires constant daylight length. Ideally this should be 12-16 hours per day. Light intensity experienced by the sow can be affected by a number of environmental inadequacies, for example, poor lighting in the first place, followed by fly faeces and dust on lamps gradually reducing the availability of light. High walls surrounding animals, or automatic feeders in front of sows producing shadows. A simple tip here is to make sure that you can read a newspaper in the darkest parts of the building at sow eye level. If not, then problems may start. Painting the roofs and walls white to increase the reflection of light is one way of improving the environment and on a number of occasions abortions have ceased after such simple improvements.

What you need to know about light
- Gilts exposed to 14-18 hours light:
  - Reach puberty earlier.
  - They are a lighter weight at puberty.
  - There is no difference in ovulation rate.
  - Both gilts and the boar are sexually more active.
- In lactation:
  - 16 hours of light increases weaning weights.
  - There is no effect on numbers weaned.
  - Milk yield is increased.
  - 16 hours is recommended at a 360 lux level.
- The weaning to service interval is reduced if 16 hours of light is given after weaning with a continuous light intensity of 250 lux
- Sows are on heat longer when exposed to more light.
- Light has no effect on litter size but absorption of embryo and foetuses may occur in poor lighting during early pregnancy.
- During the dry period a minimum of 220 lux is required for 14 hours a day.
- Fluorescent light is nearer to natural light than incandescent lighting.
- In a building 2.4m high and 4.9m wide a continuous row of fluorescent lights is necessary. As a guide 150 watts is required for every 1.5m.
- The light must be placed over the sow's heads.
- Make sure sows are not exposed to decreasing daylight lengths.
- Provided 8-10 hours of darkness after a period of light.

Anoestrus in the sow

The act of weaning the sow or even removing just 3-4 piglets increases the pressure of milk in the mammary gland and this causes the udder or relevant gland to stop production. This mechanism causes the hormones that promote milk production to cease, thus allowing the development of the follicle stimulating hormone and luteinising hormones, to bring the sow back into oestrus or heat. Provided the sow comes into heat and is served within 6 or 7 days of weaning then she is likely to have a high conception rate, good fertility and litter size. The length of the weaning to service interval is now recognised as being associated with reproductive efficiency and some sows mated 7 and 14 days after weaning are sub fertile with poor litter size and farrowing rates. A high proportion of single matings also occur at this time. If you have a reproductive problem associated with poor litter size and high numbers of repeat matings check the average weaning to first service interval across the herd (5.5 days is ideal) and analyse the results by parity or litter number. The farrowing rate loss in the sub fertile period may be as much as 10% and litter size may drop by up to a pig a litter. The first litter gilt is often a major problem in this respect and the delay in the weaning to service interval can compromise litter size by up to three pigs per litter. If the weaning to service interval is extended and associated with lowered fertility always check the newly weaned gilt, then follow through the checklist below to identify those factors that may be important on your farm.

Anoestrus in the sow - A checklist:
- Identify from records whether this relates to a particular parity.
- Make sure during lactation that the sow does not lose body weight if possible and certainly no more than 15kg. Weigh sows after farrowing and again at weaning to check this. Try to achieve weight gain.
- The most common cause of anoestrus or delayed oestrus is loss of body condition, particularly in the first two - three weeks of lactation. Feed intake here drives the weaning to service interval and subsequent fertility and stimulates the primordial follicles to determine ovulation rate into the next litter.
- Feed the sow from three days post farrowing to appetite, with a high energy diet, particularly if she is of a lean genotype.
- The diet should contain at least 14.2 MJ DE/kg, 18% protein and 1.1 lysine. A good grower type diet could be used.
- Make sure that overfeeding in lactation does not cause inappetance.
- Make sure that there is easy access to water, with a nipple flow of at least 2 litres per minute. Sows will drink up to 40 litres a day. Test the nipple drinkers and see how long it would take the sow to stand and drink. She could stand for 2 hours per day! Give the sow 4.5 litres twice daily into her trough.
- Always remove uneaten feed from the trough because in a warm farrowing house fermentation takes place within 3-4 hours.
- If there is a second litter problem, feed a weaner ration to the lactating gilts as half the daily total intake.
- If the sow is correctly fed and managed during lactation, she should come into heat in the fertile period.
- Are sows comfortable in the farrowing house? A too low temperature will cause the sow to lose weight in spite of possibly eating slightly more. Experience shows that there are no advantages to cold farrowing houses. Aim for around 20ºC (68-70ºF).
- Avoid any environmental factors that will cause the sow to lose weight, for example wet farrowing pens, high airflow and evaporative cooling, water shortage and inappetance associated with disease and spoiled feed.
- Avoid weaning more than 10% of piglets from the sow during lactation because this may stimulate oestrus and poor ovulation with delayed oestrus again at weaning and sub-fertility. Feed the sow from weaning to point of service ad libitum with the lactator diet.

> **Sows that come into heat during suckling are sub fertile. Don't serve them.**

- Do not mix first litter females with older sows if group housing is practised.
- If group housing is practised, introduce a large quiet boar into the group on the day of weaning.
- Where sows are weaned into stalls, maintain a temperature of 20ºC (70ºF), provide plenty of close nose contact with boars, check there is no evidence of mastitis at weaning time and provide a dry environment with low air flow. Assess the comfort of the sow, by her looks and posture.
- In loose-housed sows allow at least 3.4m^2 per sow at mixing and from weaning to service.
- If sows are exposed to temperatures above 24ºC (75ºF) feed intake becomes compromised. For continual temperatures above 26ºC (79ºF) it is necessary to adopt drip cooling or other evaporative cooling techniques.
- If you think a gilt or sow is on heat and she will not stand always try another boar but leave a gap of half an hour before doing so, because gilts in particular may only show a high, intense oestrus for 10-15 minute periods
- If litter size is poor in the first litter gilt it may be worth while to skip or miss the first heat after weaning and serve on the next one, particularly if such animals are coming into heat in the sub fertile period.

> **Most reproductive failure is associated with disadvantaged females**

Group 2 Losses - Ovulation and Egg Production

Refer back to Fig.5-14 to note the areas of fertility failure. Group 2 losses are related to poor egg production or poor ovulation. If there is a failure here the changes will include a low litter size, litter size variation (an increase in litters with total born of less than 9), or a possible decrease in farrowing rate as a result of insufficient embryos to maintain the pregnancy. Use the farm records to identify the group loss by referring to the factors listed in Fig.5-18. These will then indicate which group or groups are involved.

Key factors to maximising ovulation rate:
- Ensure the gilt is fed ad lib for at least two weeks prior to service.
- Keep breeding females that have the best hybrid vigour and that are from the most prolific dam lines. The pure bred female is less fertile than the cross bred. There are considerable variations in fertility between different ancestral lines and types of crossbreeds.

THE STAGES IN THE REPRODUCTIVE CYCLE ASSOCIATED WITH INFERTILITY						
Problem	Oestrus	Ovulation	Fertilisation	Implantation	Maturity	Farrowing
Litter size poor	YES	YES	YES	YES	YES	NO
Litter size * variation increased	YES	YES	YES	YES	NO	NO
Stillbirths increased	NO	NO	NO	NO	YES	YES
Mummies increased	NO	NO	NO	NO	YES	NO
Farrowing rate depressed	NO	YES	YES	YES	NO	NO
Abortions increased	NO	NO	NO	YES	YES	NO
W/S interval	YES	YES	YES	YES	NO	NO
Delayed returns increased	NO	YES Regular	YES Regular	YES Regular Irregular	NO	NO

* % of litters with total numbers < 9. Normal levels <12% in sows and 12 to 18% in gilts. W/S = Days from weaning to first service

(Fig.5-18)

- Breed from females with records of high litter size merit.
- Feed a good quality diet during lactation and in the case of the gilt for three weeks prior to mating.
- Do not serve breeding females which have any signs of disease.
- Check parasite levels. Heavy burdens can impair digestion and the uptake of nutrients and be responsible for poor body condition, catabolism and anoestrus.
- See the checklists for anoestrus in gilts, and anoestrus sows.
- Maximise feed intake in the first lactation.
- Manage the sow so that she comes into oestrus during the early fertile period. (Fig.5-19)

Group 3 Losses - Fertilisation

These are associated with failure or poor quality of fertilisation or conception. If total failure occurs then the sow will repeat on a normal cycle of 18-22 days. If however conception is poor, due for example to overworked boars, then either litter size or its variation will be affected, or a decrease in farrowing rate will be seen with increased regular returns, together with an increase in irregular returns.

Group 3 failures mean increased repeats at 18-22 days and or poor litter size.

Within an hour after service, contractions of the muscles in the womb move the sperm rapidly up to the openings of the oviducts (fallopian tubes). Once this area (the utero-tubal junction) is filled with sperm few more can enter until ovulation occurs. This suggests that the first mating may well be the important one in the ultimate reproductive performance. It then becomes an arguable point in terms of litter size whether any subsequent matings are of great value. (See single mating).

Sperm have to remain at the utero-tubal junction for about 6 hours and develop (capacitation) before they are fully able to fertilise the ova. Since the unfertilised ova can only remain viable in the oviducts for 8-10 hours it

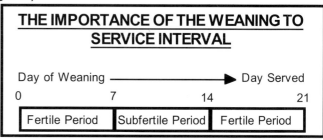

(Fig.5-19)

is important that mating is carried out at the correct time i.e. <10 hours before ovulation (egg release). Ovulation takes place two-thirds through the heat period usually about 40 hours after the true standing heat started.

Key factors in maximising fertilisation

- A complete failure will obviously occur if the animal is not served. This is not as silly as it sounds. A service house person may well think a sows has been served when infact it has not.
- To ensure maximum meeting of sperm and egg, only carry out the first mating when the sow is standing "rock hard" or completely immobile.
- Do not serve sows in the early part of the oestrus period.
- Only use a boar once every 24 hours.
- Ensure that the boar's penis is entered into the vagina and locked into the cervix. Ensure that there is no leak back of semen.
- View the boar from behind and look above his testicles to ensure that he ejaculates, by evidence of the urethra pulsating.
- Failure to place semen into the womb results in poor fertilisation.
- To ensure maximum fertility and litter size serve in the fertile period, that is, from weaning up to day 7.
- Ensure that sows are fed no more than 2kg of feed for the first 2 days post-service. High levels of feed may reduce progesterone levels and this may result in

Do not feed high levels for 48 hours post-service (>2kg) or you can expect some poor litters

higher embryo mortality. When the sow is in oestrus, she is under the influence of high levels of oestrogens. Towards the end of the heat period these drop and progesterone levels start to rise. Sows with high levels of progesterone provide a good nutritious environment for the fertilised embryo and potentially good litters. Some sows with low progesterone levels will have increased levels of embryo mortality

- The fertilised eggs remain in the oviducts for approximately 48 hours before they migrate down to the horns of the womb. It is safe to change the sow's environment during his time.
- Any management change, mixing, or movement should therefore take place in this immediate post-service period only.

A return at 18-23 days indicates either group 2 or group 3 losses or failure of implantation in group 4. If there is progressive loss in group 3, then litter size will be low, there will be an increase in litter size variation and a decrease in farrowing rates. Fig.5-20 demonstrates the effects of the timing of insemination and ovulation and subsequent results. If insemination takes place in the early part of the oestrus period, even when the sow will stand to the boar, both conception rate and numbers born are compromised. Study Fig.5-14 again because it will help you to understand how records can pinpoint the specific time of the failure. With this information the management practices and contributing factors are identified on the farm and this allows corrective action to be taken.

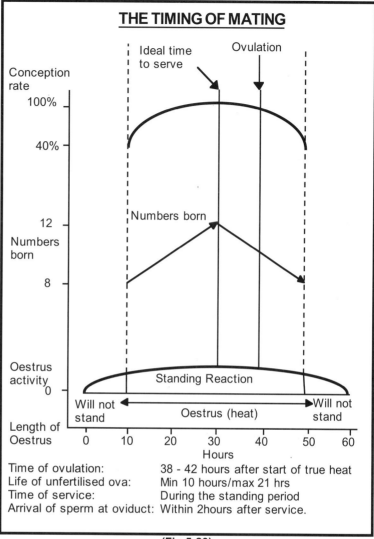

(Fig.5-20)

Fig.5-20 provides a good guide to the optimum time of mating but be aware that there is considerable variation between individual sows particularly in the time of ovulation and the time that they come on heat. Most sows come on heat in the early hours of the morning, around 4.00 am which means that the optimum time to mate them would be 30 hours later, 10 o'clock on the following day.

Repeat matings on a normal 18 - 22 day cycle

Possible causes and corrective factors for group 3 and some group 4 losses

Twenty one day repeats indicate that pregnancy failure is occurring from service to approximately 10 days post-service. An assessment of management and mating procedures are therefore necessary, particularly to identify any form of stress on the sow.

The target level of efficiency in this category would be 5-8% of repeat matings. Fig.5-21 can be used to highlight areas of importance. The role and presence of the boar is particularly important in group 3 and 4 losses. There are three golden rules relating to his use.

- Only use each boar once every 24 hours.
- Only serve a sow when she is standing absolutely "rock hard" or still.
- Ensure there is a good insemination, and quality of mating. (1 = good, 2 = moderate, 3 = poor).

A delayed return indicates progressive embryo failure starting from 4 - 30 days post-service.

Group 4 Losses - Implantation

Approximately 2 days after fertilisation, the embryos, which are now beginning to increase rapidly in size, move down into the two horns of the womb. Over the next 5-7 days they migrate from one horn to the other,

FACTORS AFFECTING REPEAT MATINGS ON A NORMAL CYCLE (18-22 DAYS)

Management of Sows/Gilts

Factors resulting in increased return rate:
- Short lactation length of < 20 days.
- Low feed intake in lactation.
- Loss of body weight in lactation.
- Weaning to service interval of 7-14 days.
- Excess stress at weaning, particularly group housed sows.
- Poor environments at weaning, dampness, draughts.
- Low light intensity after weaning.
- Short light periods after weaning.
- Breed or type of sow e.g. meishan cross breeds are highly fertile.
- Heavy parasite burden, catabolism and thin sows.
- Poor artificial insemination techniques.
- Poor checking of mating procedures.
- Old sows developing cystic ovaries.
- Failure to acclimatise gilts.
- Vulval discharges post-service.
- Bad management procedures for 21 days post-service
- High stocking density in group housed sows.
- Lack of boar contact post-service.

Actions to reduce return rate.
- Wean over 21 days.
- Consider culling all sows that return and pre-plan an increased intake of gilts.
- Maximise feed intake from days 3 to 14 of lactation.
- Consider culling sows that come into heat at 8 days post-weaning or later.
- Reduce stress at and after weaning.
- Improve post-weaning and post-service environments.
- If sows are group housed provide >2.7m^2 floor space per sow.
- Maintain high light intensity post-weaning of 14 hours per day
- Check every service to ensure it is properly done.
- Check AI techniques.
- Feed a maximum of 2kg feed for 3 days post-service.
- Feed lactation diet ad lib from 3 days post-weaning to service (at least 14.2MJ DE/kg 1% lysine).
- Feed to body condition thereafter.
- Check repeats by parity. Cull older sows that repeat.
- Cull repeat breeders
- Prevent sows loosing body weight in lactation to maintain the W/S interval at <7 days.

Management of Boars

Factors resulting in increased return rate
- Allowing the boar to serve a sow before she is fully in heat.
- Serving too early in heat.
- Do not use mature boars more than once a day every day.
- Multiple mating leading to overworked boars.
- Failure to identify and remove infertile boars.
- Using boars with low sperm counts and sperm abnormalities.
- Using young boars with poor fertility.
- Overusing young boars.
- Ill health, fever, lameness,.
- Hot environment.
- Unsupervised services in which the boar does not serve properly.
- Dirty services resulting in vulval discharges.

Actions to reduce return rate.
- Only commence mating after the sow has been fully in heat for 12 - 24 hours.
- Check that every mating is properly carried out.
- Ensure that every service is as hygienic as possible.
- Mate the sow twice only, 24 hours apart.
- * Do not use any boar twice in the same day.
- * Check the fertility records of every boar.
- Cull boars with poor fertility.
- Introduce new young boars gradually to the mating routine.
- Cross mate when using young boars for the first 4 services.
- Match the age and weight of the boar to the female.
- Examine every boar regularly for good health and physical fitness.
- Maintain boar contact for at least the first 6 weeks of pregnancy.

Diseases that can affect normal returns to heat are mentioned here but only for completeness. You are referred to chapter 6.

Diseases / Conditions
- Endometritis - womb infection.
- Infection of the fallopian tubes.
- Infection of the ovaries and surrounding tissues.
- Generalised disease and sickness.

Specific Diseases
- Erysipelas.
- Fever in the boar. This may affect sperm for a 5 week period.
- Leptospirosis.
- Porcine parvovirus (uncommon).
- Pneumonia.
- PRRS.
- Swine influenza.

* Keep a boar calendar ticking off every service against every boar. If you always cross-mate (i.e. use 2 different boars on every sow) you will have difficulty identifying infertile boars.

(Fig.5-21)

depending on numbers, so that they are spaced evenly between the horns. If the embryos die by day 4, there is no further development of the pregnancy and the sow returns on a normal cycle at 18-23 days. If less than 5 viable embryos remain in the womb at or around 12-14 days of age (the time of implantation) they are insufficient to maintain a pregnancy (Fig.5-14). In such cases there is likely to be a delayed return of between 24 and 30 days. Between days 12 and 14, the fertilised embryos become attached to the lining of the womb with the development of the placenta. Hormones are then produced which signal to the sow that she is pregnant. The corpus luteum in the ovaries increases in size and produces the pregnancy hormone progesterone. This stops the next oestrus cycle and pregnancy continues.

Irregular repeat matings occurring

Returns to heat can occur on a regular cycle every 18 - 22 days or on an irregular or abnormal cycle of 23 - 36 days or longer. Sometimes sows thought to be close to term (approaching farrowing time) are found to be not in pig. One major reason is as follows. If there are insufficient embryos to establish a pregnancy at 14 days, (less than 5) they progressively die off, are absorbed and the sow will return at an irregular interval. This could vary anywhere between 23 and 100 days post-service. However, once pregnancy has been established and embryos continue to die, then as long as one piglet remains alive the pregnancy will continue to term. Thus, if we have very small litters born of 3, 4 or 5 piglets and no mummified ones we know that there have been major problems occurring between approximately days 14 and 30 post-service. Factors that need to be considered with sows found not to be pregnant with delayed repeats are highlighted in Fig.5-22. The normal level should be less than 3% of matings.

Check the various points in Fig.5-22 for corrective action in your herd. Boar factors are usually of low priority for abnormal repeats because the failures are much more likely to be of a maternal nature. However, the

> **Examine the vulvas of sows post mating, between days 14 and 21 for any tackiness or vulval discharge. Do such sows return? If so read chapter 6.**

overuse of boars resulting in poor conception and poor viability of embryos with progressive embryo loss should not be overlooked.

Any generalised disease of the sow could result in embryo mortality. Unless there are clinical signs in the herd, such factors will usually be of an individual nature. This highlights the importance of individual records and the need to collect data on the farrowing rate loss analysis sheet.

For specific information regarding the diseases refer to chapter 6. For clarity between infectious and non infectious causes also study Fig.5-23. Pregnancy failure from point of service to the point of implantation is often due to ascending infection of the womb (endometritis). In such cases a clear or opaque light discharge of the vulva will be seen 14-21 days post-service with such animals repeating. See chapter 6 Vulval discharges.

Group 5 Losses - Foetal Death and the Mummified Pig

From approximately 30 days of age through to 115 days the foetus is maturing. This means that the skeletal system is developing and if the piglet dies, it is not completely absorbed and a mummified foetus remains. The approximate age when a mummified pig has died can be determined by measuring the length from the crown of the head to the rump or tail base. (Fig.5-24)

There are two possible causes of mummies. First, a piglet dies because there is a large litter and insufficient space in the womb. Second, there is infectious disease, usually of a progressive nature, at any stage during the period of pregnancy. In the first instance, a study of the records will show that the mummified pigs are occurring in large normal litters. For example, a litter size of 14 alive, 1 dead, 1 mummified is of no significance provided the remainder of the litter is normal and healthy. If however, the litter size is 6 born alive, 2 dead and 4 mummified, this indicates disease during the pregnancy causing mortality. By measuring the size of the mummified pigs, we can determine at what stage in pregnancy the disease occurred. Alternately, if the mummified pigs are of a variable length this is evidence of progressive disease over a period of time. Some viral infections affect the foetus from 30 days onwards and progressively spread during the period of pregnancy. Porcine parvovirus is a typical example.

Once the piglet inside the womb reaches 70 days of age it becomes immuno-competent. This means that its immune system has started to develop and therefore can respond to any infection that challenges it and attempt to protect itself. For example, if pigs inside the womb are

FACTORS AFFECTING REPEAT MATINGS ON AN ABNORMAL CYCLE (> 23 days)

Management of Sows/gilts

Factors resulting in increased return rate.
- As for those listed in Fig.5-21.
- Low ovulation rate.
- Poor conception with progressive embryo mortality.
- Implantation from day 14 with progressive embryo failure.
- No boar pheromone contact during pregnancy.
- Management induced stress from day 2-21 post-service.
- Seasonal infertility. Poor light.
- Increasing / decreasing length of daylight.
- Effects of excessive sunlight.
- Embryo loss due to high levels of feed for 72 hours post-service.

Actions to reduce return rate.
- As for those listed in Fig.5-21.
- Check feed intake in lactation.
- Provide boar contact for > 21 days post-service.
- Reduce stress from 2 - 25 days post-service.
- Provide a good intensity of light 14 hours a day.
- Reduce exposure to sunlight.
- Assess the effects of breed particularly outdoors.
- Feed well from 2 - 21 days post-service.
- Assess records and history of affected sows.
- Assess the quality of nutrition.

Management of Boars

Factors resulting in increased return rate.
- As for those listed in Fig.5-21.
- Most causes by now are due to maternal failure.

Actions to reduce return rate.
- As for those listed in Fig.5-21.
- Check boar records carefully.
- Check clinical records / observations of the boar.
- Make sure he has contact with pregnant sows from 3 - 30 days.

Diseases that can affect delayed returns to heat are mentioned here but only for completeness. You are referred to chapter 6.

Diseases / Conditions
- Endometritis - womb infection.
- Vulval discharge.
- Infection of the fallopian tubes.
- Infection of the ovaries and surrounding tissues.
- Generalised disease and sickness.
- Infection of the testes.

Specific Diseases
- Aujeszky's disease
- Brucellosis
- Erysipelas.
- Fever in the boar. This may affect sperm for a 5 week period.
- Leptospirosis.
- Porcine parvovirus (uncommon).
- Pneumonia.
- PRRS.
- Swine influenza.

(Fig.5-22)

infected with parvovirus beyond 70 days they respond by producing an immunity and thereby, no disease. By sampling the blood of such piglets at birth, before they have suckled, we can tell from presence or absence of antibodies whether indeed this event had taken place. An alternative to this would be PRRS infection, which does not affect the foetus during the mid period of pregnancy, but only as it becomes immuno-competent after day 70. In this case, the virus actually kills the pigs and therefore there will be evidence of late mummified pigs, death having occurred at any time from day 80 to the point of farrowing. Thus, by studying the numbers relative to total litter size and the time when death must have occurred, we can get a good indication as to possible disease causes.

The Significance of Mummified Pigs

- Large numbers of normal piglets born alive and a few mummified pigs - unlikely to be due to disease.
- Small numbers of piglets alive and large numbers of mummified pigs - more likely to be due to disease.

In group 5 losses, total numbers born will be the same, but numbers alive will be reduced with corresponding increases in still-births and mummified piglets. Litter size variation will be increased, with farrowing rates decreased. Abortions of course can be a major cause of loss in this group and repeats may be regular or irregular.

Detecting Pregnancy

Carrying out pregnancy testing does not influence the outcome of an infertility problem and neither does it improve it, but it does help identify problems and allow corrective actions to be taken. Pregnancy detection will assist in identifying non productive days at a much earlier stage in the pregnancy period thus allowing management action. It will also give peace of mind.

Methods of Pregnancy Diagnosis (PD)

1. Daily observation of the vulva and the behaviour of the female when a boar is present, particularly at 18-22 days post-service.
2. Amplitude depth ultrasound machines.
3. Döppler ultrasound machines.
4. Vaginal biopsy.
5. Serum analysis.
6. Ultrasound scanners.

1. Daily observations for oestrus

After the eggs are fertilised in the fallopian tubes, the embryos move around the two horns of the womb to become equally spaced. Survival of these to day 10 or 11 starts the pregnancy signal but a failure at this time results in a return to oestrus on a slightly delayed cycle of 22-26 days.

Implantation of the embryo commences during days 12-14 and a minimum of 5 embryos are required for pregnancy to continue. If the pregnancy fails at this time the return to oestrus is delayed to 23-38 days because pregnancy has already started.

INFECTIONS THAT CAN PRODUCE MUMMIFIED PIGS:	
* Aujeszky's disease virus	* Porcine parvovirus.
Blue eye disease	SMEDI viruses
Encephalomyocarditis virus	Swine fever
Erysipelas.	Swine influenza
Japanese encephalitis virus	Other one off infections
* PRRS virus	

* Common causes in countries in which they occur

CLINICAL DIFFERENTIATION BETWEEN INFECTIOUS AND NON-INFECTIOUS CAUSES OF REPRODUCTIVE FAILURE

Type of Failure		Non-Infectious	Infectious
Anoestrus		+++	+
Repeats	- at 21 days and no discharge	+++	+
	- at 21 days with discharge	+	+++
Repeats	- 23-28 days	++	++
Abortion	- sow in good health	+++	+
	- with healthy foetuses	++	++
	- with mummified or decomposing	+	+++
Sow not in pig		+++	++
Mummified pigs	- small and variable in size	+	+++
	- large	++	++
Stillbirths	- increased within a normal litter	+++	+
	- with mummified pigs	+	+++

\+ Unlikely cause +++ Likely cause

(Fig.5-23)

If pregnancy is maintained to the completion of implantation and then fails totally with absorption, the sow becomes pseudo-pregnant for a varying period and then comes through not in pig. In many cases there is a positive pregnancy test reading early on only to find the sow is negative later. The sequence of events and the results you can expect with pregnancy diagnosis are shown in Fig.5-25. **Take note that the loss of pregnancy between 15 to 35 days can give false positive test results.**

2. Amplitude tests

These machines are only of value from 28-80 days of pregnancy. Beyond this they lose their sensitivity. Also false positives can often be detected if the bladder is

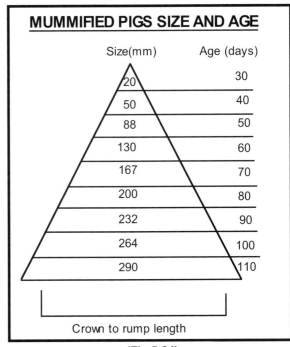

(Fig.5-24)

full and scanning misses the womb.

3. Döppler tests

Döppler ultra sound machines are more accurate and can be used over the whole range of the pregnancy period from 26 days to term. They are the most popular method with a 90% plus accuracy. The sounds detected in early pregnancy arise from the changes in blood flow that take place in the large arteries supplying blood to the womb. Movement of the foetus and the placenta can also be detected together with the foetal heartbeat. Womb infection, embryo absorption or early oestrus can give false positives and of course wrong interpretations of the sounds or inexperience can give rise to wrong interpretations. Demonstration audio tapes are available with the equipment. The technique is described in chapter 15 Pregnancy diagnosis.

4. Vaginal biopsy

This technique involves the removal of a small piece of the vaginal mucous membrane using a special instrument. The instrument is inserted into the vagina 150-300mm pressed into the membrane and the end manipulated to cut off a small piece. The sample is placed in a small container with a special preservative and posted to a laboratory for histological examinations. It is time consuming, expensive and little used.

5. Serum analysis

This can be carried out after day 22 by using a small stylette to puncture the ear vein. A thin capillary tube collects a spot of blood which is then tested for pregnancy hormones. It is time consuming, expensive and little used. Techniques are being developed to examine faeces to detect pregnancy but as yet are not perfected for commercial use.

6. Ultra sound

Scanning equipment is now available similar to that used in humans for detecting pregnancy. It is expensive but very accurate and can be justified for use on large farms.

A Practical Format for Diagnosing Pregnancy on the Farm

1. From service to 21 days maintain close boar contact. Provide boar pheromone contact throughout pregnancy.
2. Observe sows for oestrus daily and particularly on 18-22 days post-service. No oestrus indicates a pregnancy has started. Maintain daily detection throughout pregnancy.
3. Check the vulva daily for tackiness from day 14-21 and thereafter for discharges throughout pregnancy.
4. Test the sow at 28-35 post-service using a döppler machine.

INTERPRETING PREGNANCY TEST RESULTS		
Time Post-service	Observation	Outcome
2-15 days	Oestrus. Sow not pregnant.	Cystic ovaries, cull.
1-18 days	Not possible to detect pregnancy.	Sow may or may not be pregnant.
18-22 days	Sow comes into oestrus.	Sow not pregnant, embryos died at 1-10 days.
18-22 days	Sow not in oestrus. Methods 2 or 3 give -ve PD. Methods 4 or 5 give +ve PD.	Sow pregnant.
23-38 days	Sow in oestrus. Methods 2, 3, and 4 could give either +ve or -ve test results.	Sow now not pregnant, embryos died 12-18 days but pregnancy started.
28-35 days	No oestrus. Methods 2,3, and 4 all give +ve PD's.	Sow pregnant.
30-110 days	Oestrus. Methods 2,3 and 5 could have given either +ve or -ve test results previously.	Embryos died at 15-35 days, a false pregnancy due to embryo loss.

(Fig.5-25)

5. A positive test - leave the sow where she is.
6. A negative test - move the sow to the service area for close observation and boar contact.
7. A doubtful test - repeat 7 days later.
8. Pregnancy test the sow again between 40-47 days using a döppler machine. Follow as for 6.
9. Visually check the sow for abdominal enlargement, teat and mammary vein enlargement from day 80 of pregnancy.

Records help us diagnose disease

Abortion and Seasonal Infertility

Embryo loss and abortion

Embryo loss occurs when there is death of embryos followed by absorption, or expulsion. Healthy embryos grow into foetuses. Abortion means the premature expulsion of a dead or non-viable foetus.

There is often alarm when an abortion is seen but it should be remembered that there can be loss of embryos at any time during early pregnancy, which often goes unseen.

Embryo loss or abortion can be considered in three main groups:

First, during the period from fertilisation to implantation; second, during the period of implantation at around 14 days post-service to 35 days; and finally, during the period of maturation, which results in premature farrowings. It can be seen therefore that losses can take place at any stage from approximately 14 days after mating, when implantation has taken place, through to 110 days of pregnancy.

The maintenance of pregnancy

Pregnancy is maintained due to hormonal changes initiated by the implantation of embryos at day 14.

These changes allow the corpus luteum (the body from which the egg is released) in the ovary to develop and produce the pregnancy hormone progesterone. The presence of the corpus luteum is necessary to maintain the pregnancy throughout the whole of the gestation period. The loss or failure of the corpus luteum through any cause initiates the farrowing process, hence an abortion, or if near to term a premature farrowing.

Abortions and their cost

Natural biological failures of pregnancy due to a variety of causes occur across all species. In healthy normal sow herds abortions observed by the stockpeople are normally less than 1 per 100 pregnancies. The cost of an abortion can be calculated quite easily, taking into account the cost of feeding the sow during a pregnancy period and the loss of margin over feed on the loss of the piglets. For example, with feed costing £160 per tonne and 2.2 litters per sow, per year it would have cost £72 in feed to produce a litter. 10 pigs reared in the herd at a margin of £25 per pig over feed would have yielded £250, giving a total cost per abortion of £322 if it occurred near the end of the pregnancy period.

Methods of investigation

It is worthwhile monitoring the levels of abortion in your herd continually and comparing them to the normal levels. The following information should be recorded with each abortion:
- Sow number.
- Parity.
- Boar used.
- Date of service.
- Date of Abortion.
- Housing.
- Feed and amounts given.
- Clinical observations of the sow and any disease history.
- Condition of the aborted piglets - alive fresh, recently dead or mummified.

If you are using the farrowing rate loss analysis sheet illustrated earlier in this chapter you will be doing most of this anyway.

It is important to study the herd history and environment. For example, is there a seasonal effect or an association with a particular area of the housing or management practice? You should also note the clinical state of the sow at the time of abortion. Does she show other clinical signs or is she apparently normal? You should examine the aborted foetuses too. Are they fresh with no signs of any decomposition, or are they decomposing or mummified. Such observations, particularly if recorded over a period, may be of help to your veterinarian in leading to a possible diagnosis of the cause.

There are three parts to the investigations that must be carried out. First, collect information about the individual sows, then request post mortem examinations and serological tests, and finally, assess the clinical evidence and feeding procedures in the herd. The object of these is to identify the area of failure and by management studies, examination of records, clinical examinations, and laboratory tests the cause may be identified.

Post-mortem and laboratory examinations

Fresh, aborted foetuses should be submitted to a competent diagnostic laboratory where examinations can be carried out for evidence of viral and bacterial infections, together with histological examinations and toxic studies. In many cases the end results of post-mortem and serological tests do not identify any particular infectious organism, which may seem disappointing. However, it is useful in telling us what is not present.

Clinical examinations

Of all the examinations carried out, clinical observations are perhaps the most important. Look at the environmental factors in Fig.5-29. Are any of these important? By using the recorded information on individual cases and collating this to the problem group of sows, it then may become possible to differentiate clinically between an infectious and a non infectious cause. Fig.5-23 indicates the likelihood of either of these.

Non Infectious Causes

Seasonal infertility

Experiences have shown that 70% of all abortions fall into this category. Because the sow historically only produced one litter per year, with farrowings during early spring, there is an in-built tendency for the animal not to maintain a pregnancy during the summer and autumn periods. This is well recognised with summer infertility and the autumn abortion syndrome, where environmental factors are likely to cause the corpus luteum to disappear.

A catabolic state

If the metabolism of sows are allowed to progress to a negative energy or catabolic state so that they are having to use their body tissues to maintain the energy equilibrium, then individual susceptible animals may abort. Clinical examinations will identify possible changes in the environment. For example, the removal of bedding, poor quality feeds, or a drop in feed intake. The latter may simply be associated with a change in stockpeople. Outbreaks of abortion may occur when there are changes from pellet feeding to meal feeding, or where feed is presented by volume and not by weight. Wet, damp environments or high air movement cause chilling and increase demands for energy. An important feature of environmental abortions is that the sow remains normal, often eating feed in the morning, and expelling the litter in the afternoon. Some people call these "Farrowing abortions". The aborted foetuses are perfectly normal and the sow shows no signs of illness. The underlying initiating mechanism is regression of the corpus luteum.

Light

Another contributing factor is decreasing daylight length. To maintain a viable pregnancy requires constant daylight length. Ideally this should be 12-16 hours per day. Light intensity experienced by the sow can be affected by a number of environmental inadequacies, for example, poor lighting in the first place, followed by fly faeces and dust on lamps gradually reducing the availability of light. High walls surrounding animals, or automatic feeders in front of sows produce shadows. A simple tip here is to make sure that you can read a newspaper in the darkest parts of the building at sow eye level. If not, then problems may start. Painting the roofs and walls white to increase the reflection of light is one way of improving the environment and on a number of occasions abortions have ceased after such simple improvements.

Abortions, anoestrus and sows found not in pig commonly occur during the period of summer infertility when sunlight is intense and the weather is hot. This is particularly evident in outdoor sows where levels of pregnancy failure may reach 15-30%. In such cases the abortions are so early that the foetuses are either not seen or there is progressive embryo mortality and a delayed return to oestrus. Look for slight mucous discharges from the vulva and if present refer to chapter 6 "Endometritis".

The following factors are important indoors or outdoors as applicable:

- Ultra violet radiation may cause regression of the corpus luteum particularly in white breeds. The outdoor breeding female should always be derived from at least one pigmented parent.
- Provide extensive shades so that the sows can protect themselves from the sun.
- Site the arks in the wind direction so that with open ends cooling can take place.
- Provide extensive well maintained wallows suitably sited so that sows do not have too far to reach them.
- Always maintain boars within the sow groups for the first six weeks of pregnancy at least.
- Increase feed intake from days 3 to 21 after mating.
- Increase the mating programme by 10-15% over the anticipated period of infertility.
- Because boar semen can be affected follow each natural mating 24 hours later by purchased AI.

The boar

A third part of the equation involves the presence of the boar and his pheromones or male chemical hormones. Pheromones are required to maintain pregnancy in individual susceptible disadvantaged sows.

Boar presence in the dry sow accommodation is recommended from the day of service through to the day of farrowing. The boar should be mixed in or have access to the group for at least the first 21 days of pregnancy. There is clear evidence that this will improve farrowing rates particularly if they are associated with summer infertility. If sows are individually housed the boar should be allowed to move down the passages and make social contact daily.

Infectious Causes

These are referred to here for completeness but specific infectious diseases are discussed fully in chapter 6. Fig.5-26 shows those factors that contribute to abortions of either infections or management factors that cause regression of the corpus luteum (luteolysis). Infectious agents can act in several ways. They may invade and kill the foetuses, and/or they may multiply in the placenta cutting off the blood supply to the foetuses, or they may cause a generalised infection of the sow making her feverish and ill resulting in abortion.

Abortions can also be associated with mouldy feeds. To prevent this:

- Always check your feed bins. Are they water tight?
- When were they last inspected internally?
- Do they contain bridged mouldy feed?
- Are the bins filled with warm feed?
- Do you regularly treat the bins to prevent mould growth.
- Are the bags of feed kept in a dry cool or wet warm place?

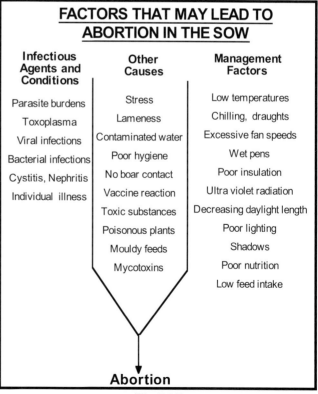

(Fig.5-26)

- If you practice home mixing and wet feeding are the tanks and pipes mould free?
- Are you ever tempted to give feed to sows that has been slightly mouldy.

If you wet feed:
- Do you check the roofs of your mixing tanks to see whether feed splashed on to them has gone mouldy.
- Do you check the pipes?
- Do you check the source materials?
- Do you let liquid components of the mix sit around in hot weather in storage tanks?

Empty feed bins monthly.
Examine internal surfaces monthly
Examine feed daily
Treat Bins regularly with a mould inhibitor.

Abortion can also result from mycotoxins in a feed component (e.g. grain). These toxins are produced by fungi growing when the feed component was itself being grown or stored. Some of them cross the sows placenta and cause abortions. Others affect the sow and result in abortion.

Infectious causes of abortion are listed in Fig.5-27 and are included here purely has a guide or checklist. See chapter 6. Other bacteria not listed here can be associated with sporadic abortion in individual sows for e.g. *E. coli*, klebsiella, streptococci and pseudomonas although if several sows are affected it can start to look like a herd problem.

Some of these other bacteria are normal inhabitants of the vagina and their identification following pathological examinations needs careful interpretation. An emerging syndrome in this category occurs when high numbers of organisms are deposited into the anterior vagina, particularly towards the end of the heat period, by the boar. A variety of opportunist bacteria may be involved including klebsiella, streptococci, staphylococci and leptospira. In such cases careful clinical examination of sows between 14 and 21 days post mating sometimes reveals a tacky discharge on the vulva which may not necessarily be very obvious. Such sows should be identified, and if they are returning out of cycle, it is likely that very early embryonic loss is occurring. See chapter 6 Endometritis. .

Low grade or chronic infections such as cystitis (infection of the bladder) and nephritis (infection of the kidneys) occasionally result in abortion. Lameness and pain, particularly coming from abscesses in the feet or leg weakness (osteochondrosis) can also cause the corpus luteum to regress due to stress. Bullying and fighting are often forgotten as predisposing factors in individual sows. Clinical examinations and study of records are important tools for investigation. The stockpersons opinions and observations are often invaluable.

A checklist is shown in Fig.5-28. If you can satisfy all these criteria you will not have an environmentally induced problem. Fig.5-29 collects together all the precipitating factors associated with the epidemiology of environmentally induced disease.

INFECTIONS THAT CAUSE ABORTION
Adenoviruses
African swine fever virus
+ *Actinobacillus pleuropneumoniae*
Aujeszky's virus (PR)
° Blue eye disease virus
Bovine virus diarrhoea virus
* Brucella suis
Chlamydia psittaci
* Encephalomyocarditis virus
Eperythrozoon suis
* Erysipelothrix rhusiopathiae
Foot-and-mouth disease virus
Influenza virus
* *Leptospira pomona*
Opportunist invaders
Porcine parvovirus (uncommon)
* PRRS
Toxoplasma gondii
Vesicular stomatitis

* In countries in which the occur.
\+ In severe outbreaks in naive herds (e.g. primarily SPF & MEW herds)
° Mexico only

(Fig.5-27)

A CHECKLIST FOR ABORTIONS	
Abortion Level. Is this more than 1.5% of sows served?	- Take action
Are sows ill?	- Probably disease
Are sows otherwise normal?	- Probably non infectious - Maternal failures
Is the problem seasonal?	- Autumn abortion syndrome
Do they occur in a particular part of the farm?	- Environmental
Are the aborted pigs fresh or alive?	- Suggests the environment
Are mummified pigs present?	- Suggests infection
Is the dry sow accommodation uncomfortable?	- Suggests the environment
Are sow pens wet, draughty, poorly lit?	- Suggests the environment
Does the ventilation system chill the sows?	- Suggests the environment
Are there factors that place the sows in a negative energy state?	e.g.: High chill factors Draughts Low feed intake A change in bedding Availability
Are sows short of food?	- Check feed intakes by volume and weight
Is the food mouldy?	- Check for mouldy feed
Do the sows experience 14 hours of good light at eye level?	
Are the lights dirty, covered in fly dirt?	
Can you read a newspaper in the darkest corner?	
Do your sows have boar contact in pregnancy?	
Are any other diseases evident in the sows?	e.g.: lameness cystitis kidney infections
Are the abortions associated with stress?	

(Fig.5-28)

Group 6 Losses - Stillborn pigs

Stillbirths are usually related to large litters, increasing age, slow farrowing or farrowing difficulties. In herds with large litter sizes stillbirth rates are higher and the target level then ranges between 5-7% of total pigs born. Increased stillbirths can also be associated with infections such as *Leptospira pomona* and PRRS.

Stillbirths - target 3 - 5%

Increases are associated with:
- Increasing age of sow.
- Fat sows.
- Individual sows. Identify by litter size - more in large litters. Monitor their farrowing progress.
- Breed - They are more common in the pure bred sows.
- Lack of exercise - poor muscle tone at parturition, associated with individual confinement.
- Prolonged farrowings. Identify these and investigate.
- Uterine inertia. Low calcium levels in the diet may be involved.
- High farrowing house temperatures.
- High carbon monoxide from old gas heaters.
- Farrowing crate and floor designs which precipitate farrowing difficulties.
- Foetal anoxia (lack of oxygen) - resulting from uterine inertia.
- Early placental separation.
- Haematoma/bruising of umbilical cord.
- Assisted farrowings.
- Diseases of the sow, fever, mastitis, etc.
- Parvovirus infection.
- The use of certain boars.

The types of stillbirth:
- Pre-partum - The piglets died a few days before parturition - no lung inflation.
- Intra-partum - The piglets died during farrowing - no lung inflation. Usually maternal failure.
- Post-partum - The piglets show evidence of some lung inflation but fail to breath properly.

Stillbirths may arise due to:
- Mechanical anoxia.
- Hypoglycaemia (low sugar).
- Hypothermia (low body temperature).
- Low viability.
- Maternal failure.

To reduce stillbirths:
- Identify the group cause by post-mortem examination.
- Do not let the age of the herd spread beyond the seventh litter.
- Identify problem sows from the previous histories and monitor their farrowings.
- Look at breed differences.
- Check sow condition.
- Check farrowing house environment.
- Check farrowing pen design.
- Monitor farrowings.

MANAGEMENT FACTORS THAT MAY LEAD TO ABORTION

Management Factors
- Low energy feed.
- Low environmental temperatures
- High air flow.
- Reduced feed intake.
- Poor nutrition.
- Wet pens.
- Poor floor insulation.
- Low back fat measurements (Breed).
- Parasitism.

↓ Energy Requirements
Variable low density lighting. No boar contact → Catabolism ← Stress
↓
Luteolysis ← Poisons Toxins
↓
ABORTION

(Fig.5-29)

- Interfere early in prolonged farrowings.
- Give good management at farrowing.
- Provide a heat source behind the sow at farrowing.
- Study herd records.
- Check haemoglobin levels in sows.
- Check parasite levels.
- Check for blood parasites.
- Check for diseases in the sow.
- Clean and service gas heaters.
- Check quality of sow feed, particularly minerals.
- Check water quality if using bore holes.

Low Litter Size

To study a problem of low numbers born alive look at the total born. Consider the following two scenarios of herds with problems. (Fig.5-30).

Herd A had a problem of embryo loss before day 35 of pregnancy. Herd B had a problem after day 35, evident from the levels of mummified pigs. An analysis of records identified a management/service problem in A and an infectious problem in B.

Examination of the farrowing records for the last 6 gilt and 2nd parity litters in herd B gave the following results. (Fig.5-31). The high numbers of stillbirths and mummies seen in the gilts is an indication of infectious disease - indicating probably parvovirus infection or PRRS. The problem relates to only gilts in this herd as evident by the good performance in parity 2. The solution was to vaccinate gilts with parvovirus vaccine after demonstrating disease in the mummified pigs by the fluorescent antibody test. Of course, in the field you should look at more than 6 litters, as this is a simplified example.

	Herd A	Herd B	Target
Born alive	9.8	10.3	11.2
Stillborn	0.3 Dead	0.8	0.4
Mummified	0.1	0.4	0.1
Total Born:	10.2	11.5	11.7

(Fig.5-30)

	Gilt litters			Parity 2		
	A	D	M	A	D	M
	8	1	-	12	1	1
	10	1	-	11	1	0
	9	2	-	12	1	0
	12	2	-	9	0	0
	2	1	3	14	1	0
	6	1	1	11	0	0
Total	47	8	4	69	4	1
Average	7.8	1.3	0.7	11.5	0.7	0.2

A = Born alive D = Stillborn M = Mummified

(Fig.5-31)

Key points to consider with a litter size problem

Sow effects
- Analyse at least 4 months of farrowing information.
- Analyse the results by born alive, dead, mummified, parity and boar used.
- Look at the distribution of good and poor litters. Is litter size generally depressed or are failures related to a few very poor litters?
- Is there anything common to those animals with poor litters?
- Determine if causes are infectious or non infectious.
- Check the breeding of the sows - do they express good hybrid vigour?
- Assess the effects of lactation length. On average 0.1 per pig is lost for each day lactation is reduced below 28 days.
- If there is a gilt problem assess the management as described previously in this chapter.
- Assess potential losses in groups 1 to 4.
- Assess key factors associated with poor fertilisation.
- Assess factors associated with normal repeats Fig.5-21 and abnormal repeats Fig.5-22.
- Check gilts are vaccinated against parvovirus.

Boar effects
- Young boars up to 9 months old produce smaller litters.
- Litter size differences exist between boars. Use records to identify.
- Check records. For each boar multiply the farrowing rate by the average total litter size. This gives a guide to numbers born per 100 services. A poor record would be 800, a good one more than 1000.
- Serve twice at 24 hour intervals.
- Always leave 24 hours between each completed boar mating.
- Check the general health of boars. Lameness or stiffness may result in poor litter size.
- Look at the timing and frequency of services. Fig.5-20. The time of mating relative to ovulation is important.
- Litter size is maximised by the time the boar is 15 - 20 months of age. This is worth up to 1.9 pigs per annum extra compared to younger boars.
- Farrowing rate is also maximised in this age of boar.
- Have sufficient boars for each to mate one sow per week.

Nutrition
- Feed the sow to appetite during lactation and to point of service with a high energy >14MJ DE/kg and >1% lysine.
- Feed gilts ad lib for 3 weeks prior to mating.
- Check the energy level of the diet relative to feed intake and to performance.
- Monitor body condition and fat depths.
- Avoid significant weight loss in the sow during lactation (>10kg).

Management and environmental effects
- Assess the dry sow house environment for draughts, wet pens, no bedding, hygiene etc. particularly from weaning to 21 days post-service.

The Boar

Anatomy and Physiology

The male reproductive system (Fig.5-32) consists of two testicles, each of which is held almost vertically with the tail of the epididymis at the top. The epididymis is the area within which all the mature sperm is stored and held until ejaculation. From each testicle a tube, the urethra, carries the sperm into the abdomen via the inguinal canal. (If this hole is enlarged an inguinal rupture will be seen). From there it enters the neck of the bladder and continues in the groin down the penis to the exterior as the urethra. Thus from the neck of the bladder to the tip of the penis the urethra can carry either sperm or urine. There are three glands called the seminal vesicles, the prostrate and the bulbo urethral glands. The seminal vesicles produce the bulk of the ejaculate (300ml) and fructose to nourish the sperm. The prostrate gland provides other nutrients and the bulbo urethral

> *There are no drugs that will increase libido or semen quality.*

gland the jelly that you often see at the end of mating

During service the sperm in the epididymis are pulsated down the urethra to be joined by the seminal fluids. This is a continuous process during the period of mating. You can see it if you stand behind the boar and you should check it when you supervise services.

The penis, which is long and rigid has a sigmoid or S - shape in its top half and an anti clockwise spiral at the end. It is 300-500mm long.

The preputial sack is filled with very smelly fluids including pheromones and it also has a very high bacterial content. The bacteria are potential pathogens and emptying the sac by squeezing at service increases the risk of infection entering the womb, particularly towards the end of the heat period.

Sperm is produced and matured under the influence of luteinising hormones (LH) and follicle stimulating hormones (FSH) and the whole process is controlled by the pituitary gland which is at the base of the brain.

Treatment for poor sperm quality is disappointing, however prostaglandins injected weekly are claimed to have some effect on libido. The evidence is not convincing.

The effects of age

Boars reach puberty around 5 months of age but the amounts and quality of semen are usually insufficient at

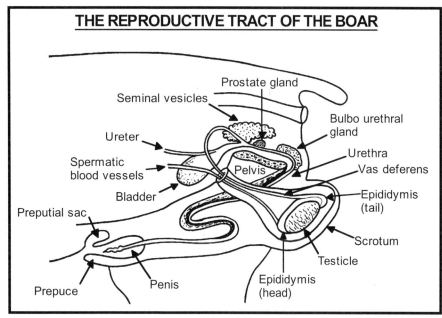

(Fig.5-32)

this age to fertilise efficiently. (Fig.5-33).

Frequency of mating

AGE: 7 - 8 months, mate twice weekly, 48 hours apart. 12 months onwards, mate 2 - 3 times weekly 24 hours apart.

Facts About Semen

- Volume - 50-400 ml, mean 250ml.
- Colour - Creamy white

> *Do not use a boar less than 7 months old. Peak fertility is reached at 15 - 20 months of age.*

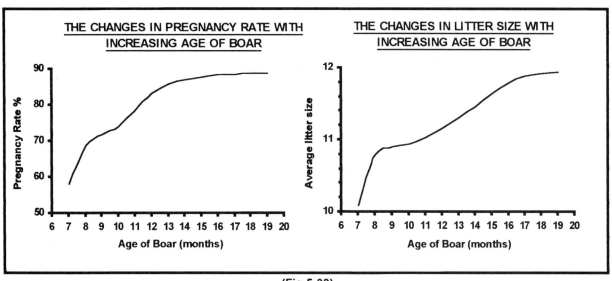

(Fig.5-33)

> *Never use a boar twice in one day.*

- A good ejaculate is very milky.
- The ejaculate becomes watery if the boar is overused. If used am/pm/am the last ejaculate will be poor.
- Temperature of sperm. 37.5°C (100°F)
- In hot weather >30°C (86°F) sperm quality is affected.
- Sperm production. This takes up to 6 weeks. High temperatures such as fevers will affect sperm production for this length of time and potentially affect fertility.
- Numbers of sperm per ml, up to 100 million.
- Sperm production time.
  Up to 4 weeks of development in the testes and 2 weeks maturing in the epididymis.
  5-20 minutes for complete ejaculation.
  Sperm remains viable in the sow for 30-48 hours

The structure and shapes of normal and abnormal sperm are shown in Fig.5-34.

Sperm consists of a head and a tail. The head has a cap or acrosome which assists it to penetrate the egg. It appears normally as a crescent shape. The tail gives the sperm mobility to penetrate the egg and thus any abnormalities will decrease the possibility of penetration. Non mobile sperm are incapable of fertilisation.

As sperm matures a small droplet - the cytoplasmic droplet - is produced just beneath the attachment of the tail to the head. However, once maturity has been reached it disappears and therefore if semen contains high numbers of sperm with droplets, fertility will be poor and it is probable that the boar is being over used. If a sample of semen is examined whilst warm under a microscope sperm appear swirling in waves. This is an indication of good viability.

Bacteria and infectious agents

Semen in the epididymis normally does not contain any bacteria or virus but during ejaculation contaminants from the prepucial sac and elsewhere can cause high numbers to be present. (Fig.5-35). Semen samples usually contain at least 100 bacteria per ml and often many more. It is common practice to add antibiotics to semen samples used for AI. These kill or incapacitate many of the bacteria but they have no effect on viruses.

At a practical level semen is not usually a cause of disease spread, nevertheless the following viral diseases may be present, particularly if the boar is ill or at the early acute stage of infection at the time of collection.

- Aujeszky's disease virus.
- Cytomegalo virus.
- Foot-and-mouth disease virus.
- Genital papilloma virus.
- Parvovirus.
- PRRS virus.
- Swine fever (HC) virus.
- Swine vesicular disease virus.

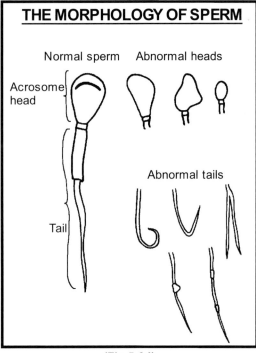

(Fig.5-34)

> *It takes 8 hours or more for sperm to mature inside the sow before they can fertilise.*

- TGE virus
- Influenza virus.

Many other viruses have been detected in semen but their significance is not known. Some important bacterial diseases can also be spread in semen during service, notably brucellosis and leptospirosis.

Fertilisation

It is important to appreciate that the mating process in the pig is a prolonged one, sometimes up to 15 minutes, during which time up to 400ml of fluid will be inseminated.

The penis spirals towards the vagina and into the cervix where it screws into the folds to become locked. This is vital because to establish an optimum pregnancy, sperm must be placed directly into the womb.

Sperm is transported from the cervix to the top of the

BACTERIA THAT COMMONLY CONTAMINATE SEMEN	
Bacillus sp.	* Klebsiella
E. suis	Micrococci
Citrobacter	Proteus
* *E. coli*	* Pseudomonas
* Haemolytic staphylococci	* Streptococcus
Various anaerobes	

* Can be important.

(Fig.5-35)

womb by contractions of the muscles and it takes up to 2 hours for them to arrive at the bottom of the fallopian tubes, the utero-tubal junction. Once the junction is filled with sperm few more enter before ovulation. It is important to appreciate this because at the first mating the quality of the semen and timing probably decide the quality and success of fertilisation and subsequent embryo survival. (Fig.5-36).

Libido

Failure of the boar to show sexual interest and activity is common in maiden boars. Some times up to 30% of animals may be affected.

Some pig farmers insist that any boar they purchase has been libido checked at least once before he arrives on the farm and some breeding organisations carry this out. It is performed either by the boar mounting a gilt in heat or encouraging the use of a dummy. In spite of this occasionally such tested boars will not work on the farm and careful coaxing and patience are required.

Now that breeding companies are tending to sell synthetic hybrid boars rather than pure bred boars libido problems should diminish.

Procedures for libido testing

- Provide a well bedded pen with a non-slip floor.
- Boars should be a minimum of 6 months old.
- Make good empathy with the boar.
- Be patient and show no aggression.
- Test boars in the morning when it is cool.
- Use a gilt firmly on heat. Always introduce the gilt to the boar pen.
- If no gilt is available use an AI stool.
- Spray the stool with urine from a sow on heat.
- If there are poor responses:
  - Move the boars to different pens.
  - Have the boars within sight of a service pen
  - Mix with a sow on heat.
  - Leave a dummy stool in the pen.
  - Inject with prostaglandin.
- Cull boars if there is no response after six weeks.

Factors and actions to consider if a boar lacks libido

- Age of the boar. Has he reached puberty?
- Breeding. Are there any hereditary problems?
- Has the boar normal testicles?
- Is he housed in a poor social environment with little contact with other pigs?
- Boars reared in a total male environment can become infertile.
- Give plenty of female exposure.
- Is the boar apprehensive?

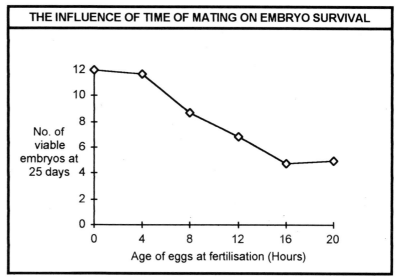

(Fig.5-36)

- Is he a timid or bullied boar? Has he been bullied by sows?
- Poor stockmanship.
- Disease
  - Look for any sign of respiratory disease, mange or sloppy faeces, pain or lameness.
  - Check for parasite burdens.
  - Lameness in particular, leg weakness or arthritis.
  - Inappetance.
  - A history of influenza or PRRS.
  - A previous history of pneumonia or rhinitis.
- Boars reared on slats in intensive conditions have poor libido.
- Is empathy with the pig poor?.
- Are lighting patterns poor? Ensure 14 hours of light per day.
- House the problem boar next to a mature good working boar.
- Allow saliva contact with working boars.
- Assess the response to an injection of prostaglandin or luteinising hormone but do not be too hopeful.
- Check for mouldy feeds (zearalenone toxin).
- Check for a damaged or defective penis. Sedate with azaperone (Stresnil) and examine.
- Provide a dry, well bedded, well drained pen.

Mating Procedures

Single Service (Supervised)

Large computer data bases show that in most herds there is no difference in litter size or farrowing rate, whether the sow is single or multiple mated.

If however records are analysed using conventional data, single services tend to show poorer litter size and farrowing rates. This is because a large proportion of single services take place in the sub fertile period i.e. weaning to service interval 7-14 days when litter size and pregnancy rates may be poor.

The advantages of single services

- Boars are only used once in 24 hours.
- Semen quality is excellent.
- Sows stand "rock hard". No continual trauma to the sow.
- The number of boars can be considerably reduced.
- There is a considerable reduction in management time.
- Extra accommodation is available.
- There is less capital cost in boars, or higher pointed boars can be purchased, thus improving performance of the progeny.
- In some herds it leads to an improvement in litter size and fertility.
- Boar usage can be facilitated by weaning half the litters one day leaving the sows in the crates and weaning the rest the next day. This will give a 24 hour gap between the two groups.
- Litter size may improve in gilts and second parity.
- There is less trauma to the reproductive tract and less likelihood of ascending womb infection.

Disadvantages of single service

- A boar may become infertile. However he will be detected earlier than with multiple matings. This is particularly so if cross mating is used, when an infertile boar may not be detected. It is uncommon for boars to be infertile. Test the semen regularly by drawing it into a syringe at service using a stomach tube placed by the cervix.
- In a few herds the results may be inferior.
- Assess the effects on farrowing rate.
- Sufficient boars must be held to allow for sudden illness or failure to work.
- The sow can be mated at the wrong time.

Procedures for single services

- Make sure the sow is fed to appetite on the day of weaning e.g. give $3/4$ of the food 3 to 4 hours prior to movement from the farrowing quarters and the other $1/4$ after movement.
- Feed the lactation diet ad lib to point of service.
- **Only serve the sow when she is standing absolutely still** i.e. only mate her when you have to almost lift her into the pen.
- Ensure the service is of good quality i.e. a good lock and long insemination.
- Never single mate if the weaning to service interval is 7-14 days - i.e. the subfertile period. The time of standing oestrus in these sows is often 12 hours or less. Always mate them am/pm.

The common failure with single serving is to mate the sow too soon. If she is weaned on a Thursday the mating will usually take place on Tuesday morning. Sows on heat on the Monday will often have a long oestrus period and still stand to the boar on the Wednesday. Thus if mating occurs on Monday, sperm will have to wait until ovulation some 48-72 hours later. Their viability could be much reduced. Many farms now do not bother to heat check on the Monday even if multiple serving.

To assess the efficiency of single service in your herd mate 15% of sows for a period of 6 weeks and compare the results to the rest of the sows.

Fig.5-37 shows the results of single services in a 200 sow herd for a 2 year period compared to a one year period of multiple matings.

There was no change in farrowing rates at 87% but there was an increase in litter size.

> **Test out single serving on a few sows first.**

Skip Services

Here the sow is not mated at the first oestrus post-weaning but at the second. This is a procedure worth considering if the second litter size is poor. Often the first parity weaning to first service interval is extended which could be the cause of the smaller second litter. However a second litter size drop may occur even if the

> **Studies have shown up to 2.6 extra pigs born (2.3 alive) in skip mated second litters and up to 2.6 pigs more (1.9 alive) in third litter females.**

RESULTS OF SINGLE MATED SOWS AGAINST DOUBLE NATURAL, OR BOAR/A.1. AT 24 HOUR INTERVALS. 200 SOW HERD.					
Parity	Alive	Dead	Mumm	Total	
GILT 1	9.7 9.9	0.8 1.1	0.1 0.2	10.5 11.0	Double mated **Single mated**
2	10.5 11.1	0.9 0.9	0.1 0.1	11.4 12.1	Double mated **Single mated**
3	10.8 11.7	0.7 1.0	0.1 0.1	11.5 12.7	Double mated **Single mated**
4	11.5 11.6	0.9 1.2	0.2 0.1	12.2 13.1	Double mated **Single mated**
5	11.0 11.4	1.2 1.6	0.2 0.1	12.2 13.1	Double mated **Single mated**
6	9.8 11.8	1.0 1.8	0.2 0.1	10.8 13.6	Double mated **Single mated**
7	10.3 11.2	1.5 1.5	0.1 0.1	11.7 12.7	Double mated **Single mated**
8	10.4 11.2	1.6 2.2	0.1 0.2	12.0 13.2	Double mated **Single mated**
9	10.5 11.3	1.2 2.1	0.2 0.2	11.6 13.4	Double mated **Single mated**
10	10.6 10.5	2.3 1.7	0.2 0.2	12.9 12.2	Double mated **Single mated**
488 litters	10.6	1.1	0.1	11.6	Double 12 months (Jan. 92 - Dec. 92)
916 litters	11.2	1.4	0.1	12.6	**Single** 24 months (Jan. 93 - Dec. 95)

(Fig.5-37)

weaning to service interval is normal (less than 7 days).
There are no economic advantages in skipping services in sows after 2 litters.

Young sows are more prone to convert both fat and protein into energy and if this process of metabolism is a negative or catabolic one, (i.e. more energy is leaving the sow than is entering via feed) the hormone control of reproduction is affected. Skipped sows will be depositing protein and fat and are therefore anabolic at the time of mating with improved reproductive efficiency.

Is it worth skip mating?

- Probably if there is a second litter size problem that cannot be solved by feed intake in lactation.
- If the increase in litter size is 2.1 pigs weaned then the 21 non-productive days lost and its consequences would be out weighed by an increase in 0.8 pigs per sow per annum.
- Practical problems such as housing and movement of the second litter female can sometimes create difficulties.
- Try the technique on a few sows first and see if it is worth while.

Multiple Services

Why should it be necessary to multiple serve the sow to establish a pregnancy? The simple answer is it is not and single mating demonstrates this, but multiple services probably ensure a better timing of fertile sperm meeting a fertile egg and provide more latitude for variable service procedures. If multiple services give you excellent results do not make any changes. If results however are poor it is worth assessing the response to both changes in the number of services and their timing on litter size and conception rates. This may be particularly advantageous in ill-defined infertility problems. As an initial guide serve am/am.

What should you do on the farm? (Fig.5-38)

- Look at the results of your existing service procedure. Is it efficient? i.e. 11.0 plus born alive and a pregnancy rate of 90%. If so don't make any changes.
- If results are poor then change the existing routine. Such a change could include:
  - Altering the number of times the sow is served (probably less than more).
  - Altering the time when the sow is first served (later).
  - Altering the frequency of the services e.g. from am/am to am/pm.
  - Mate the sow with only one boar.
  - Mate the sow with two different boars (cross mating).

If fertility is not being maximised then change your service routine. Remember however that if you have good fertility it does not matter if you serve two, three or four times, all **you do is risk continual trauma to the sow** but in your case it is not important.

Key Points to a Successful Mating

- Always introduce the sow to the boar.
- Always observe every service to completion in indoor systems. Examine boars clinically every week in outdoor systems and observe at least one service per sow as far as possible.
- Do not commence services too early.
- Make sure the sow is standing completely still and solid for the first mating.
- Match the size of the boar to the size of sow.
- Serve in a pen that is dry, with no projections and a non slip floor. The floor area should be at least $9.5m^2$. All sides should be equal in size.
- Make sure the supernumerary digits of the boar do not damage the sows back. If so use a thin carpet or other protective material over the back of the sow.
- Assist entry of the penis into the vagina if necessary by cupping a clean or gloved hand. <u>Do not handle the prepuce</u>, you will empty the preputial sac and cause heavy bacterial contamination.
- Ensure the penis is locked in and then observe between the testicles for the pulsation of the urethra to indicate that insemination is taking place.
- Observe that there is no leakage of semen from the vulva.
- Always use a fresh unused boar for the first service.
- Never use a boar that is stiff or lame, you will risk a small litter.
- Avoid using a boar for at least 14 days if he has had a temperature of more than 40°C (104°F).
- Handle the boar and sow quietly and patiently.
- Kindness and good empathy mean good fertility.
- Only serve once every 24 hours.
- Use one boar for one sow where possible and serve am and am.
- Only use each boar once every 24 hours.
- Give the boar a 48 hour rest between each complete sow mating if at all possible.
- Maintain the sow in dry warm housing for 21 days

Regimes	Time Of Mating			
	am	pm	am	pm
Single mating +	B or	B	-	-
Double mating	B	B	-	-
	B*	-	B	-
	B	-	AI	AI
	B*	-	AI	-
Triple mating	B	B	B	-
	B	AI	B	-
	B	AI	AI	-
	AI	AI	AI	-
Quadruple mating	B	B	B	B
	B	AI	B	AI
	B	AI	AI	AI

* Probably the best options.
+ Only when the sow is standing completely immobile (rock hard).
B = Same boar or different boars.   AI = Artificial insemination

(Fig.5-38)

post-service.
- Do not mix sows after day 2 post-service.
- Feed sows 2kg maximum of feed for 2 days post-service then to body condition to day 21 (minimum of 2.8kg)
- Feed a diet of at least 14.0 MJ DE/kg and 1% lysine from weaning to 21 days post-service.
- Always house the boar in a clean dry pen.

Artificial Insemination (AI)

- AI is now used extensively in many countries where it is either purchased from a commercial centre or produced on the farm. It is common practice to carry out one service, usually the first, with the boar followed up 24 hours later by AI. For herds with 300 sows or more it is cost effective to collect semen from boars on the farm daily and inseminate within one hour of collection (twice 24 hours apart). The procedures and equipment necessary are simple and described in chapter 15 Semen collection. Many herds today use only AI and produce excellent results particularly with the advent of the collapsible semen pack.

FUNGAL POISONING - MYCOTOXICOSIS

See also Chapter 13; Mycotoxins for further information.

Sometimes when moulds multiply on feeds such as wheat, barley, corn and cotton seed, mycotoxins are produced that can be poisonous. (Fig.5-39). Three factors are necessary for growth; an available carbohydrate source for energy; warm moist conditions 10-25ºC (50-77ºF) and oxygen. Other special conditions may be necessary for toxins to be produced.

An important toxin that affects reproduction is called zearalenone or F2 toxin produced by the fungus *Fusarium graminearum*.

It is an oestrogenic toxin and it is produced in high moisture environments in corn (maize) well before harvest.

Clinical signs

The most striking clinical feature is the swollen red vulva of immature gilts. The other signs are dependent up on the levels present in the feed and the state of pregnancy.

The following may be used as guidelines to the symptoms that may be observed.

Boars - Semen may be affected with feed levels above 30ppm but not fertility. At higher levels poor libido, oedema of the prepuce and loss of hair may occur.

Gilts (Pre puberty) 1 - 6 months of age - 1 to 5ppm in feed causes swelling and reddening of the vulva and enlargement of the teats and mammary glands. Rectal and vagina prolapses also occur in the young growing stock.

Gilts (mature) - 1 to 3ppm will cause variable lengths of the oestrus cycle due to retained corpora lutea and infertility.

Sows - Levels of 5 to 10ppm can cause anoestrus, which may also be associated with pseudo pregnancy due to the retention of corpus luteum. F2 toxin will not normally cause abortion however. If sows are exposed during the period of implantation litter size may be reduced. In lactation piglets may develop enlarged vulva.

Effects on pregnancy - Embryo survival to implantation does not appear to be affected at levels less than 30ppm but above this complete loss between implantation and thirty days occurs followed by pseudo pregnancies. Low levels of 3 to 5ppm do not appear to affect the mid part of pregnancy, but in the latter stages piglet growth in utero is depressed, with weak splay-legged piglets born. Some of these may have enlarged vulvas.

Effects on lactation - 3 to 5ppm has no effect on lactation but the weaning to service interval may be extended.

Diagnosis

The clinical signs are distinctive. Rations that are suspected of contamination should be examined both for the presence of zearalenone and also other oestrogen like substances.

A GUIDE TO MYCOTOXIN LEVELS IN FEED: MILD TO ACUTE DISEASE				
Fungus	Toxins	No Clinical Effect	Toxic Level	Clinical Symptoms
Aspergillus sp	Aflatoxins	< 100ppb	300 - 2000ppb	Poor growth Liver damage Jaundice Immunosuppression
Aspergillus sp and Penicillium sp	Ochratoxin and Citrinin	< 100ppb	200 - 4000ppb	Reduced growth Thirst Kidney damage
Fusarium sp	T2 DAS DON (Vomitoxin)	< 2ppm	4 - 20ppm	Reduced feed intake Immuno-suppression Vomiting
Fusarium sp	Zearalenone (F2 toxin)	< 0.05ppm	1 - 30ppm	Infertility Anoestrus Rectal prolapse Pseudo pregnancy
			< 30ppm	Early embryo mortality Delayed repeat matings
Fusarium sp	Fumonisin	< 10ppm	20 - 175	Reduced feed intake Respiratory symptoms Fluid in lungs Abortion
Ergot	Ergotoxin	< 0.05%	0.1-1.0% Ergot bodies by weight (sclerotium)	Reduced feed intake. Gangrene of the extremities. Agalactia due to mammary gland failure.

ppm - parts per million **ppb** - parts per billion.
sp - species - each of these fungi have several species only some of which are toxic

(Fig.5-39)

Removal of the suspect feed will be followed by the regression of symptoms within three to four weeks.

Treatment

☐ None is required provided the toxin source is removed.
☐ Sows that are in deep anoestrus may respond to injections of prostaglandins.

Procedures for sampling feed

- Collect 8 x 1kg quantities from separate areas of the feed.
- Mix all together.
- Take 4 x 1kg separate samples from the bulked one into clean polythene bags.
- Number 1 to 4 and date.
- Seal and witness.
- Store at 4°C (34°F) until transported to a laboratory.
- Retain two samples.
- Send two samples to the place of testing or use two separate laboratories.

Management control and prevention

Key factors leading to mycotoxicosis:

◆ The purchase of mouldy, damp or badly stored grains.
◆ The mixing of contaminated and uncontaminated grains.
◆ Holding cereals in moist, damp conditions.
◆ Allowing grains to heat.
◆ Prolonged usage of bins, feed bridging across the bin and development of moulds.
◆ Placing compounded feeds into bins whilst they are moist and warm.
◆ Poorly maintained bins that allow water to leak in.
◆ The bridging of feed in bins over long periods of time and their sudden descent.
◆ Prolonged use of automatic feeders and retention of mouldy feed.

If a problem of mycotoxicosis is suspected immediately stop using that particular feed and re-cycle it at a 1:10 dilution with other cereals into feeder pigs or destroy it. Sample all the feed ingredients and if these are required for future examinations, store in the correct conditions.

Chapter 5

6 Reproduction: Infectious Infertility

Diseases affecting reproduction... 165
Viral infertility 167
    Aujeszky's disease / pseudorabies virus (AD or PRV) 167
    Bovine viral diarrhoea virus (BVDV) and border disease virus (BDV)..... 168
    Classical swine fever virus (CSF) - hog cholera virus (HC) 168
    Encephalomyocarditis virus (EMCV)... 169
    Enteroviruses (SMEDI) 169
    Porcine cytomegalovirus (PCMV)... 170
    Porcine parvovirus (PPV) 170
    Porcine reproductive and respiratory syndrome (PRRS)....................... 173
    Swine influenza virus (SI)... 177
Bacterial infertility 178
    Abortion... 178
    Brucellosis... 179
    Endometritis and the vulval discharge syndrome 180
    Eperythrozoonosis (Epe) 184
    Erysipelas.. 185
    Leptospirosis... 186

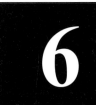

Chapter 6

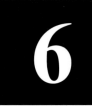

Reproduction: Infectious Infertility

Diseases Affecting Reproduction

The previous chapter has reviewed the various management and environmental factors that have an adverse affect on reproductive efficiency. The description of the diseases here concentrates on their effects on reproduction but in some of them infertility is only part of a much broader picture. In such cases references to specific chapters are given. There is often an overlap between infectious and non infectious infertility and in many cases the two are interrelated. It is important to determine if there is an infectious component to a problem in a herd because corrective measures may involve both treatment and management procedures. Fig.6-1 demonstrates a pathway that can be used to identify the causes of an infectious infertility problem. It asks the question what diseases are present in the herd, because any one of these may have an occasional effect. Such diseases are listed in Fig.6-2 and Fig.6-3. For example, if a herd is infected long term with aujeszky's disease virus, porcine parvovirus (PPV), porcine reproductive and respiratory syndrome (PRRS) or swine influenza (SI) then at varying intervals following the initial herd outbreak there may be reproductive failures, albeit in many cases at individual sow levels. If a herd is free from these infections and then become infected with one of them an acute episode of that disease will occur. This will be manifest by reproductive failure including increased numbers of abortions, repeats on a normal and abnormal cycle and in the case of those viruses that cross the placenta, there will be foetal death, mummified and stillborn piglets.

Diseases such as porcine parvovirus (PPV), PRRS and leptospirosis may infect the sow without causing other clinical signs. Usually in such cases the disease picture is sporadic (unless it appears for the first time) and a detailed examination of records helps to clarify this.

There are nine main viruses that can cause reproductive disease, but only five of these are really important in those countries where they occur. The five are:
- Aujeszky's disease (AD) virus or pseudorabies virus (PRV).
- Porcine parvovirus (PPV).
- Porcine reproductive and respiratory syndrome virus (PRRS).
- Classical swine fever virus (CSF).
- Swine influenza virus (SI).

Bovine viral diarrhoea virus (BVDV) border disease virus (BDV) and entero-virus (SMEDI) may cause sporadic reproductive problems but in most countries disease would be uncommon. Encephalomyocarditis virus (EMCV) varies in its pathogenicity in different regions of the world. In Europe it is rarely implicated in porcine disease, in the Caribbean it causes heart problems but in North America it is associated with reproductive problems

Most bacteria are opportunist invaders and usually only affect a few individual breeding females, a good example is erysipelas. The exceptions are leptospirosis and brucellosis which are herd problems.

Some of the clinical signs and pathological effects that viral and bacterial agents have on fertility are shown in Fig.6-2 and Fig.6-3.

166 Managing Pig Health and the Treatment of Disease

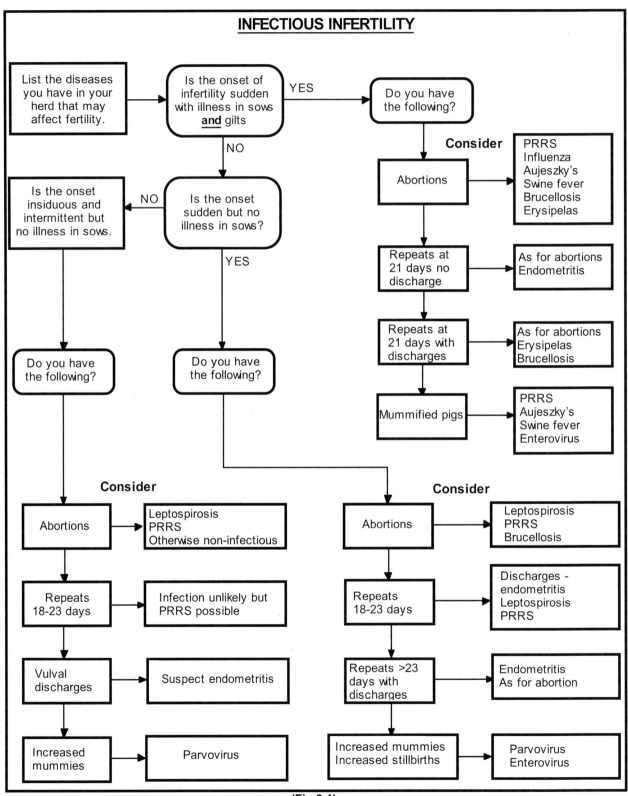

(Fig.6-1)

Chapter 6

VIRUS INFECTIONS CAUSING INFERTILITY						
	Embryo death	Foetal death	Abortion	Sows may be ill	Virus may be in semen *	Clinical signs in the breeding herd
Aujeszky's (PR)	+	+	+	+	+	+
BVDV and BDV #	+	+	+	−	?	−
EMCV	+	+	+	+	−	−
Enterovirus	+	+	−	−	+	−
Influenza	+	−	+	+	−	+
Parvovirus	+	+	−	−	+	−
PRRS	+	+	+	+	+	+
Swine fever	+	+	+	+	+	+ Severe illness

\# = Rare   + = Yes   − = No or uncommon   * In all diseases if the boar is viraemic   ? Unknown
BVDV = Bovine virus diarrhoea virus   **BDV** = Border disease virus   **EMCV** = Encephalomyocarditis virus
PCMV = Porcine cytomegalovirus   **PRRS** = Porcine reproductive and respiratory syndrome
(Fig.6-2)

BACTERIAL AND FUNGAL DISEASES CAUSING INFERTILITY						
	Embryo death	Foetal death	Abortion	Sow/boar may be ill	Spread in semen	Clinical signs in the herd
Brucellosis	+	+	+	+	+	+
Endometritis ≠	+	−	+	+	via preputial fluids	Discharges
Fungal diseases *	+	−	+	+	−	+
Eperythrozoonosis	−	+ Stillbirths	−	+	−	+ Anaemia Jaundice Weak piglets
Leptospirosis	+	+ Stillbirths	+	−	+	Weak pigs at birth
Erysipelas	+	+	+	+	−	+
Any septicaemia or uraemia	+	+	+	+	+	+

≠ = Non-specific bacterial infection of the womb   * Mycotoxicosis   + = Yes   − = No or uncommon
(Fig.6-3)

Viral Infertility

AUJESZKY'S DISEASE / PSEUDORABIES VIRUS (AD OR PRV)

See chapter 12 for further information.

This is an important disease of pigs, caused by a herpes virus. Once introduced into a herd the virus usually remains there and it can continually affect reproductive performance at varying levels. The virus can survive for up to three weeks outside the pig.

Clinical signs

Acute disease

Acute outbreaks of disease occur when virulent strains of the virus first infect an unvaccinated susceptible herd. The virus crosses the uterus and placenta and infects the foetuses. Often the first clinical signs are abortions, stillbirths and the birth of weak litters which soon die. Abortions may rise to 5% over about 6 weeks followed by reproductive failure at all stages of the cycle. Embryos are killed and absorbed and sows return to heat.

These reproductive problems may occur in up to 20% of dry sows. However these are not the only clinical signs seen in the herd. Dogs and cattle may become infected, show nervous signs and die.

Chronic disease

In an unvaccinated herd, when the early acute phase of the disease is over and the herd has developed an immunity clinical signs are sporadic and milder. The signs may also be difficult to associate with an infertility problem because of their insidious nature. Depression of reproductive efficiency across all parameters is a feature of the chronic infection with increased levels of repeats, mummification, stillbirths and piglet mortality. Young carrier females that are stressed shed virus thus maintaining infection throughout the herd. Spread of infection in the breeding herd is low with immunity and infection waning and rising over one to two year cycles.

Carrier state

After the acute phase clinical signs of disease may die out altogether and this is often seen in small herds of less than 100 sows. Sometimes the virus itself may disappear. However it is more likely to persist in a few animals sporadically.

Methods of spread between herds

- Movement of carrier pigs.
- Airborne - at least 3km (2 miles).
- Infection from feral (wild) pigs.
- The role of mechanical spread by birds is questionable.

- From contaminated carcasses.
- Mechanically on people.
- From contaminated vehicles.
- Through infected semen via AI or a carrier boar.
- From infected slurry.

Diagnosis

When a susceptible breeding herd first breaks down with this disease the clinical signs described above strongly suggest aujeszky's disease and are almost diagnostic. Laboratory tests are required to confirm the diagnosis. The common ones are as follows:

- Fluorescent antibody tests on dead piglet tissues particularly tonsils. This is reliable and results are available in few hours.
- Virus isolation from the lung and tonsils and its identification. This test is slow taking several days but may be done for added confirmation.
- Blood tests (serology) to demonstrate rising antibodies take too long to be useful.

Similar diseases

When disease is first introduced into a susceptible breeding herd there are few other diseases except possibly swine fever that would be confused with AD. Once the disease has become chronic it could be confused with PRRS and chronic swine fever. Laboratory tests would be required to differentiate them.

Treatment

- ☐ There is no treatment available but antibiotic medication to control secondary bacteria in a new outbreak could be considered such as:
- ☐ 600-800g of CTC or OTC in the breeding ration for 3-4 weeks as advised by the veterinarian.
- ☐ **Vaccination**. This is the key action to take. As soon as disease is identified all breeding stock should be vaccinated with a gene deleted vaccine to mitigate the effects and reduce spread of the virus.

Management control and prevention

- ◆ AD (PR) is a disease you cannot afford to live with.
- ◆ Gilts and boars should only be purchased from known free herds and be vaccinated before arrival or in isolation.
- ◆ Keep it out of the herd by isolating all purchased breeding stock and blood sampling them before they enter the herd.
- ◆ Only buy from AD free herds.
- ◆ If your herd is at risk, in other words within a 3km radius of large infected herds then vaccinate it to prevent disease.
- ◆ Vaccination helps to prevent the establishment of the virus.
- ◆ If you have AD, adopt strategies for eliminating disease as discussed in chapter 12.

BOVINE VIRAL DIARRHOEA VIRUS (BVDV) AND BORDER DISEASE VIRUS (BDV)

There are two viruses, which are in the same group of pestiviruses as the virus of swine fever (hog cholera) but which primarily infect cattle and sheep respectively, can get into pig breeding herds and cause reproductive problems. These include poor conception rates, a few abortions, foetal death, mummification, small litters and low birth weights. They rarely cause any other clinical signs in pigs. This disease is not a common cause of infertility in the sow and would be considered low on the list of priorities from a diagnostic point of view.

Methods by which infection may be introduced into the herd include exposure of pigs to cattle or sheep faeces, feeding of un-pasteurised cow's milk, or in contaminated live-attenuated virus vaccines.

There is no treatment and the infections are self eliminating.

CLASSICAL SWINE FEVER VIRUS (CSF) - HOG CHOLERA VIRUS (HC)

See chapter 12 for further information.

Swine fever is caused by one of the pesti family of viruses. The pig is the only natural host. The virus is spread from infected or carrier pigs via discharges from the nose, mouth and the urine and faeces and it is highly contagious.

Infection enters the pig by the mouth by direct contact of one pig with another. It gets into herds by the introduction of a carrier pig or infected meat. The virus survives in frozen carcasses for long periods of time

Clinical signs

When first introduced into the breeding herd it causes inappetance and high fevers. The virus can cross the placenta to invade the foetuses causing foetal death with mummification, abortions, malformations and increases in stillbirths.

An important characteristic is the birth of very weak pigs showing trembling like congenital tremor. In congenital tremor however there are no clinical signs of illness in the breeding females. Convulsions may occur with death within a few hours and sows may lose the use of their legs. The disease in the acute form will have dramatic effects on reproduction.

Diagnosis

CSF is a rapid spreading disease with high mortality. There are characteristic post-mortem changes with haemorrhagic lymph nodes, dead patches in the spleen, multiple small haemorrhages in the kidneys and so-called "button ulcers" in the gut.

These are all of diagnostic significance. Laboratory tests include the identification of viral antigen, isolation of the virus and the presence of antibodies in serum. In most countries CSF is notifiable.

Treatment

There is no treatment.

Prevention

The CSF virus is very persistent and survives in frozen tissues for long periods of time. In many countries there is a slaughter and eradication programme. Where there are widespread outbreaks of disease vaccination is sometimes used to control the spread followed often by slaughter policies.

ENCEPHALOMYOCARDITIS VIRUS (EMCV)

The main reservoir host is the rat although mice may also spread it. It infects and causes disease in a wide range of vertebrate animals but pigs appear to be the most susceptible of farm animal species. The virus is world-wide but differs in pathogenicity and virulence in different countries and regions. In most countries of Europe, particularly those in the EU, it tends to be relatively mild or non-pathogenic and disease in pigs is rarely diagnosed.

In Australia the strains appear to be much more virulent for pigs than those in New Zealand. Virulent strains in Florida, the Caribbean and probably Central America damage the heart and cause death whereas those in the Mid West of the US tend to cause reproductive problems.

Clinical disease in pigs tends to occur when rat numbers increase to plague levels. Pigs can be infected from rats or from rat-contaminated feed or water. It does not seem to spread very readily between pigs.

Clinical signs

In gilts and sows the first signs are often a few abortions near the end of pregnancy. Then over a period of about 3 months the numbers of mummified foetuses and stillbirths increase and pre-weaning mortality rises. The farrowing rate worsens. Affected females may go through a phase of fever and lack of appetite. In affected herds there are usually no clinical signs in weaned and growing pigs..

Diagnosis

To make a definitive diagnosis the virus has to be isolated and identified or rising antibodies demonstrated in blood samples taken two weeks apart.

Similar diseases

EMC could be confused with AD, PPV and PRRS although as you will see from Fig.6-2 there are distinguishing signs between these four. EMCV would be the last on the list of diagnostic priorities in Europe but to a lesser extent in the Mid West USA. Abortion or illness in sows or piglets due to PPV is uncommon and mummified pigs can be examined for the evidence of this infection.

Treatment

There are no methods of treatment.

Management control and prevention

◆ Check the source of incoming breeding stock for pathogenic strains.
◆ Reports of killed vaccines being effective have been documented.

ENTEROVIRUSES (SMEDI)

These are gut-borne viruses, host specific to the pig, that are described under the name "SMEDI viruses" which stands for stillbirth, mummification, embryonic death and infertility. The term is now also commonly used for parvovirus infection. Although these groups of viruses are distinct from that of parvovirus, they are often all grouped together clinically because the clinical signs are similar. The enteroviruses are subdivided into serotypes of which at least 11 are known. Four of these, serotypes 1, 3, 6 and 8, have been implicated in reproductive problems in pigs. Serotype 1 is the teschen/talfan virus which can also cause paralysis in pigs. Usually, each pig herd has an array of different serotypes which circulate in weaned and young growing pigs sub-clinically. The pigs are protected by circulatory antibodies derived from their dam's colostrum. By the time they reach breeding age they are solidly immune.

Reproductive problems only occur when a new serotype, to which the gilts are not immune, enters the herd and multiplies in the breeding females. This probably does not happen very often.

It is interesting to note that since the introduction of parvovirus vaccine and the excellent results achieved, the effects from SMEDI viruses would appear to be almost non existent, suggesting that this group of viruses are not important as a cause of reproductive failure.

Clinical signs

Natural infection of enteroviruses takes place by mouth through the ingestion of infected faeces. They multiply in the small and large intestines and in the absence of circulating antibodies escape from the intestine into the blood streams to the uterus. They cross the placenta, to produce the typical symptoms of embryo mortality, mummification and stillbirths. In some cases infertility associated with absorption of embryos also occur. If reproductive failure results there will be increases in embryo mortality, foetal deaths and mummified and stillborn piglets. Infection and disease only occur in non-immune sero-negative animals.

Diagnosis

This is carried out by serology and virus isolation.

Similar diseases

SMEDI can be confused with PPV and PRRS infection and occasionally with AD and leptospirosis.

Treatment

- There is no treatment but if a herd experiences problems with enteroviruses in incoming gilts, management practices should ensure that gilts are exposed to infection at least six weeks before breeding. See acclimatisation chapter 5.

Management control and prevention

- Expose breeding females and boars to faeces from young growing pigs 8-14 weeks of age to immunise them (feedback). This is best carried out by introducing gilts at 90kg to faeces from pigs 15-50kg weight, twice weekly for 6 weeks prior to mating.
- The practice of feeding placenta should be avoided, because it is not a good source of infection and it is a method of spreading leptospirosis, PRRS and other potentially infectious agents.
- Vaccines could be made but are not indicated.

PORCINE CYTOMEGALOVIRUS (PCMV)

This is a herpes virus found in the tissues throughout the body including the nose of newborn piglets where it causes inflammation (rhinitis). PCMV is present throughout the world and exists in most if not all pig populations but most infections are sub-clinical and clinical disease is rare. Serology carried out in the UK, for example, indicates that over 90% of herds have been exposed to infection.

The virus is excreted in discharges from the nose and eyes, urine and farrowing fluids. It is also transmitted via the boar through semen and crosses the placenta to infect piglets before birth.

The rhinitis produced by this virus is uncommon and mild and has no relationship to atrophic rhinitis caused by the toxin-producing bacteria *Pasteurella multocida*. In most herds therefore the infection is insignificant and apart from sometimes causing a mild sneeze has no major effect on the health of the pig.

Clinical signs

Clinical signs are only seen if PCMV infects a sow for the first time when she is late in pregnancy. Signs include foetal deaths, mummified foetuses, stillbirths and weak piglets. The sow may run a slight fever and be off her food. Rhinitis in newborn piglets can be severe enough to cause haemorrhage from the nose. In herds in which PCMV is endemic there are no symptoms other than mild sneezing in sucking and weaned piglets.

Diagnosis

The presence of the virus can be confirmed by serological tests, fluorescent antibody tests and demonstration of inclusion bodies in tissue sections.

Similar diseases

The disease might be confused with atrophic rhinitis or bordetella infection of the nose, however the effects are very short lived and there is no progressive atrophy or distortion of the nose.

PCMV rhinitis only occurs in newborn piglets and there is a tendency to assume that sneezing in piglets must be associated with atrophic rhinitis. Rhinitis means inflammation of the delicate tissues in the nose and is caused by dust, gases, bacteria or viruses, in fact any irritant. If toxin producing pasteurella are present the inflammation persists with damage and progressive destruction of the tissues (atrophy). This is a serious disease. It can be differentiated from PCMV by swabbing the noses of sneezing piglets and testing for the presence or absence of the pasteurella. It is important to carry this out because if the tests are negative you have no worries (or expensive treatments).

> **Do not use placenta or material from farrowed sows for feedback.**

Treatment

- None is required.
- If sneezing and poor growth occur post-weaning, the creep can be medicated with antibiotics such as CTC, OTC, trimethoprim/sulpha or tylosin for 14 days.

Management control and prevention

- Provide good environmental conditions in farrowing and weaner accommodation.
- Avoid fluctuating temperatures.
- Avoid dust.
- Maintain all-in all-out management of farrowing and weaner houses.

PORCINE PARVOVIRUS (PPV)

This is the most common and important cause of infectious infertility. Porcine parvovirus is a fairly tough virus that multiplies normally in the intestine of the pig without causing clinical signs. It is world-wide in its distribution. If you test for it in your pig herd it is almost certain it will be present. It is therefore an infection you have to live with and manage. Whereas most viruses do not survive outside the host for any great period of time PPV is unusual in that it can persist outside the pig for many months and it is resistant to most disinfectants. This perhaps explains why it is so widespread and so difficult to remove from the pig environment.

To understand the role of PPV in reproduction it is important to realise that reproductive infection usually occurs <u>without disease</u>, but sometimes there is infection <u>with reproductive disease</u>. PPV is transmitted either by mouth or through the nose passing into the intestine where it multiplies and is passed out in faeces. If a pig becomes infected for the first time when it is not pregnant there are no clinical signs. However, if the animal is pregnant and exposed <u>for the first time in the first 55 days or so of pregnancy,</u> the virus crosses the placenta killing piglets selectively. If the foetus is infected at less than 35 days of age, before there has been an opportunity for bone development, death results, followed by complete absorption and ultimately a small litter is born. If infection takes place between 30 and 55 days of pregnancy the foetuses die and they become mummified. Do not assume that all mummified pigs are caused by PPV infection. This is often not the case. It takes 10-14 days from first infection for PPV to reach the piglets inside the uterus. From 70 days of age the immune system of the piglet has started to develop and it can therefore respond and protect itself from the virus. Thus if pregnant animals are infected for the first time after approximately 55 days of pregnancy there will be little evidence of disease. This is quite different to PRRS infection, which kills the foetus only after 70 days of age inside the womb and therefore very late mummified pigs are seen in this disease. Once inside the womb PPV spreads slowly from one foetus to another and as a result the sizes of mummified pigs will vary within the litter.

Clinical signs

Acute outbreaks of disease

Infection itself causes no clinical symptoms other than the presence of mummified pigs at farrowing. In acute outbreaks of disease the following occurs:
- Small litters associated with embryo loss before 35 days
- Mummified pigs of varying size, (30-160mm).
- Increased numbers of stillbirths. These are associated with the delay in the farrowing mechanism which occurs because of the presence of the mummified piglet.
- Abortions associated with PPV infection are uncommon.
- There may be an increase in low birth weight piglets but neonatal deaths are not affected.
- The acute disease episode often lasts for up to 8 weeks then wanes for 4-6 weeks, followed by smaller bouts of mummified pigs for a further 4-6 weeks.
- The virus can take up to 4 months to infect all sows in a susceptible previously uninfected herd.

Sporadic disease in enzootic herds

This is seen in individual females which are infected for the first time. It is usually confined to gilts.

Records

Records can assist in the diagnosis of PPV disease and the differences between the normal herd and the diseased herd are shown in Fig.6-4.

In acute herd outbreaks of disease involving many animals, litter size is reduced with the percentage of litters totalling less than 9 increasing from about 10 up to 40%. The numbers of mummified pigs, particularly associated with small litters are elevated and sows not in-pig may increase from 2 to 6%. Sows found not in-pig are due to either total embryo absorption before 35 days or complete foetal death and a pseudo-pregnancy. In some cases the sow reaches the point of farrowing with normal udder development, even to the extent of producing milk, but there are no live births. An injection of prostaglandin to bring about farrowing yields mummified pigs that have been present inside the womb. These animals would not otherwise farrow because a live foetus is necessary to initiate farrowing. The above picture is only seen at this level in a susceptible herd, that is, with 50-70% of sero-negative breeding females. Such episodes are likely to occur in non-vaccinated herds every 3-4 years and arise because virus circulation ebbs and flows. During periods of low or no PPV activity a susceptible population gradually emerges.

Immunity

PPV infection results in high antibody levels in the serum which persist for long periods. You should appreciate that such levels do not necessarily mean that there is or has been a reproductive problem or a higher level of protection. For example, a titre of 1:2 will be equally as protective as a titre of 1:80,000. Blood sampling all the sows in a herd on one occasion only indicates the percentage of animals that have been exposed to parvovirus at some previous period which gives you an idea of the overall breeding herd immunity or susceptibility. Once an animal has been exposed to PPV it remains immune for the rest of its life.

From a practical standpoint the breeding herd may be in one of three phases.

- **Serologically negative.** In this situation all females

PPV INFECTION EXAMPLE OF REPRODUCTIVE DATA IN AN ACUTE OUTBREAK		
	Normal Herd PPV Infected	Acute Disease
Total litter size	Normal	Reduced
Alive and dead	11.5	< 9.5
% of litters total born < 9	< 10% sows < 18% gilts	20 - 40%
Stillbirths	4-7%	7 - 12%
Mummified pigs %	< 0.6%	1 - 4%
Sows not in pig	1.0%	2 - 6%
Delayed returns to oestrus	< 3%	> 4%
Weaning to oestrus interval	Normal	Normal
Other clinical signs	None Some disease in non-vaccinated gilts	None Disease in all parities

(Fig.6-4)

SERUM TITRES TO PPV	
	Level / Significance
Non vaccinated female	Negative - Susceptible to infection and reproductive failure
Vaccinated female	1:2 to 1:160 Protected
Gilt with maternal antibody	1:4 to 1:320 Protected but will wane
Active immunity	> 1:640 Protected

are highly susceptible to infection and reproductive failure. This is an unusual situation but can occur occasionally in small herds, from which the virus can die out. In such herds if parvovirus is introduced there is a massive outbreak of reproductive disease: repeats, mummifications, not in pig and possibly a few abortions. Such herds should be vaccinated immediately.
- **Endemic infection.** Here PPV is continually circulating and 50-90% of animals are immune. However infection can take place in the early to mid pregnancy period in any negative animals and therefore there is a variable amount of disease. This was the typical picture prior to the availability of vaccines in large non-vaccinated herds. Intermittent outbreaks of disease occur, particularly in gilts and second parity females. As viral activity increases, so does immunity across the herd. When there are large numbers of immune animals there is little infection and the herd immunity gradually drops as old immune sows are culled.
- **Disease in replacement gilts.** This is common because at least 50% of gilts at point of mating may not have met PPV and therefore are susceptible. Up to a third of such animals may become infected in the first half of pregnancy resulting in reproductive failure.

Key points to parvovirus infection
- The virus is widespread throughout all pig populations but it may disappear in small herds (<100 sows).
- Infection is endemic (present all the time) in most pig units.
- Once a pig is exposed there is a lifelong immunity.
- Reproductive problems may appear every 3-4 years in a herd if vaccination is not carried out.
- Parvovirus infection in a susceptible female can cause death of the embryo with absorption or death of the foetus with mummification.
- The major signs are therefore small litter sizes, mummified pigs of different sizes, and increases in pseudo-pregnancies and not-in-pigs.
- Abortion due to PPV is uncommon.
- Maternal immunity may persist up to 7 months of age but only in a few gilts. (This interferes with vaccine response).
- Up to 50% of gilts may be sero-negative at point of mating.

Diagnosis
In the absence of any other signs of illness in the breeding females, PPV disease can be suspected by increases in mummified pigs and small litter sizes.

The important features are disease and death in the embryo and foetus from approximately 15-70 days of pregnancy. The mummified pigs can be examined by fluorescent antibody test in the laboratory to confirm the infection. Serology will not help because many sows are positive and normal.

Key points for recognising PPV disease
- Small litters associated with variable sized mummified pigs occurring mainly in unvaccinated gilts, or gilts vaccinated while still protected by maternal antibody.
- Increased percentage of repeats.
- No other signs of ill health in the breeding female or in individual affected animals.
- Some gilts or sows progress to the point of farrowing but produce no live pigs.
- A history of no vaccination programme in gilts.
- Examine all afterbirths from sows carefully to see whether there are small mummified pigs present which vary in size.
- Submit small mummified pigs (less than 150mm) from small litters to a laboratory for fluorescent antibody tests. These will confirm whether the foetus has died from PPV infection or not.

Similar diseases
An acute outbreak could be confused with aujeszky's disease (AD) (PR), PRRS, leptospirosis or certain forms of influenza but with PPV there are no other clinical signs in adult breeding stock, newborn piglets are healthy and fully active, and there are few or no abortions. It could also be confused with SMEDI due to enterovirus infection but this is uncommon and laboratory tests can differentiate them.

Treatment
There is no treatment.

Management control and prevention
◆ In an acute outbreak immediately vaccinate the breeding herd to prevent infection in those animals that are still sero-negative. Discuss with your veterinarian. Remember it will take 10 days for the first dose of vaccine to take effect.

> *To prevent SMEDI disease vaccinate the gilt 2-3 weeks before mating.*

◆ If a sero-negative gilt is given a single dose of vaccine, the immune system is primed and a low antibody level is produced (1:64). Vaccination and stimulation of immunity by natural infection is sufficient to protect the litter from disease. It takes 10-14 days following infection for PPV to cross the placenta and infect the embryos or foetuses. If the infected breeding female has been vaccinated at some time in the past then when exposure to PPV takes place, there is rapid re-stimulation of the immune system (within 5-7 days). This is sufficient to prevent disease and to stimulate a permanent immunity.

Fig.6-5 shows the levels of disease in 69 herds over a 10 year period, prior to vaccination and over an eight year period following a single injection of suvaxyn parvo vaccine to gilts only.

These results show that disease can be controlled

by a single dose of vaccine even though serological tests demonstrated that PPV continued to circulate in all the herds. Discuss your vaccination policy with your veterinarian. Your situation may be different and he/she may advise two doses of vaccine followed by a once or twice yearly booster.

Eradication

Parvovirus cannot be eradicated from a herd.

PORCINE PARVOVIRUS Results of Single Vaccination (Suvaxyn Parvo)*		
	No. of Herds	Herds with Parvovirus SMEDI Problems
Non vaccinated herds over a 10 year period	69	58 (84%)
Gilt only vaccinated herds over an 8 year period	67	0

* Fort Dodge

(Fig.6-5)

PORCINE REPRODUCTIVE AND RESPIRATORY SYNDROME (PRRS)

PRRS is caused by a virus which was first isolated and classified as an arterivirus as recently as 1991. The disease syndrome had been first recognised in the USA in the mid 1980's and was called Mystery swine disease or blue ear disease.

The virus of PRRS has a particular affinity for the macrophages particularly those found in the lung. Macrophages are part of the body defences. They ingest and remove invading bacteria and viruses. Those present in the lung are called alveolar macrophages. In contrast to most other bacteria and viruses, macrophages do not destroy the PRRS virus. Instead, the virus multiplies inside them producing more virus and kills the macrophages.

Up to 40% of the macrophages are destroyed. This removes a major part of the bodies defence mechanism and allows bacteria and other viruses to proliferate and do damage.

A common example of this is the noticeable increase in severity of enzootic pneumonia in grower/finisher units when they become infected with PRRS virus. Another example is the alarming increase that can occur in clinical cases of meningitis in herds in which virulent *Streptococcus suis* type 2 is enzootic. This observation has been used by research workers in the experimental reproduction of streptococcal meningitis.

Once it has entered a herd the PRRS virus tends to remain present and active in the herd indefinitely.
The persistence of the virus within a herd is related to a number of factors:

1. If sero-negative susceptible gilts are regularly introduced into the herd they may enable the virus to persist.
2. Infection is maintained in recently weaned piglets once their maternal antibody disappears. Infection is transmitted to these pigs from older groups previously infected and this procedure is responsible for active enzootic respiratory disease continuing on many farms.
3. It may take up to a year for all breeding stock, particularly in large herds, to become infected for the first time and although the virus appears to spread rapidly in a herd it may be some 4-5 months before at least 90% of the sows have become sero-positive. Furthermore, it is not uncommon for sow herds 1-2 years after infection to contain less than 20% of serological positive animals. This does not however necessarily mean they are not still immune nor does it mean that they have stopped passing on immunity to their offspring.

Methods of spread

The virus is spread by nasal secretions, saliva, faeces and urine and field studies suggest it can be airborne for up to 3km (2 miles). A carrier state exists in the pig that can last for 2-3 months. In some individuals it is thought that it may last longer although the pigs may not be shedding virus. Artificial insemination can be a potential method of spread if semen is used when the virus is present in the blood (viraemia) and particularly during the first 3-4 week period following the breakdown of an AI stud. Outside this period field evidence indicates the risk of spread in semen is very low from previously infected groups of boars. In a study over a 3 year period 32,000 doses of AI, from an AI stud populated with boars from positive herds, were used in 5 large PRRS negative herds. No infection or sero-conversion occurred.

Adult animals excrete virus for much shorter periods of time (14 days) compared to growing pigs which can excrete for 1-2 months.

The following are common methods of spread.
- Movement of carrier pigs.
- Airborne transmission up to 3km (2 miles).
- Mechanical means via faeces, dust, droplets and contaminated equipment.
- Contaminated boots and clothing.
- Vehicles especially in cold weather.
- Artificial insemination but only if the boar is viraemic. This period is probably only 3-4 days.
- The mallard duck and probably other species of bird.

PRRS infects all types of herd including high or ordinary health status and both indoor and outdoor units, irrespective of size.

Clinical signs

The clinical picture can vary tremendously from one herd to another. As a guide, for every three herds that are exposed to PRRS for the first time one will show no recognisable disease, the second would show mild disease and the third moderate to severe disease. The reasons for this are not clearly understood. However the higher the health status of the herd, the less severe are the disease effects. One may be that the virus is continually mutating as it multiplies throwing up some strains that are highly virulent and some that are not.

The tendency is for any epizootic virus infections to get less virulent e.g. African swine fever and rabbit myxomatosis. Also field observations suggest that the virus destroys the macrophages and this lowers the pigs immunity. The severity of an outbreak in a herd will depend to an extent upon other viruses and bacteria already present in the herd and their capacity to cause disease. Furthermore, when the pigs' immunity is compromised, excessive stocking density and the quality of the environment also become important. For example, PRRS in a minimal diseased pig will cause no detectable pneumonia but if the pigs are already infected with respiratory pathogens and are in circumstances of poor housing and inadequate environments, severe disease may develop and persist.

Acute disease

When the virus first enters the breeding herd disease is seen in dry sows, lactating sows and sucking piglets.

Clinical signs in dry sows during the first month of infection

- Short periods of inappetance spreading over 7-14 days - 10-15% of sows at any one time.
- The body temperature may be elevated to 39-40°C (103-105°F).
- Abortions, often late term, may occur at a 1-6% level. These are often the first signs to be noted.
- Transient discoloration of the ears may be seen (2% level. Blue ear disease).
- Some sows farrow slightly early. 10-15% over the first 4 weeks.
- Increased returns occur 21-35 days post-service.
- Prolonged anoestrus and delayed returns to heat post-weaning.
- Coughing and respiratory signs.
- Transient blueing of the ears.

The inappetance may be quite short, often no longer than 12-24 hours, and the sow may eat only half her feed. Thus in the dry sow house there may be episodes when up to 10% of sows at any one time will be slightly off their food. In group housing, this inappetance may not be so noticeable. In herds where sows are subjected to wide fluctuations in environmental temperature, or if the management is poor and nutrition marginal, then the signs are likely to be more severe. Furthermore, in these types of herds, abortion levels are often elevated considerably.

Clinical signs in farrowing sows in the first month of infection

- Inappetance over the farrowing period.
- A reluctance to drink.
- Agalactia and mastitis.
- Farrowings are often 2-3 days early.

- Discoloration of the skin and pressure sores associated with small vesicles.
- Lethargy.
- Respiratory signs.
- Mummified piglets. 10-15% may die in the last 3-4 weeks of pregnancy.
- Stillbirth levels increase up to 30%.
- Very weak piglets at birth.

This chapter is primarily concerned with the effects of the disease on reproduction. Disease in piglets is discussed in chapter 8 and disease in weaners and finishers in chapter 9. The initial phase of inappetance and fever will often take 3-6 weeks to move through the breeding herd. Cyanosis or blueing of the ears is a variable finding and less than 5% of sows show it. It is transient and may last for only a few hours. Coughing occurs in some sows and a few individual cases of clinical pneumonia may occur. This acute phase lasts in the herd for up to 6 weeks, and is characterised by early farrowings, increases in stillbirths, weak pigs and an increase in the numbers of large mummified pigs that have died in the last three weeks of pregnancy.

In some herds, these may reach up to 30% of the total pigs born. Piglet mortality peaks at 70% in weeks 3 or 4 after the onset of symptoms and only returns to pre-infected levels after 8-12 weeks. The reproductive problems may persist for 4-8 months before returning to normal, however in some herds it may actually improve on the pre-PRRS performance.

Long term effects

Longer term effects of PRRS on reproductive efficiency are difficult to assess, particularly in herds of low health status. In some there are increases in repeat matings, vulval discharges and abortions, all of which may be blamed on PRRS.

The effects of PRRS on reproduction efficiency in herds in which the infection has become enzootic have been observed in the field for up to 12 months after disease has apparently settled. These are as follows:

- A 10-15% reduction in farrowing rate (90% of herds return to normality).
- Reduced numbers born alive.
- Increased stillbirths.
- Poor reproduction in gilts.
- Early farrowings.
- Increased levels of abortion (2-3%).
- Inappetance in sows at farrowing.

Some herds report that PRRS continues to be associated with reproductive failure and increases in repeats (5-10%) on a normal and abnormal cycle for as long as 6 months after the acute episode has subsided.

Field experiences show this is unusual in herds of less than 500 sows provided live vaccination has not been carried out.

Signs in boars
- Inappetance.
- Increased body temperature.
- Lethargy.
- Loss of libido.
- Lowered fertility.
- Poor litter sizes.
- Lowered sperm output.

Diagnosis

If the herd has not been exposed to PRRS then blood sampling a minimum of 12 adult animals (preferably those that have been off their food at least three weeks) provides a reliable means of diagnosis. Serological tests available include the overlay or IPMA test, the fluorescent antibody test and an ELISA test. All these tests can give rise to false positives and false negatives on individual animals, but on a group basis, they are reliable in indicating whether the herd has been infected or not. Where disease persists serum samples should be examined two weeks apart to demonstrate whether the virus is associated with a particular clinical problem. PCR tests on small blood samples taken in the early acute phase have also been developed and are available in some countries.

Similar diseases

When PRRS first enters the herd the clinical picture could be confused with AD but the absence of nervous symptoms in piglets and serological tests will differentiate the two diseases.

Treatment

There is no treatment as yet available in animals against virus infections. With PRRS however, it is essential during the acute phase to prevent the multiplication of bacteria that normally would have been destroyed by macrophages. Antibiotic treatment should be given for 3-4 weeks to all sows and boars immediately the disease is diagnosed or suspected. If necessary commence with water soluble antibiotics followed by in-feed medication. Prompt treatment usually reduces abortions, stillbirths, mummified pigs and early farrowings caused by secondary bacteria.

A control programme for dry sows during acute disease
- ☐ Raise the sow house temperature to 21° (72°F).
- ☐ Avoid night temperature drops.
- ☐ Avoid draughts.
- ☐ Medicate the sow's feed immediately with 500g/tonne of tetracycline either CTC or OTC.
- ☐ If sows are inappetent, medicate the water with OTC or CTC at the onset.
- ☐ Apply the medication to both gilts and boars.
- ☐ Maintain this for a four week period.
- ☐ Increase feed intake by at least 0.5kg per day over the four weeks.
- ☐ Inject individual sows with long-acting OTC or penicillin during periods of inappetance or as advised by your veterinarian.

A control programme for the sows in the service area during acute disease
- ☐ Apply the same procedures as for dry sows.
- ☐ Do not cull any sows for the next six weeks, (at least) to increase the mating programme.

> **When disease first appears in a herd allow at least 2 weeks before carrying out IPMA or ELISA tests.**

- ☐ Accept that you will have a 10-15% drop in the farrowing rate, and therefore plan to increase the mating programme by more gilts and retention of sows that would have been culled.
- ☐ Buy in gilts if possible from a previously exposed herd, most if not all will be immune. If home bred gilts are kept, introduce these to the infection as early as possible.
- ☐ To do this always move gilts into weaner or finisher accommodation for 3-4 days to expose them to the virus.
- ☐ Consider vaccinating incoming gilts whilst in isolation if one is available. Seek veterinary advice.
- ☐ Do not serve gilts until six weeks after exposure to infection.
- ☐ Use one dose of AI to compliment each natural mating for an 8 week period.

A control programme for the farrowing sow during acute disease
- ☐ Inject sows 2 days before farrowing with antibiotics. Continue this in succeeding sows for a period of six weeks.
- ☐ Repeat three days later or until farrowed.
- ☐ Use long-acting preparations of antibiotics. Oxytetracycline or semi-synthetic penicillins are drugs of choice.
- ☐ Top dress the sows food daily with in-feed antibiotics premixes. Use OTC, CTC or TMS. (Give 15-20g of a 10% premix per day).
- ☐ Continue this for 10-21 days post-farrowing.
- ☐ Raise the farrowing house temperature to 22°C (75°F)
- ☐ Deep bed the pens with straw, shavings or paper if this is possible.
- ☐ Provide extra heat for piglets.

Continue the above programme for 4 - 6 weeks as advised by your veterinarian.

If it is suspected that a chronic reproductive problem is associated with PRRS consider the following action plan. (Fig.6-6).

From this information the following possibilities exist :

- There is no infection taking place in the sow herd and no evidence of infection in weaners. In other words the virus has died out and PRRS is not a problem.
- The sow herd is serologically negative but there is evidence of persistent viral infection in younger growing pigs. Such animals will show evidence of rising titre levels. This continually exposes susceptible breeding stock to disease.
- Negative gilts become infected and disseminate the virus.

Because our knowledge of this disease is continually improving you are advised to discuss further controls with your veterinarian. Three procedures need to be considered:
1. Vaccination if a vaccine is available.
2. Removal of the infected group of pigs, usually the first and second stage growers from the farm to eliminate the virus.
3. Expose gilts to maintain an immune breeding herd.

Artificial insemination (AI)

Originally it was thought that artificial insemination would not disseminate PRRS but, epidemiological studies have indicated that it has been a major source of spread during acute disease. Boars may remain viraemic for 8-12 weeks after initial infection or become chronic carriers. There is, however, strong evidence to show that if young breeding boars are moved from known positive farms and held in isolation for 8 weeks with negative sentinel pigs and if the sentinels do not seroconvert the boars can be moved relatively safely into the AI stud. However sero-negative boars in the stud should be closely monitored for sero-conversion and signs of inappetance or fever. If there is any doubt semen movements should be stopped until it is sorted out. Large AI data bases have shown that semen from sero-positive, non shedding boars does not appear to transmit infection to sero-negative herds.

Immunity

Field observations show that the majority of breeding females become immune and do not succumb to further episodes of infection. However, if the virus continues to circulate in young growing pigs a few incoming negative gilts will become infected at some stage. Field experiences in the UK have shown that reappearance of disease in breeding herds is uncommon.

Management control and prevention

If your herd is in a region where it is unlikely to be infected directly from a neighbour it is important to determine by serology if your herd has or has not been exposed to PRRS. If it is found to be negative the following actions should be considered

◆ Purchase breeding stock from herds believed free of PRRS.
◆ Set up a quarantine system to hold pigs for a minimum of eight weeks.
◆ As pigs arrive in quarantine, add 6 of your own known negative pigs and mix with the incoming stock.
◆ After five weeks of direct contact, blood sample the 6 sentinel pigs and 6 of the incoming stock.
◆ Check with the donor herd that it is still believed free.
◆ Make sure lorries do not come onto your farm with other pigs already on board.
◆ Provide boots and coveralls for all visitors.
◆ Do not borrow equipment from other pig farms.
◆ Review herd biosecurity.
◆ In known infected herds one of two breeding strategies can be adopted. If the virus is not circulating it may be advisable to buy in gilts and boars from negative herds and vaccinate them in isolation. Alternatively gilts and boars from known infected sources should be purchased and acclimatised for at

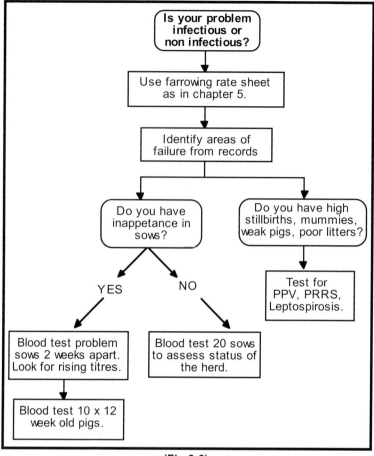

(Fig.6-6)

least six weeks before mating. The method should be determined by the performance of the gilts. Both live and killed vaccines are available in some countries and control strategies will be determined by their known safety and efficiency. Seek advice from your veterinarian.

Elimination

After a period of time the virus may disappear from the sow and finisher population but remain endemic in the first and second stage rearing in pigs 3-12 weeks of age. By blood sampling sows, weaners and finishers the status of the herd in this respect can be established. Where disease is only active in growing pigs up to 12 weeks of age they can all be removed from the farm together with the next two weeks production of new weaners. The houses are cleaned and disinfected and left empty for two weeks. PRRS disease can be eliminated by this method of partial depopulation.

PRRS free pigs can be obtained in a similar way from a herd in which the virus has become enzootic and in which herd immunity is stable and active virus infection is lower. In this process of segregated early weaning (SEW) the largest suckled piglets are weaned from the farrowing rooms at 5-10 days of age to be reared in isolated premises. The method, however, is not 100% reliable and occasionally one or more piglets in a litter may come through already infected. To reduce this happening pigs should only be taken from sero-positive mothers. To avoid all the pigs becoming infected, each group of piglets weaned should be kept in isolation until all the pigs have been tested. PCRs are coming available for this. It takes only a few days to get the results. To improve the system further, instead of farrowing the mothers on the farm they can be farrowed in temporary accommodation outside the farm (MEW). See chapter 3 Segregated weaning.

Hysterectomies can be carried out on sows from stable herds. Fostering these piglets on to sows from a PRRS negative herd is an effective method of developing PRRS negative stock. It must be remembered, though, that PRRS can cross the placenta in recently infected gilts and sows. Therefore only pregnant sows that have been sero-positive for at least 4 months should be hysterectomised. Each newborn litters should be tested for infections using a PCR. The foster sows and hysterectomy derived piglets should be kept in isolation until the results are known.

A farm can be depopulated cleaned, disinfected and repopulated with PRRS negative stock. Depopulation is very expensive and before considering this investigate how the herd became infected in the first place and assess the chances off it being re infected again. Repopulation should not be attempted in winter because as the temperature drops, the survival of the virus increases, e.g. 24 hours at 37°C (99°F), 6 days at 20°C (68°F), 1 month at 4°C (39°F). The virus is stable when frozen for long periods of time. Control of PRRS in weaners and finishers is discussed in chapter 9.

SWINE INFLUENZA VIRUS (SI)

Swine influenza is caused by a number of closely related influenza A viruses that are noted for their ability to change their antigenic structure and create new strains. SI can be introduced by infected people, carrier pigs and probably on the wind although this has not been proved. Birds particularly water fowl, are reservoirs of infection.

Each serotype is identified by surface proteins referred to as "H" and "N". The three common strains that affect the pig are described as $H_1 N_1$, $H_1 N_2$ and $H_3 N_2$. There are also different strains within these serotypes with differing pathogenicity (capacity to produce disease).

Clinical signs

The incubation period of the disease is very short, as little as 12-48 hours. When the virus first enters the herd two or three animals may be observed sick for the first two days, followed by a rapid explosive outbreak of inappetance and clinically very ill pigs. The effects on the reproductive system follow the sudden onset of a rapid spreading respiratory disease with coughing, pneumonia, fevers and inappetance. Acute respiratory distress persists over a period of 7-10 days (depending on the amount of contact between groups of sows). There are three important periods when infection causes infertility. First, if sows are ill in the first 21 days post-service pregnancy their developing embryos may not get established and an increase in 21 day returns results. If pregnancy has been established 14-16 days after mating, and it then fails returns will be delayed. Second if infection occurs in the first five weeks of pregnancy, there could be total embryo mortality and absorption with sows becoming pseudo-pregnant and not in-pig. Litter size may also be affected at this stage due to absorption of embryos. Towards the end of the pregnancy period abortions or late mummified pigs at farrowing may also be experienced. The third major effect is on the boar, where high body temperatures affect semen and depress fertility for a 4 to 5 week period.

SI in large herds may become endemic with intermittent bouts of disease and infertility and different strains may also sequentially infect the herd. Immunity to influenza viruses is often short lived (6 months) and the immunity profile in the breeding herd varies considerably with time.

At a herd level the following may also be seen:
- A sudden and rapid onset of acute illness in sows.
- Coughing and pneumonia spreading rapidly.
- A return to clinical normality over 7-10 days.
- Delayed returns to heat after post-weaning.
- Increased repeats at 21 days.
- Increased repeats outside the normal cycle.
- Increased numbers of sows coming through not in-pig.
- Increased numbers of abortions, particularly late term.

- Increased numbers of stillbirth rates and slow farrowings.
- Occasionally an increase in mummified pigs.

During the phases of high temperatures other diseases present in the herd may be triggered off. A typical example would be an increase in abortions associated with leptospira infection.

Diagnosis

This can often be made reliably on clinical grounds because there are no other diseases that are so dramatic in their onset and clinical effects. Blood samples taken at the time of onset of disease from affected sows and repeated 2-3 weeks later show rising levels of antibody to the specific virus. SIV can be readily grown from nasal and throat swabs and identified in the laboratory. This is often the best approach to confirm the diagnosis.

Similar diseases

In acute disease the spread is so dramatic across all ages that little else can be confused with it. In endemic disease however differentiation from other viral infections can be difficult, but PRRS, PRCV, AD and erysipelas should be considered (see Fig.6-2 and Fig.6-3).

Treatment

☐ Individual breeding females or boars showing acute illness, and raised temperatures, particularly with increased respiratory rate should be treated with broad spectrum antibiotics for three days.

☐ Suitable drugs would include penicillin/streptomycin, long-acting OTC or synthetic penicillins such as amoxycillin. If the illness is severe then medicate the drinking water with either CTC or OTC at a level of 25g (100% pure) per 1000kg of live weight per day, for five days.

Management control and prevention

It is important to prevent any secondary bacterial infections.
◆ Keep sows within an environmental temperature of 20-23ºC (70-75ºF)
◆ Reduce all possible stress, such as draughts.
◆ Maintain dry bedding and floor surfaces.
◆ Monitor boars carefully for evidence of illness
◆ Identify boars that have been ill and cross-serve with another boar for the next four weeks.
◆ Serve sows by AI followed by a natural mating and consider a second dose of AI (am/pm/am).
◆ Medicate the water with soluble vitamins for seven days.
◆ Medicate the feed as described above for 2 weeks.
◆ If periods of inappetance occur in boars, blood test them twice two weeks apart to establish a diagnosis.
◆ Because of the possible ways by which the virus may enter the herd it is extremely difficult to maintain populations free of infections. In some countries inactivated vaccines are available and appear to be protective. In herds in which the virus periodically circulates and causes disease this route should be explored.
◆ If you believe your herd to be free (and this can be confirmed by serological tests,) purchase breeding stock from herds that have a similar disease history and that are also serologically negative. The practicality of this however is not easy.

Bacterial Infertility

ABORTION

See chapter 5 for additional information.

The factors associated with abortion are complex, varied and often interrelated.

Fig.6-7 shows the factors that contribute to abortions of either infectious or management factors. Infectious agents can bring about abortion in three ways.
1. They can invade the placenta, cause inflammation (placentitis) and perhaps necrosis, (tissue death) cutting off the nutrient and oxygen supply to the foetus.
2. They can invade the foetus and kill it.
3. They can multiply elsewhere in the body causing fever and sometimes toxaemia (toxins in the blood).

FACTORS THAT MAY LEAD TO ABORTION IN THE SOW

Infectious Agents and Conditions	Other Causes	Management Factors
Parasite burdens	Stress	Low temperatures
Toxoplasma	Lameness	Chilling, draughts
Viral infections	Contaminated water	Excessive fan speeds
Bacterial infections	Poor hygiene	Wet pens
Cystitis, Nephritis	No boar contact	Poor insulation
Individual illness	Vaccine reaction	Ultra violet radiation
	Toxic substances	Decreasing daylight length
	Poisonous plants	Poor lighting
	Mouldy feeds	Shadows
	Mycotoxins	Poor nutrition
		Low feed intake

→ Abortion

(Fig.6-7)

Toxins from mouldy feed can cause abortions. Strictly speaking they are not infections or bacteria but for completeness are mentioned here. The fungus can be at a low level in one of the feed constituents and barely detectable by visual examination and yet produce powerful toxins. These when ingested have toxic effects which may cause abortion. This form of fungal poisoning is called mycotoxicosis. The fungus may also be readily seen growing as a mould in feed lines, bags of feed or wet feed systems and their distributing vessels and pipes.

To prevent mycotoxicosis:
- Always check your feed bins. Are they water tight?
- When were they last inspected internally?
- Do they contain bridged mouldy feed?
- Are the bins filled with warm feed?
- Do you regularly treat the bins to prevent mould growth.
- Are the bags of feed kept in a dry cool or wet warm place?
- If you practice home mixing and wet feeding are the tanks and pipes mould free?
- Are you ever tempted to give feed to sows that has been slightly mouldy.

If you wet feed:
- Do you check the roofs of your mixing tanks to see whether feed splashed on to them has gone mouldy.
- Do you check the pipes?
- Do you check the source materials?
- Do you let liquid components of the mix sit around in hot weather in storage tanks?

The major infectious bacterial diseases which spread through herds and cause abortion are brucellosis and leptospirosis. (Fig.6-8). These infectious agents affect increasing numbers of sows in the herd with typical clinical signs of the disease. There is, however, a second group of bacteria which can be described as opportunist invaders which cause embryo mortality or abortion in individual sows and sporadically in small groups of sows. They do not spread through the herd like brucella or leptospira. They are often mixed infections (i.e. several different species involved).

If, however these opportunist bacterial infections occur in sufficient numbers of sows they can become a herd problem. They are often normal inhabitants of the vagina or the boars prepuce and their identification following pathological examinations needs careful interpretation. An emerging syndrome in this category occurs when high numbers of bacteria are deposited into the anterior vagina, particularly towards the end of the heat period, by the boar. Such bacteria include klebsiella, streptococci, staphylococci and possibly leptospira. In such cases careful clinical examination of sows between 14 and 21 days post mating will sometimes reveal a tacky discharge on the vulva, which may not necessarily be very obvious. Such sows should be identified, and if they are returning out of cycle, it is likely that embryo loss is taking place.

Low grade or chronic infections such as cystitis (infection of the bladder) and nephritis (infection of the kidneys) occasionally cause abortion. Lameness and pain, particularly from abscesses in the feet or leg weakness (osteochondrosis) can also cause the corpus luteum to regress due to stress. Bullying and fighting are often forgotten as predisposing factors in individual sows. Clinical observations and examination of records are important tools for investigation and the stockperson's opinions and observations are often invaluable.

BRUCELLOSIS
See chapter 12 for further information.

This disease is caused by the bacterium *Brucella suis*, which is one of the six different species of brucella. *Brucella suis* does not exist in the UK, Ireland and in some other EU countries, but is widespread through most of the rest of the pig rearing world and is an important disease not least because some strains of it cause a

SPECIFIC BACTERIA THAT MAY CAUSE ABORTION		
Agent	Diagnosis	Treatment/Prevention
Brucella suis	Clinical picture Bacterial Isolation Serology	No vaccine available Purchase negative stock Depopulate
Leptospira	F.A.T * Isolation of the organism Serology	Vaccination Purchase negative stock? Antibiotics Avoid contaminated sources
Erysipelas	Isolation of the organism	Vaccination
Campylobacter	Culture	Antibiotics
Eperythrozoonosis suis	Blood smear (PCR)	Antibiotics organic arsenicals Needle hygiene
Chlamydia	Microscopy of smears ELISA test	Antibiotics

* = Fluorescent antibody test

(Fig.6-8)

Empty feed bins monthly.
Examine internal surfaces monthly.
Examine feed daily.
Treat Bins regularly with a mould inhibitor.

INFECTIOUS AGENTS OPPORTUNIST INVADERS	
Campylobacter	*Leptospira bratislava*
Chlamydia	Pasteurella
E. coli	Pseudomonas
E. suis	Staphylococci
Erysipelothrix	Streptococci
Klebsiella	Toxoplasma

You cannot afford to let Brucella suis contaminate your herd.

nasty disease in people. It can be spread by venereal infection and the boar is a major source either by direct contact at mating or via artificial insemination. Pigs can also be infected via the conjunctiva, through the nose or by mouth. The organism can survive outside the pig for long periods of time particularly at or near freezing temperatures. The hare in Northern Europe can also be infected where it is considered a natural host. It can be an important source of infection to the pig.

When a female becomes infected, the organism is plentiful in the blood, causing a bacteraemia, which persists over a period of 3-6 weeks. It is during this period of time that the organism establishes itself in the placenta, causing inflammation and ultimately abortion. *B. suis* infects the testicles and accessory reproductive glands, and can be excreted via semen. The disease can be transmitted to people and is serious.

Clinical signs

These include infertility and abortions which may occur at any time. If the sow is infected via the boar at mating, the abortions occur early, often before day 35 and delayed returns will be experienced. Sows aborting after day 30 may show a bloody vaginal discharge that contains high numbers of organisms. In sucking and weaned pigs, *B. suis* can infect bones and soft tissues causing paralysis of the hind legs. A carrier state persists for long periods of time.

Diagnosis

This can be readily carried out by isolation of the organism. Serology is used to detect carrier sows but cross reactions can occur quite extensively due to another organism called *Yersinia enterocolitica*. The serum agglutination test (SAT) is used and results in excess of 31 international units (iu) are considered positive. The complement fixation test (CFT) is used in conjunction with the SAT for export testing purposes within the EU.
Standards used with the EU for intra community trade.
Serum agglutination test (SAT) - More than 31iu classified as a failure.
Complement fixation test (CFT) More than 25iu classified as a failure.

Treatment

There is no effective treatment. Antibiotics give a poor response.

Management control and prevention

◆ This is based on identifying herds free from *B. suis* infection and maintaining them by purchasing pigs only from herds free of disease. In some countries eradication programmes are being carried out by identifying infected herds and removing them.

◆ Once a country is declared free of the disease,

THE VULVAL DISCHARGE SYNDROME. 1985	
Herds studied	110
Total sows	30,580
Mean herd size	278
Range	90-750
Herds affected	26 (24%)
Sows at risk	9,090

(Fig. 6-9)

serological testing of incoming breeding stock has proved highly effective in preventing disease spread.

ENDOMETRITIS AND THE VULVAL DISCHARGE SYNDROME

Since 1985 there has been a gradual reduction in farrowing rates in many herds associated with increased repeats in sows. A survey carried out at that time (Fig.6-9) indicated that up to 24% of herds may have had previously unrecognised problems with this disease.

A discharge from the vulva post-service does not automatically mean there has been a pregnancy failure, but it will in most cases indicate infection. Fig.6-10 shows the anatomy of the reproductive tract and the potential areas from which discharges could arise. These include the rectum, the vulva, the vagina, the cervix and the uterus. Discharges can also arise from infection of the kidneys (pyelonephritis) or the bladder (cystitis) with pus being passed in the urine.

It is important to record the time when discharges are first seen, their colour and composition and effects on the sow. Use the farrowing rate loss sheet as shown in chapter 5 to record the observations.

Clinical signs

Vulval discharges are common within 3-4 days of farrowing when a thick viscous material may be excreted. If the sow is healthy, the udder is normal and there is no mastitis, ignore it. It is common practice to inject such

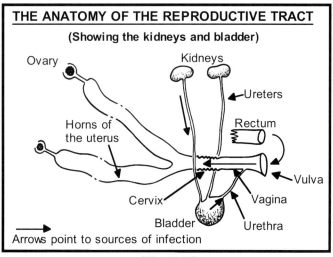

(Fig. 6-10)

sows, but this is not necessary under these circumstances. Always be mindful that with a heavy smelling bloody discharge there may be a retained piglet or afterbirth.

The time in the reproductive cycle when the discharge is seen is important particularly between 14-21 days post-service. The lips of the vulva of each sow should be parted daily and any tackiness or small discharge noted. The sow should be marked and if she repeats a problem may be developing. Note also the periods when it is quite normal for the sow to show evidence of a slight discharge. (Fig.6-11) Remember discharging sows may be pregnant and always pregnancy test before culling. The types of discharge are shown in Fig.6-12

Fig.6-13 shows the reproductive performance of 42 sows in a herd that had a discharge problem and this highlights the fact that only 28% of the sows farrowed, and 62% of them repeated. Most of the animals had 5 or more litters. It is important therefore to cull such animals because farrowing rates of only 50-60% are achieved to matings. The response to treatments is poor.

Records

The changes that take place are shown in Fig.6-14 and highlight increases in repeat matings, sows not in-pig and discharges, but a proportion of sows will discharge and remain in-pig. In these cases infection arises from either the vagina or the bladder. Doubtful or negative pregnancy tests at 30 and 40 days increase, but levels of abortions, litter size and sow health remain normal.

Diagnosis

The bacteria causing reproductive tract infections are shown in Fig.6-15. The main organisms associated with endometritis and vulval discharges are opportunist invaders. In some herds no specific organism can be identified, although bacteriological tests may show one or more bacteria predominating either in the prepuce or vagina. A precise diagnosis can be difficult.

An initial diagnosis is made from observations of vulval discharges commencing 10 days post-service and associated with a loss of pregnancy. Leptospirosis caused by *Leptospira bratislava/muenchen*, particularly in gilts, can cause discharges post-service, particularly if there is early embryo loss (14-25 days) and absorption. Brucellosis also causes vaginal discharges following absorption.

Examination of records can help in differentiating between infectious and non-infectious causes of infertility as shown in Fig.6-16.

Post mortem examinations on sows with heavy discharges are not particularly helpful. Post mortem examination of 47 discharging sows within seven days of the event showed only 12 with an infection actually in the womb. (Fig.6-17). This is because by the time sows can be slaughtered and the wombs examined they have

THE SIGNS OF VULVAL DISCHARGES IN HEALTHY SOWS	
Time of Discharge	Significance
1-4 days post farrowing	* Normal
> 5 days lactation	Abnormal
At mating	* Normal
Up to 5 days post-service	* Normal
14-21 days post-service	Abnormal
During pregnancy	Abnormal

* Unless heavy increasing and continuous

(Fig.6-11)

SOURCES AND TYPES OF DISCHARGE	
Type of Discharge	Source
Thick, white, yellow pus	Vulva Vagina Cervix Womb
Fluid, mucus, pus, blood and urine	Bladder Kidney Vulva Vagina
Chalky	Urine sediment from the kidneys and bladder
Pure blood	Internal ruptured blood vessel

(Fig.6-12)

HERD 20 The Results of Vulval Discharges Observed >5 Days Post-mating (42 Sows Untreated)		
No:	Farrowed	12 (28%)
	Died	
	Cystitis (culled)	1
	Repeated	26 (62%)
No. of pregnancies		
	Gilts	2
	2-4 litter sows	4
	5-7 litter sows	18
	8+ litter sows	18

(Fig.6-13)

VULVAL DISCHARGES > 5 DAYS POST-SERVICE		
	Problem Herd Ranges	Targets for Normal Herds
Repeats		
19-23 days	10 - 20%	< 10%
24-90 days	5 - 10%	< 3%
Sows not in pig with or without discharges	4 - 9%	< 1%
Pregnancy testing (doubtful or negative)		
% at 30 days	5 - 20%	< 5%
% at 40 days	5 - 20%	< 5%
Farrowing rate	60 - 85%	> 87%
Abortions	Normal level	< 1%
Litter size	Unaffected	
Sow health	Unaffected	

(Fig.6-14)

come into oestrus which has the effect of resolving and removing the pus from the womb. In spite of this most sows still remain infertile

Field studies have identified the following factors that do not appear to be associated with post-mating vulval discharges and infertility and these include:
- Season.
- Breed of sow.
- Source of breeding female.
- Source of boar.
- Artificial insemination.
- Cystitis pyelonephritis.
- Discharges in lactation.
- Assistance at farrowing.
- Discharge at <5 days post-mating.

Artificial insemination does not appear to be a major part of the complex because its use in problem herds does not necessarily solve the problem. Bladder/kidney infections do not cause pregnancy loss, unless the sow is ill, when abortion or death may occur. Generally, there is no relationship between discharges seen in lactation and those seen post-service with loss of pregnancy. Likewise, assistance at farrowing does not appear to affect a post-service problem.

During the period of oestrus and whilst oestrogen levels are high it is difficult to infect the womb. However, as oestrogen levels drop and the levels of progesterone rise the womb becomes susceptible to infection.

It is likely that over a period of time in problem herds, certain opportunist bacteria gradually predominate in the preputial sac of the boar, the vagina and the environment.

If matings take place towards the end of the heat period with high levels of infection persisting at the cervix, the risk of ascending infection becomes high.

The major predisposing factors leading to the development of a vulval discharge problem include:
- Herds with high numbers of old sows.
- A short lactation length (14-21 days).
- Multiple matings. Cross mating boars.
- Handling the prepuce at mating and squeezing the prepucial sac.
- No supervision at mating.
- Matings towards the end of the oestrus period.
- Wet, dirty boar pens. Poor drainage. Continual use.
- Dirty, wet sow mating pens and continual use without cleaning.
- Small stalls where the sow adopts a dog sitting posture with heavy contamination of the vulva.
- Housing maiden gilts in stalls.
- Heavy vulval contamination, for example in maiden gilts housed on slats where slurry spills over.
- Early embryo mortality.
- Re-mating discharging sows.
- Using old boars on young sows.
- Using young boars on older sows.

Management control is carried out by changing and improving the factors considered important on the farm.

Diagnosis

This is carried out in three parts:
1. Studying the records as outlined.
2. Regular observations of the vulva particularly 14-21 days post mating to identify affected females.
3. Bacteriological examinations of preputial and vaginal secretions. All boars and 10 sows that have repeated

REPRODUCTIVE TRACT INFECTIONS
Opportunist Invaders *
Chlamydia
E. coli
E. suis
Erysipelothrix
Klebsiella
Leptospira bratislava/ muenchen
Pasteurella
Proteus
Pseudomonas
Staphylococci
Streptococci

* Important in the vulval discharge syndrome.
(Fig.6-15)

CLINICAL DIFFERENTIATION BETWEEN INFECTIOUS AND NON-INFECTIOUS CAUSES OF REPRODUCTIVE FAILURE			
Type of Failure		Non-Infectious	Infectious
Anoestrus		+++	+
Repeats	- at 21 days and no discharge	+++	+
	- at 21 days with discharge	+	+++
Repeats	- 23-28 days	++	++
Abortion	- sow in good health	+++	+
	- with healthy foetuses	++	++
	- with mummified or decomposing	-	+++
Sow not in pig		+++	++
Mummified pigs	- small and variable in size	+	+++
	- large	++	++
Stillbirths	- increased within a normal litter	+++	+
	- with mummified pigs	+	+++

+ Unlikely cause   +++ Likely cause
(Fig.6-16)

VAGINAL DISCHARGES	
Results of Post Mortem Examinations of 47 sows	
No gross lesions	21
Vaginitis	2
Vaginitis and endometritis	4
Endometritis	12
Endometritis and cystitis	6
Cystitis	2
Pregnant	0
Total	47

Vaginitis = inflammation of the vagina
Endometritis = inflammation of the lining of the uterus
(Fig.6-17)

CHAPTER 6 - Reproduction. Infectious Infertility

should be tested. A swab is introduced into the prepuce either while the boar is eating, confined in a stall or just before dismounting after mating. Likewise in problem sows the lips of the vulva are cleaned with tissue, parted and a swab inserted to its full length. The predominating organisms in the herd can then be determined and antibiotic sensitivity tests carried out. Swabs from individual discharges are worth examining but the results are sometimes not helpful. However they will identify an organism such as klebsiella which is a primary pathogen in its own right. Fig.6-18 shows a typical laboratory result and some of the antibiotics that could be used. These results were obtained from a farm where 24% of served sows repeated and there was evidence of a tacky discharge 12-20 days post-service associated with some of the infertile sows. The bacteriological picture shows a high isolation rate of klebsiella bacteria from the prepuce of the boars (90%). The level in a normal herd would be less than 10%. Further examinations showed 30% of problem sows were carrying the same organism. Klebsiella is recognised as an opportunist pathogen and from the antibiotic sensitivity tests amoxycillin was selected as the drug of choice for treatment. 3ml of injectable solution were deposited into the anterior vagina of all sows 6 - 24 hours after the last mating. This was carried out for a four month period and 7ml placed in the prepuce of each boar once every three weeks, on five occasions. The conception rate improved to 88%.

Treatment of the boar

- You are advised to discuss aspects of treatment with your veterinarian but there are three methods, antibiotics installed into the prepuce, by injection into muscle or by mouth. (Fig.6-19). The latter can be best carried out using in-feed premixes and placing a small amount on the food daily for ten days. The boar could be injected with long-acting antibiotic preparations, but this should be avoided if possible because he can become needle-shy. If leptospirosis is suspected as an initiating factor injections of streptomycin should be given daily for 3 days and this repeated monthly for 5 occasions. Streptomycin is not available in some countries.

Treatment of the sow

- The most effective method is to insert an antibiotic into the anterior vagina up to the cervix (but not actually into it). A 3ml dose of most injectable antibiotics can be used the selection being dependent upon the bacteriological examinations and sensi-

PREPUCIAL SWABS			A BACTERIOLOGICAL PROFILE							
Boar No.	1	2	3	4	5	6	7	8	9	10
Bacillus	-	+	-	-	-	-	-	-	-	-
Clostridia	-	-	-	-	-	-	-	-	-	-
E. coli	+	-	+	-	+	-	-	-	-	-
Eubacterium suis	+	-	-	-	-	+	-	-	-	-
Haemolytic aerobes	-	-	+	++	-	-	-	+	-	-
Haemolytic anaerobes	-	+	-	+	-	-	-	-	+	-
Klebsiella	+	++	++	++	++	-	++	++	+	+
Proteus	+++	-	+	-	-	-	-	-	-	-
Pseudomonas	-	+	-	-	-	-	-	-	-	-
Non haemolytic staphylococcus	++	++	++	+	+	+	+	+	+	+
Haemolytic staphylococcus	+	-	+	-	-	+	-	-	-	-
Streptococcus	-	++	+	-	+	+	+	+	+	-

+ = Low numbers isolated   +++ = High numbers isolated   - = Not isolated

Sensitivity Results	P	AML	FY	N	OT	SXT	ST	CL
Bacillus								
Clostridia								
E. coli								
Eubacterium suis								
Haemolytic aerobes	R	S	S	S	S	R	R	S
Haemolytic anaerobes								
Klebsiella	R	S	S	S	S	S	R	S
Proteus	R	S	S	S	S	S	S	S
Pseudomonas								
Non haemolytic staphylococcus	S	S	S	S	S	S	S	S
Haemolytic staphylococcus								
Streptococcus	R	R	S	S	R	S	S	S

S = Sensitive   R = Resistant
P = Penicillin   OT = Oxytetracycline
AML = Amoxycillin   SXT = Compound Sulphonamide
FY = Framycetin   ST = Streptomycin
N = Neomycin   CL = Cephalexin

(Fig.6-18)

tivities. A disposable AI catheter of small diameter, or a cattle AI catheter can be used. Shorten it by approximately 150mm. Attach a syringe with an adapter. Fill the catheter and syringe completely with the antibiotic. The catheter should then be gently inserted as far as the cervix but not into it and the antibiotic can then be deposited easily. This can be carried out 6-24 hours after the last mating. It is important however, when adopting this procedure to always monitor the results for any adverse effects over the first three weeks in respect of both discharges and return rates. An alternative method of medication is to top dress the feed of the sow from weaning to 21 days post-service. In herds with major problems it may be necessary to medicate all breeding females for a period of ten days with in-feed medication using the appropriate antibiotic. Discuss these methods of treatment as outlined in Fig.6-19 and Fig.6-20 with your veterinarian.

Management control and prevention

- Monitor the vulva for evidences of discharges.
- Do not serve towards the end of the heat period.
- Do not re-serve discharging sows.
- Only mate the sow when she is totally receptive to the boar. If in doubt wait.
- Do not be eager to serve too early.
- Consider single day mating i.e. boar am AI pm.
- Consider only one service.
- Use one boar to one sow only.
- Avoid wet dirty boar and mating pens. Clean and disinfect pens regularly.
- Avoid lactation periods < 21 days.
- Increase the number of gilts available for mating.
- Serve young boars to young females only.
- Prevent heavy faeces contamination of the vulva from weaning to 14 days post-service.

EPERYTHROZOONOSIS (EPE)
See chapter 8 for further information.

This is a disease caused by a bacterium called *Eperythrozoonosis suis* which attaches to the surface of red blood cells and sometimes destroys them. The pig then may become anaemic and the products left after the destruction of the cells may cause jaundice. Clinical disease is more commonly seen in the young growing pigs. However it can also cause reproductive problems in the breeding herd. A sow may carry Epe and yet remain quite healthy, however, it can cross the placenta and infect pigs in utero causing weak piglets at birth. The disease can be transmitted by direct inoculation, through pig lice, biting house flies, mange mites and perhaps more importantly the needles that are used to inject pigs. It is also thought that Epe may enter through the mouth to the stomach and intestine and be transferred into the body this way. This is one reason why the practice of feed-back using placenta is not advised.

Epe is present in most if not all herds but the mechanisms which allow it to become pathogenic and produce disease in some populations and not in others are unknown. The incidence of disease is low.

Clinical signs
Acute disease
Affected sows are inappetent with fever 40-42°C (105-107°F) when high numbers of organisms are present in the blood. This clinical picture is seen after farrowing

---

METHODS OF TREATMENT OF THE BOAR

Sheath Treatment
Injectable antibiotics or intra-mammary mastitis preparations can be used.
7 ml doses of either -
    Penicillin and dihydrostreptomycin
    Ampicillin
    Oxytetracycline
    Trimethoprim/sulpha
    Framycetin
Instil into the sheath once every three weeks for five occasions.

Feed Medication (Top dress)
Using 10% in-feed premixes
Place 15-20g on food daily
Medicate for 10 days
Drugs available:
    Tetracyclines CTC, OTC
    Penicillin
    Trimethoprim/sulpha
    Ampicillin

Individual Injections
Use long-acting preparations if available.
Inject once every three weeks for five occasions.
Options:
    Tetracyclines
    Penicillin streptomycin
    Amoxycillin
    Trimethoprim
    Framycetin.

(Fig.6-19)

METHODS OF TREATMENT OF THE SOW

Intra Vaginal
Instil 3ml of antibiotic into the anterior vagina.
Use a disposable AI catheter.
Apply 6-24 hours after the last mating.
Monitor the results carefully.
Select antibiotics on sensitivity tests.

Feed Medication (Top Dress)
As per the boar.
Medicate for 21 days post-service.
Inject the sow on day of weaning.
Alternatively in-feed medicate all the herd for 10 days.

(Fig.6-20)

If repeat matings in the herd are high check the vulva of all sows 14-21 days post-service for tacky discharge.
DO THEY REPEAT?

and anaemia is a common symptom. Similar acute infections occur in sows at weaning time together with anoestrus.

Chronic disease

Sows become debilitated and pale with jaundice, poor conception, repeat matings and anoestrus. Signs of infertility that have been attributed to Epe include:
- Delayed returns to oestrus.
- Anaemia.
- Jaundice.
- Bleeding into tissues.
- Abortion.
- Reduced conception rates.

The carrier state

This is common and blood provides a constant source of transmission throughout the herd, particularly when females are vaccinated using common needles.

Diagnosis

This is carried out by making a blood smear on a glass slide, staining it with a special stain (Wright's stain) and looking for the organism under the microscope. The presence of Epe in a smear need not necessarily imply disease and there is still controversy over the actual role of this bacterium and its capacity to cause disease.

Treatment

☐ Arsanilic acid at a level of 90 grams to the tonne has been used to provide a dose of approximately 250mg per day to each female.
☐ If the herd is infected with mange it is important to adopt a control programme.
☐ Oxytetracycline at a level of 400g to the tonne for four weeks is claimed to have some effect but generally the response to treatment is only moderate.

Management control and prevention

There are no known methods for preventing this disease other than reducing its movement around the herd by changing needles very frequently. It is possible that infection with PRRS initiates disease.
- Take precautions when vaccinating large numbers of sows. Change needles every 2 to 3 sows and gilts.
- Wipe the needle between each animal with cotton wool and surgical spirit.
- Reduce fighting episodes.
- Take precautions to keep vice at a minimum.
- Do not carry out feed back using placenta or farrowing liquids.
- Keep stress and immuno-suppression to a minimum.
- Control mange and lice if they are present.
- Control biting insects.

ERYSIPELAS

Swine erysipelas is caused by a bacterium, *Erysipelothrix rhusiopathiae* that is found in most if not all pig farms, up to 50% of animals may carry it in their tonsils. It is always present in either the pig or in the environment because it is excreted via saliva, faeces or urine. It is also found in many other species, including birds and sheep and can survive outside the pig for a few weeks and longer in light soils. Thus it is impossible to eliminate it from a herd. Infected faeces is probably the main source of infection, particularly in growing and finishing pens.

Disease is relatively uncommon in pigs under 8-12 weeks of age due to protection provided by maternal antibodies from the sow via the colostrum. The most susceptible animals are growing pigs, non vaccinated gilts and up to 4th parity sows.

Clinical signs

The organism multiplies in the body, and invades the bloodstream to produce a septicaemia. The rapidity of multiplication and the level of immunity in the pig then determines the clinical symptoms. These are of three types:

Per-acute or acute disease

The onset is sudden, often the only sign being death. This is seen rarely in sucking pigs. In boars and sows there are very high temperatures 40°C (108°F) and they are obviously ill, although others can appear normal. It is during this acute period that the disease may cause abortion. Alternatively, if abortion does not take place one or two piglets may die inside the womb and become mummified.

The organisms block tiny blood vessels to the skin over the back and sides of the body causing thrombosis. The restricted blood supply causes small raised areas called diamonds. These become red and finally black, due to dead tissue. Often these lumps can be palpated in the early stages before anything can be seen. Sudden death is not uncommon due to an acute septicaemia or heart failure.

> *If you have a sick sow running a high temperature, always run the flat of your hand down the sides of the body and over the ham. If you find raised lumps treat with penicillin daily for 3 days.*

Sub-acute disease

The sow appears inappetent and may show characteristic skin lesions. The temperature ranges from 39-40°C (102-104°F) but in some cases the disease can be so mild as to be undetected. Some piglets may die in the womb following sub-acute disease and become mummified.

Chronic disease

This may or may not follow acute, or sub-acute disease, and the organism either affects the joints producing lameness or the heart valves producing growths.

Sporadic disease is common in sows but if one sow in a group becomes infected the exposure is high from her urine and faeces and it is advisable to inject all contact animals with penicillin.

The important effects of erysipelas on reproductive failure:
- Sick animals with high fevers.
- Abortions during acute or sub-acute disease with ill sows and dead piglets.
- The death of piglets inside the womb and mummification.
- Abortions with decomposing piglets.
- Absorption of embryos and delayed returns.
- Normal returns if infection occurs immediately post-service.
- Variable litter size.

Boars infected with erysipelas develop high temperatures and sperm can be affected for the complete development period of 5-6 weeks. Infertility is demonstrated by returns, sows not in pig and poor litter sizes.

Diagnosis

This is determined by the clinical picture and isolation of the organism which is easy to grow in the laboratory. Serology will indicate exposure to the organism but it can only be used to confirm disease if rising titres, 14 days apart, are demonstrated.

The interpretation of titre levels (hemagglutination inhibition test)
1:4 - 1:64 due to vaccination.
1:32 - 1:320 suggests maternal antibody or exposure to the organism.
> 1:640 suggests previous infection.
A rise in a titre level from 1:320 to 1:1280 would suggest active infection. Erysipelas may become a problem in herds where PRRS is endemic.

Treatment

☐ The erysipelas organism is very sensitive to penicillin. Acutely ill animals should be treated with quick acting penicillin twice daily for three days. Alternatively a long-acting penicillin, given as a single dose to cover 48 hours of treatment, could be given and then repeated.
☐ Treat by intramuscular injection 1ml per 10kg (300,000iu/ml).
☐ Medicate the feed with 200g/tonne of phenoxymethyl penicillin for 10-14 days. This is a very effective method of prevention, and can be used in major outbreaks of disease.

Management control and prevention

◆ If a boar is ill with a temperature and shows skin lesions, treat immediately and do not use for mating for a minimum period of four weeks. Alternatively, cross mate with boars that have no disease history or use AI.
◆ Vaccinate all gilts and young boars twice, two to four weeks apart (according to manufacturer's instructions) from 14 weeks of age.
◆ In herds where there is a high challenge it may be necessary to re-vaccinate gilts and boars so that a third dose of vaccine is given two months after the second often when the breeding animals arrive on the farm.
◆ Re-vaccinate sows either two weeks prior to farrowing, or at weaning time, depending on the incidence and history of disease on the farm.
◆ Make sure boars are re-vaccinated every six months.
◆ If disease breakdowns occur in spite of vaccination it is likely that the levels of challenge from the environment are high. Assess hygiene in breeding pens and move to an all-in all-out method of housing.
◆ Wet feeding systems, particularly if milk by-products are used, can become major sources for multiplication of the organism.
◆ Killed vaccines are quite safe and have no adverse effects on the sow.

> ***Do not use a boar for at least 4 weeks after infection.***

LEPTOSPIROSIS

Leptospira are long slender spiral-shaped bacteria, found in most mammalian host species. Over 160 serotypes are known, generally called serovars, with cross infections occurring between some species. Each serotype has one or more (usually only two or three) reservoir hosts which multiply up the type and maintain it. A serotype can remain as a life-long infection in its reservoir host.

The pig is a reservoir host for *Leptospira pomona*, *L. tarassovi*, *L. bratislava* and *L. muenchen*, the last two being very closely related. It is not a reservoir host for *L. icterohaemorrhagiae* but it can be infected from rats urine and become ill. It can also become infected by other serotypes from other animals urine, for example *L. canicola* from dogs and *L. hardjo* from cattle but the infections are subclinical and do not result in disease. The pig is then an incidental host i.e. does not perpetu-

Type Of Leptospira	Alternative Reservoir Host	Country	Signs
L. pomona	Skunk	USA, Asia	Abortion
L. tarassovi	Wild life	Europe Asia	Abortion
L. Icterohaemorrhagiae	Rat	World-wide	Haemorrhage and jaundice in young pigs
L. bratislava L. muenchen	Hedgehog Vole	World-wide	Stillbirths Infertility

(Fig.6-21)

ate the infection and is only responsible for minimal spread.

L. pomona causes important reproductive problems in female breeding pigs spreading slowly through the herd. It remains in the herd permanently unless steps are taken to eradicate it. It is not in the UK or Ireland and seems to have disappeared from Western Europe but is widespread throughout the rest of the pig rearing world. In America the skunk is an alternative reservoir host.

L. tarassovi causes a similar syndrome (i.e. a collection of signs and lesions) to *L. pomona* but tends to be milder and to spread more slowly. It is found in Eastern Europe and the Antipodes. It is thought that some wild animals are also reservoir hosts.

The pig is also a reservoir host for certain subtypes of *L. bratislava* and *L. muenchen* which are widespread throughout the pigs of the world. They causes a different syndrome to *L. pomona* and *L. tarassovi* and affect mainly pregnant gilts and second litter females because they will not previously have encountered it.

Once these organisms are introduced into a herd the pigs become permanent carriers with infection of the kidneys and intermittent excretion of the organism into the urine. *L. bratislava/muenchen* also permanently inhabit the fallopian tube of sows and the reproductive organs of boars and are spread in semen.

Infection can enter the herd in one of three ways:

1. Introduction of infected gilts and boars.
2. Infection brought into the herd by other animals.
3. Exposure of the herd to indirect sources of contamination, e.g.: contaminated water.

A herd can also be contaminated by *L. bratislava/muenchen* by AI if no antibiotics are used in the semen. Unless very stringent precautions are taken most herds become exposed at some stage to *L. bratislava/muenchen*. *L. pomona* and *L. tarassovi* are more easily kept out.

Leptospirosis can be a very difficult disease to diagnose because pigs are often infected but there are no clinical signs to be seen. Thus if you carry out a serological test in your herd and the result is positive, for example to *L. bratislava*, this does not necessarily mean you have disease - only that the animal has been infected and responded by producing antibodies. If you carry out a serological test with positive results for *L. pomona*, this may be a cross reaction to other non pig serotypes in the same group.

Conversely, if you have an infertility problem that clinically suggests leptospira as the cause, then such test results would support a diagnosis of disease if there were rising titres in the serum of the affected sows. However this may not be the case because pregnant females seroconvert early in the infection and by the time they abort or show symptoms the serum levels may be falling. Methods of spread within the herd are as follows:

- Infection is by mouth, through the mucous membranes.
- Most leptospira are inhabitants of the kidney and found in urine.
- Introduction and spread within the herd can occur by various forms of wildlife.
- Introduction and spread within a herd can occur through the introduction of carrier boars and gilts.
- Pig to pig transmission via urine is common.
- Venereal infection is commonplace particularly with *L. bratislava/muenchen*.
- Contaminated water, floor surfaces, pools and streams.
- Wallows used in outdoor production if there are pools of fresh water.

The most common type outside the UK, Ireland and Western Europe is *L. pomona*. The most widespread in pigs world-wide is *L. bratislava/muenchen*. All leptospira require moisture, not only for indirect transmission, but also to survive. Desiccation kills them in 48 hours. When they invade the pig for the first time, there is rapid multiplication, and antibodies become evident 5-10 days later in the blood. Titres may rise as high as 1:1000, but they gradually decline to a low point or even become negative although the animal may still carry the bacteria and excrete them.

Leptospira may become localised in the uterus during pregnancy, causing either abortions or increases in stillborn piglets. *L. bratislava* may persist in the oviduct and uterus of non pregnant sows, and in the genital tracts of boars. This may be an important medium for the maintenance of infection in the herd and be responsible for sows failing to conceive.

Clinical signs

In acute outbreaks inappetance and depression may be observed but chronic low grade disease is more common with abortions, stillbirths and an increase in poor, non-viable pigs. If abortions in a herd are more than 1% then investigations for leptospirosis should be considered. A reduction in farrowing rates and numbers of live pigs born per sow is also an associated factor particularly with *L. bratislava* infection.

Signs associated with acute *L. bratislava* disease:

- Repeat breeders are common particularly in first and to some extent second pregnancy gilts.
- This often follows embryo loss and there may be copious vaginal discharges.
- Late term abortions.
- An increase in premature piglets.
- An increase in stillbirths.
- Mixed litters of live poor pigs and dead piglets at birth.
- An increase in mummified pigs.
- An increase in repeat breeding animals.
- Often there is a two year cycle of disease.
- Reproductive failure occurs in second litter females,

rather than gilts following their introduction to older carrier boars.
- Disease is less common in older animals.
- In long standing carrier herds disease can be difficult to recognise.

Diagnosis

This is carried out by assessing the antibody levels in a cross section of breeding females and the isolation of the organism from diseased tissues. The micro-agglutination test is carried out on serum, and recently affected animals will show titres of up to 1:1000. At the onset of clinical signs a blood sample should be taken and a further one, two weeks later. If the second sample shows a rise in antibody levels at least two fold, this would be indicative of leptospira involvement. Leptospira are difficult organisms to grow, and take a long period of time. *L. bratislava/muenchen* are even more difficult to grow and very few laboratories can culture them. There is however, a method of detecting leptospira under the microscope using the fluorescent antibody test (FAT). Because of the difficulty of distinguishing between sub-clinical infection and infection with disease, an appraisal of the following will help:

- Records. Study the levels of abortions, repeats, stillbirths, week piglets and the age of occurrence in sows and gilts.
- Study the clinical picture.
- Eliminate other diseases.
- Eliminate non infectious causes of infertility.
  Blood sample suspicious animals and repeat 2-3 weeks later. Look for rising antibody titres e.g. 1st sample result 1:100, 2nd result 1:800. This would confirm active infection and indicate probable involvement.
- Blood sample ten females that have a history of infertility.
- In chronic disease however, the significance of titre levels are very difficult to assess.
- Test the aborted foetuses, urine or kidneys and fallopian tubes of slaughtered gilts by the FAT.

Similar diseases

The symptoms of leptospirosis can be mistaken for other causes of infertility including:
  Chronic PRRS.
  Endometritis.
  Non infectious causes.
  Summer infertility.
  Management failures.

A study of Fig.6-1 and chapter 5 will help in differentiating.

Treatment

- ☐ Medicate the feed with tetracycline's, either oxytetracycline or chlortetracycline at levels of 800g/tonne. Feed for a period of three weeks followed by a further course six weeks later, and repeat this for four treatment periods.
- ☐ An initial three week course of 800g of tetracycline followed by a further eight week course at 400g.
- ☐ Strategic medication. Where there is a history of periodic infertility, in-feed medication can be targeted just prior to the expected time of disease.
- ☐ Inject sows at weaning time with streptomycin if available at 25mg/kg. Boars should be treated with this drug once every six weeks. Alternatively semi-synthetic penicillins could be used.
- ☐ Introduce antibiotic into the anterior vagina post-service. This is the same procedure to that described under vaginal discharges, and involves the use of an AI catheter and the deposition of antibiotic into the anterior vagina 6-18 hours after the last mating. Ampicillin, amoxycillin, or penicillin/dihydrostreptomycin could be used. (See chapter 15). Discuss with your veterinarian.

Management control and prevention

- ◆ Control by vaccination is reasonably effective and in many countries vaccines are available that contain five or six different types of leptospira. Alternatively, where vaccines are not available, it is necessary to use antibiotic therapy.
- ◆ Whilst it can be difficult to prevent *L. bratislava/muenchen* from infecting the herd, nevertheless the more serious types such as *L. pomona* and *L. tarassovi* can be kept out of the herd by careful isolation of incoming stock, serological testing, veterinary liaison and a knowledge of the source herd.
- ◆ Once leptospira are active and present in the herd, hygiene, the constant removal of urine and good management become important methods of control. In outdoor herds, wallows could become sources of contamination especially if there are pools of fresh urine. The most effective method of control is to provide two wallows per paddock and use an electric fence which by movement will allow each to dry out and rest alternately.
- ◆ In indoor housing, poor concrete surfaces that allow the collection of urine and water are ideal sources for maintaining high levels of infection.
- ◆ If the sow is only exposed to low numbers of organisms, infection probably takes place with little disease.
- ◆ Make sure your diagnosis of disease is a correct one.
- ◆ Check the serology of your herd. Do not buy in what you don't have.
- ◆ Check your sources of boars and gilts.
- ◆ Keep rodents under control.
- ◆ Provide well drained concrete surfaces particularly in defecating areas and boar pens.

- Remove slurry regularly.
- Identify problem parities and strategically medicate.
- Vaccinate if a vaccine is available.

Eradication

This can be done but it is unreliable and is probably contraindicated for *L. bratislava*.

Chapter 6

7 Managing and Treating Disease in the Dry Period

General clinical signs of disease 193
Management and disease 193
    Records.. 193
    Reasons for sow disposal... 194
    Reasons for keeping sows beyond 6 litters 194
    Reasons for not keeping sows beyond 6 litters................................... 194
    Key points to maintaining longevity in the breeding female 194
    Nutrition and feeding 195
    Housing 196
    Hygiene.. 196
    Temperature 196
    Ventilation.. 196
    Water.. 196
    Light 196
    Stockmanship.. 196
    Stress.. 196
    The boar... 197
Diseases that may be seen in the dry period 197
Identifying problems in the dry sow 197
    Abortion - see chapters 5 and 6 198
    Abscesses 199
    Anaemia... 199
    Anthrax.. 200
    Atrophic rhinitis 200
    Aujeszky's disease 200
    Back muscle necrosis 201
    Biotin deficiency 201
    Brucellosis... 201
    Bursitis... 202
    Bush foot / foot rot... 202
    Clostridial diseases... 203
    Cystitis and pyelonephritis 203
    Erysipelas 205
    Fractures.. 207
    Gastric ulcers.. 207
    Glässers disease (*Haemophilus parasuis*)... 209
    Haematoma 209
    Jaw and snout deviation 209
    Lameness... 209
    Laminitis.. 211
    Leg weakness (osteochondrosis - OCD).. 211
    Leptospirosis.. 214
    Mange.. 214
    Mastitis.. 214
    Meningitis... 215
    Mortality.. 215
    Muscle tearing 216
    Mycoplasma arthritis (*Mycoplasma hyosynoviae* infection) 216

Peritonitis	217
Pneumonia	217
Porcine enteropathy (PE)	218
Porcine epidemic diarrhoea (PED)	218
Porcine parvovirus (PPV)	218
Porcine reproductive and respiratory syndrome (PRRS)	218
Porcine stress syndrome (PSS)	218
Prolapse of the rectum	219
Prolapse of the vagina and cervix	220
Salmonellosis	220
Salt poisoning - (water deprivation)	221
Shoulder sores	221
Streptococcal infections	221
Swine dysentery (SD)	221
Swine influenza or flu (SI)	222
Thin sow syndrome	222
Vice - abnormal behaviour	223
Vulval discharge	223
Medicines and other drugs for use in the dry sow	224

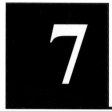

Managing and Treating Disease in the Dry Period

General Clinical Signs of Disease

During the dry period diseases may appear in individual cases, or in outbreaks involving a number of animals. Infectious diseases may attack more than one system of the body and the clinical signs then relate to the failure of that particular system and include the following.

The digestive system

- Anaemia.
- Blood or mucus in faeces.
- Colic
- Change in the faecal consistency - constipation, diarrhoea.
- Dehydration.
- Distension of the abdomen.
- Inappetance.
- Salivation.
- Variable body condition.
- Vomiting.

The locomotor system

- Abscesses.
- Fractured bones.
- Incoordination.
- Lameness.
- Paralysis.
- Swellings of joints, muscles and tendons.
- Trembling

The nervous system

- Blindness.
- Fits.
- Loss of balance, middle ear infections.
- Loss of leg function.
- Muscular tremors.
- Nystagmus (jerky eye movements), meningitis.
- Paraplegia.

The respiratory system

- Coughing.
- Discharges from the eye.
- Discharges from the nose.
- Heavy breathing - pneumonia.
- Sneezing.

The skin

- Abscesses.
- Cuts and bruises.
- Dermatitis (inflammation).
- Discoloration.
- Erysipelas lesions.
- Excessive hair growth.
- Fly bites.
- Greasy skin.
- Haemorrhage.
- Jaundice
- Lice.
- Mange.
- Paleness - anaemia.
- Rodent bites.

The urogenital system

- Abnormal discharges from the vulva.
- Abnormal oestrus.
- Abnormal urine colour.
- Abortion.
- Blood, mucus, or pus in the urine.
- Fevers.
- Mucus indicative of an early abortion.
- Oestrus, anoestrus.
- Pregnancy failures.
- Wet urine-stained vulva.

Management and Disease

To achieve profitable reproductive performance breeding males and females must be kept in good health. Each section presented below is part of the overall strategy required to achieve this. Compare the efficiency of your herd against the points raised.

Records

If productivity is to be increased it is necessary to identify those areas during the pre-mating and pregnancy period that are either inefficiently managed or adversely affected by disease. Disease and farrowing rate loss recording sheets are described in chapter 5 and they are important aids to this identification process. Records will identify why reproduction failures have occurred and also provide information about culling and mortality. They should include information on:

- Anoestrus.
- Culling policies relative to the slaughter price of the sow.
- Haemorrhage problems.
- Infertility including repeats, sows not in pig, dis-

charges etc.
- Lameness.
- Mastitis, agalactia and udder oedema.
- Mortality and its specific causes.
- Poor conformation and its effects.
- Prolapse of the vagina or rectum.
- Savaging.
- Sows with poor litters.
- Specific diseases.
- The age profile of the herd.

Compare your records to the sow disposal targets in Fig.7-1.

Reasons for Sow Disposal

Up to 50% of all sows culled from a herd are usually associated with some form of reproductive failure or poor performance. Lameness and mortality also may be significant causes of failure. By collecting and studying such information the excessive areas of loss are identified. When farrowing rates are less then 85% it should be possible to identify significant losses and take the corrective action. It has always been a point of debate how old the sow should be before she leaves the herd but the following should be taken into account when making a decision.

- Age and its effects on the individual sows' production.
- Individual record and history.
- Maintaining the mating programme.
- The availability of gilts.
- The performance of the sow compared to that of a gilt.
- Health of the sow - e.g. arthritis.
- Body condition.

With increasing age the performance of the sow will decrease as shown in Fig.7-2. On most farms sows should be culled after they have had between 6 and 10 litters, the majority after the sixth pregnancy.

Reasons for Keeping Sows Beyond 6 Litters

Using modern computer programmes it should be easy to assess farrowing rate, litter size and pigs reared by pregnancy for each sow and the herd as a whole. This assists significantly in the decision to retain a sow for further breeding including:
- To maintain the mating programme. Losses here cannot be recovered.
- No gilts may be available that week for mating.
- Records show that in this herd performance in parities 6, 7 or 8 is acceptable.
- Records show that the numbers born in older sows compare favourably with the mean of gilts and second litter females.
- Individual sow records show which sows have a good breeding and rearing history.
- Records show farrowing rates in 7th parity sows are above 86%.

Target Figures For Sow Disposal	
Reason	Percentage *
Abortion	1
Agalactia / Mastitis	1
Age only	8
Disease	4
Infertility	15
Lameness	5
Mortality	4
Miscellaneous	2
Poor production	5
Total	45

* Percentage of the sow herd per annum
(Fig.7-1)

Reasons for Not Keeping Sows Beyond 6 Litters

- Variable litter size.
- Variable piglet size at weaning.
- Variable birth weights within the litter.
- A history of agalactia or poor milking.
- Chronic mastitis.
- Vulval discharges.
- Poor genetic potential.
- Other problem areas identified with increasing age.
- Poor fertility

In indoor herds, levels of sows culled per annum should be between 38 to 45% but in the outdoor herd this often reaches 50%.

Key Points to Maintaining Longevity in the Breeding Female

- Use the correct female, that is, one expressing maximum hybrid vigour.
- Select or purchase females with sound strong legs, good teats and not too heavy hams.
- Avoid gilts showing any signs of leg weakness e.g., standing on their toes, the back legs tucked under, the front legs bent or the pasterns dropped.
- Do not breed from a female that is too lean. Maintain

PROBLEMS THAT MAY OCCUR AS THE SOW GETS OLDER
Agalactia.
Increases in small and large litters.
Increased stillbirth levels.
Increased endometritis.
Increased levels of disease, particularly cystitis and pyelonephritis.
Increased mortality.
Increased number of blind teats.
Increases in prolapses.
Mastitis.
More fostering is necessary.
More lameness and arthritis.
More pigs laid on.
Poor milking.
Reduced farrowing rates.
Reduced fertility.
Variable size and weight of piglets at birth.

(Fig.7-2)

at least 17mm of fat at the P2 measurement by point of mating, particularly in the gilt.
- Do not serve the gilt at less then 210 days of age. Gilts served too early will still be maturing into their second pregnancy. Equally do not serve too late (240 days) otherwise body size will increase.
- Do not allow excessive body weight to develop during the first pregnancy.
- Provide the pregnant gilt with exercise during the first half of the pregnancy if possible.
- Avoid mouldy feeds.
- Do not cull a sow if her first two litters have been poor. Review management procedures.
- Feed the sow from three days post farrowing, during lactation, and to point of mating to appetite.
- Do not serve maiden gilts or first litter gilts with heavy boars. This can precipitate leg problems.
- Identify sick or lame sows early and remove to a well bedded hospital pen. Many will simply recover in a better environment.
- Good nutrition is vital.

Remember that management, feeding, housing design and a comfortable well lit environment are under your control and they will have a major effect on the viability, health and production of the sow.

Nutrition and Feeding

It is beyond the scope of this book to discuss nutrition in detail, but you should keep in mind that the quality of the feeds and the way in which they are fed are important in the management of disease. Aspects relating to nutrition in the lactating sow are dealt with in chapter 8 "Nutrition". In the dry sow on the day of weaning three quarters of the daily lactation feed should be given prior to actual removal of the sow from the farrowing house and the remainder given later on that day. The sow should be given the opportunity to eat the same amount of food on the three days post weaning as she ate during late lactation. This will ensure that she does not become catabolic (a negative energy state) with an extended weaning to mating interval and subsequent infertility. Such diets should contain at least 14MJ DE/kg 16 % protein and 1.0 - 1.1% lysine, particularly if a lean genotype is being used. Immediately after mating, feed levels should be held at 2kg for the first 48 to 72 hours and then the sow fed to body condition. Provided energy levels are not excessive in the first 3 days post-mating then it is advantageous to feed the sow to body condition using a dry sow ration over the next 21 days with 3kg or more per day.

Many farms today feed separate lactating and dry sow rations. The latter with digestible energy ranging from 13 to 13.6MJ DE/kg and protein levels of 13 to 14%. It is beneficial from 3-21 days post mating to optimise feed intake relative to the sows demand since this will satisfy the nutritional requirements for the development of the placenta. This is pertinent where farms have variable weights and quality of piglets at birth. The development of the placenta in the first 12 to 25 days post mating helps to determine the quality of the piglet at the end of the pregnancy. A small placenta will contribute towards a small pig. The availability and intake of feed in this respect is important, for example where sows are fed in groups. If there is a shortage of trough space, nutritional insufficiencies can occur in the under-privileged females. During the pregnancy period the sow should be fed to body condition but also to satisfy the environmental needs. Thus it is difficult to lay down specific levels of feed intake per day, they must be determined by the stockperson. The body condition of the sow can be assessed on a numerical rating of 1 to 5 and to do this the flat of the hand should be placed over the back bone just forward of the root of the tail and rolled laterally side to side. The condition of the sow can then be scored Fig.7-3.

As a guideline sows approaching the point of weaning should score around 3. This should rise to $3^1/_2$ or possibly 4 in older sows by the time of the next farrowing. Sows scoring $2^1/_2$ or less are moving into a problem area. If more than 5% of sows at any one time score $2^1/_2$ or less then feeding levels are wrong. If sows are allowed to farrow with a score of less than 3 there will be insufficient fat reserves to maintain lactation and they will use muscle as a source of energy. Such sows are then in danger of developing the thin sow syndrome, being unable to maintain body condition with the demands of lactation.

ASSESSING BODY CONDITION IN SOWS

Condition Score: 1, 2, 3, 4, 5

Score
1. Emaciated sow, backbone very prominent.
2. Thin, backbone prominent.
3. Ideal condition during lactation and at weaning. Backbone just palpable.
4. Slightly overweight. Cannot find the backbone.
5. Body rotund, over fat.

(Fig.7-3)

In outdoor herds it is important that all sows should score over 3 before the onset of winter. It is difficult to improve body condition in cold weather. Feed levels should be higher during winter than in spring or summer.

Housing
See chapter 16 for further information.

From weaning to mating the indoor sow can be housed in one of three ways; individually confined in a stall or by a tether, mixed in groups of 2 to 15 sows or moved into a dynamic group, or introduced into a boar pen on the day of weaning for 2-4 days and then individually confined. Each of these systems has its advantages and disadvantages and they may be dictated to some extent by the welfare regulations of your country. For example in the UK, stalls and tethers are to be banned in 1999 and therefore loose housing systems will have to be used. Under such circumstances groups of sows on the day of weaning are best mixed into a large yard with a minimum of $2.7m^2$ per sow together with a large old boar. The boar's presence will have two effects, one of stimulating oestrus and the other of reducing any fighting that is likely to occur. The grouped sows should be fed ad lib from weaning to mating from at least two well separated feeders. The boar should be removed from the group on day 4 and where possible, sows should be confined to stalls over the next 48 hours during the period of oestrus. This is a welfare friendly act because it reduces riding and stress as sows come into heat. Confined sows should remain in their stalls until 21 days post mating. Loosed housed sows should be returned to the group as soon as mating is completed and a boar re-introduced until at least 21 days post mating. It is very important that the floor surfaces are dry and non slippery, the concrete not worn and there are no protrusions from sharp aggregate, especially in the mating pen. Slatted floors can be used for housing sows in the immediate post weaning period but not the mating or boar pen because they produce lameness and discomfort at mating. Remember the weight on the sows hind legs and feet is multiplied three fold during mating and slats increase the risk of damage.

Hygiene
A clean environment is important from weaning to at least 10 days post mating. In the first 2 or 3 days post weaning the mammary gland is full of milk creating pressure which may predispose to mastitis. Contamination of the teat end with faeces and urine greatly increases this risk. The housing should be washed and dried between each batch of sows weaned. If this is not possible, it should be done at least once a month. If the sows are confined individually, the rear of the pens are best slatted to allow urine to drain away. Faeces should be removed daily. The rear gates in stalls should have a 100mm gap above the floor so that faeces are squeezed out behind the sow and not allowed to build up and cause heavy bacterial contamination of the vulva. If solid floors are used they should have a fall of at least 1:20 in the last 450mm behind the sow to allow for good drainage. Alternately the pen should be well bedded with straw daily. In loose housing the pens should be well drained and a deep bed of fresh clean straw used daily.

The vagina of the sow is susceptible to ascending infection in the immediate post weaning period and for 2 to 4 days post oestrus.

Temperature
The sow at weaning is removed from a comfortable warm farrowing house at around 20°C (68°F) into what is probably one of the coldest parts of the dry sow house because there is such a low density of pigs. The environment should be controlled at an ambient temperature of 20°C (68°F) from weaning to 21 days post mating and depending on the external temperature this may involve the provision of heat or some form of evaporative cooling. This helps to maintain an anabolic (positive) energy status and provide a level of comfort necessary to achieve good reproductive performance.

Ventilation
Make sure that air flow in the mating area does not cause evaporative cooling to the animal during the critical period. A high air flow can lower the effective temperature for the sow by some 10°C or more.

Water
See chapter 3 for further information.

A water flow rate of at least 2 litres per minute should be available. A commonly undetected fault is that drinkers often fall well short of this.

Light
See chapter 5 for further information.

A minimum of 12 hours of continuous light followed by a period of darkness should be provided each day both in the mating and gestation areas.

Stockmanship
It has been scientifically demonstrated that reproductive performance and litter size may be depressed by up to 6% on farms where there is a lack of empathy between the stockperson and the pigs. This can be assessed by the way sows and boars approach people or withdraw. A calm atmosphere between the person and the pig, with a gentle pat here and there and a quiet voice, pays handsomely. The sow is a sociable animal, similar to the dog, a fact not always appreciated.

Stress
Stress is created whenever the sow has to respond to a noxious stimuli. Thus anything that causes fear or discomfort (a negative response) causes the adrenal gland

CHAPTER 7 - Managing and Treating Disease in the Dry Period

> **Walk around the farm and ask a simple question,**
> **"Is this a happy and comfortable environment for the pigs"?**

to produce hormones called corticosteroids which depress the normal protective or immune mechanisms so that the animal becomes more susceptible to disease.

The Boar

The boar is the most important animal on the farm and good management is essential to maintain health and maximise normal reproductive function. When the young boar first enters the farm allow him to make physical but not intimate contact with female pigs. He certainly must not be bullied by sows. Unless this physical contact takes place there is a risk of low sexual behaviour with poor matings, and poor shortened ejaculations. Such animals are often slow to mount and serve with reduced conception, farrowing rates and litter sizes. The same principles apply to the mature boar, he should have constant contact with females. If you find a boar is becoming less interested at mating time, change the environment into a more stimulating one by moving him to another pen (assuming there are no problems of health). Lameness, stiffness, or difficulty in rising are often pointers to early arthritis, foot lesions or leg weakness and veterinary advice and treatment can often prevent 2 or 3 months of lowered fertility. When the young boar first arrives on the farm always manage him carefully, without any aggression and be extremely patient during the first two or three matings. The boar pen should be a minimum of $9.3m^2$ and for best results provide him with a solid well bedded floor of either shavings, peat or straw. He is then less likely to develop arthritis, callous formation and become stiff and lame.

The floor surface in the mating pen is important. It should be smooth, non slippery and well drained with no projections of aggregate. The pen should be pressure-washed and disinfected at least once a month. If the floor surface becomes slippery the judicious use of dry sand can be a short term solution. Do not use too much however because it can have abrasive effects on the prepuce and penis. (Sandy soil is a major cause of the penis bleeding in outdoor boars).

> **A lame boar may produce more variable litter sizes and poorer reproductive performances**

Diseases That May be Seen in the Dry Period

If you have a problem refer to Fig.7-4 and then the index or relevant chapter. If you cannot identify the cause consult your veterinarian.

Identifying Problems in the Dry Sow

Observations and Causes

Anoestrus
  Disease
  Lack of boar contact
  Low feed intake
  Low temperature
  Metritis
  Parasites
  Poor light
  Poor nutrition
  Stress
  Thin sows

Coughing
  Ascarids (round worms) *
  App
  Aujeszky's disease
  Dust
  EP
  Flu (SI) *
  Lung abscesses
  Lung worm
  Pasteurella
  PRRS
  Swine fever
  Toxic gases

Diarrhoea
  Colitis
  Diet changes
  Over eating *
  Parasites
  Poor nutrition
  Porcine enteropathy (PE)
  Porcine epidemic diarrhoea (PED)
  Salmonellosis
  Swine dysentery
  TGE *

Haemorrhage: Faeces
  Gastric ulcers
  Ileitis
  Parasites

Haemorrhage: Vulva
  Cystitis / pyelonephritis
  Dead foetuses
  Ruptured blood vessel
  Trauma

Lameness
  Arthritis
  Biotin deficiency

Observations and Causes (Cont.)

Bursitis
Bush foot / foot rot *
Erysipelas
Foot-and-mouth disease
Fractures *
Laminitis
Leg weakness or OCD *
Osteomalacia
Poisons
Salt poisoning
Sand crack
Spinal damage
Torn muscle *
Trauma *

Mastitis

Poor hygiene
Specific bacteria
Wet floors

Nervous signs

Aujeszky's disease
Brain abscess
Meningitis
Middle ear infection *
Poisoning
Streptococcal infections
Swine fever
Talfan, Teschen diseases
Salt poisoning (Water deprivation)

Not eating - temperature normal

Constipation
Cystitis / pyelonephritis *
Faulty nutrition
Gastric ulcers *
Ileitis
Indigestion
Salt poisoning (Water deprivation)
Toxic conditions / poisoning
Unpalatable food

Not eating - temperature elevated (fever)

App
Acute cystitis
Dead foetuses
Erysipelas *
Flu (SI) *
Mastitis *
PRRS
Womb infection
Septicaemia / toxaemia *

Mortality (sudden death)

Acute cystitis (pyelonephritis) *

Observations and Causes (Cont.)

Acute stress
Anthrax
App
Clostridial diseases
Electrocution
Erysipelas
Gut torsion and rupture
Poisons carbon monoxide
Porcine enteropathy (PE)

Skin diseases

Aujeszky's disease
Dermatitis
Erysipelas
Granuloma
Jaundice
Lice
Mange
PRRS
Sunburn
Swine fever
Swine pox
Swine vesicular disease
Vulva biting

Thin sows

Epe
Cystitis pyelonephritis *
Draughts *
Low energy intake *
Low feed intake *
Low environmental temperature *
Old age
Parasites *
Poor insulation of buildings
Poor nutrition

Vomiting

Fever
Gastric ulcers
Gastritis
Over eating
Parasites
Poisons
Poor nutrition
Porcine epidemic diarrhoea (PED) *
TGE *
Torsion
Fungal toxins *

* More likely to occur

(Fig.7-4)

ABORTION - See chapters 5 and 6

ABSCESSES

Abscesses are pockets of pus that contain dead cell material and large numbers of bacteria. The bacteria normally enter the body through damage to the skin or via the external orifices. They become walled off from the body tissues, or the bacteria are disseminated by the blood stream to develop abscesses elsewhere in the body. Near the skin surface they may become painful with an inflamed appearance.

Clinical signs

They commonly arise from fighting particularly when sows are grouped at weaning. Initially there is a break in the skin which leaves a scar followed by swellings beneath. Abscesses can also arise as secondary infection to other conditions such as swine pox, PRRS, pneumonia or tail biting and if they become widespread throughout the body, the result may be emaciation followed by death or condemnation of the carcase at slaughter.

Diagnosis

This is based on the clinical signs of abnormal swellings under the skin especially with overlying scars. To confirm the diagnosis, feel and press the swelling to ascertain if the contents are fluid or solid and whether they are beneath the skin or deep seated. To examine the swelling more closely, restrain the pig by a wire noose or by heavy sedation (stresnil 1ml/10kg), and sample the contents. This is carried out using a 10ml syringe with a 18mm 16 gauge needle attached. The needle is inserted at the lowest soft point of the swelling and fluid withdrawn. If it is an abscess a white, yellow or green substance of either a watery or a cheesy consistency will appear.

Similar diseases

Haemorrhage into the tissues from a recently ruptured blood vessel or a haemorrhage of long standing is the only condition likely to be confused with an abscess. In such cases either pure blood or a very thin blood stained liquid will be withdrawn. Such pockets of blood are called haematoma and if they have been present for a long time a clot will have formed, in which case only serum or a clear liquid will be withdrawn.

Treatment

☐ This is aimed at draining the pus. Sometimes it will occur naturally after the abscess bursts but most require lancing or opening surgically. To do this make an incision approximately 15-20mm long at the lowest point particularly where it is soft and fluctuating. A sharp scalpel blade with only 15mm exposed is inserted into the abscess in a downward movement to open it up. Carry this out only when the sow is restrained. A quick controlled movement of the blade will cause little pain, far less than trying to infiltrate a local anaesthetic. The pus should be squeezed out and the interior washed using a syringe and sterile saline solution. Such a solution is made by adding 5 grams of salt to 1 litre of previously boiled water. The wound must be kept open for at least 3 or 4 days or until all the pus has drained out, otherwise the abscess may reform.
☐ See lancing an abscess or haematoma chapter 15.
☐ Most of the organisms that cause abscesses in the pig are either penicillin or oxytetracycline sensitive.
☐ If the area is badly inflamed, squeeze into the hole an antibiotic cream (a cow mastitis tube is ideal) containing penicillin/streptomycin, oxytetracycline, amoxycillin or ampicillin.
☐ Treatment should be given by intramuscular injection - if the area is inflamed or the sow is ill. Drugs that could be used include:
- Penicillin/streptomycin daily for 3-4 days.
- Amoxycillin long-acting (LA) every other day.
- Oxytetracycline (LA) every other day
- Penicillin (LA) every other day.

Management control and prevention

◆ Identify various projections and sharp objects in the environment. A typical example would be a neck abscess associated with worn and jagged metal on feeders. Long-acting antibiotic injections given at the time of damage will often prevent infection.
◆ Reduce fighting.
◆ Prevent tail biting. See vice chapter 9.
◆ Check injection procedures.

ANAEMIA

Anaemia is a condition associated with either a reduction in the number of red cells in the blood, the amount of haemoglobin they contain, or the volume of the red cells themselves.
It can arise in one of three ways:
- Loss of blood through haemorrhage. Typical examples would be gastric ulceration, trauma to the vulva or a ruptured liver.
- Lack of haemoglobin due to dietary insufficiencies, particularly iron and copper.
- Reduced numbers of red cells. These are produced in

THE COMMON CAUSES OF ANAEMIA	
Eperythrozoonosis in all ages.	The stomach worm (*Hyostrongylus rubidus*).
Fungal toxins.	The whip worm (*Trichuris suis*).
Gastric ulcers.	Umbilical haemorrhage
Iron deficiency in piglets.	Vaginal haematoma.
Mange (*Sarcoptes scabiei*)	Vulval biting.
Mycotoxins	Warfarin poisoning.
Porcine enteropathy - Bloody gut (PHE).	

(Fig.7-5)

the bone marrow and any disease, infection or toxic state affecting it may result in anaemia.

The common causes of anaemia are shown in Fig.7-5 but iron deficiency and anaemia in piglets are the most common and important. From a purely nutritional aspect anaemia in growing and adult animals would be uncommon but disease will often give rise to a secondary anaemia.

Anaemia is also common, secondary to specific diseases such as actinobacillus pleuropneumonia or glässers disease.

Clinical signs

The pig is pale and becomes breathless on exertion. The mucous membranes of the eyes are pale. They can be compared to a normal pig if there is doubt about interpretation. Haemorrhage may be obvious to the exterior or it can occur through bleeding into the tissues or the gut. Warfarin poisoning can cause severe bleeding into the tissues.

Diagnosis

Anaemia can be diagnosed on clinical grounds and by examining a sample of blood. This is tested for the red cell volume and the haemoglobin levels. (Normal levels 9-15g/100ml), anaemia <8g/100ml). A stained blood smear will also confirm the shape and size of the red cells and whether there are any bacteria present. Specific cell types are involved in the different anaemias. Iron dextran toxicity associated with vitamin E deficiency may give rise to anaemia in piglets.

Treatment

- The intestine can absorb only small amounts of iron daily which may not be enough to reverse the anaemia quickly. Nevertheless iron and copper levels in the feed should be checked. It is also helpful to give an injection of iron dextran 300-500mg depending on the age of the pig.
- Specific treatment and prevention will depend on the cause. Refer to the specific conditions in the index.
- In severe cases electrolytes can be given either by injection or by mouth.

Management control and prevention

- ◆ Carry out regular worming programmes and/or check faeces samples for parasites every 3 to 6 months and monitor iron levels in feed.

ANTHRAX

This is an uncommon disease of pigs in most parts of the world including the EU where it is notifiable. It is caused by the bacterium *Bacillus anthracis* and is characterised by acute illness, fever, respiratory distress and rapid death. Anthrax should be suspected if a sow is found dead and post-mortem examination shows copious blood tinged-mucus and large haemorrhagic lymph nodes under the skin of the neck and in the abdomen. The post-mortem examination should be discontinued immediately and veterinary help sought. Diagnosis is then confirmed by taking smears for microscopy and swabs for culture from the affected tissues. (Note that samples are not made from blood as they would be with cattle). The veterinarian should not fix the smears by flaming because this destroys the bacterial capsule which is a diagnostic feature. Smears are best fixed in Zenker's fluid. Acute infection with *Haemophilus suis* in primary MEW or SPF immunologically naive sows may result in similar signs and lesions to anthrax.

The source of the infection in sows is usually feed containing contaminated feed stuffs from a spore contaminated area, although in sows kept outdoors in such regions the source may be contaminated soil or other dead animals. The anthrax bacillus is sensitive to penicillin. Care should be taken in handling diseased pigs or carcasses because the disease is communicable to people. Effective vaccines are available in some countries for both pigs and people.

ATROPHIC RHINITIS

See chapter 9 for further information.

This is primarily a disease of the young growing pig but the mature sow can be a carrier of the organism in its nose and tonsils. The disease is caused by toxigenic *Pasteurella multocida* bacteria types A or D. The toxins damage the delicate lining of the nose of the piglet during the early growing period causing haemorrhage and distortion of the nose. If the breeding female has been infected early in life it could still show distortions of the face in adulthood. The infection rarely causes clinical disease in the mature animal and the only importance of disease in the dry sow is the sub-clinical carrier state that exists. The vaccination of breeding females is effective in reducing the carrier state and preventing establishment of infection in the young growing pig and thus removing clinical evidence of disease and the majority of its effects.

AUJESZKY'S DISEASE (PSEUDORABIES)

See chapter 12 for further information.

This disease is caused by a herpes virus and when it is introduced into the breeding herd for the first time, abortions and respiratory signs can be seen. Those females that are in the first third of pregnancy may absorb foetuses resulting in delayed returns to oestrus, but if infection occurs in the second third or the last part of pregnancy piglets are often stillborn and mummified or weak pigs are evident at farrowing. Once the acute phase of the disease has passed a proportion of sows become carriers of the virus and shed it intermittently. Few clinical signs are then seen. Vaccination of the breeding stock is effective in preventing clinical disease.

BACK MUSCLE NECROSIS

Back muscle necrosis is part of the porcine stress syndrome and in affected pigs degenerative changes take place in the back muscles along each side of the spine. It is usually seen in the young growing gilt although occasionally it occurs in the adult female.

Clinical signs

The onset is sudden with severe pain in the lumber muscles with obvious swellings. The pig is reluctant to stand and often adopts a dog sitting position. As the name implies there are muscle changes and death (necrosis) of muscle fibres with haemorrhages into the tissues themselves. The disease is relatively uncommon. It is usually initiated by sudden movement and is sometimes seen when maiden gilts are released from confinement to outdoor accommodation.

Diagnosis

There is a history of sudden lameness associated with movement and acute pain. The pig can be made to stand with difficulty but there is no evidence of fractures. Examine the lumber muscles carefully, they will be swollen and painful on pressure. The temperature is usually normal but may be elevated.

Similar diseases

These include:
    Acute erysipelas.
    Fractures.
    Mycoplasma arthritis.
    Leg weakness (OCD).
    Spinal damage.

Treatment

☐ Inject with phenylbutazone 1ml/50kg or other pain killer.
☐ Inject with corticosteroids provided the animal is not pregnant.
☐ If there is a temperature give an injection of long-acting penicillin to cover the possibility of erysipelas.

Management control and prevention

◆ Breed from pigs that are free of the stress gene.

BIOTIN DEFICIENCY

The role of biotin in nutrition and the changes that result when it is deficient are not clear. Reports from studies and field observations have highlighted the following associations:
- Diarrhoea.
- Dermatitis.
- Excessive hair loss
- Extended weaning to mating intervals.
- Haemorrhages on the solar surfaces of the feet.
- Lameness and laminitis.
- Poor litter size
- Reduce growth rates.
- Transverse cracks in hooves.

The fact that biotin is present in most nutrient sources used for pigs and that it is also produced by organisms in the gilt make a deficiency unlikely on most farms. This is supported by field experiences but very occasionally a herd is investigated for lameness problems that appear to be improved with biotin supplementation of the diet.

Clinical signs

Widespread lameness will be a constant feature particularly in sows. Detailed examinations should be carried out on at least 15-20 affected animals and the nature of the changes in the hooves documented. Examinations are best made when sows and gilts are at rest. The hooves will be soft over the walls and the soles will show slight evidence of haemorrhage. Dark transverse cracks will be seen on the hoof walls. If pigs have access to faeces biotin deficiency is unlikely. Assess trauma from poor floor surfaces as a cause.

Diagnosis

This is based on the clinical picture and the fact that the herd or a group of animals will be affected. The onset is usually gradual and this will distinguish the lameness from foot-and-mouth disease. Chronic lesions of swine vesicular disease could be confused with biotin deficiency. Levels in the ration can be determined but firm recommendations are not available. It would appear 100-200µg(mcg)kg is adequate.

Treatment

☐ Where a herd shows widespread lesions add up to 0.5-1mg/kg to the diet, any response will be slow, up to nine months but prevention gives more positive results.

Management control and prevention

◆ Add biotin to the diet as a routine.

BRUCELLOSIS

See chapter 12 for further information.

This disease, which is notifiable in some countries, is caused by a bacterium, *Brucella suis,* which causes abortion, infertility and lameness. Abortions occur at any time during pregnancy and when disease first enters the herd there will be a large percentage of sows and gilts repeating 30 to 50 days after mating. In chronically infected herds the clinical signs are ill defined and not easily recognised. Diagnosis is carried out by serology and isolation of the organism. There is no reliable treatment and the disease is best eradicated either by depopulation, or testing and elimination of individuals.

BURSITIS

Bursitis is a common condition that arises from constant pressure and trauma to the skin overlying any bony prominence. The periosteum or covering over the bone reacts by creating bone, a swelling develops and the skin likewise responds and becomes thicker, until there is a prominent soft lump. It can commence in the farrowing houses, particularly if there are bad floors but it usually starts in the weaner accommodation on slatted floors which have large gaps. As the pig increases in weight there is increased pressure on the leg bones. Swellings develop over the lateral sides of the hocks and elbows and over the points of the hocks. Such swellings are called bursa although strictly speaking they are not. The term should apply to inflammation of bursa that cover tendons. Worn and pitted floor surfaces particularly if sharp aggregate was used in the concrete, can exaggerate the trauma to the extent that the skin is broken and secondary infection develops. If this occurs on wet dirty floors major problems can arise. Under normal circumstances if there is no secondary infection the condition commercially is not important but if breeding stock is being produced then the management system needs to be adjusted, otherwise rejection rates on breeding gilts will be high.

Wire mesh, woven metal and metal bar floors can produce high levels in weaner pigs in first and second stage housing. Identify the point at which disease first appears and alter the floor surfaces or change the environment.

Clinical signs

These can develop when piglets are 1-2 weeks old particularly where farrowing crate floors are totally slatted. Metal bars are particularly bad. Most swellings commence on the hind legs below the point of the hock or on the lateral aspects of the elbow. With repeated trauma the lesions increase in size and ultimately fluid appears. This is common in pigs 30-70kg weight.

Infection with *Mycoplasma hyosynoviae* can occur and also be seen at the base of the tail over the shoulder blades and the knees.

Treatment

- ☐ There is no specific treatment that will reduce the bone reaction. Remove pigs to pens that are well bedded.
- ☐ If the swellings have become infected with bacteria inject with either oxytetracycline or ampicillin.
- ☐ If *Mycoplasma hyosynoviae* is causing infection use either lincomycin or tiamulin.
- ☐ Most lesions do not require treatment.

Management control and prevention

- ◆ Move severely affected animals onto deep bedded floors.
- ◆ Determine the point at which lesions are occurring and relate to floor surfaces.
- ◆ If the problem is arising in flat decks in breeding gilts it may be necessary to change the slats to those covered with plastic. Tri-bar or metal slats and woven mesh are bad surfaces.

BUSH FOOT / FOOT ROT

Bush foot results from infection of the claw which becomes swollen and extremely painful around the coronary band. It arises through penetration of the sole of the foot, cracks at the sole-hoof junction, or splitting of the hoof itself. It usually occurs in one foot only and is more commonly seen in the hind feet especially the outer claws, which are the larger ones carrying proportionately more weight. Infection sometimes penetrates the soft tissues between the claws and this is referred to as foot rot.

As the infection progresses inside the hoof, the claw becomes enlarged and infection and inflammation of the joint (arthritis) often develops. The condition is important because of the effect on reproductive performance of the breeding female. Foot rot involves both superficial and deep infection of the soft tissues between the claws often caused by fusiformis bacteria.

Foot pain in the boar at mating causes poor ejaculation and a shorter mating time.

> **Lame sows are less likely to conceive, have poor litters and are more likely to abort.**

Clinical signs

The pig is very lame with a painful swollen claw. Always try and examine the feet when the animal is lying down. In most cases a swelling will be visible around the coronary band which may form an abscess and burst to the surface.

Invariably only one claw is involved. With foot rot the infection will be confined to the tissues between the claws.

> **Lame boars often have poor fertility and produce small litters.**

Diagnosis

This is based on the clinical signs described above. Bush foot has to be differentiated from other forms of trauma and infection but the painful swollen claw is obvious.

Similar diseases

These include:
    Erysipelas.
    Glässers disease.
    Leg weakness or osteochondrosis (OCD).
    Mycoplasma arthritis.
    Trauma

Treatment

There is a poor blood supply to the infected tissues and therefore higher dose levels of antibiotics are required for longer periods of time.

- Antibiotics which can be used, depending on the advice of your veterinarian, include:
  - Lincocin   11mg/kg liveweight.
  - Oxytetracycline 25 mg/kg liveweight.
  - Amoxycillin   15mg/kg liveweight.
- Inject daily for 5 to 7 days.
If there is no improvement in three days change the antibiotic. Complete recovery may take 3-4 weeks.
- Anti-inflammatory injections of cortisone may be given provided the sow is not pregnant.
- An anti-inflammatory drug such as phenylbutazone may be administered either by mouth or injection.
- If there is a herd problem a foot bath containing either 1% formalin (only use in the open air) or 5% copper sulphate will help. Walk the sows through once each week on 2-3 occasions. However if there are dry cracked claws in the herd, this treatment might make them worse.

Management control and prevention

- Badly worn floor surfaces predispose.
- Sharp flint aggregates in concrete predispose.
- Pay particular attention to floors in boar pens, mating pens and loose sow housing.
- Check the quality of the floor surface around drinkers and feeders - particularly concrete slats.
- Use straw or shavings as bedding if practicable.
- Check the biotin levels in the diet.
- Wash and disinfect concrete surfaces regularly.

CLOSTRIDIAL DISEASES

Clostridia are large rod-shaped bacteria that also form spores and they persist in the environment for long periods. There are a number of different types. Disease in sows is associated with *C. novyi*, *C. chauvoei* and *C. septicum*. All these organisms produce toxins that may rapidly kill the host in a short period of time. The toxins are the main cause of disease not the bacteria so treatment must be given to prevent multiplication of the bacteria. The organism may enter the body through damage to the skin and underlying tissues and muscles. *C. novyi* spores also get carried from their normal habitat, the gut, to the liver where they may lie latent and inactive for long periods. Clostridia are also responsible for rapid decomposition of the body after death.

Clinical signs

C. septicum, often accompanied by the other two, causes malignant oedema a form of gangrene, which is characterised by the appearance of painful and discoloured swellings. Fluid and gas are often present in the tissues. The most common disease in sows is associated with *C. novyi* which causes sudden death. This occurs when some unknown event cuts off the blood supply to an area of the liver which provides a perfect medium for the *C. novyi* spores to vegetate and rapidly multiply producing toxins. These severely damage the liver and kill the sow. The course of the disease is extremely short and often the only sign is the finding of a good sow dead. A characteristic feature is the very rapid post-mortem changes particularly in the liver, which is full of gas and turns a chocolate colour. Gas bubbles may also be present throughout the carcase.

Diagnosis

Whenever sow mortality is more than 4% in the herd, death due to this disease should be considered. It is most important that post-mortem examinations are carried out as soon after death as possible (within two hours) because of the difficulty of differentiating between the lesions caused by *C. novyi* infection in the live pig and post-mortem changes.

Diagnosis is made by examining impression smears made on to a glass slide prepared from a cut surface of the liver and a fluorescent antibody test is carried out to identify the species. This disease can be a major problem in outdoor pigs and vaccination using either specific porcine vaccines or sheep vaccines containing the three clostridial organisms should be carried out. Two doses are given 3-6 weeks apart with a booster vaccination being given at each weaning time.

Treatment

Vaccines are commercially available but it may be six to eight weeks before sows are fully immune.

- Clostridia are very sensitive to penicillin.
In-feed medication using 200 grams to the tonne of phenoxymethyl penicillin can be used for 3-4 weeks to control acute outbreaks whilst a vaccination programme is established.
- Long-acting injections of penicillin given in anticipation of disease may help in the short term.

Management control and prevention

- Vaccinate all breeding stock and if necessary repeat the vaccination every six months.

CYSTITIS AND PYELONEPHRITIS

This is an important cause of mortality in all ages of

dry sows. Where disease is widespread total sow mortalities can often exceed 12% per annum. If a herd has an annual mortality of more than 5% some sows may be dying from unrecognised cystitis/pyelonephritis. In such herds post-mortem examinations of all sows that have died without apparent cause should be carried out. Urine passes from the kidneys down the two tubes (ureters) to the bladder where they enter and continue along the surface for approximately 30 to 40mm as straw like structures called the ureteric valves. As the bladder fills up pressure on them stops the urine being squeezed back towards the kidneys. In diseased sows the ureteric valves are often shortened from their normal length to as little as 10mm and if cystitis is present the bacteria can reflux back to the kidneys producing a very severe reaction. This causes the kidney function to cease (renal shunt) and death results in a matter of a few hours. Cystitis is inflammation of the bladder and pyelonephritis inflammation of the kidney and the two are often concurrent, particularly as sows get older. Occasionally it may be seen in gilts although this is uncommon unless there has been gross and prolonged faecal contamination of the vulva.

The bacteria associated with cystitis include *E. coli*, streptococci and in particular an organism called *Eubacterium suis* (originally called *Corynebacterium suis*). This latter organism is a common inhabitant of the preputial sac in the scrotum of the boar and occasionally the vagina of the sow. It has the ability to adhere specifically to the lining of the bladder and urinary tract and does not get easily flushed out with the flow of urine. It is thought that *E. suis* and sometimes *E. coli* may be deposited into the vagina at mating and when certain conditions prevail (which are not clearly understood) the organism can ascend the urethra and gain access to the bladder. Reproductive failure is not associated with this disease unless the sow is ill and as a consequence either dies or aborts.

Clinical signs

Acute disease

The sow appears very ill and off her food with the mucous membranes of the eye injected and red. The area around the vulva is wet and soiled with evidence of blood and pus in the urine. Sows showing these clinical signs often die or there will be a poor response to treatment with chronic cystitis developing. Disease can be so acute that death is the only sign. Post-mortem examinations will identify disease. It is more common in the first 21 days post mating because the urine of the sow becomes alkaline and both *E. suis* and *E. coli* will survive and multiply in alkaline urine.

Chronic disease

When nephritis caused by *E. suis* is present the disease is usually rapidly fatal but when cystitis occurs alone without progressing to nephritis the disease may be prolonged and not fatal. In these cases the appetite and the general condition of the sow can be normal, the only clinical signs being pus in the urine or a slight discharge clinging to the vulva. This should be distinguished from endometritis and vaginitis. (See chapter 6; Endometritis).

Diagnosis

This is best carried out by post-mortem examination. In the live animal, diagnosis is based upon clinical signs and evidence of blood and pus in the urine. Urine can be tested for the presence of blood, protein and the pH (acidity or alkalinity) by using paper strip tests. Urine can be collected in clean receptacles, especially if sows are made to stand 2-3 hours after feeding when they tend to urinate. Affected animals show evidence of blood and protein in the urine and a pH of 7 or more. (Normal urine is slightly acid, that is, less than the pH7.) Sows showing a pH of 8 or more have up to a 30% chance of dying in their next pregnancy.

Similar diseases

Cystitis can be confused with a vulval discharge which comes from the vagina or the womb and is usually of a salad cream consistency, whereas that from the urine contains pus and blood.

Treatment

- Antibiotic treatment is indicated to destroy the incriminating bacteria but it must be excreted in the urine.
- Lincomycin is effective at a dose level of 10mg/kg. This drug is active against *E. suis*.
- A more broad spectrum antibiotic however may be required if coliforms or other bacteria are involved. In such cases either ampicillin or amoxycillin at 10 to 15mg/kg should be given daily for 4 to 5 days.
- On a herd basis, treatment is best carried out using either CTC or OTC at levels of 600g/tonne for a period of 14 days. It may be necessary to repeat this treatment every 4 to 6 weeks.
- An alternate method is to inject the sow at weaning or at mating with a long-acting single injection of penicillin or amoxycillin.
- Sows could also be medicated from weaning to 21 days post mating during the most susceptible period by top dressing with in-feed supplements. The dose used is based on the assumption that the sow will eat 2.5kg of feed per day during this period and the amounts of top dressing should be calculated on the basis of 600g to the tonne of active antibiotic. In most cases using a 10% premix this will be between 15 and 20g of premix powder per day. In a herd with major problems the prepuces of all the boars should be swabbed and forwarded to a laboratory to determine the isolation rate of *E. suis* bacteria and its antibiotic sensitivity. In a normal herd the isolation rate would be less than 30% but

in a diseased herd this can approach 100%. In such cases attention to hygiene and management in the boar pens is required. Wet poorly drained floors accumulate urine and this is an ideal environment for *E. suis* to multiply in. Avoid shavings or sawdust as bedding.

☐ Antibiotic mastitis tubes or liquid antibiotics can be instilled into the prepuce daily for five days to reduce the weights of infection.

Management control and prevention

The sow mortality rate from nephritis may become unacceptably high, particularly in herds in which the sows are in individual confinement in stalls or tethers throughout their breeding lives. The overriding reason for this is low water intake and infrequent urination. If the stalls or tethers are (as they should be) comfortable dry and free from draughts, if the ambient temperature is constant day and night, if the sows are fed a satisfying balanced diet once a day and if they are otherwise undisturbed, most will tend to lie down for very long periods. They develop a state of what is termed 'passive withdrawal' or 'self narcosis', and become too lazy to stand up to drink and urinate. The bladder is not flushed out regularly and fills with thick turbid urine and salts. The female urethra (i.e. tube leading from the bladder to the vagina) is short and negative pressures may result in faecal matter and other contaminated material being sucked up into the bladder predisposing to cystitis. Contamination of the urethra and hence the bladder may also occur at mating. The nephritic organism, *E. suis*, is able to adhere to the lining of the urinary tract and to multiply there and it is not flushed out when the sow urinates.

Cystitis/pyelonephritis problems arise in a herd where there is a poor water supply or sows have a restricted water intake. If the disease is present as a herd problem check the points below to identify the problem areas.

◆ Ensure a good supply of clean fresh water and always check the quality if there is any doubt.
◆ Feed sows in confinement twice daily to encourage animals to rise and giving water particularly at the same time.
◆ If sows are fed in a continuous trough always put a small amount of water in first before the feed to encourage intake.
◆ Wherever possible use water troughs as drinkers, rather than nipple drinkers, particularly in loose-housed sows.
◆ If once-a-day feeding is practised in confinement or in loose housings either convert to a twice daily feeding system or scatter small amounts of feed into the trough at watering time.
◆ If there is a herd problem look carefully behind each sow daily to identify any showing clinical signs of cystitis. Treat these and check the urine as described under diagnosis. Sows that are showing blood, protein or high pH in their urine are best culled.
◆ Check that drinkers are at the correct height and provide easy access. The ideal height for sows is 800mm. In loose housing provide one nipple drinker per 10 - 15 sows with the water flow rate of 2 litres a minute . Alternatively provide water troughs with a minimum depth of 100mm.
◆ Check the water supply daily.
◆ In herds in which the sows are kept in individual confinement and in which there is a high mortality from nephritis, the most important preventative factors are to induce the sows to drink and urinate more frequently than they might otherwise do. They may be induced to drink more by increasing the salt in the ration to 0.9%. Walking a boar in front of the sow stalls daily will encourage them to stand and urinate. These actions alone usually result in a gradual decline in nephritis deaths.
◆ Reduce or prevent contamination of the vulva with faeces particularly from weaning to 21 days post mating. This occurs in stalls when solid back boards drop down to the ground level. There should be a 100mm gap between the bottom of the board and the floor to prevent faeces building up behind the sow.
◆ Sows that are too big for the stalls often adopt a dog sitting position with the vulva becoming heavily contaminated, allowing excessive bacterial multiplication.
◆ Badly drained boar and sow pens increase the risk of infection.
◆ The disease is more common in herds that have high numbers of old sows and boars.
◆ If group housing is used at weaning make sure the pens are well drained. **Do not** use sawdust for bedding and wash and disinfect pens regularly.
◆ Do not handle the prepuce at mating. Squeezing the prepucial sac increases the bacterial load transmitted to the vagina, (which may also result in increased returns to service).
◆ Always wear gloves at mating time to prevent the spread of the *E. suis* infection.
◆ Treat the boar's prepuces with antibiotic to reduce levels of *E. suis*.

Eradication

It is impossible to eradicate the organisms associated with this disease. They are present in every herd.

ERYSIPELAS

This is an important disease in the dry sow caused by the bacterium *Erysipelothrix rhusiopathiae* (syn, insidiosa). It occurs in most parts of the world where pigs are produced. The same organism also causes disease in sheep, poultry and is carried by wild birds. It also causes local skin lesions in humans but this is rare. It survives outside the pig in faeces and soil for up to six months. The most important source of infection however is the pig itself. It is estimated up to 20% of normal healthy pigs carry the organisms in their tonsils, where they are passed out in the faeces or via mucous from the mouth, thus perpetuating low level infection in the environment. Contaminated water also aids the spread of infection. Strains of erysipelas vary in their capacity to produce disease, ranging from very mild to very severe. Adverse environmental changes, poor nutrition, fluctuating temperatures and movement and mixing can activate the disease. Once a pig has been infected it will become immune and in many cases this is only associated with mild or sub-clinical disease. The organism enters the body through the tonsils, naturally occurring breaks in the integrity of the small intestine, or through wounds associated with fighting.

Clinical signs

Acute disease

The organism gains entry into the blood stream and multiplies rapidly causing a septicaemia. The onset is usually sudden and sometimes the disease will progress so rapidly that the first thing seen is a dead pig. A consistent feature of the disease is a very high temperature from 41 to 42°C (105 to 108°F). Some sows may appear very sick while others appear relatively normal. Stiffness and discomfort when walking and a reluctance to rise are common, indicating joint infection. The organisms clump together and block the small blood vessels particularly those beneath the skin. In such cases pink to dark purple areas, often diamond shaped, develop on the skin. See chapter 10. These can be palpated in the early stages even before the colour changes start. Left untreated these areas die/necrose and eventually slough off.

In non-vaccinated or inadequately vaccinated herds infected sows with high temperatures may abort. In such outbreaks up to 20% of animals in a group may be affected. Some of these animals farrow with high stillbirth rates and increased numbers of mummified pigs. Erysipelas in the boar is a serious disease because the prolonged high temperature affects the development of sperm over its period of some five to six weeks. Thus fertility can be affected by small litter sizes and increased returns to mating at both normal and variable intervals.

Usually the disease is confined to two or three animals in any one outbreak although in the non-vaccinated herd 5 to 10% of animals could be affected any one time.

Sub-acute disease

Here the animals are not as ill and the temperature is much lower, sometimes no more than 40°C (104°F) or even normal. There may be skin lesions evident and most animals will recover after three to four days.

Chronic disease

This may arise after acute or sub acute disease, or without any other clinical signs. The organism settles in the joints causing a chronic arthritis. There is a considerable amount of pain and loss of body condition but more importantly condemnations may occur at slaughter. Infection of the heart valves may result in growths and subsequent heart failure, for example during farrowing.

Diagnosis

This is based on inappetance, a very high temperature and the diamond shaped swellings which if present are diagnostic. If the diamond markings are not obvious to the eye they can be felt if the hand is run over the skin of the back or behind the back legs and over the flanks. This will assist in diagnosis. SE is easily grown in the laboratory and post-mortems and culture of the organism from the sudden deaths will confirm the diagnosis. Blood samples can be taken from the sow at the time of infection and again two weeks later and the antibody levels in the serum determined by the serum agglutination test. Titre levels of less than 1:60 would indicate sub-acute infection, low level exposure or a vaccine response. Titres of more than 1:320 would indicate recent exposure and a rising titre to tests, two weeks apart would help to confirm a diagnosis of disease. Serology however is not a reliable method of diagnosis, it only indicates exposure to the organism.

THE SIGNIFICANCE OF TITRE LEVELS Using the Agglutinating inhibition test (HI)	
< 1:10	- No exposure to infection.
1:20 - 1:320	- Either vaccine levels or long standing exposure but not necessarily disease.
> 1:60	- Exposure to infection in the past.
> 1:640	- Exposure to infection in the past and an indication of clinical disease.
A two fold rise in titre two weeks apart would indicate active infection.	

Treatment

- ❏ Swine Erysipelas is very susceptible to penicillin which is the drug of choice.
- ❏ Affected sows should be treated with long-acting preparations unless disease is acute. Usually a single injection is adequate but in severe cases it is necessary to repeat this two to three days later. The normal dose rate would be 1ml/10kg body weight.
- ❏ In acute cases a quick acting penicillin injected twice in the first 24 hours should bring about a rapid response. Continue daily injections for 3-4 days.
- ❏ Where a large number of sows are involved water medication with amoxycillin or phenoxy-methyl penicillin should be carried out. The dose level will depend upon the purity of the antibiotic powder used. (See chapter 4 Water medication).
- ❏ In prolonged outbreaks in-feed medication using 200-300g/tonne of phenoxymethyl penicillin for two weeks should control disease.

Management control and prevention

♦ In the breeding herd all the females and males should be vaccinated. Reasonably effective killed vaccines are available and two doses would normally be given 2 to 4 weeks apart. Ideally breeding gilts should be vaccinated twice from 12 weeks of age onwards and given a third dose just prior to first mating.
♦ Sows should be given a booster vaccination at each successive weaning.
♦ Boars likewise should be vaccinated twice from 12 weeks of age and thereafter given a booster every six months.
♦ Disease is sometimes seen in vaccinated animals either because the challenge has been too great, vaccination has been missed or wrongly administered, or the strain of erysipelas is not covered by the vaccine. Efficient storage of the vaccine as per the manufacturers recommendation is essential.
♦ If feed back of faeces is practised in the herd, it should be stopped immediately or it will spread the disease faster.

FRACTURES

Bone fractures are not uncommon in sows and gilts and are usually the end result of trauma and fighting although spontaneous ones occur in bone disease such as osteomalacia, associated with calcium phosphorus and vitamins A and D, and osteochondrosis.

Clinical signs

The onset is invariably sudden, the animal being unable to rise on its own without difficulty. A significant feature is the reluctance to place any weight on the affected leg. The muscles and tissues over the fracture site are often swollen and painful and the pig is very reluctant to move unless on three legs. An examination is best carried out when the pig is lying down. Crepitus or the rubbing together of the two broken ends of the bone can often be felt. Fractures of the spinal vertebra are common in the first litter female particularly during lactation and in the immediate post weaning period. The pig usually adopts a dog sitting position and exhibits severe pain on movement. Such animals should be destroyed.

Diagnosis

This is based upon the history, symptoms and palpation to detect crepitus.

Similar diseases

These include acute laminitis, arthritis, muscle tearing, bush foot and mycoplasma arthritis.

Treatment

☐ The affected pig should be slaughtered on the farm.

Management control and prevention

♦ If fractures are a recurring problem it is necessary to check that there are no diseases such as osteomalacia, osteoporosis or leg weakness (OCD).
♦ Check the calcium phosphorus and vitamin D levels.
♦ Check management procedures during the period of effect.

GASTRIC ULCERS

Erosion and ulceration of the lining of the stomach is a common condition in all pigs. It occurs around the area where the oesophagus enters the stomach (called the pars oesophagea). In the early stages of the disease the pars becomes roughened and gradually changes as the surface becomes eroded until it is actively ulcerated. Intermittent haemorrhage may then take place leading to anaemia, or massive haemorrhage may occur resulting in death. The incidence in sows is usually less than 5% but in growing pigs up to 60% may show lesions at slaughter.

The causes of gastric ulceration are multifactorial. These can be categorised as nutritional and related to the physical properties of the feed, managemental, infectious causes and miscellaneous factors.

The following need to be considered as causal or contributory:

Nutritional factors:
- Low protein diets.
- Low fibre diets. (The introduction of straw reduces the incidence).
- High energy diets.
- High levels of wheat in excess of 55%.
- Deficiencies of vitamin E or selenium.
- Diets containing high levels of iron, copper or calcium.
- Diets low in zinc.
- Diets with high levels of unsaturated fats.
- Diets based on whey and skimmed milk.

> *Consider changing from pellets to course ground meal.*

Physical aspects of the diet that increase the incidence:
- Size of feed particle - the more finely ground the meal the smaller becomes the particle size and the higher the incidence of ulcers. This is still the case if the feed is then pelleted.
- Pelleting feeds in itself increases the incidence. Feed meal.
- Particle size. Where there is a problem on the farm have the feed examined to assess the varying percentages of particle sizes. This is carried out by sifting the

meal through a series of 12 to 14 tiller screens and weighing the residual amounts remaining in each screen. Particle size is also affected by the type and moisture content of the cereals that are being used, the condition of the hammer mills and the screen and the rate of flow through the grinding system. The smaller the particle size the greater the incidence.

- Sometimes there can be problems in changing from pellets to meal and a compromise is to feed alternatively.
- If the feed is home-produced and is meal, then it is necessary to check the size and quality of the screen that is being used.
- Using cereals with a high moisture content.
- Rolling cereals as distinct from grinding them will often produce a dramatic drop in the incidence but the penalties of feed use have to be taken into consideration.

Managemental factors that increase the incidence:
- Irregular feeding patterns and shortage of feeder space.
- Periods of starvation.
- Increased stocking densities and movement of pigs. Look carefully at the environment in the pens and in finishing houses. Are there undue stresses or aggressions.
- Poor management of sows in stalls and tethers.
- Transportation.
- Poor availability of food or water.

Miscellaneous factors:
- Stress associated with fluctuating environmental temperatures.
- Adverse environmental conditions that create an unhappy environment.
- Psychological stress resulting from bad or harsh stockmanship.
- The condition is more common in castrates and boars than in gilts but the reason for this is unknown. Difference in feeding patterns may be a factor.
- Split sexing may help.
- Breed. More common in certain genotypes particularly those that have low back fat measurements and a capacity for rapid lean tissue growth.

Infectious causes:
- There is a clear relationship between outbreaks of pneumonia and the incidence of gastric ulceration.
- Ulceration may occur following bacterial septicaemias such as those associated with erysipelas and swine fever.
- In the breeding sow gastric ulceration is usually confined to the individual animal and is often secondary to a specific disease.

Clinical signs

These depend on the severity of the condition. In its most acute form previously healthy animals are found dead.

The most striking sign in these cases is the paleness

> **If ulcers are a problem then increase the screen size to 3.5mm.**

of the carcase due to internal haemorrhage.

In the less acute form the affected pig is pale, and weak, and may show breathlessness, grinding of the teeth due to stomach pain and vomiting. The passing of dark faeces containing digested blood is often a persistent symptom. Usually the temperature is normal. When the condition becomes chronic the pig has an intermittent appetite and may lose weight. The faeces vary from normal to dark coloured depending on the presence or absence of blood. Feed intake, feed efficiency and daily gain can be affected.

Diagnosis

Ulceration should always be considered in sows or pigs which are pale, lose body condition and develop a variable appetite particularly if the faeces are black and tarry.

A sample of faeces should be examined for the presence of blood and to eliminate parasites. Although the disease is usually confined to individuals or less than 5% of sows, occasionally it can become a herd problem. In such cases poor body condition is widespread through the breeding herd.

Whenever black tarry faeces are seen gastric ulceration should be suspected and in the feeding herd an examination of stomachs at slaughter should be carried out.

Similar diseases

Haemorrhage from the bowel can also arise from the intestine in cases of bloody gut (PHE) but usually this is confined to young gilts and growing pigs.

Anaemia in pigs can also be associated with eperythrozoonosis, the stomach worm *Hyostrongylus rubidus*, chronic mange and porcine enteropathy. Nutritional deficiencies particularly of minerals and vitamins can increase the incidence.

Treatment

☐ Move the affected animal from its existing housing into a loose bedded peaceful environment.
☐ Feed a weaner type diet containing highly digestible materials.
☐ Inject multi vitamins and in particular vitamin E together with 0.5 to 1g of iron intramuscularly and repeat on a weekly basis.
☐ Add an extra 100g vitamin E / tonne to the diet for two months and assess the results.
☐ Cull affected pigs.

Management control and prevention

◆ Consider the above factors and their relevance to your situation. Make alterations and adjustments accordingly.

GLÄSSERS DISEASE (*HAEMOPHILUS PARASUIS*)

See chapter 9 for further information.

This disease caused by the tiny bacteria *Haemophilus parasuis* normally affects the sucking and young growing pig, but it occasionally affects the gilt. Lameness occurs in any of the legs with slight swellings over the joints and tendons. It is rare to see this disease in the dry sow. The organism has an affinity for the smooth shiny surfaces covering the joints, tendons and other tissues, including the pericardium (heart sac) and meninges where it causes pericarditis and meningitis.

In the young gilt lameness and stiffness are the most common signs.

Diagnosis

In the living animal this is difficult, because it is similar to *Mycoplasma hyosynoviae* infection of joints and tendon sheaths. Post-mortem examinations and/or samples taken aseptically from infected joints for culture will help to differentiate.

Treatment

- ☐ *Haemophilus parasuis* is normally sensitive to injections of penicillin, synthetic penicillins, ampicillin or amoxycillin, and oxytetracycline.
- ☐ The response to a daily injection, given for at least 3 or 4 days, is usually good provided treatment is instituted early.
- ☐ Because this disease can be very difficult to differentiate from mycoplasma infection a combination of treatments using penicillin and tiamulin injections may be used daily for 3 to 4 days to cover both infections.

HAEMATOMA

A haematoma is a pocket of blood that forms beneath the skin or in muscle tissue and is associated with a ruptured blood vessel. It usually arises from trauma particularly over the shoulders, flanks or the hind quarters. Not uncommonly the ear of the sow may be damaged following fighting or head shaking and rubbing associated with mange. Once sufficient pressure has built up in the tissues the haemorrhage stops and a clot is formed which is gradually removed by the normal body repair mechanisms and the swelling disappears.

In some cases the haematoma may be infected and an abscess will develop. This should be dealt with as described under abscess. It is inadvisable in the sow to lance a haematoma if it has not developed into an abscess. Always sample the fluid first by syringe and needle. If blood is withdrawn the haematoma is of recent origin and if serum is present it is long standing. Leave both alone. Animals with large haematoma of the ear are best culled.

JAW AND SNOUT DEVIATION

This is a very common yet little recognised condition in the sow. When the jaw is at rest, a proportion of sows (often around 5%) and particularly those housed in confinement, show a malalignment of the jaw to the left or right of centre. In extreme cases this can give the appearance of rhinitis. The condition is associated with a loss in height of the vertical part of the mandible or jaw bone and as a result the jaw swings over from one side to the other. The nose is always straight.

The vertical part of the jaw bone grows in height from the cartilage that forms part of the mandibular joint. During early growth constant trauma from bar biting or the use of nipple drinkers interferes with the normal growth.

Occasional bending of the nose is seen where there has been infection of the bone as a result of faulty teeth clipping in early life. Neither condition is of significance.

There is another rare condition associated particularly with sows derived from the UK breed of Large White. It appears to result from prolonged feeding of very finely ground meal in narrow troughs which provide difficult access. The upper jaw and nose become shortened and flattened, in some cases to a grotesque degree, and the lower jaw protrudes forward several centimetres beyond the nose. There is no evidence of this condition in gilts but it gets worse with age. This is not atrophic rhinitis.

LAMENESS

Next to reproductive failure, lameness is the second most common cause of sows being culled. Most cases occur from weaning through to the point of farrowing. A lameness problem increases the culling rate, reproductive problems and the non productive sow days so reducing the litters and pigs weaned per sow per year. Often problems involve first parity gilts or second parity sows, just as they are reaching the most productive part of their life. Sows culled for severe lameness may have to be shot on the farm because on welfare grounds they should not be transported. Therefore they contribute significantly to the recorded sow mortality. In order to analyse a lameness problem on a farm it is important to keep accurate records about each sow. These should include the following:

- Sow number.
- Parity.
- Breed and genetic line.
- Date of mating.
- Date of farrowing.
- Date of weaning.
- Date of lameness.
- Type of lameness.
- Housing area.

Alternatively you could use the farrowing rate loss sheet that is used in the dry period.

The causes of lameness in breeding animals can be separated into infectious and non infectious. These are listed below.

Infectious causes
- Brucellosis.
- Clostridial diseases.
- Erysipelas.
- Foot-and-mouth disease.
- Foot rot, Bush foot.
- Glässers disease, (*Haemophilus parasuis*).
- Mycoplasma arthritis.
- Salmonellosis.
- Swine vesicular disease.
- Streptococcal infections.

Non infectious causes
- Fractures.
- Laminitis.
- Leg weakness (OCD).
- Muscle tearing.
- Nutritional deficiencies.
- Porcine stress syndrome.
- Toxic conditions.
- Trauma.

In the maiden gilt or during the first pregnancy infectious lameness is usually due to erysipelas, glässers disease, mycoplasma infections and brucellosis in those countries where it is endemic. Clostridial diseases are rare in the dry sow but infections of the claws and hock areas due to trauma (foot rot and bush foot) are common causes. Foot-and-mouth disease and the vesicular diseases are discussed in chapter 12. In such infections a number of sows in both the dry sow area, the lactating area and indeed pigs across the unit will have varying degrees of lameness and blistering around the nose, mouth and feet. If there is a herd problem use Fig.7-6 to help identify the cause.

Tissue changes that cause lameness

Apophyseolysis (OCD) - Separation of the muscle mass from the growth plate on the pelvis.
Arthritis - Inflammation of one or more joint.
Damage to nervous tissue - Clinical signs vary (e.g. partial or complete paralysis of one or more limbs) depending on the site of the damage.
Epiphyseolysis (OCD) - Separation of the head of the femur.
Fractured bones - Common in the hip, hock and elbow joints.
Haematoma - Haemorrhage into the tissues.
Laminitis - Inflammation of the tissues connecting the hoof to the bone. It is not common.
Myositis - Inflammation of muscles.
Penetrated sole - Damage due to trauma.
Periostitis - Inflammation of the membrane (periosteum)

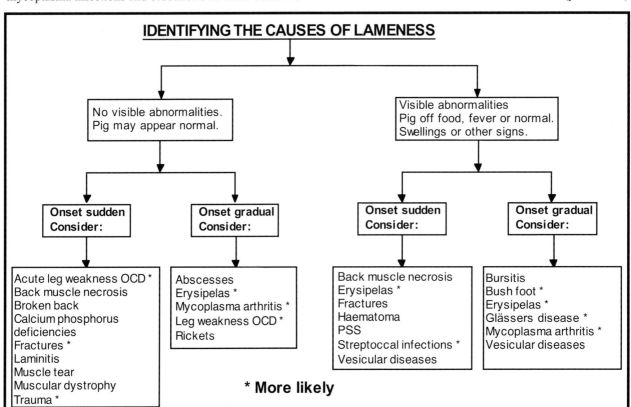

(Fig.7-6)

which covers the bone.
Osteitis - Inflammation of bone.
Osteochondrosis (leg weakness) - Growth plate and joint cartilage degeneration.
Osteomalacia - Softening of the bones due to calcium/phosphorus deficiency.
Osteomyelitis - Inflammation of all bone tissue including the spongy centre and bone marrow.
Osteoporosis - Week bones due to an imbalance of calcium and phosphorous in the diet.
Split horn - Poor hoof quality. Overgrown claws.
Torn ligaments or muscles - A common cause of lameness particularly where muscles are attached to bones.

LAMINITIS

This disease describes inflammation of the soft highly vascular structures that connect the bone to the hoof. It is an uncommon but very painful condition causing animals to walk on their knees. The cause is unknown and affected pigs should be destroyed.

LEG WEAKNESS (OSTEOCHONDROSIS - OCD)

Trauma is by far the most common cause of lameness in the dry sow from point of weaning to point of farrowing. Environmental trauma to the coronary band area and to the sole or wall of the foot results in penetration of the sensitive tissues, infection and lameness. These foot conditions are called bush foot and foot rot. Trauma however, more commonly arises indirectly from other causes within the environment that create shear forces on the muscles, tendons, bones and bone structures. Such changes associated with cartilaginous structures are referred to as leg weakness or osteochondrosis. The structure of the joint and bone is shown in Fig.7-7.

The term "Leg weakness" is also used sometimes to describe poor leg conformation or describe a clinical condition associated with lameness and stiffness. It arises due to abnormal changes in the articular cartilage and the growth (epiphyseal) plates. These plates are responsible for the growth of bones both in length and diameter. Whilst the exact mechanisms that cause these changes are not fully understood they arise due to the pressure and shear stresses that are placed upon these rapidly growing tissues. This pressure reduces the oxygen supply, causing abnormal growth and consistency of the cartilage. Damage to the cartilage tends to be progressive and irreversible. The damaged cartilage is replaced by fibrous tissue. This cartilage damage in turn produces shortening and bending of the bones near the joints and at the extremities of the long bones. Weak epiphyseal

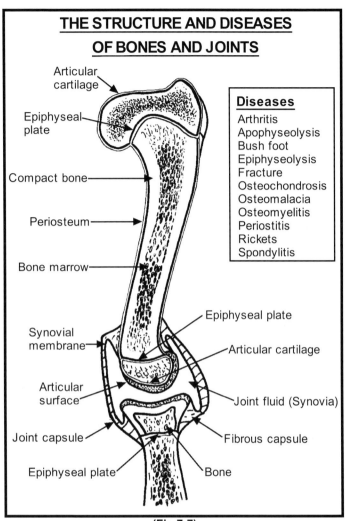

(Fig.7-7)

plates also have a tendency to fracture and cartilage covering the joint surfaces splits and forms fissures. It is important to appreciate that such changes in the cartilage take place in most if not all modern pigs from as early as two months of age. In some cases many of these can only be detected under the microscope. It is interesting to note that such changes can not be detected in the wild boar which takes up to two years to reach maturity. OCD is therefore a fact of life in modern pig production but its severity and its effects depend largely on the environment. OCD results from the many years of selecting animals for rapid growth, large muscle mass, and efficient feed conversion and therefore much greater weight on the growth plates whilst they are still immature, together with the stresses of intensive methods of production. Conversion of cartilage to bone involves the deposition of calcium and phosphorous and while the process of breaking down and reforming bone goes on throughout life, bone growth ceases when the sow is approximately 14 to 16 months of age.

212 Managing Pig Health and the Treatment of Disease

It is not uncommon in breeding enterprises for 20 to 30% of boars and gilts to be culled after completing the performance test, due to leg weakness and leg deformities.

The conformation of the pig is a predisposing factor to OCD, Fig.7- 8 shows some of these traits.

Sows with good leg conformation show angulation of the bones at the hip, knee and hock joints. The bones below the hock slope slightly forwards and the feet are well placed on the ground. Sows that are susceptible to leg weakness are straight legged with little angulation of the bones between the joints and the back tends to be arched. This alignment increases shear stresses on the growth plates.

Clinical signs

Acute disease

This is seen when there is a separation or fracture of the bones at the epiphyseal plate (epiphyseolysis) associated with sudden movement. The animal walks on three legs, the affected leg swinging freely. Crepitus or rubbing of the broken bones together can usually be felt.

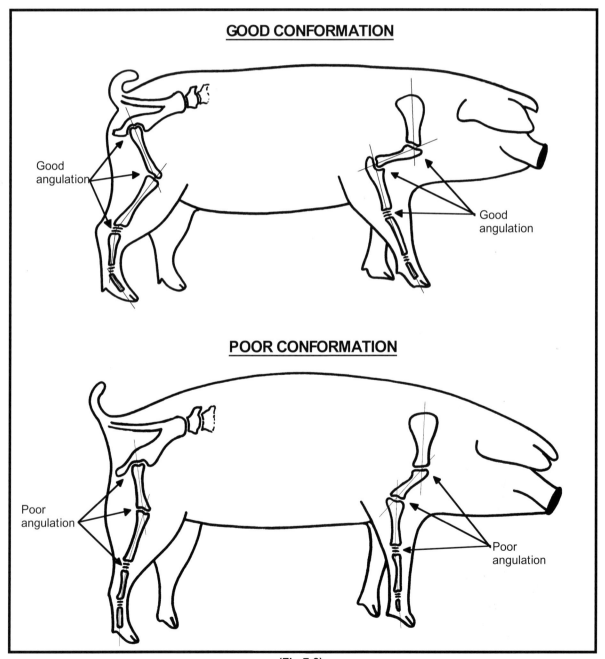

(Fig-7-8)

Sudden fractures can also occur in the knee and elbow joints, which are more common in the young growing pig. Fractures of the vertebrae in the spine occur particularly during lactation and immediately post weaning. In such cases the sow is in acute pain, often in a dog sitting position with the hind legs well forward. Animals housed in farrowing crates with slippery floors tend to slide the back legs forward and there is a risk of the hind muscles pulling away from their attachments to the pelvis (apophyseolysis). In such cases the sow will stand with assistance but it cannot pull the hind leg backwards. When it is placed on to the ground it just slides forward. Such animals should be culled immediately.

Chronic disease

The onset is gradual. The pig shows abnormal leg conformation and gait with or without stiffness and pain. The temperature remains normal and joints will not be swollen unless there are fractures.
- Front legs
  - These may be straight with the pig walking with a long step on its toes.
  - The knees may be bent inwards or flexed which causes the pig to walk with short steps.
  - The pasterns may be dropped. This is common in old sows due to shortened bones and slack tendons.
  - The feet may be rotated or twisted.
- Hind legs
  - These are straight with a swinging action from the hips as the pig moves. Avoid selecting such females for breeding.
  - The legs are tucked beneath the body.
  - The hocks turn inwards and are close together.
  - The pig walks with a goose stepping action.
  - Likewise in old sows the pasterns may be dropped. Fig.7-9.

Abnormal gaits arise either from pain in the joints or abnormal movements in the hind legs from the hips which give a swaying motion. The pain is associated with damage to the sensitive membranes around the joints resulting from either splitting or erosion of the cartilage in the joints or movement of the growth plates. Some pigs however may show severe clinical signs yet on post mortem examinations the joints appear normal and vice versa. Joints may become inflamed (arthritis), particularly in the hip, knee and elbow. OCD may be seen within three months of gilts being introduced on to the farm, during their first pregnancy, in lactation or in the first 2 to 3 weeks post weaning.

Diagnosis

OCD is diagnosed on the clinical signs described. There are no serological or other tests and post-mortem examinations may be misleading because many pigs that are found to have joint lesions may not be lame.

Similar diseases

There are two, *Mycoplasma hyosynoviae* infection and

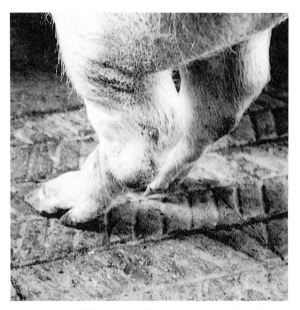

Leg weakness or OCD in a sow. Note the forward position of the legs and the dropped pasterns
(Fig.7-9)

erysipelas. In both of these the disease is usually sudden in onset sometimes with a raised body temperature and there is pain and swelling in the joints. A differentiating feature is the response to treatment. OCD does not respond to antibiotics whereas *Mycoplasma hyosynoviae* and erysipelas will respond within 24 to 36 hours, the former to lincomycin or tiamulin and the latter to penicillin.

Treatment

☐ There is no specific treatment for OCD, however, at an early stage the sow should be moved from its existing environment to a well-bedded pen where the foot can grip. If not, the lesions progress and ultimately arthritis and permanent lameness develop.

☐ Gilts that are confined in stalls or tethers, or group housed on floors that are wet and slippery should be moved as soon as clinical signs appear.

Management control and prevention

If OCD is causing a problem on your farm check through the list below and identify those points that are important in your system.
◆ Determine the time and place when OCD first becomes evident.
◆ Look carefully at surfaces that cause the foot to slip and result in increased pressure on the growth plates.
◆ If the problem is in gilts look carefully at the conformation of these animals and consider improving the selection procedure.
◆ Animals with a fine bone structure are more prone to leg weakness.

- Animals with heavy ham muscles and a disparity between anterior and posterior muscle masses, increases the horizontal pull on the growth plates. Such young gilts do not acclimatise well to stalls or tethers.
- If there is a problem in lactating gilts look at the floor surfaces in the farrowing crates. Are these slippery and causing pressure on weakened bones? The use of dry sand in these pens once or twice a week may assist in the prevention of the condition until the floor surfaces can be altered.
- The modern hybrid gilt often suckles ten or more pigs and produces a large amount of milk which is high in calcium and phosphorous. The bones are therefore more prone to calcium or phosphorus depletion and if the gilt is mixed at weaning time with older sows, damage and sudden fractures are likely to take place.
- The tethering and confinement of gilts during pregnancy can be a major contributing factor. Culling rates in such animals may rise towards 20% if the floor surfaces are very slippery.
- The design of slats can contribute to OCD. Some slats slope to the edges from the centre and are so smooth that when the animals stand, the feet slip into the gaps. This causes constant twisting and pressure on the growth plates and a high incidence of OCD may result.
- Gilts in the first pregnancy should not be housed on slippery floor surfaces.
- High levels of vitamin A (in excess of 20,000 iu/kg) particularly in the younger growing pigs can interfere with the normal growth of the epiphyseal plates. OCD lesions have been seen in piglets as young as 3 to 4 weeks of age where sows have been fed excessive levels of vitamin A.
- High lysine levels may also increase the incidence.
- High stocking densities, particularly in the growing period and where animals are housed on solid concrete floors or slats, will increase the incidence of OCD in the breeding stock. Such environments cause great stress on the legs and pens tend to be dirty and wet.
- Fat sprayed diets can make floor surfaces slippery.
- Pigs treated with porcine growth hormone tend to develop severe lesions of OCD at an early age.
- New concrete surfaces or slats during the first few weeks of use may develop slippery surfaces after contact with faeces and urine. They should be pressure washed with detergent on two or three occasions.
- Variations in nutrition within acceptable limits do not appear to influence OCD but conditions of osteomalacia and osteoporosis (soft and weak bones) occur where there is an imbalance of calcium and phosphorous in the diet or excessive withdrawal of these minerals from the bones. Soft and brittle bones in such deficiencies often fracture across the mid part of the long bones during lactation. Always check the calcium phosphorous ratios of the diet and add additional minerals during lactation, dicalcium bone phosphate could be used.
- Pain in the joints from OCD also gives rise to abnormal stresses on the muscles particularly where they are attached to the bone. Tearing of these attachments on the insides of the shoulders and legs and from the muscle masses in the pelvis is common causing severe pain and periostitis.
- Smooth concrete surfaces that have been finished with a steel float can predispose to OCD.
- The addition of 0.5% sodium bicarbonate/tonne to the ration has been shown to reduce the incidence.

LEPTOSPIROSIS
See chapter 6 for further information.

This is an important infectious disease in the pregnant animal causing abortions and pregnancy failures. Actual clinical illness is uncommon unless there are secondary infections. A prolonged carrier state exists.

MANGE
See chapter 11 for further information.

Mange which is caused by the tiny mite *Sarcoptes scabiei* is an important skin parasite and the sow once infected remains a carrier unless treatment is given to eliminate it. It is an important disease with considerable economic consequences in the growing pig.

MASTITIS
See chapter 8 for further information.

Mastitis denotes inflammation and infection of the mammary glands. It is primarily a condition seen in the lactating sow. Nevertheless it can be a problem in the dry period with new cases occurring within two days of weaning. If left untreated it can become chronic with thick fibrous scar tissue and large lumps which ultimately may ulcerate to the surface. Chronic mastitis may occur at weaning time when the udder is dried off, the gland having become infected in lactation. The disease can be caused by a number of different bacteria including streptococci, staphylococci, *E. coli*, klebsiella, pseudomonas and actinomyces.

Clinical signs
Acute disease

These are seen within 2 to 4 days of weaning. The infected glands are enlarged red and painful to pressure and the skin overlying is blanched or discoloured. The temperature is usually raised and the sow is off her food. In severe infections toxins are produced and sows may die within 24 hours.

Chronic disease

If there is a poor response to treatment or disease has not been recognised in lactation, the gland may be enlarged, often with fibrous tissue and small multiple abscesses that may ulcerate to the surface. Invariably at this stage there is permanent damage and if several mammary glands are affected the sow should be culled.

Diagnosis

This is determined by visual evidence of swellings and hard lumps in the mammary gland. The sow's udder should be examined routinely at two days after weaning and also while the sow stands at mating, to look and feel for chronic mastitis.

If the prevalence is more than 2% of the dry sow population then an investigation should be carried out to assess the reasons why and to determine where the mastitis is starting. This could be in the immediate post farrowing period, during lactation or at weaning time. Preventive measures would then be carried out relative to that period.

Treatment

- This should follow the general guidelines as for mastitis in the lactating sow in chapter 8. If the mastitis is being initiated from point of weaning a long-acting antibiotic should be given on the day of weaning.
- **Acute Disease**
  Antibiotics of value:
    - Penicillin / streptomycin.
    - Amoxycillin.
    - Trimethoprim sulpha.
    - Oxytetracycline.
    - Framycetin.

Management control and prevention

- Give long-acting injections of either penicillin, oxytetracycline or amoxycillin on the day of weaning.
- See also the procedures for the lactating sow.
- Wet dirty pens that cause heavy contamination of the udder in the first 3-4 days after weaning predispose.
- Clean and disinfect weaning accommodation regularly.

MENINGITIS

See chapter 9; Streptococcal infections for further information.

Meningitis is uncommon in the sow but it is sometimes secondary to middle ear infection or associated with water deprivation and salt poisoning. If an infectious disease enters a herd for the first time sporadic cases in sows may be seen.

Clinical signs

The sow is inappetent, trembling with an unsteady gate. The temperature is elevated, often as high as 42°C (108°F). As the meningitis develops in severity the eye moves sideways (nystagmus) fits develop and the sow ultimately cannot stand.

Diagnosis

This is based upon the signs in an individual sow, or if there are a number of cases, a specific infectious disease. It may require a post-mortem examination, including histology of the brain and demonstration of the causal organism to confirm the diagnosis.

Similar diseases

These include:
  Acute kidney infection.
  Aujeszky's disease (AD) (PR).
  Brain abscess.
  Haemophilus parasuis infection.
  Heat stroke.
  Listeriosis.
  Middle ear infection.
  Poisons.
  Water deprivation.

Treatment

- This depends upon the cause. Always consider the common ones first which include middle ear infection, brain abscess, water deprivation and in some countries aujeszky's disease. Refer to the treatment for these specific diseases.
- For bacterial infections use penicillin, penicillin/streptomycin or amoxycillin. Inject twice daily.
- Corticosteroids may also be required. Seek veterinarian advice.
- Move the affected animal to a clean warm well bedded pen.
- Provide easy access to water or dribble into the mouth three times daily by hose pipe.

MORTALITY

Sow mortality in some herds can be a cause of major economic loss. In approaching this problem first categorise the causes and in particular differentiate between those animals destroyed on welfare or other grounds and those that actually die.

Target levels: 3% - 6% deaths. Up to 2% of these may be destroyed on welfare or other grounds

The range in herds: 3% - 15%

Levels of 7-9% are not uncommon and relate to specific contributory factors on that particular farm which must be identified.

These include:

- Age of the herd.
- Culling policy.
- Welfare constraints (sows sold as culls and not recorded as deaths).
- Breed.
- Presence of the stress gene.
- Body condition - Sows in poor condition are more susceptible to disease.
- Availability of water and the incidence of cystitis - pyelonephritis.
- Susceptibility to leg weakness (OCD).
- Type of management system. Mixing of sows, fighting etc.
- Type of environment. Mortality levels are higher in poorly managed housing systems.
- Quality of the nutrition.
- Feeding system. this may predispose to ruptured or twisted intestines.

The causes of mortality

At least two thirds of all sow deaths occur in the dry period.
- Abscesses.
- Cancer.
- Chronic disease.
- Clostridial infections.
- Cystitis / pyelonephritis.
- Dead piglets. Womb infection.
- Electrocution.
- Fighting.
- Fractures.
- Gastric ulcers.
- Heart failure.
- Internal abscesses.
- Internal haemorrhage.
- Lameness.
- Paraplegia.
- Peritonitis.
- Poor body condition.
- Prolapse rectum.
- Prolapse uterus.
- Prolapse vagina.
- Strangulation associated with the environment.
- Torsion of the stomach or intestines.
- Vulval biting.

PROCEDURES FOR IDENTIFYING AND CORRECTING A SOW MORTALITY PROBLEM	
Step 1	Set up a recording system. (See chapter 3)
Step 2	Analyse the results to identify the common causes.
Step 3	Refer to the specific disease once identified.
Step 4	Apply the recommended controls and prevention.

MUSCLE TEARING

This is a common condition in sows and first litter gilts whereby the muscle fibres are torn away from their attachment to the bone and periosteum. This occurs where muscles are attached to the inner surfaces of the elbow and knee joints, and the points of attachment to the pelvis. Affected sows show considerable pain and often adopt a dog sitting position. Inflammation of bone and periosteum result (periostitis). Torn muscles arise as a sequel to OCD, trauma and fighting, slippery surfaces and weak bones. Affected sows as soon as they are identified should be moved to a solid floor area that is deep bedded where the grip for the foot is firm. Soiled or grass areas are ideal. If this is done most will recover.

MYCOPLASMA ARTHRITIS (*MYCOPLASMA HYOSYNOVIAE* INFECTION)

This is caused by the tiny organism *Mycoplasma hyosynoviae* which is ubiquitous and most, if not all herds are infected with it. It is a respiratory spread disease the organism being found in the upper respiratory tract nose and tonsils. It may be present in some herds and cause no clinical signs and yet in others cause severe disease. Infection with or without disease takes place in the young growing pig from approximately 8 to 30 weeks of age and particularly so in the gilt when first introduced onto a farm, or in the early stages of pregnancy. It is very uncommon in older sows because they develop a strong immunity resulting from repeated exposure to the organism. They pass this immunity to their offspring in the colostrum. This maternally derived immunity gradually disappears over a period of weeks. Infection then takes place as these pigs become exposed to older ones. *Mycoplasma hyosynoviae* infects joints and tendon sheaths rather than the respiratory system.

Clinical signs

Disease in the gilt is usually sudden in onset, the first signs being a reluctance to rise at feeding time. There is a considerable amount of pain and the affected pig will only stand for short periods of time. The temperature may be normal or slightly elevated. It is more common in the heavy ham straight legged animal and purchased gilts which have been reared in isolated grow out units often become diseased four to six weeks after arrival.

Diagnosis

This is based on clinical signs and the response to either lincomycin or tiamulin therapy. Joint fluid can be aspirated and examined for antibodies and isolation of the organism.

Serology is not much help because sub-clinical infection is common and so healthy animals often have antibody titres. Rising titres in blood samples taken two weeks apart together with typical symptoms strongly suggest disease.

In problem herds post-mortem examination may be necessary to reach a definitive diagnosis.

Similar diseases

These include muscle damage, leg weakness or OCD, trauma, erysipelas, glässers disease and the major vesicular diseases.

Treatment

☐ *Mycoplasma hyosynoviae* is susceptible to lincomycin or tiamulin injections.
☐ Give daily for 4 days in the early course of the disease. If the lameness is due to *Mycoplasma hyosynoviae* there should be a good response within 24 to 36 hours.
☐ Treatment is most effective if given early.
☐ Give in feed medication strategically commencing 7 days before the expected disease outbreak and continue for 14 days using 220g/tonne of lincomycin or 500-800g/tonne of OTC.
☐ An alternate strategy is to medicate the ration at half these levels and feed for 5-7 weeks.

Management control and prevention

Mycoplasma hyosynoviae can be a recurring problem in breeding gilts particularly during the first 6 to 10 weeks after introduction to the farm. Consider the following:

♦ Identify the period of onset and apply strategic preventative medication.
♦ In-feed medicate susceptible groups over the critical period with either 500-800g OTC or CTC per tonne, 110-220g of lincomycin per tonne or 100g of tiamulin per tonne.
♦ Maintain pigs on ad lib feeding during the susceptible period.
♦ Assess the quality of housing - in particular low temperatures and draughts which act as trigger factors.
♦ Remember that this is a respiratory spread disease and other factors need to be considered.
♦ Avoid mixing and fighting.
♦ Provide well bedded pens.
♦ In outdoor herds acclimatise gilts to cobs or large nuts before they are introduced into the outdoor herd.
♦ Control enzootic pneumonia and other respiratory diseases if they are a coincidental problem.

PERITONITIS

Peritonitis describes infection and inflammation of the peritoneum; the shiny membrane that covers all the internal surfaces in the abdomen. It can be caused by a ruptured gastric ulcer, a perforated bowel, penetration of the abdomen via mating, a sequel to external trauma to the abdomen and a ruptured bowel or liver.

Diseases such as actinobacillus pleuropneumonia, migrating ascarid worms, miscellaneous generalised infections may also result in peritonitis.

Clinical signs

The onset may be sudden or gradual. Signs are associated with abdominal pain. The sow is reluctant to move, loses weight and has a tucked up appearance. The mucous membranes are often pale. The most common time is 7-10 days post mating after damage by the boar at mating. A discharge from the vulva may then be apparent. The temperature may be normal or elevated and appetite normal or depressed.

Diagnosis

This is based on the clinical signs and history. A post-mortem examination may be required to confirm the diagnosis when females die or are destroyed.

Treatment

☐ This is by broad spectrum antibiotic treatments for 5 to 7 days. Inject with either OTC, penicillin, streptomycin or amoxycillin.
☐ The response is usually poor.

PNEUMONIA

See chapter 9 for further information.

Pneumonia is normally uncommon in the mature herd but occasionally occurs in the gilt if immunity levels are low. However if influenza or PRRS viruses enters the herd for the first time or herd immunity wanes, periodic outbreaks involving a small number of sows may occur. When a new respiratory pathogen is introduced into the herd for the first time, for example, a virulent strain of *Actinobacillus pleuropneumoniae*, severe pneumonia is likely to develop in all ages of animals.

PATHOGENIC ORGANISMS THAT CAUSE PNEUMONIA
Actinobacillus pleuropneumoniae
Haemophilus parasuis (Glässers disease)
Mycoplasma hyopneumoniae (Enzootic pneumonia)
PRRS virus
Respiratory corona virus (usually very mild)
Swine influenza virus

Clinical signs

These are seen at a herd level when new infections first enter. There is wide spread coughing and up to 20% or more severely ill animals. The respiratory rate is elevated with some sows showing acute respiratory distress.

In herd breakdowns with enzootic pneumonia or actinobacillus pleuropneumonia mortality can be as high as 10 to 15% if prompt treatment is not undertaken. If a clinical picture of widespread, sudden and progressive respiratory disease develops, then suspect a herd breakdown with one of the above organisms.

Diagnosis

This is based on the clinical signs of coughing, rapid breathing a high temperature and post-mortem examinations. At an individual level sows may develop pneumonia due to infectious agents already in the herd. The introduction of swine influenza into a herd is usually dramatic, with large numbers of sows off their food over a period of 3 to 7 days. Wide spread coughing and depression may be seen. In the case of a breakdown with enzootic pneumonia (in a herd that was previously free) the onset may be insidious with some inappetance but a gradual spreading cough over a period of 2 to 3 weeks. It may also appear to develop rapidly affecting sows more severely. There is likely to be severe pneumonia and some mortality if the disease is not controlled. Laboratory tests involving serology and microbiology are necessary to identify the possible causes.

Treatment.

- Usually pneumonia in the sow involves a mixed infection of viruses and secondary bacteria. Broad spectrum antibiotics such as OTC, penicillin streptomycin or amoxycillin are indicated.
- Inject individual cases daily for 3 to 4 days.
- For influenza with secondary bacteria:
  - Combine CTC or OTC in the water at the onset together with in-feed medication at a level of 600g/tonne.
  - Antibiotic cover is required for at least 14 to 21 days.
- Enzootic pneumonia - If there is a herd breakdown, drugs specifically effective against mycoplasma are indicated
  - Lincomycin   - In feed, water, or by injection.
  - Spectinomycin   - Injection.
  - Tiamulin   - In feed, water, or by injection.
  - Tylosin   - In feed, water, or by injection.
  - Chlortetracycline - In feed, or water.
  - Oxytetracycline - In feed, water, or by injection.
- It is important in the early stages of a breakdown to control the levels of infection, particularly in the numbers of organisms excreted into the air, until an immunity has developed. This can be achieved by using 600-800g/tonne of OTC or CTC in feed for two weeks reducing this to 200 to 300g over the next 3 to 4 weeks.
- Actinobacillus pleuropneumonia. If there is a herd breakdown early treatment of individuals is necessary together with preventative medication in-feed or water. Individuals should be injected with either OTC, penicillin/streptomycin, ceftiofur or sulphonamides.

PORCINE ENTEROPATHY (PE)

See chapter 9 for further information.

This disease is associated with changes in the intestines. PE is seen in four forms, bloody gut or porcine haemorrhagic enteropathy (PHE), intestinal adenopathy (PIA), necrotic enteritis (NE) and regional ileitis (RI). All are uncommon in the mature female but outbreaks of PHE are not uncommon in maiden and pregnant gilts.

PORCINE EPIDEMIC DIARRHOEA (PED)

See chapter 8 for further information.

This is caused by a corona virus which affects all ages of pigs. When it is first introduced into the breeding herd the clinical picture in the dry sow area can vary considerably from very mild "cow pat" type faeces through to a watery diarrhoea. Sows normally recover over a period of about a week, usually without after affects. The virus is widespread throughout Europe and as a result it is uncommon to see disease in the breeding side of the herd due to the strong immunity that develops. The disease is much more important in the sucking pig.

PORCINE PARVOVIRUS (PPV)

See chapter 6 for further information.

This virus is ubiquitous and present in almost all sow populations. Once exposed the sow becomes immune. The virus itself has no clinical effects on non pregnant sows when infection takes place. If however a sow or gilt is exposed for the first time in the first half of pregnancy the virus will cross the placenta and selectively kill off the developing foetuses in the womb. Good control is achieved by vaccinating the gilt.

PORCINE REPRODUCTIVE AND RESPIRATORY SYNDROME (PRRS)

See chapter 6 for further information.

The effects of this disease in the sow are severe when infection is first introduced into the herd. The virus causes inappetance, abortions, late mummified piglets, high stillbirths and neonatal mortality.

PORCINE STRESS SYNDROME (PSS)

This term covers a group of conditions associated with an autosomal recessive gene. It includes acute stress and sudden death (malignant hyperthermia), pale soft exudative muscle (PSE), dark firm dry meat, and back muscle necrosis. Heavy muscle pigs are more likely to carry the gene. The pig is either homozygous recessive (susceptible) heterozygous, or free of the gene.

The gene can be identified by the pigs response to the anaesthetic gas halothane but recent developments have produced gene probes using blood, that identify both the homozygous and heterozygous carriers.

Clinical signs

When the homozygous state is present and following

a period of muscle activity, there is a change in muscle metabolism from aerobic to anaerobic and biochemical abnormalities develop. The body tissues become acid with a marked rise in temperature 42°C (107°F).

The onset is sudden with muscle tremors, twitching of the face and rapid respiration. The skin becomes red and blotched. Death usually occurs within 15-20 minutes. PSS is often precipitated by sudden movement. Back muscle necrosis is a more localised form. Whilst the gene produces a leaner carcase, growth rates are slower and the levels of sudden death increase.

Diagnosis

This is based on the sudden onset, symptoms, breed, susceptibility and the known presence or absence of the gene in the pig.

In many cases the pig is just found dead and a post-mortem examination is necessary to eliminate other disease. Rigor mortis (stiffening of the muscles after death) within 5 minutes is a striking feature.

Similar diseases

These include the other causes of sudden death, twisted bowel, internal haemorrhage, mulberry heart disease and pyelonephritis. Hypocalcaemia in the lactating sow although uncommon can give identical symptoms to PSS.

Treatment

This is usually ineffective but the following are worth adopting:

- ☐ Spray the pig with cold water to control the temperature rises.
- ☐ Inject 50-100ml of calcium gluconate (used in cows for milk fever) by intramuscular injections at two separate sites. Seek veterinary advice.
- ☐ Sedate the pig with stresnil.
- ☐ Do not move or cause undue muscle activity.
- ☐ Give an injection of vitamin E 2iu/kg.

Management control and prevention

- ◆ Remove the gene from the population.
- ◆ Use a homozygous or heterozygous male on stress gene free females if the gene is to be used to improve carcase quality.
- ◆ Maintain a gene free herd.

PROLAPSE OF THE RECTUM
See chapter 9 for further information.

This is not uncommon in sows and occasionally outbreaks occur in herds. Whilst the exact mechanisms are not fully understood the following should be considered as contributory to the problem.

- A prolapse may occur following oestrus, associated with levels of oestrogenic hormones that are present at this time.
- It maybe associated with constipation.
- Penetration of the rectum at mating is a common cause with prolapse occurring 24 to 48 hours later.
- Cases develop if sows are confined in stalls or tethers where there is an excessive slope towards the back of the floor. Up to 8 % of sows have been affected where sows are confined to stalls or tethers with sloping floors to the rear.
- Rectal prolapses are seen occasionally in sow stalls or farrowing crates where the retaining gate at the back consists of parallel bars. If these are of such a height that the sow can sit or rest with the tail over the back, pressure is placed on the anal sphincter. This causes a partial relaxation of the sphincter itself, poor circulation, swelling and ultimately the sow strains to prolapse.
- A small lying area with a step down to the defecating area causes increased abdominal pressure if the sows lay over it. This predisposes to prolapse.
- Prolapsed rectum may occur whenever there is an increase in abdominal pressure.
- Abnormal fermentation in the gut and the production of gas in the large bowel may predispose. In such cases the components of the feed and the method of feeding should be investigated.
- Mouldy feeds or straw can be important causes of rectal prolapses due the present of mycotoxins.
- Low fibre diets can lead to constipation and rectal prolapse.
- When environmental temperatures drop, sows that are loose-housed group together to keep warm, thus increasing abdominal pressure.
- A water shortage may predispose.
- There is no evidence to suggest that genetic factors have a part to play in the disease.

Clinical signs

At the onset, the red coloured mucosa of the rectum protrudes from the anal sphincter and then may return on its own. After a short period however it remains to the exterior and becomes swollen and filled with fluid. It is prone to damage and haemorrhage and where sows are loose housed cannibalism often results with evidence of blood on the skin.

Treatment

- ☐ This consists of replacing the prolapse and retaining it with a suture around the rectum. The procedure for carrying this out is described in chapter 15. Sometimes the prolapse is very swollen and it is necessary to gradually reduce its size by gentle pressure using hands covered in obstetrical lubricant. This can sometimes take up to 15 minutes.
- ☐ Where outbreaks occur a change in ration or the inclusion of 200g of CTC in feed for a short period will often be sufficient to control the condition. The CTC suppresses those organisms that cause

fermentation and gas production in the large bowel.

PROLAPSE OF THE VAGINA AND CERVIX

Prolapse of the vagina and cervix is more common prior to farrowing and may be seen in the last third of pregnancy including the pre-farrowing period in the farrowing house. It occurs normally in about one pregnancy in 200, usually in older sows from 5th parity onwards. It is a response to increased abdominal pressure together with a relaxation of the internal structures that support the cervix or the neck of the womb. Older sows that are heavy in pig, with large litters and in very good condition are also more likely candidates.

The following factors need to be considered as causal or contributing to the problem:

- It is much more common in older sows than young ones.
- Sows housed on tethers on slippery floors are more prone.
- When sows lie down there is an increased abdominal pressure which tends to force the cervix or vagina to the exterior.
- Fat sows are more prone as are those carrying large litters.
- It is common in sows that are lying in confinement on a floor that slopes too steeply to the rear.
- High levels of feed intake, particularly food containing high starch materials, produce abnormal fermentation, excess gas formation and an increase in abdominal pressure.

Clinical signs

In the early stages the protruding tissues appear between the lips of the vulva and return to their normal position when the sow stands. However with advancing pregnancy the prolapse may remain to the exterior and as soon as this occurs the animal should be removed from it's existing environment and loose-housed. The tissues become swollen with time.

Diagnosis

The clinical signs are obvious but occasionally can be confused with vaginal polyps that may protrude from the vulva, and eversion of the bladder. Handling the tissues will differentiate.

Treatment

◻ Remove the sow to loose housing.
◻ If the prolapse remains when the sow is standing replace and pass a tape suture across the vulva.
◻ If the sow is at point of farrowing, the farrowing crate floor should be raised to slope towards the feeding trough by using raised floor boards. When the sow then stands or lies down the weight of the piglets inside pulls the womb forward to hold the vagina in. Under such circumstances the sow usually farrows normally.
◻ If the vagina remains prolapsed as farrowing approaches, the cervix will not open fully and both the sow and the litter are likely to be lost. In such cases a tape suture should be placed across the lips of the vulva to hold the prolapse in. As the sow reaches the point of farrowing it can be relaxed. This technique is described in chapter 15.

Management control and prevention

◆ Consider the factors outlined above.
◆ Consider the factors predisposing to rectal prolapse.

SALMONELLOSIS
See chapter 9 for further information.

Salmonella bacteria are widespread in human and animal populations. Some of them cause food poisoning in man or disease (salmonellosis) in animals. Salmonellosis is mainly a problem in the growing pig. The organisms are found in the intestine including sows and they are excreted for long periods of time with little or no disease. Salmonella in the gut of the pig can contaminate carcasses during the slaughter process and their presence creates potential public health risks.

There are two types commonly found in the pig, *Salmonella typhimurium* and *Salmonella choleraesuis*. *Salmonella derby* is also fairly common in some regions. Other so called exotic types may also be detected without causing disease. Infection is usually by mouth from contaminated faeces and the sow may continue to shed the organism for several months.

Disease is dose dependent, that is, a minimum number of organisms are required before clinical signs occur. *Salmonella typhimurium* in the adult sow is mainly confined to the intestines whereas *Salmonella choleraesuis* spreads throughout the whole system causing septicaemia, pneumonia, meningitis arthritis and diarrhoea.

Clinical signs

Salmonella typhimurium disease occurs in pigs less than 6 months of age and only rarely are clinical signs seen in the sow. When it does occur it is associated with diarrhoea.

With *Salmonella choleraesuis* infection however the sow has a high temperature as the organisms spread throughout the body with pneumonia, coughing and diarrhoea following 2 to 3 days after the onset of clinical disease. Death may occur in the acute phase of the disease.

Diagnosis

This is carried out by culturing the organism either from the diarrhoea, or in the case of dead pigs, from the internal organs. Control and treatment of this disease is dealt with in chapter 9.

Treatment
- This is rarely necessary in the sow.

Management control and prevention
- The most important control mechanism for preventing spread from sow to piglet is the maintenance of all-in all-out procedures in farrowing houses. Recent work suggests that during sucking maternal antibody prevents infection being established in the piglet and provided weaned piglets are not infected from older carrier ones good control can be achieved.
- A vaccine is available against *S. choleraesuis* that has proved effective.

SALT POISONING - (WATER DEPRIVATION)

Salt poisoning is common in all ages of pigs and almost without exception is related to water shortage either caused by inadequate supplies or complete loss. The normal levels of salt in the diet (0.4-0.5%) become toxic in the absence of water.

Signs develop within 24 to 48 hours.

Clinical signs
The very early stages of disease are always preceded by inappetance and whenever a sow or groups of pigs are not eating always check the water supply first. The first signs are often pigs trying to drink from nipple drinkers unsuccessfully. Nervous changes are the major signs and in more advanced cases involve fits, with animals wandering around apparently blind. Often the pig walks up to a wall, stands and presses its head against it in a characteristic position. One symptom strongly suggestive of salt poisoning is nose twitching just before a convulsion starts.

Diagnosis
This is based upon the clinical signs and lack of water. Examination of the brain histologically at post-mortem confirms the disease.

Similar diseases
Aujeszky's disease, swine fever, streptococcal meningitis and glässers disease all produce nervous signs. The condition might also be confused with middle ear infection but this only affects one individual rather than a group of pigs.

Treatment
- The response to treatment is poor but involves rehydrating the animal. At a practical level this can be achieved by dripping water into the mouth of the pig through a hose pipe or alternatively via a flutter valve into the rectum where it is absorbed. (See chapter 15 Flutter valve).
- Discuss the possibility of administering sterile water into the abdomen with your veterinarian.
- Corticosteroids may also help.

Management control and prevention
- It must be a daily routine to check that all sources of water are adequate free flowing and available.

SHOULDER SORES

They arise due to constant trauma over the bony prominences on the shoulder blade. Ultimately the skin breaks, there is an erosion and a large sore develops. It is associated with totally slatted flooring and individual sows that have a prominent spine to the shoulder blade. It is first noticed in the farrowing crates where the floors are slippery and the sow has difficulty in rising, thus constantly bruising her shoulder. Such sows should not be kept for future breeding.

Clinical signs
At the highest point on the spine of the scapula or shoulder blade a reddening of the skin first appears, which gradually forms into an ulcer. In severe cases the lesion may extend to 40-70mm in diameter with the development of extensive granulation tissue. Often both sides of the shoulder are affected.

Treatment
- As soon as the condition appears move the sow into a well bedded pen. Feed ad lib for 2 to 4 weeks.
- Cut a hole slightly larger than the sore in a 70mm square piece of foam or thick carpet and place over the shoulder sore. Hold it in place with contact adhesive such as evostik. This pad will then protect the sore and allow it to heal.
- Large granuloma that sometimes develop can be surgically removed.
- Watch for cannibalism by sucking pigs. If this occurs wean the sow.

STREPTOCOCCAL INFECTIONS
See chapter 9 for further information.

As disease causing organisms streptococci are not important in breeding females. However they are prolonged carriers of potential pathogens both on the tonsils and in the respiratory tract. The skin and vagina are also other sources. Streptococci cause diseases in the sucking pig including meningitis, arthritis and septicaemia's and ascending metritis in the female.

SWINE DYSENTERY (SD)
See chapter 9 for further information.

Swine dysentery is caused by a small snake-like bacterium called *Serpulina hyodysenteriae*. This organism causes a severe inflammation of the large intestine with a bloody mucous diarrhoea (i.e. dysentery). It is a major disease in the young growing pig but the breeding female however can become a carrier of the organism for a long period of time and therefore acts as a potential source of infection to the sucking pig. Clinical disease is unusual except where the organism is first introduced into the herd, when a mild sloppy or severe acute dysentery may be seen. In very severe cases the diarrhoea may also extend to the litter. The stress at farrowing can activate disease to produce sloppy "cow pat" faeces which expose piglets to infection.

SWINE INFLUENZA OR FLU (SI)
See chapter 6 for further information.

This is caused by one of 4 or 5 different strains of influenza virus which cause respiratory disease and infertility. If a new strain is introduced into the breeding herd and there is no immunity, the respiratory disease that follows can be quite dramatic. Within 2 to 3 days up to 40 to 50% of animals may be off their feed looking very ill. This can be quite alarming but the rapidity of the clinical signs are almost exclusively confined to this disease. The major risk to the pregnant sows are the high temperatures which cause abortions, embryo or foetal loss, or high stillbirth rates. Widespread coughing and pneumonia may also be seen and individuals should be treated with broad spectrum long-acting antibiotics.

To prevent secondary infections causing complications such as abortions and stillborn piglets it is advisable to treat the breeding herd at the very onset with water soluble antibiotics, OTC or CTC, for a period of 48 to 72 hours. The course of the disease in individual sows is usually 4 to 7 days and within 14 days most animals in the herd have returned to normal. In large herds SI can become endemic with disease appearing every 3 to 6 months. A vaccine is available in some countries

THIN SOW SYNDROME

The thin sow syndrome occurs over a period of months, with gradual declining body condition until 10 to 30% of the animals have a condition score between 1 and 2. The syndrome arises due to inadequate nutrition or poor quality feeds failing to satisfy the bodily needs of the sow in that environment. During lactation the sow is unable to maintain her body condition due to either an insufficient intake of energy, or increasing demands due to low temperatures or high milk output. The sow therefore uses her body fat to maintain the supply of energy and once this is used muscle protein is degraded. This process continues over successive lactations. It is exacerbated in sows kept outdoors in cold weather and by heavy worm burdens. In sows kept permanently outdoors the stockman should ensure that all the sows have a high body score before the start of cold weather.

Clinical signs

These will be evident by the appearance of a number of very thin sows. Each week during the clinical observations of the herd, an assessment of the overall body condition of sows in the dry sow area should be carried out. If there are more than 5% of sows scoring body condition less than 2 then the herd might be moving into problems. In such cases a more specific examination should be made of body condition at farrowing and at weaning time, the feed intake during lactation and pregnancy, the quality of the feed itself and evidence of any specific diseases.

Treatment

☐ This should be aimed at increasing the nutritional intake of the sow during the various key periods of production and attending to any disease situations.
☐ Immediately raise feed intake across the whole herd by 1 to 2kg a day for a period of 10 to 14 days.
☐ Sows that have become very thin should if possible be moved from their dry sow accommodation and housed in warm deep straw pens in an environmental temperature of at least 20°C (70°F) and ad lib fed for 3 to 4 weeks using a lactating diet because the appetite in such animals is often depressed. It is essential to do this to reverse the catabolic or negative energy state and allow the sow to lay down body fat again. If the sow has become too lean (body score 1) the condition can become irreversible.

Management control and prevention

◆ Check the feed used per sow per year. This should be a minimum of 1.1 tonnes per annum for an indoor herd and for an outdoor herd 1.4 tonnes per annum.
◆ Check the quality and energy content of the ration in relation to the feed intake.
◆ Check the energy content of the ration during lactation. For the lean genotype this should be at least 14.2MJ DE/kg of feed and 1.1% lysine.
◆ Sows should be fed at least twice daily to appetite during lactation commencing three days post farrowing.
◆ Assess the body condition of sows coming into farrow and at weaning time.
◆ Monitor temperatures in the dry sow accommodation. For indoor sows in stalls or tethers with no bedding it should not drop below 17°C (63°F), preferably higher and should not vary greatly day and night, otherwise it will be necessary to increase feed intake to compensate.
◆ Select at least twelve faeces samples from thin sows. Submit them to a laboratory for examination

to eliminate coccidiosis, blood (from gastric ulcers) and parasites.
- Always carry out an immediate investigation if the body condition of sows is dropping because if it is not corrected there will be infertility, poor litter sizes, increased disease and mortality.
- Assess the comfort of sows last thing at night or first thing in the morning, particularly during severe spells of cold weather. Always increase feed intake when external temperatures drop significantly.
- Damp floors or draughts will increase the energy requirement of the dry sow. Once the body condition of the sow has dropped then it becomes more susceptible to a variety of diseases, including gastric ulceration, cystitis and pyelonephritis, PRRS and other respiratory viruses.

VICE - ABNORMAL BEHAVIOUR
See chapter 9 for further information.

Vice in the dry sow is confined to vulval biting particularly in the last 3 to 4 weeks of pregnancy. This can be a major problem in loose-housed sows and in badly managed systems there may be 80% of all sows in a herd with the vulva completely bitten off. During the process of damage there can be severe haemorrhage with loss of life in a few animals.

Clinical signs
The vulva is a highly vascular tissue and trauma results in haemorrhage which further attracts sows. Extensive lacerations are common and evidence of blood on the skin and noses of the sows must highlight the possibility of the condition. Severely traumatised vulva heal with scar tissue and this can cause constrictions and difficulties at farrowing.

Diagnosis
This is obvious from the clinical evidence but an examination should be carried out to ensure the haemorrhage is not arising from the vagina, womb or bladder.

Treatment
- Because sows continue to traumatise an already damaged vulva it is most important that affected sows are removed from the group at the onset.
- In most cases once the sow is isolated the haemorrhage will stop and the tissues will shrink and heal.
- Occasionally it is necessary to stem the haemorrhage. To do this sedate or restrain the sow and apply pressure using bandage as a tourniquet.
- If haemorrhage continues infiltrate local anaesthetic into the vulva and place two or more mattress sutures behind the bleeding points. (See chapter 15).

Management control and prevention
- It usually occurs towards the end of pregnancy. The reasons for this are unknown but may be associated with the increased demand for food and perhaps the swollen vulva becomes attractive.
- Increase the feed intake and assess the response.
- Increase the salt levels to 0.9% per tonne.
- It is more likely to occur if the stocking density is high.
Allow a minimum of $2.7m^2$ per sow particularly in the latter part of pregnancy.
- There is usually one offending sow in the group. If she can be identified remove her.
- Where floor feeding is practised and the feed is placed in small areas sows group together to feed. Any sow that is excluded quickly learns a simple way to get in is to bite a vulva.
To prevent vulval biting therefore it is important to spread the feed as widely as possible over the floor area, even to the extent that where automatic drop or dump feeders are used spread some feed manually as well over the feeding area.
- Vulva biting is also common when electronic feeder systems are used. It requires careful stockmanship and good pen design to prevent it occurring during the waiting periods outside the feeders and as sows leave them.
- There is a relationship between feed intake, the size of the feed pellet, the type of floor surface and the bedding used.
A change from a small to a larger pellet or vice versa will often improve the situation because it allows a better feeding system on the floor surface. This needs to be carried out by trial and error.
- Vulval biting is much more common in pens that are long and narrow rather than those that are wide. There is less competition at feeding time in a wide pen.
- Where there are severe problems within a group move them to a different type of pen with more floor area. Sometimes this will solve the problem, particularly in the last 4 weeks of pregnancy.

VULVAL DISCHARGE
See chapter 6; Endometritis for further information.

In the dry sow any evidence of discharge from the vulva must be viewed with suspicion as this could be due to a potential loss of pregnancy or evidence of cystitis or pyelonephritis.

Develop a management routine to examine the vulvas of sows to identify any tacky discharge. In such cases the sow should be identified and an assessment of the pregnancy state monitored.

Medicines and Other Drugs for use in the Dry Sow

Common generic medicines that are used in the dry sow are shown in Fig.7-10. Because trade names for these medicines can vary from one country to another the right hand column can be used to categorise these for comparison of price and availability.

MEDICINES AND OTHER DRUGS FOR USE IN THE DRY SOW
* A Guide to Doses and Availability.

Drug (Concentration mg/ml)	Some Trade Names	Short Acting Injections	Long Acting Injections	Available Orally	Available In Feed g/tonne	Trade Names of your Available Drugs
Amoxycillin (150)	Clamoxyl	1ml / 20kg	1ml / 10kg	✓	300 - 500	
Ampicillin(150)	Penbritin	1ml / 20kg				
Apramycin	Apralan			✓	100	
Baquiloprim (33) Sulpha (175)	Zaquilan	1ml / 20kg				
Ceftiofur(50)	Excenel	1ml / 25g	1ml / 16kg			
Chlortetracycline	Aureomycin			✓	400 - 900	
Cephalexin(180)	Ceporex	1ml / 25kg				
Chloramphenicol	Chloramphenicol	1ml / 25kg				
Doramectin (Parasites)	Dectomax	1ml / 33kg				
Enrofloxacin (100)	Baytril	1ml/40kg		✓		
Erythromycin	Erythrocin			✓		
Flunixin (50) (anti toxic effects)	Finadyne	1ml / 45kg				
Framycetin (150)	Framomycin	1ml / 30kg				
Gentamycin (50)	Pangram	1ml / 10kg				
Intagen (oral *E. coli* vaccine)	Intagen				✓	
Lincomycin (100)	Lincocin	1ml / 10kg		✓	110 - 20	
Lincomycin spectinomycin	Linco-spectin				44 / 44	
Ivermectin 1% (Parasites)	Ivomec	1ml / 33kg		✓	✓	
Neomycin	Neobiotic			✓	163	
Oxytetracycline (100)	Terramycin	1ml / 10kg	1ml / 10kg	✓	300 - 900	
Phenoxymethyl penicillin	Potencil			✓	200 - 300	
Phosmet 20% (mange)	Porect	Topical 1ml/10kg				
Procaine Penicillin (300)	Depocillin	1ml / 20kg				
Procaine(150) + Benzathine Penicillin (150)	Duphapen LA	1ml / 30kg	1ml / 30kg			
Penicillin(250) Streptomycin(250)	Duphapen + Strep	1ml / 25kg				
PG 600 injection, oestrus	PG 600	1 injection				
Phenylbutazone (200)	Phenyzene	1ml / 50kg		✓		
Spectinomycin (100)	Spectam	1ml / 5kg		✓		
Streptomycin (250)	Devomycin	1ml / 10kg				
Sulphadimidine (333)		1ml / 3kg		✓	100 - 300	
Tiamulin (200)	Tiamutin	1ml / 20kg		✓	40 - 100	
Trimethoprim (40) /sulpha (200)	Trivetrin	1ml / 15kg		✓	✓	
Tylosin (200)	Tylan	1ml / 50kg		✓	100	

* Consult your veterinarian.

(Fig.7-10)

8 Managing and Treating Disease in the Farrowing and Sucking Period

How to achieve low pre-weaning mortality 227
Using records to identify problems 227
Understanding and maximising the role of the sow 229
    Breed and selection 229
    Age 229
    Parturition - farrowing 230
    Controlled farrowings 233
    Udder 234
    Udder oedema and failure of milk let down 236
    Mammary hypoplasia - undeveloped udder 237
    Agalactia - no milk 237
    Mastitis - inflammation of the mammary glands 237
Management at farrowing 239
    Farrowing house design 239
    Preparing the farrowing house 241
    Preparing the sow 241
    Maternity management - supervising the farrowings 241
    Acclimatising the newborn piglet to the creep area 242
    Maximising colostrum intake 242
    Fostering piglets 242
    The stillborn pig 244
Nutrition 246
Diseases of the farrowing and lactating sow 247
Identifying problems in the lactating sow 247
    Atrophic rhinitis (AR) 248
    Aujeszky's disease (AD) 248
    Clostridial diseases 248
    Cystitis / pyelonephritis 248
    Eclampsia 249
    Electrocution 249
    Enzootic pneumonia (EP) - *Mycoplasma hyopneumoniae* 249
    Erysipelas 250
    Fever 250
    Fractures 250
    Gastric / intestinal torsion 251
    Gastric ulcers 251
    Leg weakness - osteochondrosis (OCD) 251
        Osteomalacia (OM) 251
    Metritis - inflammation of the womb 252
    Porcine enteropathy (PE) 252
    Porcine parvovirus (PPV) 252
    Porcine reproductive and respiratory syndrome virus (PRRS) 253
    Prolapse of the bladder 253
    Prolapse of the rectum 253
    Prolapse of the uterus (womb) 254
    Prolapse of the vagina and cervix 254
    Salt poisoning - (water deprivation) 255
    Savaging of piglets (cannibalism) 255

- Shoulder sores 256
- Vulva haematoma 256
- Diseases and problems in the sucking pig 257
- Identifying problems in the piglet 257
  - Actinobacillosis 258
  - Anaemia - iron deficiency 259
  - Arthritis - joint infections 260
  - Atresia ani - (no anus or no rectum) 261
  - Atrophic rhinitis (AR) 261
  - Aujeszky's disease (AD) 262
  - Brucellosis 262
  - Bursitis 262
  - Clostridial diseases 263
  - Coccidiosis (coccidia) 263
  - Congenital tremor (CT) - shaking piglets 264
  - Cryptosporidiosis 265
  - Diarrhoea or scour 265
  - Enzootic pneumonia (EP) - (mycoplasma infections) 267
  - Eperythrozoonosis (Epe) 267
  - Epitheliogenesis imperfecta - (imperfect skin) 269
  - Erysipelas 269
  - Glässers disease (*Haemophilus parasuis* HPS) 269
  - Greasy pig disease - (exudative epidermitis) 270
  - Hypoglycaemia - low blood sugar level 271
  - Leptospirosis 272
  - Mange mites (*Sarcoptes scabiei*) 272
  - Middle ear infections 272
  - Navel bleeding / pale pig syndrome 272
  - Porcine epidemic diarrhoea (PED) - scour 273
  - Porcine reproductive and respiratory syndrome (PRRS) 273
  - Porcine respiratory corona virus infection (PRCV) 274
  - Rotavirus diarrhoea 274
  - Salmonellosis 275
  - Splaylegs 275
  - Streptococcal meningitis 276
  - Swine dysentery (SD) 276
  - Swine influenza (SI) 276
  - Teat necrosis 276
  - Tetanus 277
  - Thrombocytopaenic purpura - bleeding 277
  - Transmissible gastro-enteritis (TGE) 277
  - Vomiting and wasting disease / ontario encephalitis 279
  - Vitamin E deficiency and iron toxicity 279
- Summary - 12 key points to piglet survival 279
- Medicines and other drugs for use in lactating sows and sucking pigs 280

Managing and Treating Disease in the Farrowing and Sucking Period

How to Achieve Low Pre-Weaning Mortality

(Indoor production unless otherwise stated)

An efficient and well managed farrowing house should be able to achieve an average pre-weaning mortality of between 5 and 8%. One objective of this chapter is to discuss those key factors that will achieve such targets. Fig.8-1 identifies the major components of the management system that are relevant to low pre-weaning mortality. A good recording system to identify the problem areas or areas of failure is a prerequisite.

Good planning

The planning and control of the mating programme, which ultimately dictates the farrowing programme, are important for disease control because they determine the rate at which pigs move in and out of the farrowing rooms and indeed the whole of the farm. The quality and breeding of the dam and its health status also contribute significantly towards reducing piglet mortality, but the greatest influence arises from management techniques that are adopted around farrowing and during the first 72 hours after birth. A healthy viable piglet with a good birth weight must interact with a good farrowing house environment. Maximising the numbers of piglets reared per breeding female per annum is a major contributing factor to ultimate economic viability of the unit. "Without pigs you can not sell pig meat" is an obvious but little appreciated statement. Fig.8-2 shows the effect on cash flow by increasing the pigs per sow per year from 18 to 25 and most of this economic output will be net profit because the overheads of the unit are not increased by any significant amount.

Pigs sold per sow per year multiplied by the weight of pig leaving the farm determines the kilograms of meat sold per annum and economic output. It is important to maximise this by achieving the maximum biological efficiency of the breeding female on the farm. However over production initiated by too many matings in a given period of time, can have a depressant effect on both health and the efficient use of feed and a study of Fig.8-3 highlights the progression of events that can take place. (See also chapter 3 Management of mating). Note the hidden effects that over use of boars and excessive numbers of matings may have on disease throughout the whole of the production system.

THE 7 KEY POINTS RELEVANT TO ACHIEVING LOW PIGLET MORTALITY.
Good planning.
Using records to identify problems.
Understanding and maximising the role of the sow.
Farrowing house design.
Maternity management - Supervising farrowings.
Good pig viability.
Nutrition.

(Fig.8-1)

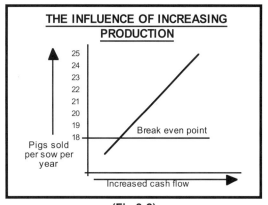

(Fig.8-2)

Using Records to Identify Problems

Records should provide two types of information, end data which identifies what is being achieved, and epidemiological data which gives the detailed components that have been responsible for this achievement. End data on its own is not of great value in understanding a problem. There must be the facility to collect, examine and learn from the components. For example, 3% piglet mortality due to diarrhoea is of little value in helping to decide action without the knowledge of the sows involved, their parity and the age of the deaths. Within the management system of the farrowing house, detailed observations and time scales should be recorded on the sow and litter cards. Such information will help you to understand a problem if it arises. Records identify achievements that can be assessed against target levels of efficiency.

Fig.8-4 shows targets that should be achieved using a modern breeding female in an indoor system.

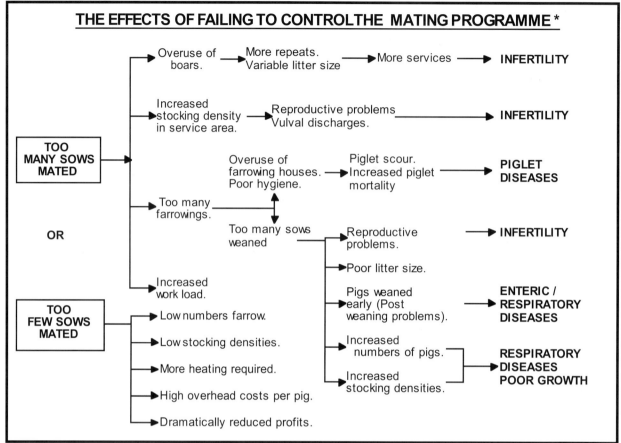
(Fig.8-3)

SUGGESTED TARGETS IN THE FARROWING HOUSE	
Total litter size	11.8
Stillbirths	< 5%
Born alive	11.2
Piglet mortality	7%
Pigs weaned	10.4

(Fig.8-4)

CAUSES OF PIGLET MORTALITY AND ACHIEVABLE LEVELS		
Cause of Death	The Old Technology %	The New Technology %
Stillborn	8	4
Crushed	7	< 3
Poor viability	1.5	1
Starvation	2	1
Scour	3	0.5
Defects	0.5	0.5
Miscellaneous	2.5	1.5
Total mortality	up to 24.5	11.5
Born live / litter	10.5	11.2
Weaned / litter	8.8	10.4

(Fig.8-5)

If a 7% piglet mortality is to be achieved it is necessary to both identify and document the reasons for the losses. Fig.8-5 shows the type of results that can be achieved in herds using management principles described in this chapter, compared to herds that are not applying them. The major differences are the higher stillbirth rates and more piglets that are crushed or laid on. A good management system also produces lower mortality associated with poor viable piglets, starvation and in particular it controls losses from scour and miscellaneous conditions.

Information from indoor production (Fig.8-6) shows that piglets laid on and those of poor viability account for major losses followed by miscellaneous causes and scour. However piglet mortality must also include deaths that occur both pre-farrowing and during the farrowing period.

Fig.8-7 shows the total distribution of pre-weaning mortality and Fig.8-8 the time scale when this occurs. It is a sobering thought that 30% of the pigs that die do so before or during birth and 44% within the first two days of farrowing. This information highlights the importance of management inputs immediately before and for the first 48 hours after farrowing.

The categorisation of piglet mortality as shown is

based on observations, but accurate figures on born dead are difficult because some die in utero and others during farrowing. On some farms however, despite considerable efforts, piglet mortality remains high and in these cases it is necessary to carry out a piglet mortality survey. This involves the post-mortem examinations of all the piglets that die over a period, for example one month, with each piglet being documented back to the dam the litter size and the fostering carried out. Clinical observations recorded on the sow and litter card together with the post-mortem findings then help in determining corrective action. It is also helpful to differentiate between a poor viability or a low birth weight pig and one that has the capability of surviving with assistance. If a sucking reflex can be felt by placing the little finger at the back of the tongue the piglet has a chance of survival.

PIGLET MORTALITY. FIELD DATA *			
Causes of Piglet Deaths as a % of Total Deaths		% of Pigs Born Alive that Die	
		Actual	Target
1. Laid on	38	4.1	< 3
2. Poor viability	18	1.9	1
3. Miscellaneous	15	1.6	1.5
4. Scour	10	1.1	0.5
5. Starvation	7	0.75	0.5
6. Not recorded	5	0.5	0.5
7. Savaged	2	0.2	0.2
8. Deformed	5	0.5	0.5

* Easicare data and field experiences

(Fig.8-6)

44% of all the piglets that die do so within the first two days of farrowing.

Understanding and Maximising the Role of the Sow

Breed and Selection

The breed of sow has a vital role in the successful rearing of piglets and the selection of a good female is paramount. Breed from a hybrid or multiple breed female that through her mothering ability exhibits good hybrid vigour and one that is supported by historical data from the genetic base. This should show good milking ability, number of pigs reared and low mortality. The larger the sow the more difficult it becomes for her to rear pigs, maintenance costs increase and there is a relationship between girth size and piglet mortality. A large girth results in bad teat placements at farrowing and inadequate or delayed intake of colostrum in individual pigs. Increased body size may also produce sows too large for existing farrowing crates.

Age

The age profile of the herd is important in relation to fertility as discussed in chapter 5 and the same comments are equally true of the performance of the sow in the farrowing house. Fig.8-9 shows typical results expected in gilts, and older parities in terms of litter size, mortality and pigs reared per sow per year. Stillbirth rates should be noted with increasing age of the sow and piglet mortality which will often exceed 12% from parity 8 onwards. Also with increasing age, birth weights and litter sizes become more variable and there are greater losses associated with poor viable pigs. However older sows may have to be retained to maintain the mating programme and they can be useful in rearing surplus piglets. It should be noted that there are four distinct groups of breeding females in the herd, gilts, second parity, parities

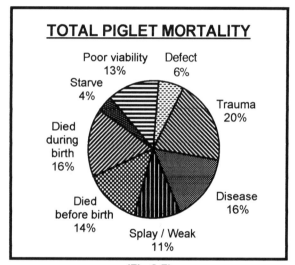

(Fig.8-7)

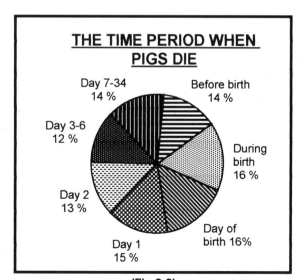

(Fig.8-8)

Managing Pig Health and the Treatment of Disease

3 to 8 and old sows, all with different performance levels. Each can become a specific problem associated with management and disease.

Parturition - Farrowing

To appreciate the intricacies of the farrowing process it is necessary to understand the anatomy of the pelvis and the reproductive tract at farrowing. As farrowing approaches the vulva becomes enlarged, together with the vagina that leads to the cervix or opening into the womb. A small lubricated hand and arm can be inserted into the vagina to just beyond the cervix without damage. The neck of the cervix opens into the two long horns of the womb that contain the piglets. (Fig.8-10). The umbilical cord of the piglet terminates at the placenta which is attached to the surface of the womb. Nutrients pass from the blood of the sow across the placenta and into the developing piglet. The placenta also extends around the piglet as a sac which contains fluids and waste materials, produced by the piglet during its growth. The placenta and the sac are referred to as the afterbirth.

How does farrowing start

This is an intriguing mechanism activated by the piglet once it reaches its final stage of maturity, at approximately 115 days after mating. The sequence of events is depicted in Fig.8-11. The piglet activates its pituitary and adrenal glands to produce corticosteroids. These hormones are then carried via its blood stream to the placenta. The placenta then produces prostaglandins which are circulated to the sow's ovary. As you will have seen earlier, the corpora lutea in the ovaries are responsible for the maintenance of pregnancy. Prostaglandins cause them to regress, thus terminating the pregnancy and allowing the hormones that initiate farrowing to commence.

Length of pregnancy

The mean length in the sow is between 114 - 115 days with a range from 111-120. Gilts tend to have a shorter pregnancy. The variation within the range is influenced by the herd, environment, breed, litter size (it tends to be shorter in larger litters and longer in smaller litters) and the time of year.

The farrowing process

This can be considered in three stages, the pre-farrowing period, the farrowing process and the immediate post-farrowing period when the afterbirth is expelled.

Stage 1 - The pre-farrowing period

The preparation for farrowing starts some 10 to 14 days prior to the actual date, with the development of the mammary glands and the swelling of the vulva. At the same time teat enlargement occurs and the veins supplying the udder stand out prominently. The impending signs of farrowing include a reduced appetite and restlessness, the sow standing up and lying down and if

AN EXAMPLE OF THE EFFECTS OF AGE ON REPRODUCTIVE EFFICIENCY *				
		Litter Number		
	Gilt	2	3 - 5	8+
Pigs Born	10.7	11.3	11.7	12.2
Alive	10.2	10.6	11.0	10.4
Dead %	5	5.5	6	15
Fostered (essential ones) %	3	4	8	10
Mortality				
Laid on %	3	3	3	5
Starvation %	1	1	1	2
Other	5	5	4	6
Total mortality %	9	9	8	13
No. weaned	9.3	9.5	10.1	9.1
Farrowing rate %	85	87	90	83
Litters/sow/year	2.3	2.28	2.4	2.25
Pigs reared/ sow/year	21.4	21.6	24.3	20.5

* Based on studies of field records

(Fig.8-9)

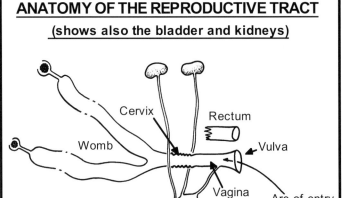

(Fig.8-10)

bedding is available chewing and moving this around in her mouth. If she is loose-housed on straw she will make a bed. Within 12 hours of actual delivery of piglets, milk is secreted into the mammary glands and with a gentle hand and finger massage it can be expressed from the teats. This is one of the most reliable signs of impending parturition. A slight mucous discharge may be seen on the lips of the vulva. If a small round pellet of faeces is seen in the mucous and the sow is distressed, farrowing has started and it is highly likely the first piglet is presented backwards. This small pellet is the meconium or first faeces coming from the rectum of the piglet inside. **An internal examination is immediately required.** The final part of stage 1 is the opening of the cervix to allow the pigs to be pushed out of the uterus, through the vagina and into the world.

Stage 2. The farrowing process

This can range from 3 to 8 hours and piglets are usually delivered every 10 to 20 minutes but there is a wide variation. Consult the sow and litter card to see if there have been any previous problems at farrowing. For example if a sow has had high stillbirth rates, monitor her more closely and take any necessary actions. There is often a gap between the first and second piglet of up to three quarters of an hour. The majority of pigs are born head first but there are more pigs presented backwards towards the end of the farrowing period. Immediately prior to the presentation of a pig the sow lays on her side, often shivering and lifting the upper back leg. This is an important point to take note of because it may indicate the presence of a stillborn pig. Twitching of the tail is seen just as a pig is about to be born.

Stage 3. Delivery of the placenta

This usually takes place over a period of one to four hours and is an indication that the sow has finished farrowing although some afterbirth will sometimes be passed during the process of farrowing. Once the sow has completed the farrowing process there are certain signs that should be observed.
- She appears at peace, grunts and calls to the piglets.
- **The shivering and movement of the top hind leg ceases. If this is still occurring it is likely that a pig is still presented**.

After the placenta has been delivered there will be a slight but sometimes heavy discharge for the next 3 to 5 days. Provided the udder is normal, the sow is normal and eating well ignore it, it is a natural post-farrowing process. Occasionally a pathogenic organism enters the uterus causing inflammation (endometritis). This may cause illness, requiring treatment.

What to do when there are farrowing problems

Step 1. Recognise that the sow is in difficulty. This is shown either by lack of piglets being born, the sow panting heavily and obviously in distress or blood and / or mucus at the vulva.
Failure to deliver the piglets can be due to the following:
- A large litter and inertia of the womb.
- Very large piglets and a small pelvis.
- Two or more pigs presented in the birth canal at the same time.
- Illness of the sow, for example acute mastitis.
- Rotation of the womb.
- Failure of the cervix to relax and open.
- Dead pigs inside the womb.
- Mummified pigs.
- Failure of the womb to contract (uterine inertia).
- Nervousness of the sow, excitation and distress.
- An over fat sow.

Step 2. Investigate. Never carry out an internal examination without a container of clean warm water containing a mild antiseptic and use a soft soap or preferably a special obstetrical lubricant. Do not use detergents, they are irritant and **never** be tempted to try and force a dry arm into the vagina of the sow.

Step 3. Wash the hands and arm well and in particular ensure the finger nails are short. It is preferable to use

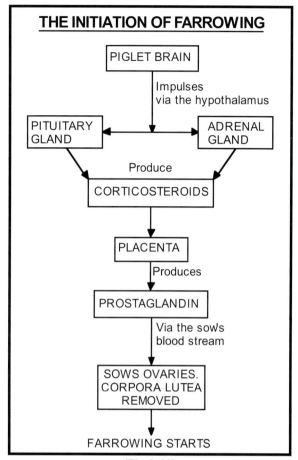

(Fig.8-11)

a plastic arm sleeve because this reduces contamination from the hands.

Examine the sow as she is lying down on her side. It is easier to use your left hand if she is on her left hand side and your right hand if she is on her right side. Occasionally you may have to examine the sow in a standing position.

Hold the fingers of the hand together and introduce the arm into the vagina in an arc as shown in Fig.8-10. Progress to the cervix and beyond so that you can feel the entrance to each horn of the womb. To do this your arm will have to enter up to the armpit.

Problems at farrowing

Uterine inertia - This is where the womb has just stopped contracting. Usually there will be two or three pigs waiting just beyond the cervix. If they are in an anterior presented position place the hand over the head with the first and second fingers around the nape of the neck. (Fig.8-12). If the piglet is presented in a breech or backward position raise both hind legs and clamp the hands around using the first and second fingers as leverage around the points of the hock. (Fig.8-13).

Difficult presentations - Occasionally (particularly in gilts) a large piglet is presented that is too big, but in most cases with gentle traction such a pig can be delivered. The best method is to use a piece of cord, 2 metres long (clean disinfected nylon cord is satisfactory) and loop the centre of it around the end of the third finger. Using plenty of lubricant pass the cord into the vagina to approximately 50mm behind the head of the piglet. The cord is then placed behind the left and right ears and finally brought down beneath the jaw. Twisting it lightly under the piglets chin may help to secure it. Traction can then be applied in a downward movement to bring the pig out. This is an excellent and simple technique and I would recommend that you familiarise yourself with it by cutting off the end of a wellington boot, place a dead piglet inside with its head presented to you and practice placing the cord around the neck. (See Fig.8-14).

Rotation of the horns of the womb - This sometimes occurs when very large litters are present. One horn crosses over the other. This distorts the cervix so that piglets cannot be pushed through and 2, 3 or 4 pigs form into a pouch below the cervix itself (many are presented backwards). When the hand is passed through the cervix (which has become elliptical) the pigs can be felt by reaching downwards and back towards yourself. In such cases it is necessary to take the arm full length into the sow (sow standing) and work hard to bring three or four piglets up. Once the piglets have been removed with the sow standing use a closed hand on the side of the abdomen, swing it to try and realign the piglets and horns of the uterus. If the sow has not passed further piglets within half an hour re-examine.

Stimulating a piglet to breath - If a piglet is delivered and it fails to breath take a small piece of straw and poke it up the nose. This will in many cases elicit a coughing reflex and remove mucus that has blocked the windpipe. Alternatively place the third finger across the mouth of the piglet with its tongue pulled forward. Place the rest of the hand around the head and hold the back legs. Swing the pig with a firm downward movement to propel any mucous from the back of the throat and the windpipe. (Fig.8-15).

Step 4. If after a manual examination you suspect some degree of uterine inertia, (through fatigue or some other reason the uterus has stopped contracting strongly) or the sow appears to have given up trying, a small injection of oxytocin (0.5ml) may be given. Normally it is not necessary because the pressure of the arm in the vagina stimulates further contractions. Well grown piglets passing through the vagina have the same effect but small mummified piglets do not, hence a stillborn piglet may follow after a mummified piglet. Piglets suckling the sow's teats also stimulate uterine contractions so gentle massage of the udder and teats with your hand may be helpful.

Step 5. If an internal examination has been necessary and the farrowing process has been completed an injection of antibiotic should be given. A injection of long-acting penicillin (10-15ml) should be adequate to prevent

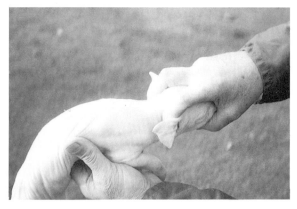

Assisting the piglet in anterior presentation.
(Fig.8-12)

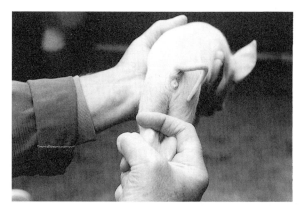

Assisting the piglet in a breech presentation.
(Fig.8-13)

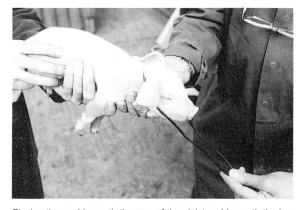

Placing the cord beneath the ears of the piglet and beneath the jaw.
(Fig.8-14)

any potential infection.

If there have been dead possibly infected piglets present two antibiotic pessaries should be deposited through the cervix at the end of the third stage.

Step 6. Always monitor the sow frequently over the next 24 hours to make sure that infection is not developing in the udder or womb, that the placenta has been expelled and the sow is suckling her litter normally.

Controlled Farrowings

If a sow is injected intramuscularly with the correct dose of prostaglandin from 112 days onwards farrowing will take place approximately 20 to 30 hours afterwards. The use of such drugs can be used to make the time of farrowing in an individual sow or a group of sows more predictable and allow better farrowing management.
- To carry this out on a group basis determine the mean gestation length in the herd.
- Inject the sows on either day 113 or 114 depending on the herd gestation length, by intramuscular injection with the precise recommended dose. The vulva is a common site.
- Always check the mating and farrowing date of each sow.
- Assess the udder of each sow to ensure that she is close to farrowing in case mistakes have been made with the mating date. A good pointer here is that the back quarters of the udder tend to swell and fill up last.
- Inject the sows 24 hours before the required time of farrowing, which is usually early in the morning so that the sow commences farrowing predictably from mid morning the following day. The normal distribution of farrowings and the results following injections are shown in Fig. 8-16 and Fig.8-17.

There are a number of advantages to synchronising farrowings:
- It is possible to prepare the farrowing pens at a more predictable time and increase throughput.
- The sow can be supervised before, during and immediately after farrowing.
- There can be a better use of labour particularly during the evening, nights and the weekends.
- The sow can be managed throughout the whole of the farrowing process and thus any difficulties, stillbirths, savaging or history of previous problems can be monitored.
- The sow can be treated as an individual.
- A considerable amount of care can be given to the piglets immediately after birth, particularly those not breathing well or of low viability.
- All the various management procedures to reduce piglet mortality can be carried out. Gilts which savage their litters can be identified and preventative action taken.
- There can be better use of farrowing houses.

If these advantages are to be gained it is important that people are present to supervise and carry out the management tasks.
There are disadvantages to using prostaglandins:
- Mistakes can occur and the sow can farrow early with weak pigs.

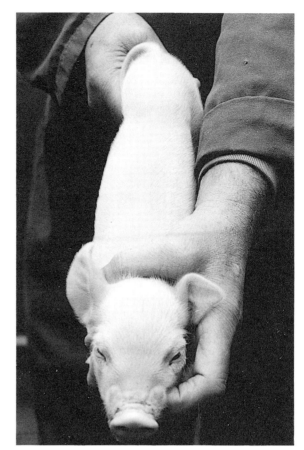
Swinging the piglet to remove mucous at birth.
(Fig.8-15)

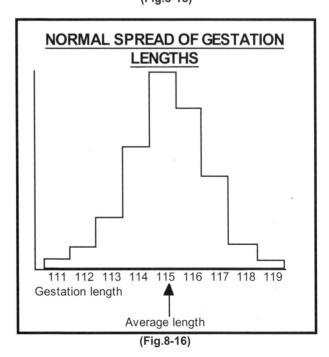
(Fig.8-16)

- In some herds there maybe an increase in navel bleeding.
- Wrong timing of the injection may cause problems.
- If there is lack of quiet supervision mortality may be worse, because sows are farrowing during the daytime when there are a considerable number of distractions.

There is also a risk to the pig attendants of accidental self injection which could result in abortion in pregnant women or temporary adverse side effects in non-pregnant women and men. In some countries, prostaglandins can only be used under the supervision of a veterinarian and on veterinary prescription. They should be stored in a locked cupboard under the managers control and pregnant women should not be allowed to handle them. Procedures for the safe use of prostaglandins are described in chapter 4: Hormones.

The decision whether to use prostaglandins or not must be an individual one based on veterinary advice and the results assessed on each farm. The economics are based on the fact that if one pig is saved per 10 litters farrowed (and this is easily attained by reducing stillbirths by 1 piglet) then the cost of the injections alone will be recovered. The important criterion however is that the extra time and effort should reduce piglet mortality by at least $1/2$ pig a litter.

Udder

A healthy functional well-formed udder is vital to piglet survival not only to provide colostrum and milk but also to give all the piglets easy teat access.

Teat and udder conformation

There are two fundamental factors that decide whether a sow can rear 12 or more pigs; first whether all piglets are able to get access to teats and second whether they can suck milk freely from them. These may seem obvious but how seriously are they considered when the gilt is being selected? It is not uncommon to see a gilt at farrowing with no functional teats at all, or a sow farrowing with say, five viable teats and the remainder non functional. But selection for good teats and udders is not as easy as it sounds, particularly if the number of females to choose from is small. Some teats that appear small and inverted at selection may develop and be fully functional at parturition and vice versa. Fortunately, in large herds the odd mistake can usually be mitigated by cross-fostering. Nevertheless, if you are a farmer who selects gilts from your own herd you should not forget that successful rearing of litters starts at gilt selection.

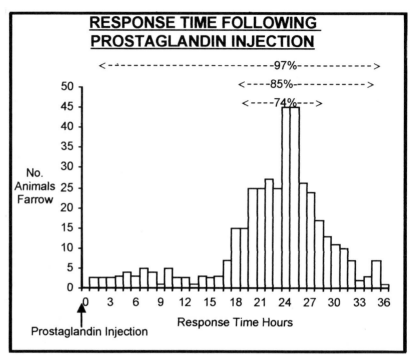

(Fig.8-17)

Teat conformation

A basic understanding of the anatomy of the teat is helpful if good functional ones are to be selected and their conformation can be classified from 1 to 5 (Fig.8-18). The perfect teat is elongated and pointed with two teat canals opening to the exterior. A class 2 teat will not be so elongated but the teat end protrudes well down. Class 3 is the cut-off point for selection and this is where the teat sphincter (often appearing as a black dot) can still be seen when viewed at eye level. A class 4 teat is one where the teat sphincter is not visible, in other words the teat canal is shortened resulting in an inverted teat. Such a teat should be considered non viable. A proportion of inverted teats will be drawn out by the piglet at suckling, but at least 50% of them will remain blind. Why take the risk? A class 5 teat is usually one where the teat has been scrubbed off in the first 48 hours of birth. (Teat necrosis).

Teat numbers

The optimum or minimum number of functional teats on the breeding gilt is a debatable point.

The ideal would be 16 teats, but this may represent only 5% of the gilt population, with around only 25% having 14 - so the commercial choice is 12 good teats with 14 or 16 in the Meishan cross breed. If however, you are selecting gilts from your own herd, select 14 or more if possible.

Teat placement

The position of the teats on the udder is equally as important as teat conformation. It is no use having 14 perfect teats if their placement results in poor accessibility at birth. Teats should be equally spaced with no

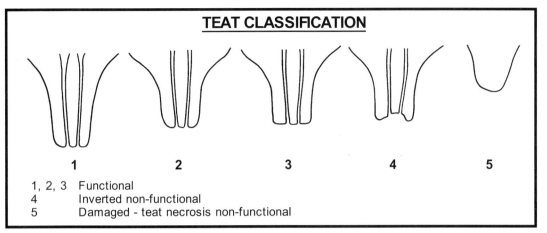

(Fig.8-18)

supernumerary ones and be in two parallel lines. When teats diverge they are poorly presented to the piglet at birth. Animals with large girths also exaggerate the teat placement. (Fig.8-19).

Bad teat conformation is one of the major reasons why a breeding female will not rear 11 or 12 pigs. There may be a history in a herd of good litters born yet by the time the pigs are five days of age, two or three begin to show signs of lack of milk they loose condition and have to be fostered. Two pigs can survive on one teat in the first 12-24 hours after farrowing but eventually the stronger pig takes over and the other is left with the teat that has now become accessible but it has started to dry off.

The placement of good teats on the boar that is used to produce breeding females should also be given due emphasis at selection.

Reputable breeding companies selling replacement breeding stock are fully aware of the importance of teat conformation, teat numbers and teat placement and make their examination an important part of the selection process. However, demand for gilts may be variable and selection rates (e.g. 50%, 60%, or 70%) have a bearing on profitability. As a commercial producer buying gilts you should always check their underlines on arrival.

Teat necrosis

It has been recognised for a number of years that within 18 hours of birth some of the teat sphincters on those teats in front of the umbilical cord are traumatised by the floor surfaces. This causes the sphincter to become necrotic (die). It is most likely to occur in piglets born with swollen, oedematous teats and glands which results from the sow's female hormones crossing the placenta. Such damage occurs on most floor surfaces but is obviously worse on rough floors and is almost complete within 24 hours of birth. If gilts are to be selected, their teats should be protected from this trauma as soon as possible after birth. In some circumstances this can be helped by maintaining a deep bed of straw or shavings beneath the sow but in many cases this is not practical.

The alternative is to protect the teats by painting them with cow gum, (which is a rubber solution, often used for attaching photographs to paper), contact adhesive or covering them with adhesive zinc oxide elastoplast for up to 36 hours.

Selection technique

Gilts for breeding can be selected initially at five days of age (and ear notched) for conformation and 12 to 14 good pointed well placed teats. This will give an indication of the number of animals that are potentially available for selection at a determined future date and with a simple computer programme details of availability at that date can be predetermined. Up to 90% (but allow for no more than 75%) of these animals should be finally selected at 90kg weight.

Potential breeding animals should be examined first in a confined space such as a weigh crate to check the teats. If a five day selection has been carried out you will know that most gilts will have 12 to 14 teats. The ideal is to set a weigh crate on a ramp so that the gilts udder is 0.9-1.2m from the ground. The observer can then carry out a detailed examination and at the same time assess the lateral displacement of teats. The final selection should be based upon a normal vulva, overall conformation and ease of movement to reduce the risk of leg weakness.

Recognising impending disorders and possible lactation failure

These must be determined at the onset and the following procedures will help:
- The udder of every sow at farrowing and 12 to 24 hours afterwards should be palpated. The palm of the hand is placed over each gland with the teat in the centre and pressure applied to a normal gland to the point at which the sow just responds. This standard is then used to detect any abnormal pain and changes in texture to the other glands.
- The presence of oedema or fluid in the vulva or in the surface tissues between the legs should be noted.

- A finger should be pressed hard into a gland to see whether a small impression is left behind. If so this is further evidence of the very early stages of oedema.
- The first detectable changes are usually seen 4 to 6 hours after farrowing but occasionally severe mastitis or infection of the gland would be evident before farrowing in which case inappetance and failure to suckle are observed.
- The experienced stockman or the veterinarian will recognise lactation failure by behavioural changes in the sow, lack of alertness and failure to lie over and suckle.
- Affected glands may be discoloured and swollen.
- The sow may be off her food with a fever and laid on her belly.

The first indication of lactation failure is shown in the piglets by raised hair, hollow flanks and they actively seek food.

Disorders associated with the udder can be grouped into four conditions;
1. Udder oedema and failure of milk let down.
2. Mammary hypoplasia.
3. Agalactia.
4. Mastitis.

UDDER OEDEMA AND FAILURE OF MILK LET DOWN

This presents itself as a failure of milk let down associated with excess fluid in the mammary tissues and is a condition seen in both gilts and sows. It is characterised by a clinically normal animal with no fever or loss of appetite. The distinguishing features are a firmness of all the glands, discomfort on high pressure but no actual pain. The oedema or fluid can be both in the skin and deep in the udder tissue. The pressure produced in the glands once farrowing has ceased prevents a good milk flow and there is a reduction in both the quantity and quality of the colostrum which means a lowered immune status of the piglet. Severe oedema, particularly in the rear glands may result in poor accessibility of teats at sucking time. Such glands often dry off. When piglets eventually find the teat they will not thrive but waste away.

Clinical signs

Usually there is a history on the farm of poor milking amongst all ages and one or two pigs per litter having to be fostered at around 5 to 7 days of age due to poor growth. Scouring problems can sometimes be related back to udder oedema and a poor intake of colostrum. Palpitation of the udder shows fluid either just beneath the skin or deep in the gland and often extending between the legs towards the vulva. The vulva is also often involved.

Diagnosis

This is based on the demonstration of oedema of the udder, by appearance and palpation and the appearance of the litter. Oedema and congestion can lead to mastitis.

Treatment)

- ☐ Recognise the condition early and medicate.
- ☐ Treat the sow with small doses of oxytocin ($1/2$ to 1 ml) every 4 to 6 hours on four occasions.
- ☐ Supplement the piglets with artificial milk and make water available in dishes.
- ☐ Give a preventative injection of long-acting antibiotic either penicillin, amoxycillin or OTC if there are any signs of mastitis.

Management control and prevention

Whilst udder oedema usually occurs in individual animals it can become a problem at a herd level. If this is the case the following actions should be considered:

- ◆ Look at feed levels and the development of the udder 7 to 10 days pre-farrowing. Excessive tissue growth can be associated with high feed intake, particularly high energy levels.
- ◆ Maintain sows on the same bulk level of feed pre-farrowing and from the time of entering the farrowing house to two days post-farrowing.
- ◆ Use the same ration pre-farrowing until two days post-farrowing and then change to a lactation ration.
- ◆ Low water intake 2 to 3 days before farrowing can also predispose. Add water to dry feed.
- ◆ Constipation can be a predisposing factor. Bacterial toxins become absorbed from the gut and interfere with the circulation in the udder tissue. In some cases a response will be obtained by feeding

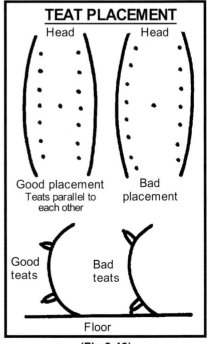

(Fig.8-19)

CHAPTER 8 - Managing and Treating Disease in the Farrowing and Sucking Period

- increased levels of fibre before farrowing to increase bulk and reduce constipation.
- ◆ Alternatively the levels of feed can be reduced but it is important to increase the fibre content with bran or other available fibre source. A typical example would be 2kg of breeding diet with 0.5 - 0.75kg of bran. This is better fed wet in the trough to improve palatability.
- ◆ A change from straw yards into farrowing houses is associated with a marked reduction in fibre intake. In such cases give the sow straw for the first 3 to 4 days pre-farrowing.

MAMMARY HYPOPLASIA - UNDEVELOPED UDDER

This term defines failure of udder development and is relatively uncommon. It can occasionally be seen in gilts because the hormones that are responsible for the development of the udder have not been produced in sufficient quantity. Such animals should be culled. Occasionally herd problems are seen where poor nutrition, heavy worm burdens, chronic disease or mycotoxins may be implicated. The most likely mycotoxin to cause it is from ERGOT poisoning in pregnant gilts running in grass paddocks. Shortage of water is a common cause. Rarely, hypoplasia may be due to a genetic mutation in the affected gilts ancestors.

AGALACTIA - NO MILK

Agalactia describes a shortage of milk supply in an otherwise healthy lactating animal. It is relatively uncommon as a prime condition but common as a sequel to extensive oedema of the udder and mastitis. It is also seen in older sows where hormone outputs are reduced. The major cause however is associated with inadequate water supplies.

MASTITIS - INFLAMMATION OF THE MAMMARY GLANDS

Mastitis is inflammation of one or more mammary glands caused by a variety of bacteria species or secondary to other diseases. It is a common condition that occurs sporadically in individual sows or sometimes as a herd outbreak associated with a specific infection. Disease starts at or around farrowing and becomes clinically evident up to 12 hours later. It can arise as a primary infection, that is, bacteria getting into one or more mammary glands for the first time around farrowing or it may be a flare-up of a sub-clinical latent infection, possibly present in one or more small abscesses, activated by the development of the gland and the flush of milk. It sometimes arises as a sequel to udder oedema possibly due to poor milk flow.

The route of entry of the bacteria is thought to be the teat orifice or injection into the gland by sharp piglets teeth. Very occasionally mastitis may arise from a septicaemia. Unfortunately, there has been much less research into sow mastitis than into mastitis in the dairy cows so knowledge of the disease is fragmentary and empirical.

The bacteria considered to cause mastitis in the sow can be grouped into three broad categories: coliform bacteria, staphylococci and streptococci, and miscellaneous bacteria. Limited surveys suggest that coliform mastitis is the most common and usually most serious, staphylococcal and streptococcal mastitis fairly common and usually less serious, and miscellaneous bacteria uncommon and varying in seriousness in the individual sow.

Coliform mastitis - Coliform bacteria are bacteria that are related to *E. coli*. The two commonest in sow mastitis appear to be *E. coli* itself and klebsiella species. These organisms can be responsible for severe acute necrotising mastitis. They release a toxin (endotoxin) which results in reduction in milk yield, a very ill sow and poor "doing" piglets. Marked discoloration of the skin over the udder and dark blueing of surrounding skin, ears and tail is a feature of the condition.

Major herd problems can develop because the normal habitat is the pigs intestine and faeces, and bacteria may also be present, particularly klebsiella, in sows' urine. Consequently, they are everywhere in a piggery and can survive and build up in water bowl, pipes and header tanks. They can multiply rapidly in stagnant contaminated pools or films of liquid on the farrowing room floors and in wet bedding under the sow. Coliform mastitis may thus be regarded as environmental in origin.

Staphylococcal and streptococcal mastitis - These are usually less acute and less severe than coliform mastitis. They tend to occur sporadically in individual sows in one or two or sometimes several glands and usually do not make the sow ill. The exception is an acute severe staphylococcal infection usually in a single gland which becomes swollen, hard and discoloured. In the majority of cases however the sow remains normal with a hard gland which has reduced milk supply.

Unlike coliform bacteria the source of these organisms is not usually the contaminated environment but the skin and possibly orifices of the sow herself. There is some evidence to suggest that as in the dairy cow and sheep some of these bacteria may persist sub-clinically in the udder and then flare up at or after farrowing

Miscellaneous bacteria - These include organisms such as pseudomonas which can produce a serious mastitis and toxaemia and which are often resistant to antibiotic treatment. Fortunately such infections are rare.

Clinical signs

Acute disease

The sow is inappetent at farrowing, or before if mastitis is already developing, she is obviously ill and the mucous membranes of her eyes are brick red. There may be discoloration of the ears and the whole of the udder but particularly over the affected glands. In the early stages, palpation as described earlier will identify the infected quarters but observation alone is often enough to detect swollen glands without carrying out an examination. The temperature ranges from 40 - 42°C (104 -107°F).

Chronic disease

This follows acute episodes at farrowing or at weaning. The mammary tissue is infiltrated with abscesses and hard lumps that are usually not painful when palpated. They may ulcerate to the surface and thereby become a potential source of infection to other sows.

Diagnosis

The clinical signs are usually sufficient to diagnose mastitis. However if there is a herd problem with a number of sows affected, you should examine all animals clinically at farrowing and again at weaning, to determine the starting point of the mastitis. A sample of the secretions from the infected quarters should be submitted to a laboratory for examination. This is carried out by wiping the teat end with cotton wool soaked in surgical spirit, injecting the sow with 0.5ml of oxytocin and once there is a good flow squirt the milk on to a sterile swab. The swab should be immersed in a transport medium. It is very important that mastitis is diagnosed early and that prompt treatment is given.

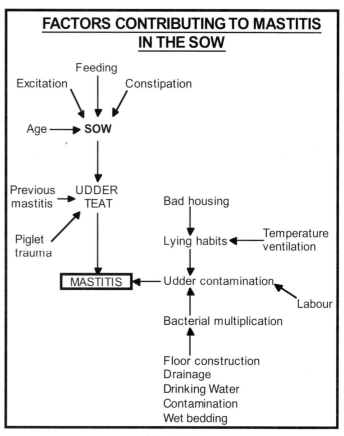

(Fig.8-20)

Treatment

Treatment should consist of the following:
- Oxytocin to let milk down (0.5ml).
- Antibiotics as prescribed by your veterinarian depending on the organism and its sensitivity.
- The following could be used: OTC, penicillin and streptomycin, trimethoprim/sulpha, semi-synthetic penicillins such as amoxycillin; framycetin, tylosin, enrofloxacin and ceftiofur.
- In very severe cases the sow should be injected twice daily.
- If the sow is toxic an injection of flunixin could be given.
- Corticosteroids may also be prescribed.
- In severe outbreaks the sow can be injected 12 hours prior to farrowing with an appropriate long-acting injection.
  If sawdust is used as bedding stop using it because when soaked with urine it is an ideal medium for bacterial growth.
- Top dress sows' feed with antibiotic commencing 3 to 5 days pre-farrowing. Use OTC, trimethoprim/sulpha, amoxycillin or CTC depending on the antibiotic sensitivity.

Management control and prevention

There are two fundamental requirements for the development of mastitis. The first is the presence of the causal organism and secondly an ideal environment at the teat end for the organism to multiply and gain access to the mammary gland. Occasionally mastitis will arise from a blood borne infection associated with the farrowing process.

The following factors predispose to mastitis and require remedial action:
- The continual use of farrowing houses.
- Poor farrowing pen hygiene, bad drainage, inadequate bedding, poor quality bedding.
- The use of saw dust or shavings for bedding that become soaked in water or urine.
- A warm temperature for the organisms to multiply.
- Worn pitted farrowing house floors.
- Wet farrowing house floors.
- Contaminated drinking water.
- Adverse temperatures and ventilation in the farrowing houses that cause abnormal lying habits in the crate.
- A build up of faeces behind the sow associated with shortage of labour or failure to carry out normal hygienic tasks. Faeces behind the sow in the crate should be removed every day.

Additional measures are as follows.
- If a klebsiella infection is the cause of a herd out-

break it may be necessary to clean out the watering system.

- If floor surfaces are poor these can be improved by brushing them with lime wash containing approximately 1oz to the gallon of a phenolic disinfectant. This should be allowed to dry for 48 hours or so before the sow enters the crate to farrow.
- The udder can be sprayed daily with an iodine based dairy teat dip, commencing 24 hours before expected farrowing. This spraying should continue once a day for the first two days post-farrowing. If a specific organism is identified and its antibiotic sensitivity is known, the sows feed can be top-dressed from day of entry into the farrowing houses until three days post-farrowing with the appropriate in-feed antibiotic or injections of appropriate long-acting antibiotics at farrowing.
- Cull chronic infected sows.

If you have a mastitis problem on your farm and have read this section now study Fig.8-20 and Fig.8-21 which summarise the various predisposing factors.

Management at Farrowing

Farrowing House Design

The control of piglet diseases is dependent upon the design of the house and the way it is managed. Key features of a good farrowing house:

- The design should enable an all-in all-out management system to be operated with complete cleaning, disinfection and drying of pens between groups. This prevents the build up of infection and reduces the expo-

LACTATION FAILURE. SUMMARY			
Udder Change	Aetiological Factors	Management / Action	Treatment
Udder oedema and failure of milk let down (congestion)	Constipation Excitement Fear High levels of feed Lack of exercise Lack of roughage Oedema of udder Too much fall on farrowing crate floor	Correct the cause Reduce feed level	Electrolytes for litter Oxytocin Penicillin
Mammary hypoplasia	Age Breed Hormonal Individual animal Mycotoxins Water shortage	Correct aetiology Cull affected animals	Foster litters
Agalactia	Age Excess body condition Poor crate design Sequel to congestion Sequel to oedema Water shortage	Correct the cause Foster / cull Reduce feed level	Oxytocin Supplement milk
Mastitis, metritis and toxic agalactia	Assisted farrowings Contamination of udder Cystitis Diet change farrowing High feed levels predispose Lack of roughage Metritis / vaginitis Nephritis Previous mastitis Prolonged farrowings Septicaemia Sequel to toxic agalactia Sequel to udder oedema and congestion Stress	Assess aetiological factors Carry out bacteriology of farrowing houses Check feed Check feed levels given See under mastitis	Antibiotics as for mastitis.
Acute mastitis	Bad drainage Continuous antibiotic usage Faulty drinkers Piglet teeth damage Poor farrowing house hygiene Poor floor surfaces Presence of pathogenic organisms Shavings, sawdust as bedding Teat trauma Wet floors	Assess aetiological factors Check teat damage Check udder contamination Farrowing house hygiene / floor quality Keep individual records Lime wash pen floors (+ disinfectant) Look at all management procedures Water supplies	Antibiotics Corticosteroids Diuretics Flunixin Framycetin Medicate pre-farrowing Neomycin Oxytetracyclines Oxytocin Penicillin Streptomycin Synthetic penicillin Tylosin

(Fig.8-21)

sure to viruses, bacteria and parasites.
- To achieve an efficient all-in all-out system the farrowing houses should be of a size appropriate to the number of the sows in the herd and the number of farrowings planned for each week. Thus, ideally, in a family farm of 300-500 sows farrowing houses should contain about 10 crates and in smaller herds about 6. In large herds of 1000 or more sows it is useful to have farrowing houses of two or more different sizes, say, 10 to 12 crates and 20 to 24 crates. If rooms are bigger than this the farrowing spread becomes too large to operate an efficient all-in all-out system.
- The floor and work surfaces should be made of non-porous easily cleaned materials that dry quickly.
- The floors should be well constructed and drained so that no pools of liquid occur and they should be free from cracks and fissures that harbour infections.
- The rooms should be adequately insulated and the ventilation system should maintain even temperatures with no draughts around the sows or piglets. In temperate and colder climates the system should be mechanically operated.
- There should be passages in front of the farrowing pens as well as behind them for easy access to the piglets, without climbing from one pen to another. This is particularly important when outbreaks of piglet diarrhoea occur.

Examples of farrowing house layouts are given in Fig.8-22.

Farrowing crate and pen design are important in the management of the sow and litter. Pig producers are nothing if not resourceful and ingenious and it is not surprising that over the 25 to 30 years of the development of the modern industry a variety of pen and crate designs have been developed, some good, some not so good, none perfect. Numerous pens have been designed that avoid total confinement of the sow in a crate or which confine the sow for the first few days of lactation and then allow her free

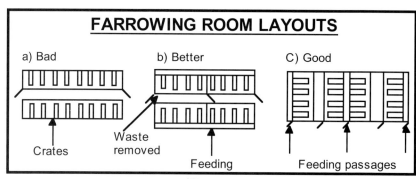

(Fig.8-22)

movement (e.g. multi suckling systems) but they have all been found wanting and some have been disastrous. There is, as yet, no system more productive and welfare friendly to the piglets as well as the sow and safe for the attendant, than full confinement in a farrowing crate for most or preferably all of lactation, provided weaning is at less than $4\frac{1}{2}$ weeks.

An example of a satisfactory farrowing pen layout is shown in Fig.8-23.

The pen area is a minimum of 1.8m wide by 2.4m

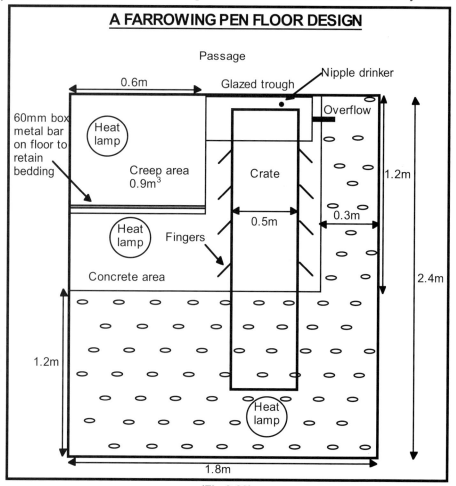

(Fig.8-23)

with the crate offset to one side with a side creep to the larger side close to the front passage. Provided the management is good there seems to be little difference in piglet mortality whether the creep is in front of the sow (as in the Camboro crate), to one side of the head of the sow (as in Fig.8-23) or further back, level with the udder. The position of the creep in Fig.8-23 gives the piglet contact to the sows head, fostering a maternal bond. It encourages the piglets to remain at the head of the sow rather than at the udder where they may be laid on. In hot climates a heated front creep may prevent the sow cooling herself and drip cooling procedures become necessary.

Crate designs vary widely and serve several purposes.
- Safety for the stockperson.
- Ease of management for such procedures as clipping teeth and tailing, examining the piglets and the sows udder.
- Treating the piglets or the sow, feeding, changing creep feed and general hygiene.
- Provision of a simple safe creep close to the sow for the piglets.
- Reducing piglet mortality from crushing and disease.
- Economy of space in the farrowing room.

One guide to the efficiency of the design is the level of mortality achieved but other factors should also be assessed, such as the comfort and contentment of the sow, whether the crates are big enough for the biggest sows and the availability of both rows of teats to the piglets. To facilitate this (and to reduce crushing against the bottom bar) "fingers" are incorporated as in Fig.8-23 instead of a low bottom bar. Various gadgets have been developed to reduce crushing when the sow lies down:
- Adjustable bottom rails for different size sows.
- A hinged bottom bar that drops inwards when the sow stands up making it difficult for her just to drop down when lying again.
- Bottom bars that operate on an hydraulic ram (the proctor crate) so that the sides swing in when the sow stands and will only swing out slowly again when the sow starts to lie down. Such crates are expensive and elaborate but they do help to reduce mortality.
- Crates with a fan that automatically turns on when the sow stands and blows cool air around her feet (blowaways) encouraging the piglets to return to the creep.

The floors of farrowing crates are important to piglet survival and health. If solid they should be insulated, smooth enough not to cause abrasions on the piglets legs but not too smooth and slippery to make it difficult for the newborn piglet to get to the udder and creep area.

Floors may be fully perforated, partly perforated as in Fig.8-23 or only perforated at the back end of the sow. They may be raised to various heights above the passage level to help in manipulation by the stockperson, to deter the stockperson from climbing in, and to raise the piglet away from draughts at floor level.

Whilst crate design is important in assisting the sow to lie down gently, nevertheless its impact on pigs laid on is low if the management and the design of the house encourages the piglet not to lie in the danger dropping zone. The day by day management of the pen, the bedding and good drainage of the floor are vital components for success.

Good management in the farrowing house is the key to the successful rearing of healthy pigs and low pre-weaning mortality.

If your mortality is 9% or more then consider in detail the following outlines. If you are achieving all of these you should reach the target of between 5 and 8%.

Preparing the Farrowing House

- Sows should be moved into a dry warm house about three days before the expected farrowing date.
- The house should have been completely emptied, cleaned, disinfected and more importantly dried.
- As farrowing approaches a second heat lamp should be placed opposite the sows udder (if it is a side creep) to attract the piglet away from the sow.
- If the farrowing crate floor is slatted and the sow is likely to farrow at night time, a lamp should be hung at the back of the crate.
- If a sow is farrowing on slats, the areas behind and to the side of her should be covered over with solid material during the actual period of farrowing, and kept dry with shavings.
- Make sure there are no draughts or high air flow across the house.
- Make sure all nipple drinkers are working correctly.
- Check the floors for any wear or tear or any loose panels if slatted. (Failure to carry this out frequently results in the loss of a litter in the slurry).

Preparing the Sow

- Make sure that all health routines have been carried out, for example vaccinations, mange treatment and worming.
- Check the feeding of the sow.
- Regularly examine the udder as farrowing approaches.
- Examine the vulva of the sow twice a day for any abnormal discharges.
- Make sure the faeces is removed twice a day from behind the sow until two days post-farrowing, then once daily for eight days.

Maternity Management - Supervising the Farrowings

The greater the management input from point of farrowing and for the next two days then the lower the piglet mortality. Remember most mortality occurs in the first 48 hours. Prostaglandin can be used to synchronise farrowings. Monitor the progress of the farrowings as previously described.

Acclimatising the Newborn Piglet to the Creep Area

This is a vital component of farrowing management and is the one procedure that dramatically reduces the number of pigs laid on. It is possible to teach the piglet within 4 to 6 hours of birth that the creep area is the most attractive and best place to lie. This is achieved by:

1. Removing the piglet as soon as it is born into a well bedded comfortable creep area. (At least 50mm of shavings is ideal). The piglet is fastened in the creep area for approximately 20 minutes then introduced to the udder of the sow, so it is necessary to have a barrier to hold the pigs into the creep area for this period of time. Watch out for damaged navels and bleeding. If so use navel clips.
2. Once the piglet has had sufficient colostrum and has finished suckling it is placed back into the creep area for up to 1 hour.
3. Piglets during the period of farrowing when they are not suckling are gently moved and fastened in the creep area for up to 1 hour.
4. At any period of time thereafter if any piglets are seen lying next to the sow and not suckling they are immediately fastened in the creep for a short period.
5. As soon as the sow has finished farrowing, with the piglets fastened in the creep area, she is made to stand. She will often drink and then lie down, after which the litter is allowed out again. The following morning when the sow is fed the piglets should be fastened into the creep for 40 minutes.
6. To carry out these acclimatisation procedures it is necessary to design the creeps with a simple and practical method of confining the piglets.
7. This system of management allows split suckling, whereby the larger pigs in the litter can be held in the creep area and the smaller ones given uninhibited access to the udder and then the procedure reversed.
8. A second creep lamp should be provided for 24 to 36 hours post-farrowing opposite the sows udder.
9. Provide bedding beneath this lamp to attract piglets to it.

Maximising Colostrum Intake

- Maximising the intake of colostrum in the first 6 hours is vital to piglet survival.
- Once each pig has stopped suckling for the first time it should be marked and fastened into the creep area.
- Split suckling will increase the availability and intake of colostrum.
- As soon as piglets are born or have received adequate colostrum they maybe split amongst other farrowing sows by number and even weights.
- Weak or poor viable piglets can be given colostrum by a syringe into the mouth. The colostrum is withdrawn from the sow as she is farrowing, into a small dish. (See management of the poor viable pig). A minimum of 10ml of colostrum should be given to underprivileged small pigs.
- Assist weaker pigs to a teat.

Fostering Piglets

Post-mortem surveys carried out to investigate high levels of piglet mortality have shown that over 30% of the piglets that die have no milk in their stomachs.

> *Provide a warm comfortable well bedded creep area. Both you and the piglet will be rewarded.*

> *The newborn piglet is a very vulnerable animal.*

The baby piglet is usually born in a fairly precarious state with limited energy reserves and with no acquired immunity. It undergoes a marked drop in environmental temperature from 39°C (102°F) often down to as low as 18°C (65°F). It has no fat insulation, very little hair and poor thermo-regulating mechanisms. It is therefore very sensitive to temperature changes and is heavily dependant on a high environmental temperature to maintain its own body temperature. It has a disparity in size to the sow of approximately 1:200, which is rather an unbalanced situation to be presented with at birth.

It therefore has to satisfy three very important requirements.

1. The intake of antibodies from the colostrum, in particular IgG (immunoglobulin G) and IgA (immunoglobulin A). Without these it will die, having no protective mechanisms against the environmental organisms.
2. It must conserve heat to be able to utilise its scant energy resources to compete with litter mates and gain access to a teat.
3. It requires an immediate digestible source of energy (i.e. sows milk).

Clinical abnormalities of the piglet at birth.
- Low birth weight. - immature
- Hypoglycaemic. - low blood sugar.
- Anoxic - short of oxygen.
- Defective - e.g. splay leg, cleft pallet.
- Anaemic.
- Diseased e.g. PRRS, *E. coli*.
- Traumatised.

Fostering the piglet implies removing it from its own natural mother to another sow so that it is able to gain access to a teat, suckle and thereby survive. There are a number of reasons why it is necessary to carry this out.

Reasons for fostering

Too many piglets - Some herds have the luxury of having too many pigs born alive and these surplus pigs if they are to survive must be given a new dam. The fostering of such pigs is a vital component of increasing output and when we see records of herds weaning 11 piglets per sow farrowed, invariably they are fostering to create new litter groups.

Variable birth weight - The mortality within any litter group is dependent in part upon the variation in birth weights. The greater the variations, then the higher the mortality in those piglets of low birth weight.

Fostering pigs at birth between sows is an important procedure in reducing piglet mortality.

Weak or poor viable piglets - As with small pigs, poor viable weak piglets are likely to die if left unattended. The grouping of eight or ten of these together onto a sow with good teat access is a part of efficient farrowing house management and increases the survivability of these piglets by some 80%.

Mastitis or diseases in the sow - These may result in little milk being available. It may be necessary to foster the whole litter onto other good milking sows.

Savaging - This is common in intensive environments. Occasionally if a gilt or sow does not respond to sedation it is necessary to foster the whole litter.

Delayed weaning - Pigs that are held back from weaning because they are small or unthrifty are often moved to a foster sow. Be careful not to move sick pigs back to younger ones. The ideal is to have separate small farrowing rooms for such procedures. Foster sows should not be moved to the next room where sows are due to farrow (see "culled sows" below).

Starved piglets - These are often seen at 3 to 5 days of age because one or more quarters of the udder have stopped producing adequate milk.

Death of a sow at farrowing - Occasionally this occurs and it is necessary to foster the complete litter. This can also arise if an emergency hysterectomy is carried out on the sow due to farrowing difficulties.

The rules of fostering

If fostering is to be successful then there are certain ground rules which should be followed closely.

Timing - The ideal time to foster a pig is as soon as it is born or within six hours and this is the procedure often adopted to even up numbers across litters and birth weights when a number of sows are farrowing at the same time. Provided piglets are moved within this period onto another sow that is at a similar stage then there are no problems with incompatibility or intake of colostrum. The second time period is when surplus pigs are being collected together to make a fresh litter. In this case they should **not** be moved from the sow until at least 6 to 8 hours after farrowing, when they have had a minimum four 40 minute periods of uninhibited access to the teat. This is to ensure maximum colostrum intake because the fostered pigs are going to be moved forward to a sow that will be suckling a litter approximately 4 to 5 days of age and there will be no colostrum.

This age factor is important if the establishment of a new litter is to be successful. Furthermore it is essential that only the biggest pigs are fostered forward to make up a fresh litter.

Procedures

1. Mix the sow's own litter and the foster one in the creep and hold there for approximately 30 minutes.
2. Move the sow's 5-day-old litter forward to a sow suckling a litter of 10 days of age and repeat the mixing process. This acclimatisation is a valuable technique because it allows the piglets to inter-mingle and make the foster litter much more acceptable to the sow.
3. Repeat 2 and the 10 day old litter is moved to a sow suckling at 15 days of age.
4. The 15 day old litter is weaned early and there is no loss in non-productive days or increase in lactation length.
5. Fostering can also be carried out with poor piglets between one and seven days of age. It is important to identify these pigs early because they tend to lose their suckling reflex and die. Again the technique is similar. Find a sow that is suckling a litter 5 to 7 days of age, moving her litter forward and foster on the poor pigs. For disease control purposes isolated farrowing pens are best used.

Give such piglets a 0.5ml injection of long-acting oxytetracycline at the time of movement because they are disadvantaged and susceptible to infections.

Selection of the sow and management - The success of fostering, particularly whole litters, depends on the number of days the foster sow has been suckling and keeping the age disparity between the foster litter and the sow's own litter to within 4 to 6 days. Always select a docile sow with a good teat profile, particularly if a litter of poor viable pigs are collected together. The gilt or second parity animals are best.

The sows udder - Look carefully at the foster sows udder and the quality of the piglets that are suckling. For example, if there are ten good pigs suckling then that sow will receive ten foster pigs. However, if there are only eight good suckling and two poor pigs then do not expect ten pigs to survive. Only foster eight.

Availability of water - Whenever a litter is fostered always make sure there is clean, fresh water available for the piglets. In some cases the sow may be reluctant and slow to accept the fostered litter and piglets quickly become dehydrated.

The movement of foster pigs - Wherever possible always foster within farrowing houses, or into a farrowing house with older pigs. It is bad policy to move piglets back into younger age groups due to the risk of spreading disease.

Culled sows - It is a useful technique to have a number of farrowing crates set aside so that sows due for culling can be used for extra suckling. By removing them out of the mainstream of the farrowing houses they do not interfere with the important all-in all-out procedures.

If you have a litter size of a least 10.5 born alive and are only weaning nine pigs per sow, I suggest you read this section again and look at the advantages that can be gained from fostering.

The Stillborn Pig

Stillbirths are usually recorded as such when they are found dead behind the sow. However this can be an erroneous assumption because there are three possible causes:
1. Death before farrowing.
2. Death during farrowing.
3. Death after farrowing.

If the pig dies before farrowing, then depending on how long before, it will show varying degrees of post mortem or degenerative changes including discoloration of the skin and loss of fluids. If death occurs in the early stages of pregnancy a fully-formed mummified pig will be seen.

A pig that dies during the process of farrowing or immediately afterwards will be fresh and normal. The two can be differentiated easily. The chest is opened and the lungs and the trachea examined to determine whether the pig had breathed, i.e. born alive and then died. The lungs of the true stillborn pig are a dark plum colour, showing none of the pink areas associated with inflation and breathing. Pigs that attempt to breath during the process of farrowing will also show evidence of mucous obstructing the wind pipe.

Ask your veterinarian to show you the differences.

A good target level for stillbirths is 3 to 5 % of total pigs born. At this level there is no point in carrying out investigations because it is unlikely that external inputs can alter the situation. However once the level reaches beyond 7% it is worthwhile carrying out an investigation by records and post-mortem examinations. The following factors need to be considered as causal or contributory to the problem:
- Stillbirths increase with the increasing age of the sow and beyond 5th parity may reach 20%.
- Individual sows may be regular offenders and these can be identified by the sow litter card. The farrowing process should then be monitored.
- Stillbirths occur in larger litters.
- They are more common in pure breeds.
- Sows that have prolonged farrowings will have a higher number of stillbirths.
- Farrowing house temperatures above 24°C (75°F) increase the risk of stillbirths due to the difficulties of the sow panting and resting during delivery.
- Sows with uterine inertia and particularly if it is associated with calcium deficiency produce high numbers of stillbirths. One sow can make the average look bad.
- High carbon monoxide levels in the air associated with faulty gas heaters can raise stillbirth rates significantly.
- Pigs found dead behind the sow can sometimes be related to specific farrowing crates in certain rooms, associated with draughts behind the sow, the pig dying shortly after birth due to hypothermia.
- An examination of records both by parity and total numbers born per individual litter, will clarify whether the problem is one of individual sows or there is an infectious or common environmental component.
- Stillbirths are raised where there is a long gestation period and in such cases prostaglandin injections can be used. In some herds the use of prostaglandin has reduced stillbirths and yet in others it has increased.
- Lack of exercise may have an effect on the stillbirth rates.
- Diseases of the sow such as fever, mastitis, septicaemia, acute stress or haemorrhage.

Diseases associated with the stillborn pig
- Anaemia.
- Aujeszky's disease.
- Enteroviruses.
- Eperythrozoonosis.
- Erysipelas.
- Leptospirosis.
- Mycotoxicosis.
- Parvovirus (sequential to the delivery a mummified pig).
- PRRS.
- Toxoplasmosis.

Where stillbirth levels are high it is necessary to eliminate disease as a possible cause and then identify the predisposing factors and their relevance. Most stillbirths in the absence of diseases or environmental faults are related to age, individual sows and large litters.

To reduce stillbirths
- Do not let the age of the herd spread beyond the seventh litter.
- Identify problem sows. Observe farrowing behaviour.
- Look at breed differences.
- Check farrowing house environments.
- Check farrowing pen designs.
- Monitor farrowings.
- Interfere early in prolonged farrowings.
- Give good management at farrowing.
- Provide a heat source behind sow at farrowing.
- Study herd records.
- Check haemoglobin levels in sows.
- Check parasite levels.
- Check for blood parasites.
- Check for diseases in the sow.

The poor viable pig (often called low viable)

Poor viable pigs are usually classified as being small and less than 800g in weight, but they can also include those of good birth weight that are weak and lacking vitality. It is necessary to differentiate between the poor viable and the non-viable one. The latter is the pig considered, on that farm with that management, to have no possibility of survival. The rule of thumb is simple, when the body temperature has been brought up to normal and if the pig has no suckling reflex when the little finger is placed inside the mouth, it is unlikely to survive and therefore management time should not be wasted on it.

The size of the piglet is in part determined very early on in its life at around the time of implantation. While we do not understand all the mechanisms that are likely to produce a large or small placenta and thereby a large or small piglet, nevertheless, several contributing factors can be identified.

- Breed is important and in particular hybrid vigour. This is clearly seen in the difference between breeding from a pure-breed or pure line and a cross-bred female. There are different levels of hybrid vigour between different hybrid and breed combinations. The selection of a good breeding female should include the capacity of that animal to produce good even birth weights.
- Nutrition during the early part of pregnancy, particularly around implantation, may play a role. Unidentified growth factors contribute to the establishment of the placenta. Field experiences have shown that major problems of poor viable piglets (up to 40%) tend to occur more in herds where milk by-products such as whey, have been fed in the first three weeks post-mating. In such farms when the ration was changed to a cereal diet, the problems went away. The reasons for this are not known and one can theorise that dietary insufficiencies or unknown growth inhibiting substances might be present in some diets.
- Some authorities recommend increasing the daily ration during the last 3 to 4 weeks of pregnancy in order to increase the birth weight of all the pigs in the litter, particularly for outdoor sows in winter. This however, will not reduce the variation within the litter.
- As the age of the sow increases so do the numbers of poor viable pigs and there is a greater disparity in birth weights

Diseases such as swine flu, PRRS, swine fever and parvovirus (in fact any disease that can cross the placenta), can produce marked increases in poor viable pigs. If there is a herd problem, it is necessary to assess the

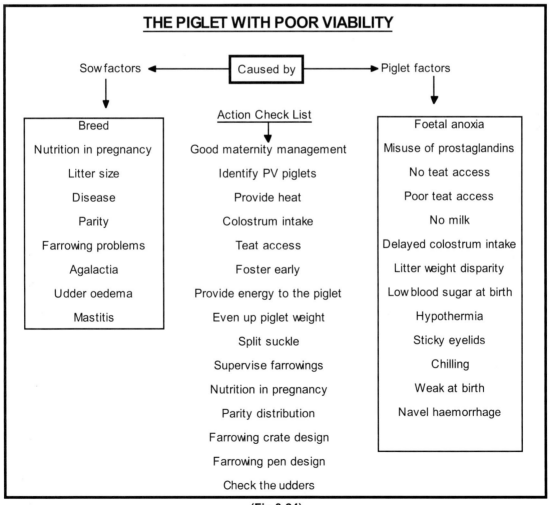

(Fig.8-24)

overall clinical picture to identify any diseases that might be associated. Fig.8-24 shows the factors that contribute to poor viability.

Key points to managing the poor viable piglets
- Immediately place the piglet in a draught free environment at a temperature of at least 30ºC (86ºF), ideally in a well bedded box with an infra-red lamp above.
- Make sure that the lamp is not too far down to burn the skin.
- Poor viable pigs rapidly deplete their minimal energy resources if they are allowed to dry off in the normal farrowing house environment.
- Always make sure that the eye lids are prised open because some are born with eye lids stuck together.
- Provide the piglet with a rapid source of energy. Sows colostrum is ideal, obtained at farrowing and given to the piglet by syringe.

> *If there is a poor viable problem consider lifting feed intake from 3 to 21 days post-mating.*

- Do not use a stomach tube because it does not stimulate a suckling reflex and the sooner this is established the better. Do not syringe colostrum into the piglet until a suckling reflex is felt by the little finger placed in the mouth. Cow or goat colostrum collected soon after parturition and stored deep frozen can be used as an alternative source. It is thawed out in warm water (do not microwave) as and when required. Poor viable pigs should be given between 5-10ml as soon as the body temperature has returned to normal and this again repeated 4 to 6 hours later. Commercially produced artificial colostrums are available but they are expensive and no better than the natural products.
- A poor viable pig has a much less chance of survival if it is left within the litter to compete with the bigger piglets. Where a number of sows are farrowing at the same time collect all the small pigs together to form a new litter so that they are given special attention and a much warmer more comfortable environment. A newly farrowed sow with easy teat access should be selected to suckle these under privileged animals.

> *A creep temperature of 35ºC (95ºF) is required immediately at birth provided the air flow is less then 0.15m/sec. If the air flow is doubled the temperature required by the piglet could rise by up to 6ºC (10ºF). A wet creep area and an uninsulated or unbedded floor could also increase the required temperature by 5 to 10ºC.*

- Split suckling is useful if poor viable piglets have to be left on the sow. The litter is divided into two weight groups and the smaller weaker ones given uninhibited access to the udder on at least two separate occasions, as soon as they can be collected together after birth.

Nutrition

Modern lactating sows are leaner than their contemporaries of 10 to 15 years ago and they produce large amounts of milk. They also have a larger body weight relative to age and are more immature and still growing at the times of mating, farrowing, lactating and weaning as a gilt. These females therefore have higher maintenance requirements together with reduced feed intake in lactation. These changes make it particularly difficult for the gilt to consume sufficient energy to meet the demands, of growth and maintenance, foetal growth and then milk production. As a result there may be a breakdown of body tissues (catabolism) to meet these requirements. Although mature sows are not growing, they often have larger litters and an increased demand for milk products. The following factors need to be considered when assessing gilt and sow nutrition, feed intake, production and disease.

- The breeding female should ideally not loose more than 10kgs of weight during lactation.
- Losses above this will extend the weaning to mating intervals with fewer animals in heat within 10 days of weaning. Animals that have become catabolic may have poorer farrowing rates and litter sizes.
- Low feed intake during lactation can have a significant effect in depressing subsequent reproductive performance.
- With a high feed intake body condition is maintained and milk production is increased.
- Growth rate in the piglet is maximised by converting feed into milk.
- The lean genotype female requires a high intake of lysine and the lactating ration should contain 1.1 to 1.2% lysine with a protein level of 17-18%. Energy levels should range from 14 to 14.5MJ DE/kg.
- Remember the sow is an individual and the feed intake will vary from one animal to another.
- The first litter gilt is a particular problem because it has a restricted appetite and its energy and lysine requirements are greater than those of the sow. This can be satisfied by feeding an early grower diet (up to 1.3% lysine 14.8MJ DE/kg) or giving it as half of the daily ration.
- Managing the feed intake is an art and sows from three days post-farrowing should be fed a lactation diet of the above specification to appetite but not to cause indigestion.
- Sows should be fed twice daily with sufficient amounts that are eaten within an hour and a half.

- Water flow should be a minimum of 2 litres per minute.
- There is considerable variation in feed intake between different genotypes during lactation. Manage your own herd to maximise feed intake but do not cause inappetance.
- Many sows will show a drop in their feed intake during the second and third week of lactation. This dip reduces milk production and hence weaning weights. Make sure that it is not due to inadequate or slow water supply. Recent work suggests that controlling feed intake on a set rising scale improves weaning weights. This is a contentious area however and is dependent on the diet quality. You are advised to determine your own response in this respect.
- Maximising energy and lysine intake in the first two weeks of lactation stimulates the development of the primordial follicles in the ovary and ovulation rate in the next oestrus.
- Sows prefer to eat in the early morning and late in the evening. It is debatable whether sows will eat anymore by feeding them more than twice daily.

Factors that affect feed intake during lactation
- High environmental temperatures. Above temperatures of 24°C (75°F) feed intake may be reduced by up to 80g per day for every increase of one degree.
- Some breeding females eat more than others.
- Sows eat more wet feed rather than dry.
- Heat lamps placed too near the sow increases the temperature.
- Low-nutrient-density high-fibre diets will reduce the availability of nutrients to the sow.
- Litter size.
- Lactation length.
- Fat depths at farrowing. If a sow has been fed too heavily for the 3 to 4 weeks pre-farrowing this will depress appetite during lactation.
- Floor surfaces. Slatted floors are cooler than solid floors. Air flow, humidity and efficiency of insulation of the house can also affect the temperature of the environment.
- Sow health - It is important to ensure that the preventative routines have been carried out, particularly worming, so that damage to the digestive tract does not impair the use of food.
- Palatability - A small pellet (5mm) is more palatable than a large one.

Nutrition during lactation is ideal if:
- Sows maintain good body condition throughout.
- Average total litter size born is 12 or more.
- The farrowing rate is 90%.
- Weaning weights at 21 days average over 6kg.

Do not make any changes if you are achieving this performance.

Diseases of the Farrowing and Lactating Sow

If you have a problem refer to Fig.8-25 and then the index or relevant chapter. If you cannot identify the cause consult your veterinarian.

Identifying Problems in the Lactating Sow

Sows: Observations and Causes
Blown up abdomen
Constipation
Excess gas in large bowel *
Faulty nutrition
Too much food *
Torsion stomach or intestines
Haemorrhage: Faeces/urine
Acute cystitis *
Gastric ulcer *
Porcine enteropathy - bloody gut
Ruptured blood vessel
Haemorrhage: Nose
Rhinitis
Ruptured blood vessel
Trauma *
Haemorrhage: Vagina
Dead piglets
Ruptured blood vessel *
Haemorrhage: Vulva
Haematoma *
Trauma
Head on one side or nervous signs
Brain abscess
Eclampsia
Haematoma of the ear
Meningitis
Middle ear infection *
PSS
Salt poisoning (water deprivation)
Inappetance over the farrowing period
a. Temperature normal
Constipation
Cystitis pyelonephritis
Gastric ulcers
PRRS
Water shortage *

(Fig.8-25) - continued next page

> **Sows: Observations and Causes** (Cont.)
>
> **b. Temperature elevated and/or the sow is toxic or ill**
>
> Dead piglets inside the womb *
> Erysipelas *
> Flu
> Kidney infection
> Mastitis *
> Metritis (womb infection) *
> PRRS
> Torsion of the womb
>
> **Lameness, stiffness, paddling**
>
> Acute stress
> Arthritis
> Bush foot / sandcrack
> Erysipelas
> Fractures
> Glässers disease in gilts
> Leg weakness or OCD *
> *M. hyosynoviae* in gilts
> Torn muscles *
>
> **No milk/ sow will not suckle**
>
> Age
> Discharges
> Excitation
> Fever *
> Flu
> Mastitis *
> Metritis (womb infection) *
> PRRS
> Shortage of water
> Sow ill or toxic *
> Trauma to teats
> Udder oedema
>
> **Mortality (sudden death)**
>
> See dry sow
>
> * More likely to occur
>
> (Fig.8-25)

ATROPHIC RHINITIS (AR)
See diseases and problems of the sucking pig.

AR (progressive disease) is associated with the presence of toxin producing strains of a bacterium *Pasteurella multocida*. Clinically it is not important in the sow unless infection as a growing gilt had stunted her growth. However the sow might become a carrier, particularly if infected as an adult, and might spread it to other breeding animals and possibly to her litter. AR is controlled by vaccination, usually two doses 4 to 6 weeks apart. The sow is then re-vaccinated once approximately 2 to 3 weeks prior to each subsequent farrowing.

AR is only spread by close droplet contact and if the organism is not present in the herd the main method of entry will be by the carrier pig. However, nasal mucus from pigs with acute AR contains large numbers of organisms and these may be brought into a herd on a visitors clothes or equipment. Replacement breeding stock should be selected from herds that are known to be free of this disease. Such herds are monitored by regular examination of snouts at slaughter when the degree of damage to the turbinate bones is assessed; and also by nasal swabs taken from young growing pigs and breeding stock, cultured to demonstrate the absence of the organism.

AUJESZKY'S DISEASE (AD)
See chapter 12 page for further information.

Clinical signs are only seen in the lactating sow when the disease is introduced into the herd for the first time. In such cases sneezing and coughing are often the first signs with fever, inappetance, vomiting and nervous signs. The incubation period is usually 2 to 3 days. Deaths in suckling sows can occur in acute disease. The major clinical signs are in piglets.

CLOSTRIDIAL DISEASES
See chapter 7 for further information.

Clostridial infections in the sow during lactation are not common but occasionally do occur and the only sign is sudden death. If mortality is high detailed post-mortems must be carried out within 1 to 2 hours of death. The dead sow should be removed immediately from the farrowing house into a more cooler environment, otherwise differentiation between disease and post-mortem changes becomes impossible. Diagnosis is by post-mortem examinations and fluorescent antibody tests performed on impression smears from the cut surface of the liver made onto glass slides. Sows can be vaccinated against the disease.

CYSTITIS / PYELONEPHRITIS
See chapter 7 for further information.

The stress of farrowing can activate a chronic infection.

Clinical signs

Bladder and kidney infections are very common in the sow but disease is usually seen in the early pregnancy period. The stress of farrowing can occasionally activate disease and in such cases the response to treatment is usually poor. The disease is usually acute, the sow is very sick, toxic and continually passing blood stained urine, which often dribbles out from the vulva. Occasionally the more chronic form will be seen where the sow passes urine containing small amounts of pus, mucus and occasionally blood. Mortality can be high.

Diagnosis

This is based on the clinical signs and in particular the changes in the urine. The disease can be life threatening in the lactating sow. Remember that a dead piglet in the womb may give similar symptoms.

Treatment

- Antibiotic therapy must be given immediately by injection twice daily for a period of at least 4 to 5 days.
- The best drugs to use are: trimethoprim/sulpha, semi synthetic penicillins such as amoxycillin, lincomycin, oxytetracycline or penicillin/streptomycin.
- The dose will vary from 7 to 10mls depending on the body weight of the sow and the strength of the preparation used.

Management control and prevention

- Once a sow has shown clinical signs of cystitis or pyelonephritis and lactation has ceased it is advisable to cull her.

ECLAMPSIA

This is an uncommon condition associated with low levels of calcium in the blood stream (hypocalcaemia) and it may occur at any stage during pregnancy but more likely within seven days either side of farrowing.

Clinical signs

These are sudden in onset with the sow becoming distressed and panting heavily. There is muscle trembling and shaking of the body. The sow is also reactive to external stimuli, both touch and sound.

Diagnosis

This is based on the sudden onset and the clinical signs presented but it can be confused with the porcine stress syndrome (PSS). The response to calcium injections if given early enough help to differentiate. Most animals with PSS die regardless of treatment.

Treatment

- This involves giving up to 100mls of 40% calcium boroglucinate by injection (this is the drug used for treatment of the analogous condition in the dairy cow which is very common).
Ideally the injection should be given intravenously but this can be difficult. Alternatively 25mls should be given by intramuscular injection at four separate sites in the neck. The muscles in the rump can also be used.
- Cool the sow by spraying with cold water.

ELECTROCUTION

Electrocution of sows and litters occurs sometimes in farrowing houses where electricity is used for heating. Farrowing crates are often connected together throughout the house by various pieces of metal and because of this several animals maybe killed - including piglets when they make contact with the sow.

Clinical signs

A large number of animals suddenly found dead in one house should immediately raise a suspicion of electrocution.

The skin will often be burned at the points where it has made contact with the metal, although piglets in contact with the sow may show no external signs. Blood and froth are commonly seen around the nostrils and mouth. Bones may fracture.

Diagnosis

Post-mortem examinations are necessary to differentiate electrocution from other causes of sudden death although the circumstances are almost diagnostic. Veterinary certification is usually required for insurance claims.

Prevention

- Trip out switches should be provided in the electricity circuits and the electricity lines and switches well maintained.
- A common cause however is damage by sows that escape from farrowing crates. Make sure that gates into crates are secure.

ENZOOTIC PNEUMONIA (EP) - *MYCOPLASMA HYOPNEUMONIAE*

See chapter 9 for further information.

Clinical signs of enzootic pneumonia occur in the lactating sow only if the disease has been introduced into a fully susceptible herd for the first time. In such cases acute pneumonia may develop with severe respiratory embarrassment and sometimes high mortality. The breakdown of disease usually takes place over 6 to 8 weeks with sows coming into the farrowing house continuing to be affected. During this time it is advisable to inject all animals at the point of farrowing with long-acting OTC. For the treatment of acute pneumonia injections of either lincomycin or tiamulin are advised daily for 4 to 5 days. There is a widely held but erroneous belief that the sows and gilt will become carriers and pass this infection to their next litters. They may do so

---

If you go into your farrowing house and find large numbers of dead animals STOP and THINK ELECTROCUTION or TOXIC GASES.

to their present litter when they are in the early acute stage of the disease and their piglets may cough but by the time they farrow again 4 to 5 months later most sows and gilts will have eliminated the infection and will provide a solid immunity to their piglets via colostrum. If weaning is at 3 to 4 weeks, subsequent litters are not likely to become infected until after weaning.

ERYSIPELAS
See chapter 7 for further information.

It is unusual to see clinical signs of erysipelas in the lactating sow but when it does occur there is a high fever and sometimes but not always skin lesions. In a susceptible herd the piglets may also be affected. If sows are ill with very high temperatures first check that there is no mastitis or womb infection. In the absence of specific symptoms treat with penicillin or amoxycillin and assess the results of this.

Previous infection with erysipelas can cause growths on the valves of the heart (valvular endocarditis) resulting in circulatory problems at farrowing or in some cases heart failure and sudden death. All breeding stock should be vaccinated against this disease and where it is recognised early prompt treatment with penicillin over a period of 4 to 5 days should be given to prevent such chronic lesions developing.

FEVER

Fever means a high body temperature. It may occur with little or no other symptoms. The causes will in most cases be associated with bacterial or viral infections or, rarely stress. Consider the following conditions in order of importance:
- Mastitis or metritis.
- Retention of a dead pig.
- Retention of afterbirth.
- A bacterial septicaemia (e.g. erysipelas).
- Flu or PRRS
- Secondary bacterial infections associated with flu or PRRS.
- Cystitis/ pyelonephritis.
- Acute stress or eclampsia.
- Heat stroke.

Clinical signs
Usually the sow appears dull and sometimes shows a reddening of the skin. The respiratory rate may be raised. Clinical examinations will often indicate a cause and always look for the obvious first. Temperatures will range from 39-40ºC (103-109ºF).

Diagnosis
Examine the animal closely to see if any of the above conditions can be detected. If not and there are a number of animals involved, veterinary advice should be sought.

Bear in mind depending on where in the world your herd is located, fever may be the first clinical sign in such diseases as classical swine fever (hog cholera), African swine fever and aujeszky's disease (pseudorabies)

Treatment
- In most cases fevers in sows will be associated with bacterial infections and a broad spectrum antibiotic should always be used. Check the temperature at and 24 hours after treatment.
- Broad acting antibiotics include, oxytetracycline, trimethoprim/sulpha, amoxycillin and penicillin / streptomycin.

FRACTURES

Bone fractures are not uncommon in sows and gilts and are usually the end result of trauma and fighting although spontaneous ones occur in bone disease such as osteomalacia, associated with calcium phosphorus and vitamins A and D, and osteochondrosis.

Clinical signs
The onset is invariably sudden, the animal being unable to rise on its own without difficulty. A significant feature is the reluctance to place any weight on the affected leg. The muscles and tissues over the fracture site are often swollen and painful and the pig is very reluctant to move unless on three legs. An examination is best carried out when the pig is lying down. Crepitus or the rubbing together of the two broken ends of the bone can often be felt. Fractures of the spinal vertebra are common in the first litter female particularly during lactation and in the immediate post weaning period. The pig usually adopts a dog sitting position and exhibits severe pain on movement. Such animals should be destroyed.

Diagnosis
This is based upon the history, symptoms and palpation to detect crepitus.

Similar diseases
These include acute laminitis, arthritis, muscle tearing, bush foot and mycoplasma arthritis.

Treatment
- The affected animal should be slaughtered on the farm.

Management control and prevention
- If fractures are a recurring problem it is necessary to check that there are no diseases such as osteomalacia, osteoporosis or leg weakness (OCD).
- Check the calcium phosphorus and vitamin D levels.
- Check management procedures during the period of effect.

GASTRIC / INTESTINAL TORSION

Torsion of the stomach or the small intestine is one of the major causes of death in adult breeding stock. The twist can involve the stomach the spleen, part of the liver or the intestine. The condition occurs more often in the dry sow, initiated by excitement or anticipation of feeding particularly in sows held in confinement. Agitation and jumping up at the bars when large volumes of feed and water are present in the stomach causes the rotation. Torsion of the intestines is also common because the complete digestive tract is suspended by the mesentery from a single point of the back. It is associated with abnormal carbohydrate fermentation in the small or large bowel, high levels of feed intake and the production of gas. This is seen commonly in sows which are fed liquid waste products such as milk, beer waste, fats and whey. If there is a problem change feeding practices and feed constituents. Large amounts of feed eaten during lactation will predispose. Early signs include a bloated abdomen but in most cases the sow is found dead. A post-mortem is necessary to confirm diagnosis.

GASTRIC ULCERS

See chapter 7 for further information.

Gastric ulceration in the lactating sow is probably common but difficult to diagnose. Many chronic ulcerated lesions are activated during lactation because of the high and continual intake of feed.

Clinical signs

These vary according to the severity of the ulcer and whether it is bleeding or not. The feed intake can be variable with occasional vomiting. If haemorrhage is occurring there will be dark coloured faeces, the animal will have a tucked up appearance, sometimes grinding its teeth indicative of pain and appear anaemic.

Diagnosis

Suspect ulceration from the clinical signs.

Treatment

- With such clinical signs and in the absence of anything more specific it is worthwhile feeding the sow on a high milk diet such as a first stage diet and assess the results.
- Cull such animals at weaning.

LEG WEAKNESS - OSTEOCHONDROSIS (OCD)

See chapter 7 for further information.

This is more common in first and second litter females and it is also described under the term osteochondrosis (OCD). Leg weakness may result in separation of the head of the femur or tearing of the muscles from the pelvis to the leg bones. Fracture of the growth plates of the vertebrae may cause pressure on the spinal cord or on nerves leaving the spinal cord resulting in loss of leg function and acute pain. Major predisposing factors are sloping farrowing crate floors or very slippery ones. When the young sow tries to stand up the front legs are moved backwards and the back legs slip underneath. This creates enormous shear stresses on the young growth plates in the long bones causing changes in the bone structure or even fractures. The lameness in many cases may only become evident at weaning time when sows are mixed and they fight and ride each other, or at mating due to the weight of a heavy boar. Thus if there are lameness problems in the post-weaning period check and examine sows in the farrowing crates carefully and in particular the relationships of the feet to the floor surfaces. The judicious use of fine dry sand on the floors daily can often significantly improve the situation in the short term until floor surfaces can be changed. Alternatively, because first and second parity sows are most susceptible, a small proportion of farrowing crate floors can be altered and used specifically for these animals.

OSTEOMALACIA (OM)

Osteomalacia is a condition responsible for the "downer sow syndrome". Fractures of the long bones at the mid shaft and fractures of the lumber vertebrae are common, with the sow becoming paraplegic. The condition is due to inadequate levels of calcium, phosphorous and vitamin D in the ration. Sometimes sows cannot absorb sufficient micro-nutrients in spite of there being adequate levels in the diet. OM is also associated with immature skeletons, an imbalance of calcium and phosphorus and vitamin D and/or a failure of the sow to consume adequate feed and satisfy her nutritional requirements. Large amounts of calcium and phosphorus are excreted into milk from the bones resulting in weaker less dense bone which predisposes to fractures. Bone mass is also lost due to lack of exercise during confinement in the farrowing crate.

Clinical signs

The condition is common in first litter animals and up to 30% of such animals may be affected. The history is one of sudden acute lameness often with the animal completely off its legs. The lameness is usually precipitated when the sow is moved from the farrowing crate, during mixing or when the boar mounts at mating. Other symptoms include a stiff gait, difficulty in rising, discomfort in the hind legs and a dog sitting position.

Diagnosis

This is based upon history clinical signs and examinations.

Treatment

- In the early stages move the sow to well bedded loose housing.

- If there are no fractures inject with calcium and vitamin D_3
- If there is a problem in first litter females inject them with vitamin D_3 after farrowing and 7 days later.
- Supplement the diet with dicalcium bone phosphate 30g day of sterilised bone flour.
- If there are fractured bones affected sows should be culled or destroyed.

Management control and prevention

Once OM has developed treatment is of minimal effect although injections of calcium phosphorus and vitamin D may help. If your herd has a problem consider the following:

- Feed a high dense diet in lactation 14.5MJ DE/kg and 18% protein.
- Check the levels of calcium and phosphorus (minimum 0.9% and 0.75%). In first litter animals it may be necessary to raise the levels to 1.2% and 1%.
- Give up to 100,000iu vitamin D_3 by injection 10 days before farrowing.
- Keep gilt litters to ten piglets or less.
- Top-dress the feed in lactation with calcium/phosphorus.
- Bone ratios of calcium/phosphorus in affected sows are often 3:1 (normal < 2:1).
- Mate gilts younger 210 to 220 days.
- Use a good lactation diet and feed through to 21 days post-mating.
- Provide non slip floors in farrowing crates.
- Wean first litter females singly and use a light weight boar.
- Provide exercise to the pregnant gilt.
- Check parasite levels to ensure no dietary insufficiencies arise.

METRITIS - INFLAMMATION OF THE WOMB

Metritis in the immediate post-farrowing period is fairly common. During the process of farrowing a large amount of fluid, a varying number of piglets and afterbirth have to be expelled from the womb. At the end of this process the two horns of the womb contract and squeeze the final contents out through the vagina. This process can continue for up to 3 to 4 days after farrowing and therefore it is not unusual or abnormal to see a slightly mucoid to white discharge from the vulva. However discharges can also indicate the presence of an active infection requiring treatment. Metritis is more likely to occur where farrowings are prolonged or where there has been manual assistance. It can also be common in association with mastitis so that whenever discharges are evident carefully examine the udder. (Mastitis, metritis, agalactia syndrome).

Clinical signs

If the discharge is not heavy, disappears after 3 to 4 days, the sow is eating well and there is no mastitis, ignore it. It is a normal biological process and no action is required. Alternatively if there are signs of mastitis, the sow's temperature is above 39°C (102°F) or the sow is off her food with bright red mucous membranes around the eyes, then treat her.

Diagnosis

This is based on a sow not eating and a fever, evidence of a discharge from the vulva usually a white or brown colour and sometimes associated with mastitis.

Treatment

- Give twice daily injections of antibiotics together with 0.5ml of oxytocin each time.
- Treatment should be given for 2 to 3 days.
- If the sow has been assisted at farrowing then an injection of long-acting penicillin is advised at the time to prevent infection.
- Antibiotics that can be used include OTC, penicillin/streptomycin, amoxycillin, ampicillin, framycetin, trimethoprim/sulpha.

PORCINE ENTEROPATHY (PE)

See chapter 9 for further information.

In lay terms this condition is often described as bloody gut because there is acute haemorrhage into the lower part of the small intestine and, occasionally into the upper part of the large intestine (also called porcine haemorrhagic enteropathy PHE). Bloody gut is common in maiden gilts after selection or when they are moved to new premises but it can occur in pregnant gilts and very occasional in first litter lactating gilts. The disease is caused by a bacterium, recently named *Lawsonia intracellularis*, which cannot be cultured on common bacterial media but only in the living cell cultures, so your local diagnostic laboratory may not be able to confirm the diagnosis. The gilt with bloody gut may appear pale and weak with bloody or dark faeces or found dead. Post mortem examination showing massive haemorrhage in the lower intestine is strongly suggestive of this disease. PHE and its related syndromes porcine intestinal adenopathy (PIA), necrotic enteritis (NE) and regional ileitis (RI) are grouped under the heading of porcine enteropathies (PE).

PORCINE PARVOVIRUS (PPV)

See chapter 6 for further information.

The clinical outcome of infection is seen at farrowing where the presence of numbers of mummified pigs of varying size indicate infection had taken place in the first third of pregnancy in a non immune animal. PPV is of no significance to the lactating sow other than the fact that colostrum contains a very high antibody content and will protect the piglet from infection for up to 5 to 6 months of age. The presence of mummified piglets however may predispose to increased stillborn pigs.

PORCINE REPRODUCTIVE AND RESPIRATORY SYNDROME VIRUS (PRRS)

See chapter 6 for further information.

Clinical signs

When first introduced into a herd PRRS virus infection has a marked affect on all lactating sows over a 6-8 week period. They show varying degrees of inappetance and mild illness but the most striking sign is agalactia, not necessarily with oedema of the udder or mastitis, but just a very poor milk flow. In part this is associated with inappetance and reluctance of the sick sow to drink. The temperature may be normal or elevated. Mastitis or urinary infections may occur as secondary effects. Typical signs in the sucking piglets are also evident (these are given later in this chapter under problems in disease in piglets). Stress at farrowing may activate latent infections and this is a common experience 6 to 12 months after the initial outbreak of PRRS.

Diagnosis

When disease first appears in the herd the most striking picture is the high mortality in piglets that are weak at birth and the poor milking and agalactia in sows. Antibodies become evident in serum 10-14 days after exposure and virus isolation can be carried out during the clinical phases.

Treatment

- ☐ Medication in acute outbreaks should include long-acting injections of OTC 2 to 3 days prior to farrowing.
- ☐ Alternatively top dress the sows feed for 4 days before and 10 days after farrowing or during the total period of lactation with either CTC, OTC or trimethoprim/sulpha. Use 15-20g per day of 10% premixes (or pro-rata).
- ☐ Medication during an acute outbreak should be maintained for a period of up to 6 to 8 weeks.
- ☐ Once a herd immunity has developed it is uncommon to see disease again at a herd level however if the virus continues to circulate in the breeding herd in individual animals and in particular the incoming pregnant gilts, top dress the feed with CTC, OTC, or TMS for 4 days pre and 3 days post-farrowing.
- Also assess acclimatisation procedures for replacement gilts in the breeding herd as a whole.

Management control and prevention.

◆ Consider vaccination and/or acclimatisation of incoming gilts.

PROLAPSE OF THE BLADDER

This is an uncommon condition but rather confusing when it appears, the bladder turns inside out and protrudes from the lips of the vulva. It arises when there is a large urethral opening at the floor of the vagina and complete loss of muscle tone in the sphincter.

Clinical signs

The inside of the bladder appears as a large red mass about the size of an orange. It can be confused with an early prolapse of the uterus but examination will show that is like a small balloon.

Treatment

- ☐ The everted bladder can usually be returned to its former position using obstetrical fluid. The tissues are gently pushed back into the vagina and the bladder returned. This may be a task for your veterinarian.
- ☐ Give antibiotic cover by injections for 3 days.

PROLAPSE OF THE RECTUM

See chapter 9 for further information.

This is not uncommon in sows and occasionally outbreaks occur in herds. Whilst the exact mechanisms are not fully understood the following should be considered as contributory to the problem.

- A prolapse may occur following oestrus, associated with levels of oestrogenic hormones that are present at this time.
- It maybe associated with constipation.
- Penetration of the rectum at mating is a common cause with prolapse occurring 24 to 48 hours later.
- Cases develop if sows are confined in stalls or tethers where there is an excessive slope towards the back of the floor. Up to 8 % of sows have been affected where sows are confined to stalls or tethers with sloping floors to the rear.
- Rectal prolapses are seen occasionally in sow stalls or farrowing crates where the retaining gate at the back consists of parallel bars. If these are of such a height that the sow can sit or rest with the tail over the back, pressure is placed on the anal sphincter. This causes a partial relaxation of the sphincter itself, poor circulation, swelling and ultimately the sow strains to prolapse.
- A small lying area with a step down to the defecating area causes increased abdominal pressure if the sows lay over it. This predisposes to prolapse.

Provide antibiotic cover at farrowing

- Prolapsed rectum may occur whenever there is an increase in abdominal pressure.
- Abnormal fermentation in the gut and the production of gas in the large bowel may predispose. In such cases the components of the feed and the method of feeding should be investigated.
- Mouldy feeds or straw can be important causes of rectal prolapses due the present of mycotoxins.
- Low fibre diets can lead to constipation and rectal prolapse.
- When environmental temperatures drop, sows that are loose-housed group together to keep warm, thus increasing abdominal pressure.
- A water shortage may predispose.
- There is no evidence to suggest that genetic factors have a part to play in the disease.

Clinical signs

At the onset, the red coloured mucosa of the rectum protrudes from the anal sphincter and then may return on its own. After a short period however it remains to the exterior and becomes swollen and filled with fluid. It is prone to damage and haemorrhage and where sows are loose housed cannibalism often results with evidence of blood on the skin.

Treatment

☐ This consists of replacing the prolapse and retaining it with a suture around the rectum. The procedure for carrying this out is described in chapter 15. Sometimes the prolapse is very swollen and it is necessary to gradually reduce its size by gentle pressure using hands covered in obstetrical lubricant. This can sometimes take up to 15 minutes.
☐ Where outbreaks occur a change in ration or the inclusion of 200g of CTC in feed for a short period will often be sufficient to control the condition. The CTC suppresses those organisms that cause fermentation and gas production in the large bowel.

PROLAPSE OF THE UTERUS (WOMB)

This involves the complete eversion of both horns of the womb which turn completely inside out. It usually takes place within 2-4 hours of the completion of farrowing but sometimes up to 24 hours afterwards. Prolonged straining causes a small part of the tube to be propelled outwards by uterine contractions.

Clinical signs

The prolapse occurs over a period of approximately one hour and commences with the appearance of the red congested lining of the womb. This rapidly increases in size until the large everted mass is presented.

Diagnosis

This is obvious from the appearance.

Treatment

☐ This involves replacing the womb inside the sow. It is often impossible or the sow dies from internal haemorrhage.
☐ The technique for carrying this out is discussed in chapter 15.

In most cases on welfare grounds the sow should be destroyed. Uterine prolapses are uncommon but usually occur in old sows with large litters or where large piglets have been born. The supporting structures of the uterus become weak or the uterine wall becomes flaccid.

PROLAPSE OF THE VAGINA AND CERVIX

Prolapse of the vagina and cervix is more common prior to farrowing and may be seen in the last third of pregnancy including the pre-farrowing period in the farrowing house. It occurs normally in about one pregnancy in 200, usually in older sows from 5th parity onwards. It is a response to increased abdominal pressure together with a relaxation of the internal structures that support the cervix or the neck of the womb. Older sows that are heavy in pig, with large litters and in very good condition are also more likely candidates.

The following factors need to be considered as causal or contributing to the problem:

- It is much more common in older sows than young ones.
- Sows housed on tethers on slippery floors are more prone.
- When sows lie down there is an increased abdominal pressure which tends to force the cervix or vagina to the exterior.
- Fat sows are more prone as are those carrying large litters.
- It is common in sows that are lying in confinement on a floor that slopes too steeply to the rear.
- High levels of feed intake, particularly food containing high starch materials, produce abnormal fermentation, excess gas formation and an increase in abdominal pressure.

Clinical signs

In the early stages the protruding tissues appear between the lips of the vulva and return to their normal position when the sow stands. However with advancing pregnancy the prolapse may remain to the exterior and as soon as this occurs the animal should be removed from it's existing environment and loose-housed. The tissues become swollen with time.

Diagnosis

The clinical signs are obvious but occasionally can be confused with vaginal polyps that may protrude from the vulva, and eversion of the bladder. Handling the tissues will differentiate.

Treatment

- Remove the sow to loose housing.
- If the prolapse remains when the sow is standing replace and pass a tape suture across the vulva.
- If the sow is at point of farrowing, the farrowing crate floor should be raised to slope towards the feeding trough by using raised floor boards. When the sow then stands or lies down the weight of the piglets inside pulls the womb forward to hold the vagina in. Under such circumstances the sow usually farrows normally.
- If the vagina remains prolapsed as farrowing approaches, the cervix will not open fully and both the sow and the litter are likely to be lost. In such cases a tape suture should be placed across the lips of the vulva to hold the prolapse in. As the sow reaches the point of farrowing it can be relaxed. This technique is described in chapter 15.

Management control and prevention

- ◆ Consider the factors outlined above.
- ◆ Consider the factors predisposing to rectal prolapse.

SALT POISONING - (WATER DEPRIVATION)

Salt poisoning is common in all ages of pigs and almost without exception is related to water shortage either caused by inadequate supplies or complete loss. The normal levels of salt in the diet (0.4-0.5%) become toxic in the absence of water.

Signs develop within 24 to 48 hours.

Clinical signs

The very early stages of disease are always preceded by inappetance and whenever a sow or groups of pigs are not eating always check the water supply first. The first signs are often pigs trying to drink from nipple drinkers unsuccessfully. Nervous changes are the major signs and in more advanced cases involve fits, with animals wandering around apparently blind. Often the pig walks up to a wall, stands and presses its head against it in a characteristic position. One symptom strongly suggestive of salt poisoning is nose twitching just before a convulsion starts.

Diagnosis

This is based upon the clinical signs and lack of water. Examination of the brain histologically at post-mortem confirms the disease.

Similar diseases

Aujeszky's disease, swine fever, streptococcal meningitis and glässers disease all produce nervous signs. The condition might also be confused with middle ear infection but this only affects one individual rather than a group of pigs.

Treatment

- The response to treatment is poor but involves rehydrating the animal. At a practical level this can be achieved by dripping water into the mouth of the pig through a hose pipe or alternatively via a flutter valve into the rectum where it is absorbed. (See chapter 15 Flutter valve).
- Discuss the possibility of administering sterile water into the abdomen with your veterinarian.
- Corticosteroids may also help.

Management control and prevention

- ◆ It must be a daily routine to check that all sources of water are adequate free flowing and available.

SAVAGING OF PIGLETS (CANNIBALISM)

This is a common condition in first litter gilts that may account for a 1 to 3% increase in piglet mortality.

It occurs from time to time in many mammalian species (including young women), when giving birth for the first time and is thought to be related, in part at least, to the major hormone changes that take place around parturition.

In the gilt a number of factors seem to predispose to it, including a harsh or alien environment, poor empathy between the gilts and the stockperson, nutritional deficiencies and the effect of being placed in total confinement for the first time. It may also be related to temperament and breeding. It seems to be more prevalent in some breeds than others. For example, it is more common in pure-bred large white gilts than Landrace or Duroc, possibly their overlapping ears reduce visibility.

Major outbreaks have been experienced in new gilt herds where large numbers of the pregnant animals have been reared in extensive straw yards. In such environments (100-150 animals) no pecking order develops and one animal sees another as its enemy. In one particular herd a dramatic reduction occurred when the gilts were moved from the yards to sow stalls for three weeks prior to farrowing. During this period the gilt learned to recognise another pig and become familiar with individual confinement. Sometimes a change of farrowing room attendants reduces the incidence.

Clinical signs

Offending gilts can often be identified by their nervousness and apprehension at the onset of farrowing. Such animals have a wild eyed look. A careful watching brief therefore should be taken.

Treatment

- Try and identify potential gilts before farrowing.
- Constant supervision is required to identify animals at the onset of farrowing. To make this more feasible, prostaglandin injections on the 113th day

could be used on gilts, to give a more predictable time of farrowing.
- ☐ Watch all gilts carefully for the first 2 or 3 piglets and if there is any sign of savaging, inject with azaperone (stresnil) at a dose level of 1ml/12kg weight. All the piglets should be confined to the creep area away from the sow for at least 20 minutes following injection until she has settled down and rolled over on her side. The piglets should then be reintroduced. Most farrowings will continue normally thereafter.
- ☐ Discuss with your veterinarian the possibility of treatment with mysoline. This drug is available in tablets containing 250mg of a drug called primidone which is an anti-convulsant drug but has the effect of reducing hysteria and nervousness. 3 to 4 tablets may be given twice daily 24 to 48 hours prior to farrowing.

Management control and prevention

- ◆ Assess the gilts when they come into farrow.
- ◆ Try where ever possible to have a sow in a crate next to a gilt.
- ◆ Give the gilt plenty of straw to eat pre-farrowing.
- ◆ If there is a major problem hold the gilts in sow stalls for at least 7 days prior to entry into the farrowing crates.
- ◆ Consider a different breeding female. Where there is a breed factor very often the savaging will progress into the second and sometimes even the third litter.
- ◆ Document any savaging episode on the sow card so that this can be noted into the next litters.
- ◆ Ensure that the farrowing houses are dimly lit, warm and comfortable and with no draughts.
- ◆ Play background music during the farrowing period, talk to all the gilts, stroke them and develop a good empathy starting 3 to 4 weeks before farrowing.
- ◆ With "the wild eyed gilt" test her reaction to a two week old pig placed in the pen before farrowing.
- ◆ Cut the top off a rubber boot and fasten this over the mouth of the gilt, using a retaining string fastened behind the ears.
- ◆ Try introducing a rabbit into the gilt farrowing pen for 48 hours prior to farrowing.

SHOULDER SORES

They arise due to constant trauma over the bony prominences on the shoulder blade. Ultimately the skin breaks, there is an erosion and a large sore develops. It is associated with totally slatted flooring and individual sows that have a prominent spine to the shoulder blade. It is first noticed in the farrowing crates where the floors are slippery and the sow has difficulty in rising, thus constantly bruising her shoulder. Such sows should not be kept for future breeding.

Clinical signs

At the highest point on the spine of the scapula or shoulder blade a reddening of the skin first appears, which gradually forms into an ulcer. In severe cases the lesion may extend to 40-70mm in diameter with the development of extensive granulation tissue. Often both sides of the shoulder are affected.

Treatment

- ☐ As soon as the condition appears move the sow into a well bedded pen. Feed ad lib for 2 to 4 weeks.
- ☐ Cut a hole slightly larger than the sore in a 70mm square piece of foam or thick carpet and place over the shoulder sore. Hold it in place with contact adhesive such as evostik. This pad will then protect the sore and allow it to heal.
- ☐ Large granuloma that sometimes develop can be surgically removed.
- ☐ Watch for cannibalism by sucking pigs. If this occurs wean the sow.

VULVA HAEMATOMA

This is a condition where shortly after farrowing blood vessels inside the vulva rupture, due to stretching, pressure or trauma to the tissues. The vulva fills with blood. When this occurs the tissues become very fragile and if they are crushed the vulva splits with severe haemorrhage. Vulval haematoma can also arise where a gilt has to be assisted at farrowing and damage occurs from a large arm.

Clinical signs

The vulva becomes swollen and very dark blue. If it ruptures it may bleed continuously. Blood clotting is poor and the animal becomes anaemic and ultimately bleeds to death. Always consider this as a serious condition that is life threatening and requires frequent monitoring over 24 hours.

Treatment

- ☐ The animal should be sedated using stresnil and local anaesthetic injected around the tissues nearest the body of the sow just forward of the bleeding area. Three methods are then used for control:
  1. A piece of band or bandage is placed between the lips of the vulva and behind the bleeding tissues. It is then tightened to produce a tourniquet. This should be left for 24 hours.
  2. If this does not stop the bleeding then a series of mattress sutures should be passed through the vulva and tied to the exterior. See chapter 15.
  3. If the haemorrhage still does not stop, the haematoma must be opened by a veterinarian who will

use a pair of artery forceps to clamp the ruptured blood vessels and tie them off.
- ☐ Observe the effectiveness of the measures taken by placing a paper bag beneath the vulva so that any subsequent haemorrhage can be observed.
- ☐ Cover the tail gate of the crate with a bag of straw or other suitable protective material to stop further crushing.

Diseases and Problems in the Sucking Pig

Whilst there are a large number of diseases that affect the sucking pig only a few are important. Recognition of different conditions is not easy sometimes but Fig.8-26 highlights disease associated with clinical observations.

Identifying Problems in the Piglet

If you have a problem refer to Fig.8-26 and then the index or relevant chapter. If you cannot identify the cause consult your veterinarian.

Piglets: Observations and Causes

Diarrhoea   0-5 days of age

Clostridial diseases
E. coli infections *
Low colostrum intake *
Mastitis *
PRRS *
Rotavirus
TGE *
Udder oedema and poor milk supply *

Diarrhoea   6-21 days of age

Clostridia
Coccidiosis *
Cryptosporidia *
E. coli infections *
Low colostrum intake *
Low immunoglobulin A in milk *
Porcine epidemic diarrhoea (PED) *
PRRS
Rotavirus
Salmonellosis
Strongyloides
TGE

Laid on / trauma

Inadequate temperatures
Poor crate design
Poor environment
Poor farrowing house management
Poor farrowing house design

Observations and Causes (Cont.)

Splayleg

Lameness (arthritis)

Actinobacillus suis
Faulty teeth clipping and or tailing *
Glässers disease
Poor environment particularly floor surfaces
Specific infections
Splayleg
Staphylococci
Streptococci *
Trauma to knees, tail etc.
Vitamin E / Iron

Mortality   Diarrhoea

See diarrhoea

Mortality   Generalised infection

Actinobacillus suis
E. coli infections *
Erysipelas
Flu
Glässers disease *
Meningitis
PRRS

Mortality   Poor viability

Age or breed of the sow
Flu infection during pregnancy
Hypoglycaemia (low blood sugar)
Low birth weight
Navel bleeding
Poor environment *
Poor nutrition / starvation (see below)
PRRS infection in the sow
Purpura (bleeding)

Mortality   Trauma

Laid on *

Nervous symptoms

Actinobacillosis
Aujeszky's disease
Congenital tremor *
Glässers disease
Hypoglycaemia *
Middle ear infection
PRRS
Streptococcal meningitis
Swine fevers
Tetanus
Trauma

Observations and Causes (Cont.)

Sneezing / coughing

Ammonia
Actinobacillus pleuropneumonia
Atrophic or progressive rhinitis *
Aujeszky's disease
Bedding (dusty, mouldy)
Bordetella infection *
Cytomegalovirus
Dust *
EP
Flu
Glässers disease *
PRRS
Rhinitis non progressive *
Virus infections of the nose

Starvation / wasting

Actinobacillus suis
Anaemia
Arthritis
Chronic diarrhoea *
Coccidiosis
Congenital tremor
Eperythrozoonosis
Low birth weight
No milk available *
Pneumonia
Poor colostrum intake *
Poor teat access *
PRRS *

* More likely to occur

(Fig.8-26)

The sucking pig is potentially exposed to all those disease producing organisms that are present in the herd. The source of most of these infections is occasionally the sow, but more often the source is other diseased piglets or clinically healthy, usually older, piglets that become infected as the maternal antibody wanes. The levels of disease experienced in any one herd are dependent upon the management practices, the attention to detail and the various important predisposing factors that are listed under each specific disease. An over view of the diseases in the sucking pig is shown in Fig.8-27. Fig.8-28 highlights some of those diseases that may be controlled by vaccination of the sow to raise the level of antibodies in the colostrum. It is now recognised that provided the sow is not diseased and is passing antibodies via the colostrum, many of the above diseases will not be transmitted to the piglet. However once maternal antibodies disappear the piglet becomes susceptible.

ACTINOBACILLOSIS

This is caused by a tiny bacterium called *Actinobacillus suis* or sometimes *Actinobacillus equuli*. The

THE MAJOR INFECTIOUS DISEASES THAT MAY BE TRANSMITTED FROM SOW TO PIGLET

Viruses	
Aujeszky's disease	(V)
Classical swine fever	(V)
African swine fever	
Transmissible gastro-enteritis	(V)
Swine vesicular disease	
* Epidemic diarrhoea	
Foot-and-mouth disease	(V)
* Swine influenza	(V)
* Porcine parvovirus	(V)
PRRS	(V)
Swine pox	
Bacteria and Mycoplasma	
* Enzootic pneumonia	(V)
* Streptococcal infections	(V)
* Atrophic rhinitis	(V)
* Haemophilus infections	(V)
Salmonella choleraesuis	(V)
* Swine dysentery	
Porcine enteropathy	
Brucellosis	

(V) Vaccines available in some countries.
* Diseases unlikely to spread from the sow if the piglet is weaned at less than 21 days of age.

(Fig.8-28)

first of these is present in most herds and lives in the tonsils of older pigs, particularly sows. It may enter the piglet via the respiratory system or via cuts and abrasions. It occasionally produces a septicaemia, that is, it invades and multiplies in the blood stream and settles out in various parts of the body, particularly the lungs and the joints. Here it produces multiple small abscesses. During the acute septicaemic phase of the disease sudden death is often the only symptom. It can be precipitated by PRRS. It is not a common disease

Clinical signs

Sudden death in otherwise apparently healthy pigs is common, involving only one or two litters and only one or two pigs per litter. In less acute cases there may be discoloration of the skin, a very high fever, coughing and pneumonia. Occasionally skin lesions are seen that can resemble erysipelas. Some piglets may develop arthritis and lameness.

Diagnosis

If there is a history in the herd of sudden death then laboratory examinations are necessary to demonstrate the presence of the organism.

Similar diseases

Meningitis, acute *E. coli* infection, erysipelas, clostridial diseases and pigs that have been laid on can produce very similar symptoms.

Treatment

☐ The organism is sensitive to most antibiotics but

Disease or Condition	Born Dead	Low Viability	Enteritis (scour)	Lameness	Respiratory Signs	Skin Lesions	Nervous Signs
Actinobacillosis suis infection				✓	✓		
Arthritis				✓	✓		
Aujeszky's disease	✓	✓			✓	✓	✓
Bordetellosis					✓		
Brucellosis	✓	✓					✓
Clostridia			✓			✓	✓
Coccidiosis			✓				
Colibacillosis			✓				✓
Congenital tremor							✓
Enterovirus infections	✓	✓					
Eperythrozoonosis	✓	✓			✓		
Epidemic diarrhoea			✓				
Erysipelas	✓	✓		✓	✓	✓	✓
Exudative epidermitis						✓	
FMD disease				✓	✓	✓	
Glässers disease (*Haemophilus parasuis*)				✓	✓		✓
Iron deficiency	✓	✓			✓	✓	
Leptospira	✓	✓					
Listeriosis					✓		✓
Mange						✓	
Mycoplasma infections				✓	✓		
Mycotoxicosis	✓				✓		
Parvovirus	✓	✓					
Pasteurellosis					✓		
PRRS	✓	✓	✓		✓	✓	
Salmonellosis			✓	✓	✓	✓	✓
Streptococcal meningitis				✓	✓		✓
Swine dysentery			✓				
Swine influenza.					✓		
Tetanus					✓		✓
TGE			✓				
Thrombocytopaenic purpura						✓	
Toxoplasmosis	✓	✓					
Vitamin E deficiency	✓			✓	✓		

(Fig.8-27)

in particular amoxycillin or ampicillin injected at 5mg per kg or procaine penicillin, 1ml/20kg.
- Other antibiotics that can be used include OTC, lincomycin, ceftiofur, cephalexin and trimethoprim/sulpha.
- In persistent outbreaks if the appearance of the disease is predictable then preventive measures can be taken by giving long-acting preparations of the above drugs to all litters over a period of 3 to 4 weeks after which the preventative medication then ceases and the situation is then further assessed.
- In-feed medication with phenoxymethyl penicillin at 200g/tonne to the sow for the first 3 weeks of farrowing has proved successful in problem cases.

Management control and prevention
- In persistent herd problems the point of entry may be associated with teeth clipping or de-tailing, scrubbed knees from poor concrete, or respiratory spread from the sow. Assess the significance of these.
- Where there are rough concrete floors it may help to brush these over with lime wash containing 28ml phenolic disinfectant to 4.5 litres of lime wash.

ANAEMIA - IRON DEFICIENCY

The piglet is born with limited supplies of iron and if it had been born in the wild would depend on supplementation to its diet from iron bearing soils. Indoors the pig has no access to iron other than to the sows' milk (which is deficient) until it starts to eat creep feed. It is necessary therefore to give extra iron either by mouth or by injection. The pig is born with a normal level of haemoglobin in the blood of 12-13g/100ml and this rapidly drops down to 6-7g by 10 to 14 days of age. A shortage of iron results in lowered levels of haemoglobin in the red cells, (anaemia), a lowered capacity for the carriage of oxygen around the body and an increased susceptibility to disease.

Clinical signs

Piglets appear pale from 7 days onwards, sometimes but not always with a slight check in growth. The colour of the skin may take on a slight yellow or jaundiced appearance. In severe cases breathing is rapid particularly with exercise and there may be a predisposition to scour.

Diagnosis

This is based on the clinical signs, the lack of any supplemental iron and the haemoglobin level in the blood. If this is less than 8g/100ml the piglet is becoming anaemic.

Treatment

☐ Inject piglets with 200mg of iron dextran.

Management control and prevention

- The easiest method is to give the piglet an injection of 150- 200mg of iron dextran in either a 1 or 2ml dose.
- Iron is best given from 3 to 5 days of age and not at birth. A 2ml dose at birth causes considerable trauma to the muscles.
- The sites of injection are either into the muscles of the hind leg or into the neck. Use a 21 gauge $^5/_8$" needle.
- Iron can also be given orally but this method is time consuming and the pig must be treated on 2 or 3 occasions at 7, 10 and 15 days of age.
- Oral pastes available ad lib have been used but the uptake within any litter is variable and a few piglets remain anaemic.

ARTHRITIS - JOINT INFECTIONS

See chapter 9 for further information.

Joint infections in the sucking piglet are very common. They are invariably infectious in origin, the sources of infection either being respiratory spread from the sow, or through the skin as a result of some form of trauma, which allows the organisms to enter the system. The common bacteria include *Actinobacillus suis*, *Haemophilus parasuis*, (glässers disease), very occasionally mycoplasma infections, staphylococci, but most commonly *Streptococcus suis* serotypes. Most of these respond well to antibiotic therapy but treatment must be given early at the onset of disease.

Clinical signs

They are seen from 2 to 10 days of age. At the early onset the pig is laid on its belly, shivering slightly and with its hair stood on end. Stiffness or lameness involving one or more legs is evident. It is a common belief that the infection enters through the navel at birth, but this is unlikely. It is most likely to have gained entry via the tonsils. If the claws are involved infection has probably arisen from damage by the sow, bad slats or poor floor surfaces. The hock and elbow joints are often visibly swollen. Whilst lameness is the most common symptom, if the organism gains access to the blood stream and a septicaemia results death may occur before the arthritis develops.

Diagnosis

This is by clinical observation of lameness and the swollen joints. In well managed herds the numbers of piglets requiring treatment should be less than 2%. Where there are problems this could rise to as high as 10 to 15%. *Streptococcus suis* type 14 can cause severe sudden outbreaks of arthritis with acute pain.

Treatment

☐ Treatment of the infected pig could include one of the following antibiotics: lincomycin, penicillin and streptomycin, oxytetracycline, amoxycillin, ampicillin, trimethoprim/sulpha, enrofloxacin and framycetin. Inject daily for five days. Long-acting preparations can also be used and these should be injected every other day. Antibiotic penetration of the joint is slow. The choice will depend on the organism, the antibiotic sensitivity and the best response obtained.

☐ Cortisone or other anti inflammatory drugs can be of value.

Management control and prevention

- Check the mouths of the piglets to see that they are not infected following teeth clipping.
- Check the teeth clippers. Hold them to the light to make sure the edges are not damaged. If light is showing through abandon them and use a new pair.
- Make sure the teeth clippers are washed in warm soap and water between litters.
- Do not use the same instrument for removing both teeth and the tails.
- Preferably remove tails either by scalpel blade or sharp scissors to produce a clean cut to the surface. This will bleed a little but it will clot over with a minimum risk of infection.
- Check that iron injections are carried out hygienically with a sharp needle.
- Check for trauma to the piglet, particularly scrubbed knees, legs or tail.
- If there is a problem on the farm submit samples to the laboratory to identify the organism.
- In severe cases preventative medication of the sow pre-farrowing may help particularly if the organism

- is spread by the respiratory route.
- ◆ Where there are bad floor surfaces brush these over with hydrated lime.
- ◆ Preventive medication - Administer a long-acting antibiotic injection 3 to 4 days prior to the expected onset of disease. Oxytetracycline, amoxycillin, ampicillin, ceftiofur or penicillin could be used. Most streptococci are sensitive to penicillin.
- ◆ Sometimes the skin of the sow is a source of infection. In such cases spray a skin antiseptic onto the udder one day before and two days after farrowing. Iodine dairy teat dips are ideal.

ATRESIA ANI - (NO ANUS OR NO RECTUM)

The piglet is born with no anus externally because it has developed a blind end to its rectum 5-10mm from the exterior, inside the pelvis. The incidence in the mature herd is usually less than 0.5% but it can be much higher in newly established gilt herds. The condition is heritable but of low penetrance. In a problem herd records will indicate whether there is an incriminating boar involved. The condition is self limiting in that death invariably ensues. It is not worth attempting surgical repair because the artificial opening closes again. Make sure the female is mated to a different boar for the next litter.

ATROPHIC RHINITIS (AR)
See chapter 9 for further information.

Rhinitis is inflammation of the tissues inside the nose and in its mild form it is very common. Progressive atrophic rhinitis (PAR) however is a serious condition both in sucking and growing pigs. The term atrophy indicates that the tissues inside the nose, which become infected or damaged, shrink and become distorted. There are two forms of the disease: mild and non-progressive where the infection or irritation occurs over a period of 2 to 3 weeks. The inflammation does not progress and structures in the nose called turbinate bones repair and return to normality.

The serious disease is progressive atrophic rhinitis (PAR) where toxin producing strains of the bacterium *Pasteurella multocida*, cause a continual and progressive inflammation and atrophy of the tissues and nose distortion. All herds will show some degree of non-progressive atrophic rhinitis, the inflammation being of short duration. Organisms such as bordetella, haemophilus, non toxigenic pasteurella, other environmental organisms and dust or gases can produce this type of rhinitis in the nose.

For a herd however, to have PAR toxigenic pasteurella must be present. They are carried in the nose and tonsils of the adult pig and there is always the risk therefore of buying them into the herd. This is the most common method of entry.

> *Always make sure that breeding stock is purchased from herds checked and believed free from toxigenic pasteurella.*

Clinical signs

They include sneezing, runny eyes, discharges from the nose sometimes containing blood and early signs of distortion of the face, with shortening or twisting of the upper jaw becoming evident at weaning time. It is important also to appreciate that sneezing is a common occurrence in the sucking pig and need not necessarily be associated with PAR. PAR affects most of the piglets present. However, individual piglets may also develop distortion of the nose from trauma or some other cause but this is not PAR.

Diagnosis
This is carried out by:
1. The clinical signs in the sucking piglets and nasal distortion in growing pigs.
2. Sectioning the snout of pigs at slaughter and examining the degree of turbinate damage in the nose.
3. Isolating the organism from sucking or rhinitic pigs by swabbing the nostrils and submitting to a specialist laboratory for examination.

Similar diseases

The most common would be non progressive rhinitis and sneezing caused by cytomegalo virus, bordetella and haemophilus organisms or environmental irritants. A significant differentiating feature here is that if these organisms are causing sneezing in the sucking pigs then by 4 weeks after weaning sneezing will have disappeared with no facial distortions.

Treatment
- ☐ Once toxigenic pasteurella have been identified the complete breeding herd should be immediately vaccinated six weeks apart using a vaccine made from toxigenic pasteurella. It takes approximately four months for a total herd immunity to develop and it may be nine months or more before the disease is brought completely under control. In the early stages of a herd breakdown the following could be recommended:
- ☐ In-feed medicate sows with trimethoprim/sulpha or sulphadimidine from point of entry into the farrowing house through to weaning. (500g/tonne)
- ☐ Inject all piglets with 0.25 to 0.5ml of long-acting OTC or amoxycillin on days 3, 10 and 15 during sucking.
- ☐ Inject pigs similarly at weaning time with 0.5 to 1ml of long-acting antibiotic. This treatment programme should continue for a period of at least 2 months after all sows have been fully vaccinated.

- ☐ Medicate the creep rations with OTC or CTC 800g/tonne or trimethoprim/sulpha combinations for 4 weeks post-weaning.
- ☐ Sows should be given a booster dose of vaccine 2 to 3 weeks prior to each subsequent farrowing.

Management control and prevention

Management can play an important part in controlling the disease. If there is a problem in the herd consider the following predisposing factors:
- ◆ Disease is more common in young herds particularly those containing large numbers of gilts.
- ◆ Large permanently populated farrowing houses are ideal for the maintenance and spread of disease therefore split the houses into small modules of 6-10 crates only.
- ◆ Operate an all-in all-out system with pressure washing and disinfection between batches.
- ◆ If multi suckling is practised then convert this to single suckling. The more pigs noses that make contact with each other the greater is the spread of disease.
- ◆ Make sure that divisions between farrowing pens are solid and at least 0.6m high to reduce the risk of droplet infection.
- ◆ Outdoor rearing reduces the risk of PAR.
- ◆ Poor ventilation and low humidity together with dusty atmospheres and toxic gases predispose to the disease.
- ◆ Poor colostrum management or udder problems such as agalactia result in piglets with poor immunity.

Eradication

It is possible by vaccination, segregated early weaning or segregated disease control, to eradicate the organisms from a breeding weaning herd. This is carried out by vaccinating the sows and after approximately 12 months of vaccination and no evidence of clinical disease, a segregated disease control programme is carried out as discussed in chapter 3.

Problems however arise in the breeding finishing unit where the organism persists in the continually populated finishing houses and it is necessary to depopulate the weaning, growing and finishing houses. Total herd depopulation and repopulation is also successful.

AUJESZKY'S DISEASE (AD)

See chapter 12 for further information.

Usually disease is only seen in piglets when the virus first enters the herd. The incubation period is short, only 2 to 3 days, after which sucking pigs become acutely ill, hairy, wander around aimlessly and listlessly and stop sucking their dam. Nervous signs are common. Piglets go into fits and often paddle on their sides. Some piglets may adopt a dog-sitting position and develop vomiting and diarrhoea. During acute disease mortality is very high, approaching 100%. For a period of up to 3 months after the virus enters the herd, sows produce weak pigs at birth and there are high levels of mummification. Vaccination should take place as soon as the disease is diagnosed to boost immunity and mitigate the effects. Clinical signs in the sucking pigs ultimately disappear.

Treatment has no effect on the course of the disease.

BRUCELLOSIS

See chapter 12 for further information.

This disease is caused by the bacterium *Brucella suis*. Infection of the pregnant sow may result in abortion. Generally it has no affect on sucking pigs that are born viable and healthy at full term except that some may develop infection of the spinal column (spondylitis) leading to posterior paralysis.

BURSITIS

Bursitis is a common condition that arises from constant pressure and trauma to the skin overlying any bony prominence. The periosteum or covering over the bone reacts by creating bone, a swelling develops and the skin likewise responds and becomes thicker, until there is a prominent soft lump. It can commence in the farrowing houses, particularly if there are bad floors but it usually starts in the weaner accommodation on slatted floors which have large gaps. As the pig increases in weight there is increased pressure on the leg bones. Swellings develop over the lateral sides of the hocks and elbows and over the points of the hocks. Such swellings are called bursa although strictly speaking they are not. The term should apply to inflammation of bursa that cover tendons. Worn and pitted floor surfaces particularly if sharp aggregate was used in the concrete, can exaggerate the trauma to the extent that the skin is broken and secondary infection develops. If this occurs on wet dirty floors major problems can arise. Under normal circumstances if there is no secondary infection the condition commercially is not important but if breeding stock is being produced then the management system needs to be adjusted, otherwise rejection rates on breeding gilts will be high.

Wire mesh, woven metal and metal bar floors can produce high levels in weaner pigs in first and second stage housing. Identify the point at which disease first appears and alter the floor surfaces or change the environment.

Clinical signs

These can develop when piglets are 1-2 weeks old particularly where farrowing crate floors are totally slatted. Metal bars are particularly bad. Most swellings commence on the hind legs below the point of the hock or on the lateral aspects of the elbow. With repeated trauma the lesions increase in size and ultimately fluid appears. This is common in pigs 30-70kg weight. Infection with *Mycoplasma hyosynoviae* can occur and also be seen at the base of the tail over the shoulder blades and the knees.

Treatment

- There is no specific treatment that will reduce the bone reaction. Remove pigs to pens that are well bedded.
- If the swellings have become infected with bacteria inject with either oxytetracycline or ampicillin.
- If *Mycoplasma hyosynoviae* is causing infection use either lincomycin or tiamulin.
- Most lesions do not require treatment.

Management control and prevention

- Move severely affected animals onto deep bedded floors.
- Determine the point at which lesions are occurring and relate to floor surfaces.
- If the problem is arising in flat decks in breeding gilts it may be necessary to change the slats to those covered with plastic. Tri-bar or metal slats and woven mesh are bad surfaces.

CLOSTRIDIAL DISEASES

Clostridia are large gram-positive spore-bearing bacteria that are present in the large intestine of all pigs. There are several species but one in particular, *C. perfringens*, types A, B or C, can under certain conditions produce a severe diarrhoea with very high mortality. Type C is by far the most important and if it gets into the small intestine and becomes established before colostrum is taken in, disease can result. Piglets are normally infected under 7 days of age and more typically within the first 24 to 72 hours of life.

Clinical signs

These are sudden in onset. Piglets rapidly develop a rotten smelling diarrhoea which is often blood coloured. Many piglets die. The lining of the small intestine sloughs off (necrosis) and this may also be observed in the scour. The disease caused by *C perfringens* type A tends to be milder less dramatic and more prolonged but it can look similar to that caused by type C. Clostridial disease is common in outdoor herds.

Diagnosis

In typically acute cases the clinical signs and post-mortem lesions are diagnostic. If the abdomen of a dead piglet is cut open the middle portion of the small intestine is often claret wine coloured and this can usually be seen without cutting into the intestinal wall. Bubbles of gas may also be seen in the wall of the intestine. In less striking cases, confirmation of the diagnosis must be carried out in a laboratory. It is necessary to submit preferably a live or very recently dead pig to the laboratory (within 3 to 4 hours) because the causal organisms multiply after death and cause rapid post-mortem changes.

Treatment

- In acute outbreaks lamb dysentery antiserum can be injected into the piglets at birth.
- Oral antibiotics and in particular amoxycillin should be given at birth and again at day 2 or 3.
- The sows ration can be medicated with 200g/tonne of phenoxymethyl penicillin or the feed top dressed daily with the premix, from 5 days pre-farrowing and during lactation.

Management control and prevention

- This is carried out by vaccinating the sow herd using either sheep vaccines made from *Clostridium perfringens* type C toxoids or pig vaccines containing these toxoids. At the onset of an outbreak sows should be given 2 doses about two to three weeks apart, the last one at least 7 days before farrowing. The general principles of control of diarrhoea in the sucking piglet should also be considered as contributory factors.

COCCIDIOSIS (COCCIDIA)

Coccidiosis is caused by small parasites called coccidia that live and multiply inside the host cells, mainly in the intestinal tract. There are three types, Eimeria, Isospora and Cryptosporidia. Disease is common and widespread in sucking piglets and occasionally in pigs up to 15 weeks of age. Diarrhoea is the main clinical sign.

The life cycle

Tiny-egg like infected structures called oocysts are passed out in the faeces into the environment where they develop (sporulate). This takes place within 12-24 hours at temperatures between 25°-35°C (77°F-95°F). Oocysts can survive outside the pig for many months and are very difficult to kill. They are resistant to most disinfectants but OO-CIDE (Antec) is effective. The oocysts are eaten and undergo three complex developments in the wall of the small intestine to complete the cycle. It is during this period that damage occurs. Sows faeces are one source of infection and it is important that they are removed daily from the farrowing house. The life cycle in the piglet takes 5-10 days and disease therefore is not seen before five days of age.

Clinical signs

Coccidiosis causes diarrhoea in piglets due to damage caused to the wall of the small intestine. This is followed by secondary bacterial infections. Dehydration is common. The faeces vary in consistency and colour from yellow to grey green, or bloody according to the severity of the condition. Secondary infection by bacteria and viruses can also result in high mortality, although mortality due to coccidiosis on its own is relatively low. Occasionally disease is seen in young boars and gilts that are housed in permanently populated pens and floor fed.

Diagnosis

Coccidiosis should be suspected if there is a diarrhoea problem in sucking pigs from 7-21 days of age that does not respond particularly well to antibiotics. Diagnosis however is not easy in some outbreaks because identifying oocysts in the faeces of infected pigs can be difficult. In other outbreaks however clear signs are evident at post-mortem examinations. The oocysts do not pass out into the faeces until approximately 3-4 days after diarrhoea is seen, by which time the pig may have recovered. Faeces samples for laboratory examination should be taken from semi-recovered pigs rather than pigs with scour. Diagnosis is best made by submitting a live pig to the laboratory for histological examination of the intestinal wall. *Isospora suis* is the most pathogenic of the three types of coccidia.

Treatment

- For this to be effective it must be given just prior to the invasion of the intestinal wall. Once clinical signs have appeared the damage has been done.
- Medicate the sow feed with either amprolium premix 1kg/tonne, monensin sodium 100g/tonne or sulphadimidine 100g/tonne. Feed from the time the sow enters the farrowing house and throughout lactation.
- Inject each litter with a long-acting sulphonamide at six days of age.
- Medicate small amounts of milk powder with a coccidiostat such as amprolium or salinomycin and give small amounts daily to the piglets from three days of age onwards top dressed on the creep feed.
- One or two doses of Toltrazuril (Baycox Bayer) at a level of 6.25mg/kg is effective in controlling disease. It is prepared by mixing 250ml of glycerol, 125ml water and 125ml of Baycox together. A 2ml dose may be given once at 4, 5 or 6 days of age, the exact time determined by the response, and repeated again at ten days of age. If there is no response it is unlikely that coccidiosis is the problem. Specifically discuss this method of treatment with your veterinarian who may prepare this for you.

Management control and prevention

- Once the oocysts have become established in an environment the sow plays only a minor role. The oocysts contaminate the environment by other means such as flies, dried faeces, dust and faeces contaminated surfaces. Hygiene and insect control are important.
- Remove sow and piglet faeces daily.
- Improve the hygiene in farrowing houses, in particular farrowing pen floors and prevent the movement of faeces from one pen to another.
- Ensure as far as possible that slurry channels are completely emptied between farrowings.
- Thoroughly wash and disinfect the farrowing houses with OO-CIDE (Antec) or other substances that are active against oocysts.
- If farrowing crate floor surfaces are made of concrete and pitted, brush these over with lime wash and allow it to dry before the next sow comes into farrow. See chapter 15.
- Keep pens as dry as possible and in particular those areas of the floor where the piglets defecate. An effective method is to cover the wet areas with shavings and remove them daily.
- If creep is fed on the floor stop creep feeding until piglets are at least 21 days old.
- Control flies. See Flies chapter 11.
- In outdoor herds control can be difficult. Always move farrowing arcs to new ground between farrowings and burn bedding.
- If floor boards are used in farrowing arcs disinfect these with OO-CIDE (Antec).
- Wallows can be an ideal focus of infection particularly during lactation. Increase the amount of shade and provide sprays. Provide alternating wallows.
- Site wallows well away from the source of food.

CONGENITAL TREMOR (CT) - SHAKING PIGLETS

This is a sporadic disease seen in newborn pigs, evident by tremors and shaking of the muscles, of the head and body. Usually there is more than one pig involved in a litter but the tremor is only seen when piglets are walking around and not when they are asleep. The condition decreases with age but if the tremors are too great for the piglets to find a teat and suckle then mortality maybe high. Mortality in an affected litter or in a herd outbreak could increase above the norm by 3-10%

The causes of the condition are varied and classified into 4 groups based on brain histology.

Group 1 - associated with a classical swine fever.
Group 2 - possibly associated with a recently recognised circovirus. Most of the problems in the field are found in this group.
Groups 3 and 4 - associated with either hereditary disorders seen in the Landrace or Saddleback breeds or with organophosphorus poisoning.
Group 4 - includes aujeszky's disease and Japanese encephalomyelitis virus.

It would be unusual to find a pig farm that sometime in its history had not experienced one or more litters of trembling piglets. The circovirus or perhaps also other viruses are therefore widespread among most if not all pig populations, yet little disease is seen in most herds, presumably because an immunity is established in the sow herd. In gilt herds however, there can be major outbreaks involving up to 80% of all litters during the first parity. The reasons for this are not fully understood.

Diagnosis

This is based on clinical evidence although histological examinations in the laboratory can help to differentiate the groups.

Treatment

- ☐ There is no specific treatment for affected piglets but careful management will greatly reduce mortality.
- ☐ Ensure that piglets are given colostrum at birth and assisted to a teat.

Management control and prevention

- ◆ Attempts to immunise breeding stock should be carried out. The following may assist and the results should be documented for further studies where litters are continually affected.
- ◆ If there is a history of the disease on the farm expose incoming maiden gilts to faeces from older animals and boars for 4 to 6 weeks prior to mating.
- ◆ At the time of mating use tissue paper to wipe around the prepuce of the boar and the vulva of the mated sow. Expose the group of maiden gilts to the tissues. Do this 2 to 3 times weekly.
- ◆ Maintain a continually populated gilt pen when gilts first enter the farm to ensure continual exposure to any viruses. (You would need to make sure however there is no build up of parasites in this pen).
- ◆ Assess the results of using a vasectomised boar from one your affected litters for a period of 6 weeks prior to full mating.
- ◆ Move all maiden gilts into the main mating area for a period of 7 days commencing at least 4 weeks before mating is due to start to expose them to any possible infectious agents.

CRYPTOSPORIDIOSIS

Cryptosporidia are parasites similar to coccidia that can also cause diarrhoea but at a slightly older age of 10 to 21 days. They can infect the human and this may be serious in immuno-suppressed people. They are also found in other species such as rats and mice which can become a source of constant infection.

Diagnosis

This is made by examining faeces in the laboratory.

THE MAIN CAUSES OF PIGLET DIARRHOEA					
	Early Period Days		Late Period Days		Mortality Level
	0-3	3-7	7-14	15-21	
Agalactia	✓	✓	✓	✓	Moderate
Clostridia	✓	✓	✓		High
Coccidiosis			✓	✓	Low
Colibacillosis (E. coli)	✓	✓	✓		Moderate
PED	✓	✓	✓	✓	Low
PRRS	✓	✓	✓	✓	Variable
Rotavirus			✓	✓	Low
TGE	✓	✓	✓	✓	High

(Fig.8-29)

If the organism is associated regularly with diarrhoea the management control procedures recommended for coccidiosis control should be adopted. There is no recognised treatment and the condition is not common.

DIARRHOEA OR SCOUR

Of all the diseases in the sucking piglet, diarrhoea is the most common and probably the most important. In some outbreaks it is responsible for high morbidity and mortality. In a well run herd there should be less than 3% of litters at any one time requiring treatment and piglet mortality from diarrhoea should be less than 0.5%. In severe outbreaks levels of mortality can rise to 7% or more and in individual untreated litters up to 100% (in TGE it may reach 100% overall). The causes of diarrhoea are shown in Fig.8-29. Four of these are viruses, transmittable gastro-enteritis (TGE), rotavirus, porcine epidemic diarrhoea (PED) virus and PRRS virus. The main bacterial causes are *E. coli* and clostridia and the main parasite is coccidia. This section deals principally with *E. coli* diarrhoea. Clostridial diarrhoea, coccidiosis, TGE and PED are dealt with in more detail in other sections in this chapter.

At birth the intestinal tract is micro-biologically sterile and it has little immunity to disease producing organisms. Organisms begin to colonise the tract quickly after birth, among them potentially pathogenic strains of *E. coli* and *Clostridium perfringens*. Immunity is initially provided by the high levels of antibodies in colostrum (IgG, IgM, IgA). After the colostral antibodies have been absorbed into the blood stream, the immunity is maintained by the antibody (IgA) which is present in milk. IgA is absorbed into the mucous lining of the intestines. It is essential that the newborn piglet drinks sufficient colostrum soon after birth to prevent potentially pathogenic organisms multiplying against the intestinal wall and causing diarrhoea. It is also essential that the piglet continues to drink milk regularly after the colostrum has gone so that its intestines continue to be lined by protective antibodies.

The antibodies acquired passively from the colostrum and milk are finite and can be overwhelmed by large doses of bacteria present in the environment. The higher the number of organisms taken in, the greater the risk of disease. Environmental stress such as chilling also plays a role because it lowers the piglets resistance. There is thus a delicate balance between the antibody level on the one hand and the weight of infection and stress on the other.

Clinical signs

Scour in the piglet can occur at any age during sucking but there are often two peak periods, before 5 days and between 7 and 14 days.

Acute disease

The only sign may be a perfectly good pig found dead. Post-mortem examinations shows severe acute enteritis, so sudden that there may be no evidence of scour externally. Clinically affected piglets huddle together shivering or lie in a corner. The skin around the rectum and tail will be wet. Look around the pen for evidence of a watery to salad cream consistency scour. In many cases there is a distinctive smell. As the diarrhoea progresses the piglet becomes dehydrated, with sunken eyes and a thick leathery skin. The scour often sticks to the skin of other piglets giving them an orange to white colour.

Prior to death piglets may be found on their sides paddling and frothing at the mouth.

Sub acute disease

The symptoms are similar but the effects on the piglet are less dramatic, more prolonged and mortality tends to be lower. This type of scour is often seen between 7 to 14 days of age manifest by a watery to thin salad cream consistency diarrhoea, often white to yellow in colour.

Diagnosis

The overall picture must be considered when making a diagnosis. Sudden outbreaks of scour involving large numbers of litters with acute diarrhoea and high mortality suggest TGE, epidemic diarrhoea or PRRS. It always helps in differentiating these infections to know whether the herd had previously been exposed to any of these diseases or not. If exposure is for the first time the outbreak is likely to be explosive.

Rotavirus diarrhoea appears in waves in individual litters or groups of litters and normally in the second half of lactation. Coccidiosis has an incubation period of 6 days and is usually involved in diarrhoea complexes from 7 to 14 days of age. At less than 5 days of age the most common cause is *E. coli* with acute diarrhoea particularly in gilts' litters because they pass on poorer levels of immunity. Clostridial infections also occur at this age.

Diagnosis is based on the clinical examinations, the response to treatment (viral diseases do not respond to treatment) and laboratory examination of the scour. Submit a rectal swab or a live pig to the laboratory for cultural examinations and antibiotic sensitivity tests.

Treatment

- Some antibiotics available are shown in Fig.8-30. Most of these are active against *E. coli* and clostridia but not the virus infections.
- In severe outbreaks of *E. coli* disease the sows feed can be top dressed with the appropriate antibiotic daily, from entry into the farrowing house and for up to 14 days post-farrowing. This can be effective in reducing bacterial output in the sows faeces.
- Observe litters for the presence of diarrhoea both night and morning.
- Study the history of the disease on your farm. Is it sporadic, in one piglet in a litter, or total litters?
- In the light of the history either treat the individual pig or on the first signs of disease treat the whole litter.
- If a litter is badly scoured dose night and morning for a minimum of two days.
- Assess the response to treatment. If there is no change within 12 hours then change to another drug as advised by your veterinarian.
- Always treat piglets less than 7 days of age by mouth.
- For older pigs where the disease is less acute injections are equally effective and easier to administer.
- Provide electrolytes in drinkers. These prevent dehydration and maintain body electrolyte balances.
- Cover the pen, the creep area and where the pigs defecate with straw, shredded paper, shavings or sawdust.
- Provide an additional lamp to provide an extra source of heat.
- Use binding agents such as chalk, kaolin or activated attapulgite to absorb toxins from the gut.

Management control and prevention

◆ Adopt procedures to prevent the spread of the scour.
- Disinfect boots between pens.

SOME ANTIBIOTICS AVAILABLE TO TREAT PIGLET DIARRHOEA		
Drug	Method of Dosing	
	Oral	Injection
Amoxycillin	✓	✓
Ampicillin	✓	✓
Apramycin	✓	
Ceftiofur		✓
* Chloramphenicol		✓
Enrofloxacin	✓	✓
Framycetin		✓
* Furazolidone	✓	
Neomycin	✓	
Spectinomycin	✓	
* Streptomycin	✓	✓
Sulphonamides	✓	✓
Trimethoprim/sulpha	✓	✓
Tylosin		✓

* Banned in some countries

(Fig.8-30)

- Use a disposable plastic apron when dosing piglets to prevent heavy contamination of clothing.
- Wash hands after handling a scoured litter.
- Disinfect brushes and shovels between pen.
- ◆ Ensure that farrowing houses are only used on an all-in all-out basis with a pressure wash and disinfection between each batch.
- ◆ Farrowing pens must be dry before the house is repopulated. Remember that moisture, warmth, waste food and faeces are ideal for bacterial multiplication.
- ◆ Pen floors should be well maintained. Poor pen hygiene associated with bad drainage predisposes to scour.
- ◆ Look carefully at the part of the pen floor where there are piglet faeces. Is this poorly drained? Do large wet patches develop? If so cover them with extra bedding daily and remove. This is a most important aspect of control.
- ◆ Check nipple drinkers and feeding troughs for leakages.
- ◆ Ensure that faeces are removed daily from behind the sow from the day she enters the farrowing crates until at least 7 days post-farrowing if the floors are slatted. Also remove faeces daily throughout lactation if they are solid concrete.
- ◆ Maintain creep environments that are always warm and comfortable. Fluctuating temperatures are a major trigger factor to scour particularly from 7 to 14 days of age.
- ◆ Do not penny-pinch on your heating costs. Many cases of scour are precipitated by attempts to save on costs of energy.
- ◆ Check for high air flow and draughts. They predispose to scour.
- ◆ Consider vaccinating against *E. coli* (make sure first that this is the cause of the problem however). *E. coli* vaccines only protect the piglet for the first 5 to 7 days of age.
- ◆ Assess the environment of all the farrowing house. Poor environments allow heavy bacterial multiplication and a much higher bacterial challenge is likely to break down the colostral immunity.
- ◆ Check the sow's health. Animals affected with enteric or respiratory disease, lameness or mastitis predispose the litter to scour.
- ◆ Avoid the use of milk replacers where possible. Their routine use, particularly if they are allowed to get stale or contaminated, may increase the incidence.
- ◆ Where farrowing house floors are very poor, pitted and difficult to clean, brush them over with lime wash containing a phenolic disinfectant. See chapter 15.
- ◆ Scour is more common in large litters. Split suckling should be adopted.

Colostrum management

It is vital that the piglet receives the maximum amount of colostrum within the first 12 hours of birth. High levels of antibody are only absorbed during this period. Factors such as poor teat access, poor crate design, and particularly the development of agalactia in the sow, associated with udder oedema, reduce intake.

In an outbreak of scour it is important to establish if udder oedema is present. It is more common in gilts and second parity than in older sows. If *E. coli* diarrhoea is a problem in younger aged females this suggests that immunity levels are low and vaccination should be considered. Inject the sow twice 2 to 4 weeks apart the second injection at least two weeks before farrowing, but these times are variable depending upon the vaccine used. With good management it should not be necessary to vaccinate the sows, only the gilts.

Eradication

It is not possible to eliminate organisms such as rotavirus *E. coli* and coccidiosis from the herd and most if not all pigs will be infected with them. Herds can be maintained free of TGE, PED and PRRS. All herds carry clostridia but other factors are required to cause disease.

A summary of the management factors associated with disease is shown in Fig.8-31.

ENZOOTIC PNEUMONIA (EP) - (MYCOPLASMA INFECTION)
See chapter 9 for further information.

This is caused by *Mycoplasma hyopneumoniae*. The disease is not normally a problem in the sucking pig, because in herds in which it is endemic immunity from the sow via the colostrum protects it. If however a herd has been free of the organism and becomes infected for the first time, severe disease may be seen in sucking pigs until the sows have had sufficient time to develop immunity. In such cases it may be necessary to inject the piglets for a period of 6 to 8 weeks with antibiotics that are active against mycoplasma, such as oxytetracycline, tiamulin, lincomycin or tylosin. Depending on the severity of the disease these injections would be given on day 3, 10 and 21 and if necessary at weaning - if this is later than 21 days.

EPERYTHROZOONOSIS (EPE)

Eperythrozoonosis is caused by a small ricketsial bacterium called *Eperythrozoon suis* (Epe) which attaches itself to the red cells in the blood, damaging them and

---

Are piglets getting sufficient colostrum?

causing them to break apart. This causes an anaemia associated with a reduction in the number of red blood cells and haemoglobin the substance by which oxygen is transported around the body. When large numbers of red cells are damaged, jaundice may result.

The disease is somewhat of an enigma because the organism can be identified both in normal animals and in those severely affected with disease. It is likely that Epe is very widespread and most sources of pigs examined (varying health status) have shown evidence of the bacteria.

In the majority herds where it has been identified there have been no clinical problems and the significance therefore of the organism in relation to infection in these cases must be in doubt. However, in the past two years a positive diagnosis associated with disease has become more common. Epe can cross the placenta and be responsible for poor pale pigs at birth and high pre-weaning mortality.

Clinical signs

Epe affects all classes of pigs from sows and piglets through to weaners and growers. Clinical pictures vary, particularly if there are secondary infections involved. It is useful however, to look at the clinical symptoms in acute and chronic disease. In piglets and weaners the acute disease is manifest by primary anaemia and secondary infections, whilst the more chronic picture appears related to slow growth, variable growth rate and poor-doing pigs. The chronic symptoms in sows are associated with reproductive failure and if there is stress at farrowing, fevers and agalactia may be experienced.

If pale anaemic pigs are evident during sucking or in the immediate post-weaning period and an injection of iron has been given, the possibility of Epe should be considered.

Diagnosis

The presence of the organism does not necessarily confirm disease. The following need to be considered to clarify the relationship between Epe and disease.
- The presence of pale and anaemic pigs.
- The identification of the organism in blood smears stained with Wright's stain. Fifty microscopic fields should be examined before a negative diagnosis is arrived at.
- The clinical picture on the farm should include lowered reproductive performance.

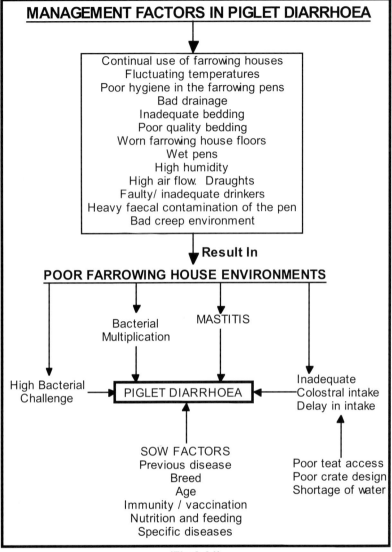

(Fig.8-31)

EPERYTHROZOON SUIS - CLINICAL SIGNS		
Sows	**Piglets**	**Weaners/Growers**
Abortion	Jaundiced	Anaemia
Agalactia	Increased scour	Ear necrosis
Anaemia, jaundice	Pale pigs	Enteritis
Fever	Pneumonia	Fever
Increased repeats	Weak at birth	Pneumonia
Reduced conception		Poor doers
Reproductive failure		Pot-bellied pigs
		Scour

- Jaundice, particularly in young growing pigs from 7 to 21 days of age.
- Serological tests are being developed including an ELISA but at the time of writing they are still unreliable.
- Eliminate other causes of anaemia.
- Blood samples should be examined for packed cell volume (PCV) and haemoglobin levels. In normal

pigs the mean PCV would be around 35% and in clinically affected pigs 24%. Haemoglobin levels would normally range from 9 to 14g per 100ml but in anaemic pigs they would be as low as 3 to 7g per 100ml.

Similar diseases

Actinobacillus pleuropneumonia.
Chronic respiratory disease complexed with PRRS and influenza.
Glässer's disease - *Haemophilus parasuis*.
Iron / copper anaemia.
Leptospirosis (*L. icterohaemorrhagiae* and *L. canicola*).
Malabsorption and chronic enteritis.
Pale piglet syndrome - haemorrhages.
Porcine enteropathy (PE, NE, PHE and PIA).

Treatment

Consider the following and discuss with your veterinarian:
- The response to treatment is not very good.
- Inject piglets with oxytetracycline at 10mg/kg daily for 4 days or use long-acting preparations, three injections each two days apart.
- In-feed medicate sows at 800gms/tonne of OTC for 4 weeks and repeat again 4 weeks later.
- Arsanilic acid in-feed at 85gms/tonne is reported to have an effect but in many countries there is no licensed product in food producing animals. Where it is available it is probably the drug of choice.
- The response to other drugs is poor.

Management control and prevention

Epe suis is spread by inoculation (including inoculation by insects). In a problem herd it is important to eliminate possible methods of spread including:-

Sows
- Vaccinating sows with the same needle - Wipe the needle between inoculation with cotton wool well dampened with surgical spirit and change every third sow.
- Tagging gilts - Wash the applicators between animals or hold three pairs in an antiseptic solution and rotate.
- Eliminate lice or mange mites.
- Prevent or control fighting, vulval and tail biting etc.
- Do not feed back placenta or farrowing house material.
- Control biting insects.
- Control internal parasites.
- Wear plastic arm sleeves when attending a farrowing.

Piglets
- Spread occurs during tailing, teething and iron injections.
- Control as for sows.

Weaners and growers
- Prevent fighting at weaning. Reduce mixing.
- Prevent tail biting and vice.
- Reduce mixing and use Stresnil to prevent fighting.
- Prevent spread through vaccination and inoculations between pigs.
- Control biting insects.
- Control respiratory diseases.

> *Do not let the infection get out of control and cause disease.*

EPITHELIOGENESIS IMPERFECTA - (IMPERFECT SKIN)

See chapter 10 for further information.

The piglet is born devoid of areas of skin that have failed to develop correctly. If these areas are small they will gradually heal but if they are more than 15mm in diameter it will be necessary to infiltrate local anaesthetic, loosen the skin and stitch it together. (See chapter 15). This will depend on the availability of skin and whether the loss is over the flanks where there is plenty of skin, or over the legs where there is little. In severe cases the piglet should be destroyed.

ERYSIPELAS

See chapter 7 for further information.

This disease is uncommon in the piglet because it is protected from infection by colostral immunity but it occasionally occurs in gilt litters and the only sign may be a good piglet found dead from septicaemia. The skin extremities are often blue and post-mortem examinations show minute haemorrhages in the drainage lymph glands, the liver and the kidneys. A laboratory diagnosis to demonstrate the organism is necessary to confirm disease. Treatment consists of injecting the whole litter with long-acting penicillin (sometimes piglets vomit when using procaine penicillin but this is not of any consequence). All breeding herds should be vaccinated for erysipelas.

GLÄSSERS DISEASE (*HAEMOPHILUS PARASUIS* HPS)

This is caused by the bacterium *Haemophilus parasuis*, a small organism, of which there are at least fifteen different types. It is ubiquitous, found throughout the world and is present even in high health herds. If such herds are set up using SPF or MEW techniques and are free from Hps it can be devastating when they first become contaminated, producing an anthrax-like disease with high mortality in sows. In the majority of herds in which the bacterium is endemic, sows produce a strong maternal immunity which normally persists in their offspring until 8 to 12 weeks of age and as a result, the effects of the infection in weaners are usually nil or very minimal. The pigs become sub-clinically infected when still protected and then stimulate their own immune response. If however the maternal immunity wears off before they become infected they may develop severe disease. It can however become a secondary organism where there are other major pathogens and in particular enzootic pneumonia. Outbreaks of disease are sometimes experienced in sucking pigs, particularly in gilt herds.

Clinical signs

Acute disease

Pigs with glässers disease become rapidly depressed, with an elevated temperature, stop eating and are reluctant to rise. Hps attacks the smooth surfaces of the joints, coverings of the intestine, lungs, heart and brain. In young growing pigs meningitis or middle ear infections are common together with pneumonia, heart sac infection, peritonitis and pleurisy. Hps also causes individual cases of arthritis and lameness with acute pain, fever and inappetance. It is respiratory spread and a characteristic feature is a short cough of only 2-3 episodes. Sudden death in good sucking piglets is not uncommon in herds with a problem and in particular when immunity in gilt litters is low.

Chronic disease

Sucking piglets are often pale and poor growing and 10-15% may be affected in a litter. Such pigs then continue into the growing period with poor growth. When long standing pericarditis is a feature sudden deaths occur.

Diagnosis

This is confirmed by clinical observations, post-mortem examinations and isolation of the organism in the laboratory but it is not an easy one to grow.

Similar diseases

These would include:
Actinobacillus suis.
App.
Mulberry heart disease.
Streptococcal meningitis.
Streptococcal septicaemias.
Post-mortem and bacteriological examinations are required to differentiate.

Treatment

- Hps has a wide antibiotic sensitivity including amoxycillin, ampicillin, OTC, sulphonamides, penicillin and ceftiofur.
- Look for the very early signs of huddling and shivering and identify clinical cases.
- Treatment must be given early, particularly if cases of meningitis are occurring. It is important to differentiate this disease from streptococcal meningitis and this can only be done by isolating the respective organisms from the brain.
- Identify the onset of disease in sucking pigs and inject 3 to 4 days prior to this to prevent disease, with long-acting penicillin.
- Treatments are best, using injections of either penicillin/streptomycin, trimethoprim/sulpha or synthetic penicillins.
- Treat for 2 to 3 days.
- Medicate the water with amoxycillin or phenoxymethyl penicillin for 4-5 days over the period of risk.

Management control and prevention

- Where the disease is a problem in sucking pigs the sows feed can be top dressed daily 7 days before and 7 days after farrowing with phenoxymethyl penicillin.
- Alternatively sows can be injected with long-acting penicillin at point of farrowing.
- Autogenous vaccines can be produced and given to the sow to stimulate an immunity but the response is serotype specific and in any one herd there may be a number of different serotypes. The vaccines need to be multivalent.
- The lactating and creep rations can be medicated with 200-300g of phenoxymethyl penicillin.
- Apply the relevant general principles discussed for the control of respiratory disease in chapter 9.

GREASY PIG DISEASE - (EXUDATIVE EPIDERMITIS)

This is caused by the bacterium *Staphylococcus hyicus* which invades abraded skin causing infection. The *Staphylococcus* produces toxins which are absorbed into the system and damage the liver and kidneys. The disease is also called exudative epidermitis which describes the oozing of fluid from the inflamed skin. In the sucking piglet disease is usually confined to individual animals, but it can be a major problem in new gilt herds and weaned pigs.

It has been shown recently that during the days immediately preceding farrowing the bacterium multiples profusely in the sows vagina. Piglets are frequently infected during the birth process or soon after. The sharp eye teeth often damage the cheeks during competition for a teat, or the knees are traumatised when seeking to suck milk. These may trigger the disease. In severe cases where the liver becomes damaged the piglet will die. Often only 50% of piglets affected during suckling will survive.

Clinical signs

These usually commence with small, dark, localised areas of infection around the face or on the legs, where the skin has been damaged. The skin along the flanks the belly and between the legs changes to a brown colour gradually involving the whole of the body. The skin becomes wrinkled with flaking of large areas and it has a greasy feel. A more localised picture is seen if the sow has passed some immunity to the piglet, with small circumscribed lesions approximately 5-10mm in diameter that do not spread. In weaned pigs disease may appear 2-3 days after weaning with a slight browning of the skin that progresses to a dark greasy texture. In severe cases the skin turns black. Such cases usually die due to the toxins produce by the staphylococci organisms. In nurseries up to 15% of the population may be involved.

Diagnosis

This is based on the characteristic skin lesions. (See chapter 10). In an outbreak it is important to culture the organism and carry out an antibiotic sensitivity test. A moist wet area should be identified, the overlying scab removed and a swab rubbed well into the infected area. This should be returned to the laboratory in transport medium to arrive as soon as possible, certainly within 24 hours.

Treatment

- Determine the antibiotic sensitivity and inject affected piglets daily for 5 days, or on alternate days with a long-acting antibiotic to which the organism is sensitive to.
- Antibiotics include; amoxycillin, OTC, ceftiofur, cephalexin, gentamycin, lincomycin or penicillin.
- Topical application of antibiotics can also be of use. Novobiocin, an antibiotic used for treating mastitis in dairy cows, can be mixed with mineral oil and sprayed onto the skin or the piglets dipped into a solution of it.
- Piglets become very dehydrated and should be offered electrolytes by mouth.
- Ensure there are no mange problems in the herd. The mange mites damage the skin and allow *Staphylococcus hyicus* to enter.
- Long-acting injections can be given 2 to 3 days before the first signs are likely to appear as a method of prevention. Use either long-acting amoxycillin or OTC if indicated.
- In severe outbreaks an autogenous vaccine can be prepared from the organism and sows injected twice 4 and 2 weeks prior to farrowing to raise immunity in the colostrum. This has proved successful on a number of farms where disease has appeared in both the sucking and weaned pigs.
- If the problem is occurring in gilt litters, cross suckling these piglets using older sows at birth for 4 or 5 hours can be of value.

Management control and prevention

- Examine the pigs to see where abrasions are taking place. For example, these may be arising from new concrete surfaces or rough metal floors.
- If concrete surfaces are poor, brush these over after cleaning with hydrated lime that contains a phenol disinfectant.
- Check the procedures for removing tails and teeth. Jagged edges of teeth can damage the gums leading to infection around the cheeks particularly when piglets fight for teat access and during mixing after weaning.
- The skin of the udder is one reservoir of infection. This should be sprayed daily 3 days before and after farrowing with a iodine based skin antiseptic (cow teat dip is ideal).
- Disinfect floors well between farrowings.
- Make sure that sharp needles are used for iron injections and change these regularly between litters.
- If mange is present in the herd treat the sow prior to entering the farrowing house.
- Extremes of humidity and wet pens can encourage the multiplication of the bacteria.
- Metal floors and side panels, in particular woven metal flooring, can cause severe abrasions particularly around the feet and legs. In such cases the first signs of greasy pig will be in these areas. Damage to the face by metal feeding troughs can precipitate disease.
- Check the humidity of the weaning accommodation. High levels above 70% and high temperatures provide an ideal environment for the multiplication of the bacteria on the skin.
- Adopt an all-in all-out policy in the weaning accommodation. Have the pens bacteriologically checked after they have been washed out and disinfected.

HYPOGLYCAEMIA - LOW BLOOD SUGAR LEVEL

The newborn piglet can be born with low glycogen reserves in the liver and during the first few days of life it is unable to mobilise this to provide adequate levels of glucose in the blood. It is therefore dependent for energy on a regular intake of lactose from the sows milk. If a piglet cannot obtain sufficient to maintain its energy output, the body temperature drops and it ultimately goes into a coma and dies.

Clinical signs

These progress from an animal laid on its belly, shivering and becoming very cold to eventually lying on its side, paddling, frothing at the mouth and becoming comatosed. The eyes are sunken and the head bent backwards.

Diagnosis

Hypoglycaemia occurs in the first 12-24 hours of

birth and the clinical picture is characterised by the symptoms. Examine the eyes to see that there is no evidence of lateral movements (nystagmus) which would indicate meningitis.

Treatment
- ☐ The condition must be recognised early if treatment is to be successful.
- ☐ Immediately remove the piglet to a warm draught free environment to achieve 30°C. A box well bedded in shavings with an infra-red lamp above is ideal.
- ☐ Feed the piglet with sow or alternatively cows colostrum or 20% dextrose solution by syringe or stomach tube every 20 minutes until it has returned to normal. Then introduce the piglet to a newly farrowed sow.

Management control and prevention
- ◆ Identify potential piglets at birth and treat as describe under poor viable piglets.

LEPTOSPIROSIS
See chapter 6 for further information.

Leptospira occasionally affect the sucking piglet, infection coming from the urine of rodents or the carrier pig. The main type involved is *L icterohaemorrhagiae*. Piglets become ill, inappetent with jaundice and blood in the urine. Severely infected pigs die. Leptospira are sensitive to oxytetracycline, penicillin and streptomycin antibiotics. The disease can also be spread to humans if infected urine makes contact with broken skin or mucous membranes.

Disease is uncommon in the sucking pig and would only involve individuals.

MANGE MITES (SARCOPTES SCABIEI)
See chapter 11 for further information.

Mange is caused by a small skin parasite *Sarcoptes scabiei*. The life cycle of the mite is at least 3 weeks and disease therefore will be rarely seen in the sucking piglet but infection is often picked up from the carrier sow at this time. However it is a common disease in the weaned and growing pig and adult animals. Control is by treating the sow pre-farrowing.

MIDDLE EAR INFECTIONS
See chapter 9 for further information.

This disease occurs occasionally in the sucking pig from 7 to 10 days of age. The middle part of the ear is responsible for balance and infection causes the piglet to hold its head on the affected side and to lose its balance. Infection arises as a sequel to joint infections or septicaemia and the common organisms involved include;
Haemophilus parasuis, streptococci, and staphylococci. Early identification of the condition is essential to allow prompt treatment. This should be carried out using daily antibiotic injections of penicillin/streptomycin, OTC or amoxycillin. It is more common in the weaned pig.

NAVEL BLEEDING / PALE PIG SYNDROME
At birth or within a few hours the piglet becomes extremely pale and in many cases dies. The condition arises in one of three ways:
1. Anoxia or shortage of oxygen inside the womb during farrowing causes the piglet to pool its blood into the placenta. If it is born and the cord separated at this point, then it will be born very pale and anaemic. This picture is seen when piglets are delivered by hysterectomy and they are removed from the womb at a critical time before the piglet has time to recall its blood from the placenta. Affected piglets are more likely from old sows and in large litters.
2. Pigs are sometimes born with a haemorrhage or a haematoma in the cord itself. The cause of this is unknown but in some cases it is related to premature removal of the piglet from behind the sow at farrowing. The blood vessels in the cord bleed.
3. Continual bleeding from the navel during the first 3 to 4 hours after birth.

Clinical signs
Fresh blood on the floor of the pen arising from the end of the navel is diagnostic.

Treatment
- ☐ Early recognition of a bleeding navel is essential. The cord should be clamped approximately 13mm from the skin using an umbilical clip. (See chapter 15). Those used for babies are ideal. Nylon or plastic ties used to bind together electrical wires are also good
- ☐ As an alternate and in an acute emergency the navel can be tied in a knot.
- ☐ A ligature can be applied around the umbilicus but it shrinks and the bleeding often continues. The cord should be bent back on itself and re-tied in the shape of a "U".

Management control and prevention
- ◆ Navel bleeding is associated with the use of wood shavings as bedding. The reasons for this are unknown but wood preservatives or other substances may be responsible.
  Change the shavings to an alternate source or use straw for bedding.
- ◆ Warfarin poisoning can be responsible for haemorrhage.
- ◆ Vitamin C was thought to be involved and im-

provements by feeding sows with 1g/day have been reported. Experiences however with this vitamin have been disappointing.
- Do not move pigs away from the sow immediately at farrowing. Allow the piglet to break the cord naturally. There is a particular part of the cord where separation takes place naturally without any haemorrhage. The navel cord is always slightly longer than the birth canal so that when the newborn piglet starts to rise and walk the cord is stretched, breaks and recoils to block the blood vessels. It should not be cut.
- Supplementing the diet with vitamin K can sometimes help.
- Mycotoxins from contaminated feed have been implicated.
- A riboflavin deficiency has been implicated.
- In some herds there appears to be an association with the use of prostaglandin to synchronise farrowings.
- Do not allow excessive trauma to the cord within 3 hours of birth. This may occur if too many piglets are fastened in the creep area.

PORCINE EPIDEMIC DIARRHOEA (PED) - SCOUR

Porcine epidemic diarrhoea is caused by a coronavirus somewhat similar to that which causes TGE. This virus is widespread in Europe particularly. The virus damages the villi in the gut thus reducing the absorptive surface, with loss of fluid and dehydration. After introduction into a susceptible breeding herd, disease is followed by a strong immunity over two to three weeks. The colostral immunity then protects the piglets. The virus disappears spontaneously from small breeding herds but tends to be maintained in finishing farms due to the repeated introduction and subsequent infection of susceptible pigs.

Clinical signs

Acute disease

This occurs where the virus is introduced into a susceptible population for the first time. In such cases up to 100% of sows may be affected, showing a mild to very watery diarrhoea. Two clinical pictures are recognised: PED Type I only affects growing pigs where as PED Type II affects all ages including sucking pigs and mature sows. The incubation period is approximately 2 days and the disease episode lasts for 7 to 14 days. In sucking pigs the disease can be mild or severe with mortalities up to 40%.

Endemic disease

In large breeding herds, particularly if kept extensively, not all the females may become infected first time round and there may be recrudescence. This only occurs in piglets suckling from sows with no maternal antibodies and it is therefore sporadic.

Diagnosis

This can be suspected on the clinical signs but it cannot be differentiated from TGE. If acute diarrhoea is occurring in weaned and older animals on a growing/finishing farm with no symptoms in sucking piglets then this would suggest PED Type I. PED Type II would affect piglets. Virus particles from diarrhoea samples can be identified under the electron microscope but this would not differentiate PED from TGE. Blood tests can be carried out to look for rising antibody titres. An ELISA test is also available for examining diarrhoea samples or intestinal contents.

Treatment

- Because this is a virus infection there is no specific treatment but often secondary bacteria complicate the picture and these can be treated by broad spectrum antibiotics such as neomycin, framycetin, apramycin or trimethoprim/sulpha.
- If the virus enters the herd for the first time it is important to ensure that all the adult animals become infected at an early stage to allow an early immunity to develop. This can be achieved by exposing sows to the diarrhoea three times, two days apart via the drinking water. Mix scour or contaminated material into a bucket of water and use this as the source.

PORCINE REPRODUCTIVE AND RESPIRATORY SYNDROME (PRRS)

See chapter 6 for further information.

Disease is normally only a problem in piglets when the virus infects the herd for the first time. It may continue infecting litters for up to 12 weeks until all sows have had sufficient time to develop an immunity and pass this protection on through the colostrum.

Clinical signs

In the early stages of acute disease piglets are born in a very weak condition and rapidly become hypoglycaemic because they are unable to get to the teat and suckle. Together with weak pigs there are a high numbers of stillbirths and late mummified ones. Newborn piglets show sticky brown material over the eyelids and very occasionally small blisters on the skin. Scour, pneumonia and coughing are commonly observed but with increasing time the quality and survivability of the piglets improves.

Diagnosis

This is based on the herd history, clinical signs both in piglets and sows and serological and virological tests.

Similar diseases

Aujeszky's disease (AD) when it first enters the herd

can be confused with PRRS but nervous signs are present with AD but not with PRRS. A serological test will differentiate between the two.

Treatment

- [ ] This is aimed at preventing secondary infections, usually either respiratory or enteric until an immunity builds up.
- [ ] Piglets should be injected with either long-acting OTC or amoxycillin on days 3, 7 and 14 after farrowing.
- [ ] Electrolytes should be given to counteract dehydration.

Management control and prevention

- ◆ Raise the farrowing house temperature during the period of farrowing and whilst disease is active to 23ºC (75ºF).
- ◆ Provide extra bedding. Use shavings or other suitable materials to create the best environment for the piglet.
- ◆ Provide an extra heat lamp by the side of the sow.

PORCINE RESPIRATORY CORONA VIRUS INFECTION (PRCV)

See chapter 12 for further information.

PRCV is a relatively new virus that first appeared in pigs some ten years or more ago in Europe. It is related to but distinct from TGE virus, which is another corona virus.

PRCV is respiratory spread and believed to travel long distances and because of this it is extremely difficult to maintain herds free from it and very few countries have not been exposed.

Clinically it is totally non-pathogenic and field experiences have shown that herds exposed for the first time have no symptoms of disease.

It has been suggested however that it may have an effect on lung tissue when other respiratory pathogens are present in chronic respiratory disease complexes.

PRCV does however cross react with the serological test for TGE and it therefore can confuse the diagnosis. A differential test is available.

PRCV has no clinical effect on the sucking pig but infection often takes place at 2 to 3 weeks of age from the sow or airborne from weaned pigs. It is not of importance.

ROTAVIRUS DIARRHOEA

These viruses are widespread both in pig populations and most other mammals and there are a number of different types or groups.

Group A is probably the common pig one, but B, C and E also occur. However the frequency with which different ones occur is unknown and from a practical view point it is probably academic.

Rotaviruses are ubiquitous and they are present in most if not all pig herds with virtually a 100% sero-conversion in adult stock. A further epidemiological feature is their persistence outside the pig, where they are resistant to environmental changes and many disinfectants. Maternal antibodies persist for 3-6 weeks after which pigs become susceptible to infection but exposure does not necessarily result in disease. It is estimated that only 10-15% of diarrhoeas in pigs are initiated by a primary rotavirus infection.

The fact that the virus persists in the environment accounts for widespread infection and therefore a constant risk of disease.

Clinical signs

In a mature herd disease appears after piglets are 7 to 10 days of age, with a watery profuse diarrhoea in younger animals. It becomes progressively less important with age. However if pathogenic strains of E. coli are present severe disease can occur with heavy mortality. Villus atrophy is a consistent feature with dehydration and malabsorption and diarrhoea usually persists for 3-4 days. Pigs look hollow in the abdomen the eyes are sunken and the skin around the rectum is wet.

The role of rotaviruses in the post-weaned pig is probably less important although they are often identified when acute E. coli diarrhoea occurs in the first 7-10 days after weaning.

Diagnosis

Whenever there is a diarrhoea problem in pigs from 10 to 40 days of age rotavirus infection either as primary agents or secondary must be considered. Laboratory examinations are required by electron microscopy and ELISA tests. Try the litmus test by soaking scour in litmus paper, E. coli infections turn blue, virus infections red.

Treatment

- [ ] There are no specific treatments for rotavirus infections.
- [ ] Provide antibiotic therapy either by injection, by mouth or in the drinking water, to control secondary infections such as E. coli.
- [ ] Apralan, amoxycillin, neomycin, framycetin and enrofloxacin could be used.
- [ ] Provide dextrose/glycine electrolytes to counteract dehydration.
- [ ] Provide dry warm and comfortable lying areas.

Management control and prevention

- ◆ Reduce the levels of virus in the environment by all-in all-out procedures and effective disinfection. Leave the house empty for 2 to 4 days before pigs are moved in.
- ◆ Disinfect with peroxygen based disinfectants such

as Virkon S or chlorine based ones.
- Reduce the spread of virus between infected and non infected pigs. Use foot dips and clean clothing and wash hands after handling sick pigs.
- Apply control procedures outlined for coliform infections.
- If a persistent problem is diagnosed in sucking pigs expose sows to piglet scour by collecting it in wet saw dust, or mix the faeces in waters. Feed the contaminated material via the watering systems or into troughs two to three times weekly. Carry this out in weeks four and three before farrowing.
- Modified live vaccines are available in some countries.
- In the weaned pig adopt all-in all-out procedures with cleaning and disinfection in first stage flat decks. Pay particular attention to environmental stress and temperature fluctuations.

SALMONELLOSIS
See chapter 9 for further information.

Disease would be uncommon in the sucking pig due to passive immunity provided via colostrum. If the piglets are infected with PRRS virus salmonella may become secondary invaders. Control procedures are similar to those adopted for diarrhoea and *E. coli* infections.

SPLAYLEGS

This is a condition where the newborn piglet is unable to hold the front and/or (more commonly) back legs together and up to 2 % of piglets can be affected. The mobility of the piglet is impaired which makes teat access difficult. It is more common in the Landrace breed and males. Disease is caused by immaturity of the muscle fibres in the hind legs, over the pelvis and occasionally in the front legs.

Clinical signs

The piglets are unable to stand with the hind legs deflected laterally and as a result they often adopt a dog sitting position. The condition is exaggerated when piglets stand on very smooth or wet slippery floors. Death usually ensues either due to starvation or crushing, because the pig cannot move away from the sow.

Diagnosis

This is based upon the clinical signs.

Treatment

- As soon as the affected pig is identified use 25mm wide elastoplast and tape the hind legs together leaving a gap of 50-80mm. The same procedure can be applied to the fore legs. The sticky tape should be passed around the legs just above the supernumerary digits. Never use string it will stran-

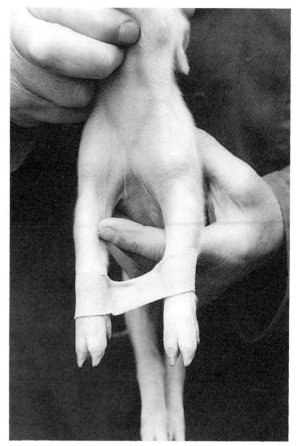

Taping the legs of a splay leg piglet.
(Fig.8-32)

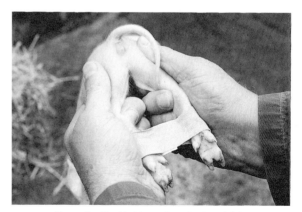

Massaging the hind legs of a splay leg piglet.
(Fig.8-33)

gulate the legs if not removed. Fig.8-32.
- Hold the piglet up by both its hind legs and vigorously massage the muscle masses over the pelvis and the front and rear of the hind legs. Repeat this 3 or 4 times during the first day. Fig.8-33.
- Assist the piglet to suckle 2 to 3 times daily.
- Dose the pig with 10mls of sows colostrum or

- cows colostrum immediately after birth.
- Confine the strongest mobile pigs into the creep area for a period of one hour to allow splay leg pigs uninhibited access to the teats.

Management control and prevention
- If floor surfaces are smooth these can be roughened by covering with lime wash or increase the use of bedding, particular by sawdust, shavings or newsprint.

STREPTOCOCCAL MENINGITIS
See also chapter 9; Streptococcal infections for further information.

Meningitis denotes inflammation of the meninges which are the membranes covering the brain. In the sucking piglet it is usually caused by *Streptococcus suis, Haemophilus parasuis,* or sometimes bacteria such as *E. coli* and other streptococci. *S. suis* has many serotypes. In most countries *S. suis* type 1 is the main one in sucking piglets, but this may not be true in other countries. For example in Denmark it is type 7. *S. suis* also causes joint problems particularly types 1 and 14. *S. suis* is carried for long periods in the tonsils and may be transmitted to the sucking piglet from the sow or from other piglets. The sow also provides a variable level of immunity in the colostrum. Streptococcal meningitis in sucking piglets is sporadic occurring occasionally in individual piglets. *S. suis* type 1 occasionally cause meningitis but more commonly joint infections. Meningitis in piglets is more commonly caused by *Haemophilus parasuis* or glässers disease.

Clinical signs
These are rapid in onset, the piglet lying on its belly and shivering. When presented with such symptoms also consider scour or joint infections from a septicaemia.

Meningitis is characterised by a continual movement of the eyes from one side to the other (nystagmus) and this is an early diagnostic symptom together with shivering and shaking, paddling and convulsions. In acute cases the piglet may just be found dead. Streptococcal meningitis may be worse in sucking pigs when the organism has been introduced into the herd for the first time, or where it is secondary to infection with PRRS.

Diagnosis
The organism must be isolated from the meninges of clinically affected pigs and identified in a laboratory.

Treatment
- If your herd has a problem always examine the at risk pigs twice daily to identify and treat affected pigs early.
- *Streptococcus suis* is usually sensitive to penicillin, synthetic penicillin's or sulphonamides.
- Injections of penicillin should be given twice daily.
- Good nursing is equally important because the condition is very painful. Remove the piglet during the first 3 to 6 hours from the litter to a warm environment and carefully supplement it with milk via a stomach tube.

Similar diseases
Consider joint infections, glässers disease, generalised septicaemia, salt poisoning, aujeszky's disease and hypoglycaemia.

Management control and prevention
- It is possible to vaccinate the sow using an autogenous vaccine to improve the colostral immunity.
- The sow can be injected with long-acting penicillin just before farrowing.
- The litter can be injected with long-acting penicillin in anticipation of disease.

SWINE DYSENTERY (SD)
See chapter 9 for further information.

This is a very important disease in the growing and finishing pig but not so in the piglet. It is unusual to see SD in sucking pigs except when the organism *Serpulina hyodysenteriae,* first enters the herd. In such cases there may be sloppy faeces in the sow often containing some blood and mucus and a similar type of diarrhoea in piglets. In rare cases it may be much more dramatic with very bloody faeces. In herds in which the organism is endemic the lactating sow may be a carrier and infect the older piglet, but there will be no disease in the piglet until maternal antibodies disappear.

SWINE INFLUENZA (SI)
See chapter 6 for further information.

It would be unusual to see any signs of swine flu in the sucking pig unless disease entered the herd for the first time. Colostrum prevents infection during the sucking period. SI is manifest by coughing and short periods of illness and secondary pneumonia. Usually no treatment is required unless the pneumonia is severe. Good nursing, increasing farrowing house temperatures and bedding are important during the acute period. The disease becomes active in the young growing pig and periodically in the sow as immunity rises and falls.

TEAT NECROSIS
Teat necrosis describes a condition where constant rubbing and pressure on the end of the teat causes the teat sphincter and delicate tissues to die (necrosis) and slough off. It is of no consequence in commercial herds which are buying in replacement gilts but it is a very important condition where breeding stock are being produced.

Clinical signs

It first becomes evident 12 to 24 hours after birth. The teat end appears bright red gradually becoming black. Trauma to the teats occurs on all floor surfaces but to a lesser extent on those that are well bedded with shavings or straw. The teats in front of the umbilicus are the ones at risk because these have the greatest contact with the floor during sucking.

The damage to the tissues can be severe resulting in a blind or inverted teat.

Treatment

☐ There is no treatment for this condition and prevention is necessary.

Management control and prevention

◆ As soon as the female piglets are born and have dried off they should be held by the hind legs and the teats anterior to the umbilicus coated with a protective compound. Such compounds could include copydex, a white rubbery glue used for sticking carpets, cow gum which is a rubberised solution often used for sticking photographs into albums or a contact adhesive such as evostik. These compounds gradually disappear over the next 3 to 4 days but protect the teats during the susceptible period

TETANUS

Tetanus is caused by the bacterium *Clostridium tetani* which produces toxins that affect the central nervous system. The organism, which can form spores, lives in the large intestines and faeces of many mammals, including pigs and in certain soils. It must enter through a dirty abrasion or a cut. In the sucking pig the most common source is castration. Tetanus spores are found in the soil and this disease can be a problem in outdoor pigs. The incubation period is from 1 to 10 weeks. It would be uncommon to see disease in the sucking piglet under 2 weeks of age. The affected piglet is hypersensitive, shows stiffness of legs and muscles, an erect tail and muscular spasms of the ears and face. A multivalent clostridium vaccine containing tetanus toxoid is highly efficient in preventing disease and could be used in pregnant sows if a herd has a problem. Castration techniques should also be checked because unhygienic methods can lead to infection and tetanus 2-8 weeks later.

THROMBOCYTOPAENIC PURPURA - BLEEDING

This is an uncommon condition seen only in young piglets from approximately 7 to 21 days of age. It arises when the sows colostrum contains antibodies that destroy the piglets blood platelets (thrombocytes). The immune system of the sow during the period of pregnancy recognises the platelets as foreign protein and produces antibodies against them. The formation of these antibodies is also related to the boar that is used. Disease commences 7 to 10 days after the intake of colostrum.

Clinical signs

These can be sudden and are indicated by good pigs found dead. Look closely at the skin of these and you will see haemorrhages wherever there as been bruising, teeth marks or trauma.

Haemorrhages are evident throughout all body tissues. The piglet dies through the failure of normal blood clotting mechanisms. The disease is very sporadic but up to half the litter may be affected. Invariably the pigs die.

Treatment

There is no known treatment other than good nursing. In the early stages of the disease it is worthwhile cross-fostering litters to remove exposure to any lingering antibodies in the sows milk.

Management control and prevention

◆ Where a sow has produced such a litter make sure she is mated with a different boar at the next pregnancy or cull her.

TRANSMISSIBLE GASTRO-ENTERITIS (TGE)

TGE is a very important and highly infectious disease in the piglet caused by a corona virus. It is similar in structure but quite distinct from the corona virus PRCV that infects the respiratory system.

TGE virus enters the pig by mouth and multiplies in the villi (finger like structures in the small intestine) and destroys them. This takes place in 24 to 48 hours and is followed by vomiting and a very severe acute diarrhoea with high mortality. When the virus enters the herd for the first time mortality in piglets up to 14 days of age may be 100%. This decreases in pigs over 3 weeks of age but morbidity is high.

The virus multiplies in the intestine and is shed in large numbers in the faeces. Pig faeces therefore are the major source of transmission either directly through the purchased carrier pig or indirectly through mechanical transmission.

The virus is killed by sunlight within a few hours but will survive for long periods outside the pig in cold or freezing conditions. It is very susceptible to disinfectants particularly iodine based ones, quaternary ammonia and peroxygen compounds.

Dogs and cats may shed the virus in their faeces for 2 to 3 weeks.

Birds and in particular starlings may transmit the disease and management should ensure that feed is not exposed to attract these birds.

Read chapters 2 and 3 on biological control of diseases entering the farm and the precautions necessary to prevent diseases spreading by faeces.

Clinical signs

Acute disease

The most striking feature of TGE when it is first introduced into the herd, is the rapidity of spread. It affects all classes of pig on the farm with evidence of vomiting and diarrhoea. Adult animals show varying degrees of inappetance and usually recover over a 5 to 7 day period. In the sucking piglet the disease is very severe and under 3 weeks of age there is a very acute watery diarrhoea with almost 100% mortality within 2 to 3 days in piglets under 7 days of age due to severe dehydration and electrolyte imbalance. There is no response to antibiotic therapy. The most striking feature is the wet and dirty appearance of all the litter due to the profuse diarrhoea. Disease will persist in the farrowing houses over a period of 3 to 4 weeks until sows have developed sufficient immunity to protect the piglets.

Chronic or endemic disease

In herds less than 300 sows the virus is usually self eliminating provided there are good all-in-all-out procedures in farrowing houses and grower accommodation. In some herds however the virus will persist in the growing herd because piglets at weaning time, still under the influence of the maternal antibody, move into houses where the virus still persists. Once the antibody disappears the pigs become infected allowing the virus to multiply. The pigs then shed the virus, contaminating the weaner rooms and infecting pigs being weaned after them. TGE can become endemic in herds in a mild form with high morbidity but low mortality.

Diagnosis

The clinical picture in acute disease is almost diagnostic. There are no other enteric diseases that would spread so rapidly across all pigs. The ultimate diagnosis of TGE must be made in the laboratory from the intestine of a fresh dead pig using fluorescent antibody tests. Isolation of the virus is also carried out.

Similar diseases

In the acute form epidemic diarrhoea could give a similar picture but it would be less acute and with less mortality in sucking pigs. Where TGE has become chronic then differentiation from the other causes of diarrhoea must be carried out in a laboratory. If the herd has been infected previously with TGE and there are scour problems persisting it is necessary to determine whether the virus is still present or not.

Treatment

- There is no specific treatment for TGE.
- Antibiotic treatment by mouth in individual piglets may reduce secondary infections.
- Provide easy access to water containing electrolyte and an antibiotic such as neomycin. Make this available to the litters twice daily.
- Improve the nursing and environment of the litter by providing extra heat and deep bedding to reduce the weights of infection from the diarrhoea.

Management control and prevention

- As soon as disease is suspected isolate those farrowing houses not infected, by using separate personnel boots and coveralls. This is particularly important in piglets under 14 days of age. The longer the disease can be kept away the more pigs will be reared and mortality reduced.
- If it is possible move sows that are within 3 weeks of farrowing from the farm before they become infected so that they could farrow down in an isolated building or outside in arks and escape disease.
- It is essential to develop immunity in the dry sows as soon as possible.
- There are two methods, either squeeze the piglets abdomen and collect the diarrhoea into a bowl or use sawdust or shavings in the areas where the piglets are scouring. Paper towels can also be used to soak up piglet faeces. This material is then mixed with a bucket of water and fed to the pregnant sows, (feed back).
- A further method is to collect the small intestines from a number of pigs that have died and macerate them in a food blending machine. The liquid provides a rich source of virus and this can if required be preserved by deep freezing.
- The disease should be spread as soon as possible across the whole farm. The object is to get a good immunity developed in the shortest possible period of time. It will take approximately 3 to 4 weeks to achieve this.
- Once the infected period is over ensure an all-in and all-out management system of the farrowing houses, weaner and finisher accommodation.
- Disinfection of pens between batches should be carried out using an iodine based disinfectant or one highly active against viruses
- This cleaning process is an important one to ensure the virus does not linger on the farm and become endemic.
- If your herd as become infected with TGE ask the question why and how? Look at all your prevention procedures and biosecurity as discussed in chapter 2. (Do this before you get TGE).
- Always provide boots and protective clothing for any one entering your farm.
- Provide disinfectant foot dips at all entrances.
- Keep starlings and migrating birds away from the farm by not exposing them to feed.
- Do not borrow equipment from another pig farm.
- Site all bins to the exterior of the unit and always

have your own feeder pipes to your own feed bins. This is a high risk source for the spread of enteric diseases.
- Vaccination - live modified and killed vaccines are available in some countries. The results in the field are very variable. The objective is to maintain immunity in the colostrum. This can only be carried out by stimulating the gut of the sow to produce antibodies in the milk. Intra-muscular vaccines give a very poor response.

VOMITING AND WASTING DISEASE / ONTARIO ENCEPHALITIS

This is caused by a coronavirus called haemagglutinating encephalomyelitis virus (HEV). The virus is widespread in the pig populations of North America and is probably world-wide but is unimportant because clinical disease is rare. This is because most sows have been infected and are immune. They pass their immunity to their piglets in colostrum which protects them through the vulnerable period. Although the virus can infect susceptible pigs at any age it only causes clinical disease in newborn piglets.

Clinical signs

Although there is only one antigenic type of the virus there is a variation in virulence between strains resulting in two different disease syndromes. Both start at around 4 days of age, are sudden in onset and affect whole litters. The piglets are huddled and hairy. They vomit bright green-yellow vomitus which is often mistaken for acute scour. Infact they are constipated.

In the typical vomiting and wasting disease syndrome they lose their ability to suck or swallow, become very thirsty and stand with their heads over water but are unable to drink. They rapidly waste away, become severely emaciated and die.

In the typical encephalitis syndrome they froth and champ at the mouth, develop blueing of their extremities, their abdomens become bloated and they tremble. They have a stilted gait which rapidly progresses to partial paralysis of the legs. They lie down, go into convulsions, roll their eyes and die within two to four days of onset.

Diagnosis

The clinical picture in 4 day old piglets of vomiting and constipation is characteristic of the disease. If you open up their abdomens the appearance is typical, gas in the stomach and intestine but no food, only some brightly coloured liquid. Firm faeces and sometimes brightly coloured crystals in the kidneys. A blood test is available.

Treatment

None is available.

Management control and prevention

- All the affected pigs will die so they are best destroyed. This is a one-off phenomenon which tends to occur in small herds in the litters of sows which have no immunity. The virus will circulate and immunise the herd. The disease will not occur again in these sows' litters or any others.

VITAMIN E DEFICIENCY AND IRON TOXICITY

See chapter 14 for further information.

Iron toxicity occurs when the sow is deficient in vitamin E and piglets are born as a consequence with low levels. The routine iron dextran injections become toxic and cause severe muscle reactions at the injection sites. Vitamin E deficiency in the sow occurs when fats in the diet become rancid or cereals or corn have fermented and spoiled and the vitamin E is destroyed.

Clinical signs

Two to four hours after injection most of the litter become acutely lame on the legs that have received the iron. the muscles are swollen and the piglets develop heavy breathing and look pale. Death occurs within 24 hours. At post-mortem the muscles are coagulated and appear like fish tissue due to necrosis of the muscle fibres.

Diagnosis

This is based upon the history of deaths within 24 hours of iron injections and swollen muscles at the site of the injections.

Treatment

☐ Inject sows due to farrow over the next 3 weeks with a vitamin E selenium preparation.
☐ Alternatively use water soluble vitamin E.
☐ Inject all litters for a 3 week period with vitamin E or dose by mouth at least 2 days before iron injections are given.

Management control and prevention

- Clean out the cereals at the bottom of the storage bins.
- Assess cereals and corn for spoilage.
- Supplement the sow feed with 150g/tonne vitamin E.

Summary - 12 key points to piglet survival

Piglet survival is increased by:

1. Maintaining a healthy sow.
2. Providing good hygiene at farrowing.
3. Providing extra heat lamps both at the side and behind the sow during farrowing.
4. Good observation at farrowing.

5. Maintaining a warm farrowing house without draughts and with good insulated floors.
6. Ensuring the piglet dries off quickly after farrowing.
7. Immediate removal of the piglet to the creep area for acclimatisation.
8. Maximising early colostrum intake.
9. Giving prompt assistance to weak pigs.
10. Fostering and even up of weights at birth.
11. Removing eye teeth promptly.
12. Cross fostering early.

> *All the above procedures require a good stockperson. Remember that their qualities include a sound knowledge, a recognition of the individual animals needs, patience, awareness, ability to organise their work, immediate attention to detail and the most important, a sense of achievement.*
> *If you have one look after him or her!*

Medicines and Other Drugs for use in lactating sows and sucking pigs

Common generic medicines that are used in the lactating sows and sucking pigs are shown in Fig.8-33. Because trade names for these medicines can vary from one country to another the right hand column can be used to categorise these for comparison of price and availability.

CHAPTER 8 - Managing and Treating Disease in the Farrowing and Sucking Period

INJECTABLE ANTIBIOTICS AND OTHER DRUGS FOR USE IN THE LACTATING SOW
* A Guide To Doses And Availability.

Actual Drug (Concentration mg/ml)	Some Trade Names	Short Acting Injections	Long Acting	Available Orally	Available In Feed g/tonne	Trade Names of Your Available Drugs
Amoxycillin (150)	Clamoxyl	1ml / 20kg	1ml / 10kg	✓	300-500	
Ampicillin (150)	Penbritin	1ml / 20kg				
Apramycin	Apralan			✓	100	
Baquiloprim (33) Sulpha (175)	Zaquilan	1ml / 20kg				
Calcium boroglucinate 40%	Same	1ml / 4kg				
Ceftiofur (50)	Excenel	1ml / 25kg	1ml / 16kg			
Chlortetracycline	Aureomycin			✓	300-900	
Cephalexin (180)	Ceporex	1ml / 25kg				
Chloramphenicol (100)	Same	1ml / 25kg				
Cortisone (2) (anti inflammatory)	Various	See data sheet				
Erythromycin	Eryterocin	1ml / 25kg		✓		
Flunixin (50) (anti toxin effects)	Finadyne	1ml / 45kg				
Framycetin (150)	Framomycin	1ml / 30kg				
Gentamycin (50)	Pangram	1ml / 10kg				
Intagen (oral scour vaccine)	Intagen				✓	
Ivermectin 1% (Parasites)	Ivomec	1ml / 33kg		✓	2-6	
Lincomycin (100)	Lincocin	1ml / 10kg		✓	110-220	
Neomycin	Neobiotic			✓	163	
Oxytocin (milk let down) 10iu/ml	Oxytocin	$1/2$ to 1ml				
Oxytetracycline (100)	Terramycin	1ml / 10kg	1ml / 10kg	✓	300-900	
Pessaries various			Per vagina			
Phenoxymethyl penicillin	Potencil			✓	200-300	
Phosmet 20% (mange)	Porect	Topical 1ml/10kg				
Primidone 250mg tablets	Mysolin (anti savaging)			15 - 30 mg/kg		
Procaine Penicillin (300)	Depocillin	1ml / 20kg				
Procaine(150) + Benzathine Penicillin (150)	Duphapen LA	1ml / 30kg	1ml / 30kg			
Penicillin(250) Streptomycin(250)	Duphapen strep	1ml / 25kg				
Prostaglandin	Planate	2ml				
Phenylbutazone (200)	Phenyzene	1ml / 50kg		✓		
Spectinomycin (100)	Spectam	1ml / 5kg		✓		
Streptomycin (250)	Devomycin	1ml / 10kg				
Sulphadimidine (33.3%) Sulphamezathine	Same	1ml / 3kg		✓	100-300	
Tiamulin (200)	Tiamutin	1ml / 20kg		✓	40-100	
Tilmicosin	Pulmotil			✓	200 - 400	
Trimethoprim (40) /sulpha (200)	Trivetrin	1ml / 16kg		✓	✓	
Tylosin (200)	Tylan	1ml / 50kg		✓	100	

* Consult your veterinarian

(Fig.8-33)

9 Managing and Treating Disease in the Weaner, Grower and Finishing Period

Managing the weaner for health and maximum productivity 285
Managing the growing pig for health and efficient production 288
Diseases of the weaned and growing pig 295
Identifying problems in the post-weaning period - 5-20kg weight 296
Identifying problems in the growing period - 20-110kg weight 298
    Abscesses 299
    Actinobacillus pleuropneumonia (APP) 299
    Anthrax 301
    Arthritis 301
    Atrophic rhinitis (AR) - progressive disease (PAR) 301
    Aujeszky's disease (AD) or pseudorabies (PR) 303
    Back muscle necrosis 304
    Bordetellosis 304
    Bursitis 304
    Bush foot / foot rot 304
    Classical swine fever (hog cholera), African swine fever 305
    Clostridial diseases 305
    Coccidiosis 305
    Coliform infections and post-weaning diarrhoea 306
    Colitis 307
    Enteric diseases 308
    Enzootic pneumonia (EP) or *Mycoplasma hyopneumoniae* infection 308
    Eperythrozoonosis (Epe) 311
    Erysipelas 312
    Foot-and-mouth disease (FMD) 313
    Fractures 313
    Gastric ulcers 314
    Glässers disease (*haemophilus parasuis* HPS) 315
    Greasy pig disease - (exudative epidermitis) 316
    Haematoma 317
    Lameness 317
    Leg weakness - osteochondrosis (OCD) 318
    Leptospirosis 319
    Mange mites (*Sarcoptes scabiei*) 319
    Middle ear infection 319
    Mortality 319
    Mulberry heart disease (vitamin E / selenium) 320
    Mycoplasma arthritis (*Mycoplasma hyosynoviae* infection) 321
    Oedema disease (OD) - bowel oedema 322
    Parasites 323
    Pasteurellosis 323
    Porcine epidemic diarrhoea (PED) 323
    Porcine enteropathy (PE) 324
    Porcine reproductive and respiratory syndrome (PRRS) 325
    Porcine respiratory coronavirus (PRCV) 326
    Porcine stress syndrome (PSS) 326
    Prolapse of the rectum 327
    Rectal stricture 328

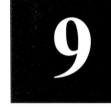

Managing Pig Health and the Treatment of Disease

- Respiratory diseases and control strategies 328
- Rotavirus.. 333
- Ruptures or hernias.. 334
- Salmonellosis... 334
- Salt poisoning - (water deprivation)... 336
- Spirochaetal diarrhoea 336
- Streptococcal infections 336
- Swine dysentery (SD) 338
- Swine influenza (SI)... 341
- Torsion of the stomach and intestines 341
- Transmissible gastro-enteritis (TGE) 342
- Tuberculosis 342
- Vice - abnormal behaviour (tail biting, flank chewing, ear biting).......... 342
- Yersinia infection 344
- Medicines and other drugs for use in weaned and finishing pigs 344

Managing and Treating Disease in the Weaner, Grower and Finishing Period

Managing the Weaner for Health and Maximum Productivity

The production of healthy weaners is a complex interaction between disease, the environment and management. Management decisions and procedures however are the initiating factors that cause abnormal conditions in the immediate post-weaning phase. These factors include:

- The production and maintenance of a healthy sucking pig.
- An adequate weaning weight for the weaning system.
- An optimum age of pig for the weaning system.
- An environment with the necessary temperature, ventilation and humidity for the age and weight of the pig.
- A correct diet for the age of the pig.
- Good feeding procedures.
- An all-in all-out system.

Key points to producing a healthy sucking pig

- Use a hybrid or cross bred female.
- Satisfy the nutritional requirements of the sow both in pregnancy and lactation.
- Bring a healthy sow into the farrowing house.
- Achieve good birth weights.
- Ensure each pig receives maximum colostrum at birth.
- Use a high energy and lysine diet in lactation to provide maximum nutrition for the litter.
- Provide good farrowing house management and hygiene. (Chapter 8).
- Vaccinate the gilt and sow against *E. coli* diarrhoea.
- Maintain an even creep temperature.
- Provide fresh uncontaminated creep feed pre-weaning.

Age and weight of the pig at weaning

Successful weaning requires a combination of both minimum age and weight at the time of weaning to suit the weaning system. Weaning ages generally range from 14 to 28 days with most intensive farms having a mean between 21 and 26. As weaning age is reduced it is important to appreciate the potential effects this might have, not only on the pig but also on the sow.

The effects of reducing weaning age

- The younger the pig the poorer its appetite at weaning.
- Poor feed intake results in lower daily liveweight gain.
- The younger the pig is weaned the less efficiently it will adapt to and digest solid food.
- Highly specialised diets are required.
- More weaning accommodation is required.
- A more exacting weaning environment is required; more supplementary heat, more labour, more costly housing and higher creep costs.
- The piglet is more susceptible to enteric diseases.
- There is often an increase in post-weaning mortality.
- A shorter lactation may reduce subsequent litter sizes and conception rates.
- The days from weaning to first mating interval may be increased with more sows showing vulval discharges and found not pregnant.
- Pigs produced per sow per annum or pigs weaned per crate can be increased.
- Pigs may be healthier if weaned away from the farm (SEW).

The question is "How do you determine the best age at which to wean on your farm"?
This is dependent on:

- The number of farrowing crates.
- The milking capabilities of the sows, the breed and reproductive efficiency.
- Litter size.
- A good weight for age at weaning.
- The health of the piglets at weaning time.
- The quality and digestibility of the creep feed.
- Weaning accommodation that will satisfy the pig's requirements.
- A weaning age that results two weeks later in a healthy weaner which has achieved maximum daily liveweight gain. (Fig.9-1).
- A weaning age that does not depress efficient reproductive performance in the sow.
- The use of segregated early weaning techniques to improve health status.

Feed intake after weaning

Optimum levels of feed intake post-weaning maximise daily gain and feed conversion efficiency and reduce costs per kilogram of liveweight gain and energy requirements.

The heavier the pig at weaning the more efficient is the growth and feed conversion during the next four weeks and the quicker it reaches slaughter weight.

Changes in the intestine of the pig at weaning

Fig.9-2 shows the cross section of the small intestine of the weaned piglet to consist of many thousands of finger like projections called villi, which increase the absorptive capacity of the small intestine. During suckling they are continuously bathed by sows milk which contains the immunoglobulin IgA. This becomes absorbed into the mucus covering the villi surfaces and prevents *E. coli* and other organisms attaching to the fingers. If they are unable to attach they are unable to cause disease. The secretory IgA also helps to destroy bacteria. After weaning time however no more IgA is available, the levels rapidly decline and bacteria damage the villi causing them to shrink. This atrophy reduces the absorptive capacity of the gut and the ability of the pig to use its food. The enzymes produced by the cells of the villi are likewise reduced. The changes result in malabsorption of food and poor digestion with or without the development of scour. The villi normally regenerate within 5 to 7 days after weaning from cells at their base called enterocytes, which multiply and migrate upwards causing the villi to return to their normal length. The rate of multiplication and regeneration is in part an environmental temperature and energy dependent phenomena. If the pig is weaned in an environment below its lower critical temperature (LCT), the rate of regeneration of the villi is reduced and in some cases ceases. (This results in the hairy pig that doesn't grow). Feed intake is a crucial part of the equation.

Before weaning the piglet receives milk as a liquid feed at regular intervals. As a result the bacterial flora of the gut, although relatively simple compared with that of a mature pig, is stabilised.

At weaning cessation of milk removes secretory IgA and there is a period of starvation, followed by irregular attempts to eat solid feed. This results in a dynamic disruption of the bacterial flora of the gut which may last for 7 to 10 days before stabilising. This bacterial disruption may also contribute to poor digestion and possibly scour, particularly when high levels of pathogenic strains of *E. coli* are involved.

Before weaning the piglets led an ordered life, being "called" with their litter mates to suckle and obtain small amounts of milk at regular intervals, sleeping between meals in a warm creep. All this suddenly changes at weaning, the pigs finding themselves in strange surroundings with strange piglets, and only solid feed. Psychological trauma is inevitable and is likely to affect some pigs more than others, resulting in impaired digestibility and lowered resistance to disease. The more this psychological stress can be minimised the better

If poor growth is evident in the first seven days post-weaning the following options or variables need to be considered:
- Check that the weights of all pigs at weaning are to the target level.
- Check the ages of the pigs at weaning.
- Heavier but younger pigs will have a more immature digestive system.
- Group the pigs by weight or keep them in their litter groups.
- Use a highly digestible and palatable diet and mix and soak this for the first day or two with water.

SUGGESTED WEIGHTS FOR AGE AT WEANING	
Age (average days)	Weight kg
21	6
28	9
35	12

SUGGESTED TARGETS FOR 3 WEEK WEANING *			
Day	kg	ADG Previous Week (g)	FCE
21	6.0	—	—
28	7.0	140	1.25
35	9.5	357	1.33
42	11 - 12	420	1.38
49	14 - 16	571	1.40
56	18 - 21	714	1.41

SUGGESTED TARGETS FOR 4 WEEK WEANING *			
Day	kg	ADG Previous Week (g)	FCE
28	8.5	—	—
35	9.25	142	1.28
42	12.9	520	1.38
49	17.0	580	1.40
56	22 - 23	714	1.49

* Assuming no environmental challenges.

(Fig.9-1)

The greater the villus atrophy the poorer the growth rate of the pig.

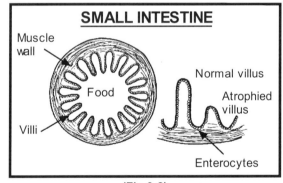

(Fig.9-2)

- Use different diets according to body weight and age.
- Use open dishes for feeding for the first three days at least, instead of troughs.
- Feed small quantities of creep four to five times daily and remove uneaten stale feed.
- Provide easy access to fresh clean water.
- Use in-feed medication for the first ten days post-weaning.
- Check that the environmental temperature is constant and satisfies the pigs requirements particularly in the first four days post-weaning.
- Maintain a dry house without draughts.
- Reduce any form of stress.
- If pigs are housed on slatted floors provide solid comfort boards for them to lie on for the first few days.

CHAPTER 9 - Managing and Treating Disease in the Weaner, Grower and Finishing Periods

- Remove the smallest piglets from each pen after 7 to 10 days and place them together in one pen in the same room. Their diet can then be adjusted accordingly.

Key factors that dictate the degree of villus atrophy
- Age of the pig at weaning.
- Weight of the pig at weaning.
- The environmental temperature and its fluctuations.
- Feed intake and availability of feed.
- Digestibility of the feed.
- Quality of the proteins.
- Levels of milk proteins.
- Levels of bacterial and viral challenge.

Nutrition

Only minimal amounts of solid food are eaten during the suckling period and very little before 10 days of age.

Key points to maximising feed intake
- Pigs at weaning time will eat a warm gruel better than a solid food.
- Gruel feeding reduces the degree of villus atrophy and dehydration.
- Pigs need to be encouraged to feed in the first 2 to 3 days post-weaning because the maternal discipline of suckling every 40 minutes is lost.
- Provide creep feed for the first 72 hours in open dishes 5 to 6 times a day. This will encourage the pigs to eat and avoid over eating. Piglets naturally "root" pellets from the floors rather than a trough. Recently washed metal troughs have unattractive smells.
- By experiment place the feeders in the most attractive part of the pen.
- A small pellet or crumb will increase intake. Pellet size should be 2mm or less.
- Examine the piglets mouths at weaning time to ensure there has been no damage to the gums during teeth removal. Pigs with sore infected gums will not eat.
- Use a highly palatable diet.

Creep feeding / options

The term "creep feed" here means the pre-starter diet offered to piglets before and just after weaning until they can be changed to a cheaper starter diet. When sows were loose-housed in farrowing pens the pre-starter had to be placed in a "creep" where the sows could not get to it. Now that sows are farrowed in crates or tethers the creep is placed outside the warm creep area in a cooler part of the pen to keep it fresh but the term "creep feed" is still used.

There are a number of options:
- No creep given pre-weaning.
- Different creeps given pre and post-weaning.
- Mixed creeps given post-weaning.
- A high dense diet used pre-weaning and a low one post-weaning.
- A low dense diet used pre-weaning and a high one post-weaning.
- Restricted feed for varying periods of time.
- Choice feeding.

By trial and error determine the best methods that produce a healthy rapid growing weaner.

On most farms the best method is to offer very small quantities of fresh creep feed several times a day for the last 7 to 10 days before weaning and to continue this for one to three days after weaning while gradually changing to starter rations.

Nutritional components of a good creep diet

Whilst it is not the purpose of this book to discuss nutrition in detail nevertheless Fig.9-3 shows the effects on growth rate of a simple diet compared to a complex one. A complex diet could consist of the following:

Cooked cereals 38 %, maze oil 11%, milk products 45%, Glucose and sugars 5% plus minerals and vitamins, MJ DE/kg 16.4, Protein 21 to 23%, lysine 1.3 to 1.4%, oil 20%.

Water

At weaning time the pig's diet changes abruptly from milk as its source of nutrients to water and solid feed and it should therefore be given encouragement to drink. Water is best provided in open cube drinkers, poultry drinkers or water bowls for the first 3 to 4 days. If nipple drinkers are the only source of water many pigs may take up to 24 hours before they drink adequate amounts and if the drinkers are not functioning correctly some may never get enough.

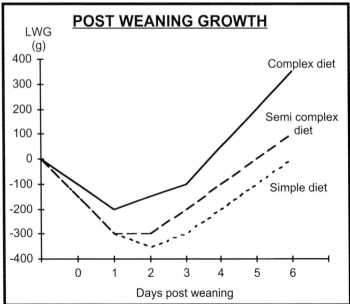

Complex diet - Cooked cereals and skim milk
Semi complex and simple diets - Wheat, barley, soya.
Courtesy of Frank Aherne

(Fig.9-3)

WATER REQUIREMENTS FOR THE WEANED PIG		
Weeks Post-weaning	Liveweight kg	Approximate Usage / Day Litres
Week 1	6 - 7	1.0
2	8 - 9	1.4
3	11 - 13	2.0
4	14 - 16	2.5

GUIDES TO LOWER CRITICAL TEMPERATURES					
Weight of Pig		Straw		Slats	
kg	(lbs)	°C	(°F)	°C	(°F)
5	(11)	27	(81)	30	(86)
6	(13)	25	(77)	29	(84)
7	(15)	22	(72)	28	(82)
8	(18)	21	(70)	26	(79)
9	(20)	20	(68)	25	(77)

(Fig.9-4)

Housing

Good weaning accommodation should satisfy the following criteria;
- Be easy to clean, disinfect and be dry.
- Provide good observation.
- Require minimum handling of waste (faeces, slurry) and separate the pig from its faeces.
- Have a simple feeding system that is adaptable for the first 3 to 4 days.
- Provide a draught free, well insulated environment that satisfies the needs of the piglets.
- Segregate one weeks pigs from another, ideally at least 10m apart, with no direct air or faeces contact.
- Segregated disease control or segregated early weaning principles should be adopted. (See chapter 3).
- In flat decks and mechanically ventilated housing a fail safe and alarm system should be in operation.
- Weaner kennels, deep bedded in straw, provide an ideal post-weaning environment in temperate climates.
- If slats are used these should preferably be made of plastic and self cleaning.

Temperature requirements

Satisfying these is essential if a pig is to be weaned successfully. (Fig.9-4). These requirements are dependent upon the weight of the pig, the feed intake, the quality of the feed, the floor type and the air flow. Whilst guidelines can be given for any particular age and group of pigs these should never be relied upon totally, but rather the temperature of the building adjusted to the observed requirements of the pig. A pig in its thermo-neutral zone (its comfort zone) lies on its side making little bodily contact with its contemporaries.

Temperature requirements of the pig are increased in wet draughty pens, or where there is high air flow. Always measure the temperature at pig level using a maximum minimum thermometer or computer monitoring equipment, placed in a guarded position.

Stocking density

The stocking density for pigs weaned on fully slatted or partly slatted floors is approximately $0.1m^2$ per 10kg liveweight. This should provide sufficient room for all pigs to lie down in the pen without body contact. No more than 40 pigs should be housed in each pen, ideally less (this can be doubled in deep straw accommodation) with a maximum of 200 pigs per room. Pens of pigs may be split after 10 to 14 days or the smallest pigs removed and placed together. Do not mix different ages of pigs in one room.

Problems of over stocking:
- There is a greater risk of disease developing, particularly greasy pig disease, post-weaning diarrhoea, PRRS, SI and EP.
- Growth rates are reduced.
- Vice increases including ear and tail biting.
- Ventilation problems arise.

Ventilation

Observe the pigs at the end of each day. If they are huddled and lying on their bellies the environment is wrong. If they are laid apart on their sides it is correct

This is critical in the first 24 hours of weaning. Draughts must be avoided otherwise the pig loses energy and becomes catabolic with a predisposition to the development of disease. (Fig.9-5).

Fig.9-6 highlights the major diseases of the weaned pig and the major contributing factors. Take particular note of the importance of an adverse environment and bad management.

Managing the Growing Pig for Health and Efficient Production

To maintain efficient production in the growing pig it is necessary to understand the complex interactions that are involved. There are five important areas:

1. Management. The quality of this contributes to the health and biological efficiency of the pig.
2. Feed. This is the major cost component of the growing pig. The efficiency of use is vital and the nutritional value versus price is very important. How it is delivered and made available to the pig can increase feed intake and maximise feed efficiency.
3. The type of housing used and the quality of the environment.
4. The levels of disease and their economic effects. These are significantly demonstrated by the very marked improvements in daily gain and feed conversion achieved when pigs are segregated and early weaned, or produced under segregated disease control conditions.
5. The genetic potential of the pig.

CHAPTER 9 - Managing and Treating Disease in the Weaner, Grower and Finishing Periods

The differential diagnosis of poor growth

How do we identify problems of poor growth?

This is a most difficult area to clarify and understand. Up to 75% of the total feed purchased is used from weaning to slaughter and it is surprising that so little emphasis is placed upon the efficiency of its use. The starting point is to identify those points along the pig's growth curve where targets are not met.

First of all the factors that affect the growth and feed efficiency of the pig in an intensive production system must be considered and these are listed in Fig 9-7. Study these in relation to the factors that affect profitability in Fig.9-8. In many respects they have a great deal in common. Note that planning and the use of records are considered two of the main factors because these are the starting points for the identification of poor growth rate, followed by clinical observations of the pigs on the farm. The results of any tests or post-mortem examinations, either for monitoring purposes or disease investigations, must also be appraised. Fig.9-9 collects these together at farm level for practical use.

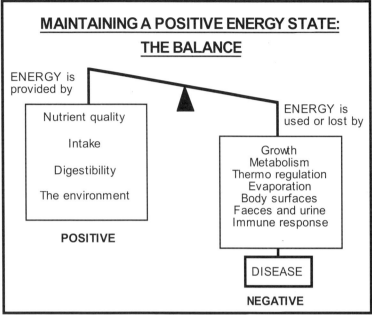

(Fig.9-5)

> *The pig must balance its energy requirements during the first 72 hours post-weaning. If not, disease is likely to occur.*

The pig

Profit comes from the margin between the price paid for the carcase and the costs that are incurred to produce it. The major cost is feed. The more feed required to produce a kg of meat then the less the profit. The genetic make up of the pig is vital in this respect. To produce 1kg of lean meat requires approximately 1.25kg of feed, whereas, to produce 1kg of fat requires approximately 4kg of feed. An animal that can convert more of its feed into lean meat therefore is much more profitable than one that converts it into fat. How often this obvious factor is neglected. Furthermore excess fat at slaughter may be severely penalised. The rate of deposition of lean meat is dependent on the sex of the animal, its genetic background, the type of feed used, the quantity fed and the disease and its effects on growth rate. A lean pig

DISEASES OF THE PIG DURING THE FIRST 28 DAYS POST-WEANING					
Condition	Important Precipitating Factors				
	Stocking Density	Infection	Nutrition	Adverse Environment	Bad Management
Atrophic rhinitis *		✓		✓	✓
Aujeszky's disease *		✓		✓	✓
Streptococcal meningitis *	✓	✓		✓	✓
Swine dysentery *		✓	✓	✓	✓
Actinobacillus pleuropneumonia	✓	✓	✓	✓	✓
Enteritis		✓	✓	✓	✓
Glässers disease		✓		✓	✓
Greasy pig disease		✓		✓	✓
Internal Parasites - uncommon		✓		✓	✓
Lice		✓		✓	✓
Malabsorption			✓	✓	✓
Mange		✓		✓	✓
Oedema disease		✓	✓	✓	✓
Porcine enteropathy		✓		✓	✓
Salmonellosis	✓	✓		✓	✓
Transmissible gastro-enteritis		✓			

* Prolonged carrier state

(Fig.9-6)

FACTORS INFLUENCING GROWTH RATE		MANGEMENT FACTORS THAT MAY INFLUENCE FCE (MEAN 2.7)	
		(↑ Worse by up to. ↓ Better by up to)	
Disease	Diseases present Management of disease Therapy / prophylactics	Multiple sources of pigs (disease)	↑ 0.2
Environment	Airborne dust Air speed Humidity Micro-organisms Noxious gases Temperature Toxins Ventilation	Increasing sale weight to 113kg	↑ 0.2
		> 500 pigs per air space	↑ 0.2
		Cubic capacity per pig < 0.7m^3 (80ft^3 /100kg)	↑ 0.1
Feed and intake	Ad lib / restricted Availability Growth promoters Palatability Trough / floor feeding Wet feeding Water availability	Continuous Production	↑ 0.25
		Feed waste	↑ 0.5
		Mixing pigs	↑ 0.2
Housing	All-in all-out management Floor type / bedding Floor space / stocking density / group size Insulation/ temperature Method of waste disposal Moving, mixing, stress	Temperature < 16°C (60°F)	↑ 0.01 per °C
		Temperature > 30°C (85°F)	↑ 0.01 per °C
		Add 1% fat	↓ 0.05
Management	Direction Education People quality	Add a growth promoter	↓ 0.07
Nutrition	Amino acid / lysine levels Energy levels Protein levels and quality	Reduce backfat by 10%	↓ 0.05
Pig	Age / weight / sex Genetics	Increase protein in diet by 10%	↓ 0.1
		Boars	↓ 0.1

(Fig.9-7)

however is more susceptible to environmental change and disease.

During the past 15 years in many pig producing countries across the world there has been considerable emphasis on the selection of pigs with high lean tissue deposition that will continue through to the slaughter weight. The unimproved pig 15 years ago would maximise its lean tissue growth at around 40kg. The pig of today will maximise its lean tissue growth at the expense of fat at 60-90kg, the boar being more efficient. Always use the best sires available i.e. those with rapid growth, good feed conversion efficiency, good killing out percentage or yield and high levels of lean tissue deposition. All these traits are highly heritable.

Records

The growing period is the most difficult section on the farm from which to gather useful information. It requires the extra burden of weighing, identifying pigs, recording feed usage and objective analysis of these in relation to the cost of feed, (including medication) and carcase grading. However, such information is highly cost effective because it determines how the pig is growing during the different phases on your farm and identifies the inefficient and weak points. Monitoring is best carried out by tattooing a number in the ear for each week of birth, from which weight for age is easily determined. Alternatively a minimum of ten males and ten females

---

SOME FACTORS AFFECTING THE PROFITABILITY OF GROWING AND FINISHING PIGS

Price of feed
Quality of feed.
Method of feeding.
Feed conversion.
Price of pig meat.
Grading or carcase quality.
Genetic potential of the pig.
Growth rate / throughput / pen utilisation.
Housing - Type / Design / Stocking densities.
Environment - Quality / Control.
"Disease" - Prevention / Control / Medication.
Welfare/ freedom from stress / comfort.
Planning. Use of records.
Management - Decisions / Work / Detail.
Education.

(Fig.9-8)

---

should be randomly selected every one to four weeks at point of weaning and each batch tagged with different coloured tags. Such selected groups of pigs can then be weighed and assessed against age at predetermined points. It is then possible to build up a growth curve and assess both the efficient and inefficient points. A typical example is shown in Fig.9-10, where there is increasing variability in the weight of pigs as age increases. There are two distinct dips in the growth curve, one at 80 to 90 days of age and another at 130 to 140. This graph identifies two problem areas that can then be investigated further.

CHAPTER 9 - Managing and Treating Disease in the Weaner, Grower and Finishing Periods

The use of a modern computer programme has taken a lot of hard work out of compiling information but the following are necessary to assess the efficiency of growth.
- Average liveweight gain per pig from weaning to point of sale.
- Daily gain related to age.
- Average numbers of days from weaning to point of sale.
- Amount of feed consumed per pig per day.
- Food conversion efficiency
- The price of feed.
- Feed cost per kg of liveweight gain.

Efficient growth is dependent on many factors most of which have been listed in Fig.9-7. Fig.9-11 shows growth curves that might be achieved under good conditions on the farm.

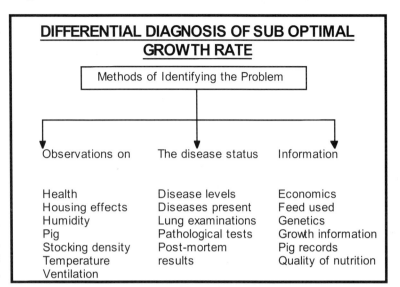
(Fig.9-9)

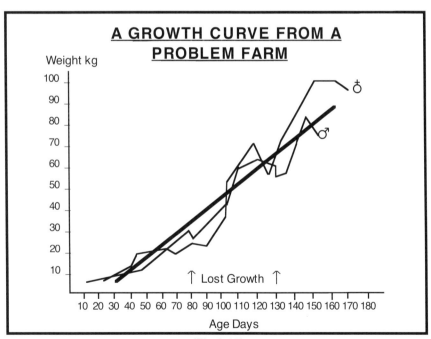
(Fig.9-10)

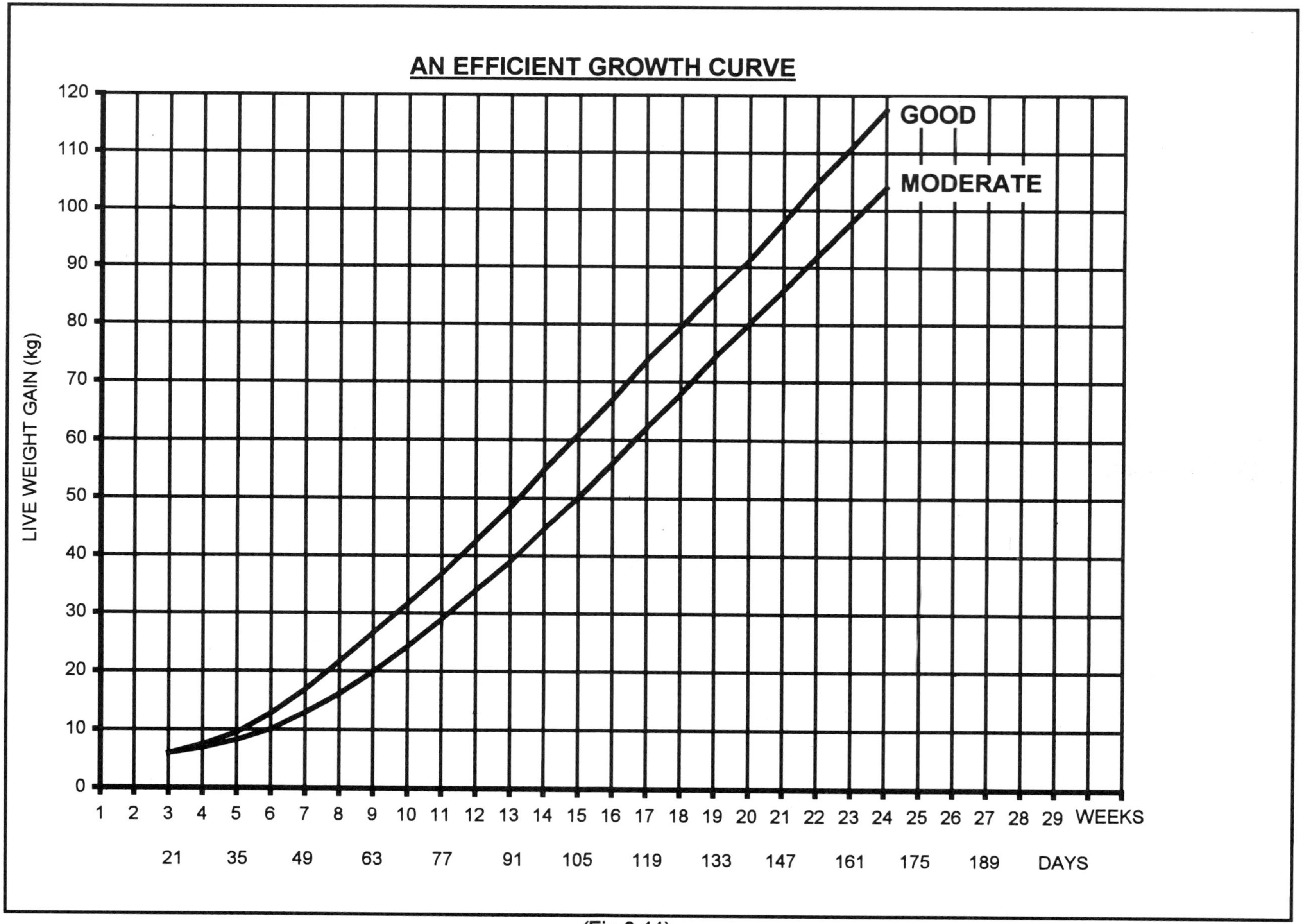
AN EFFICIENT GROWTH CURVE
GOOD
MODERATE
LIVE WEIGHT GAIN (kg)
0
10
20
30
40
50
60
70
80
90
100
110
120
1 2 3 4 5 6 7 8 9 10 11 12 13 14 15 16 17 18 19 20 21 22 23 24 25 26 27 28 29 WEEKS
21 35 49 63 77 91 105 119 133 147 161 175 189 DAYS

(Fig.9-11)

CHAPTER 9 - Managing and Treating Disease in the Weaner, Grower and Finishing Periods

SUGGESTED REFERENCE DATA FOR EFFICIENT GROWTH (LEAN GENOTYPE, HIGH HEALTH STATUS)											
Age	Weeks	Live Weight		DLWG (g/day)		DLWG at age	FCE		Protein %	Energy (MJ DE/kg)	Feed Intake kg/day
		(kg)	(lbs)	From Birth	From 21 days		At age	From 21 days			
At Birth		1.20	2.7								
Weaning at											
21 days		5.75	12.7	216		230	0.9		23.0	15.0	
28 days	4	7.00	15.4	242	178	202		1.1			0.22
35 days		9.50	20.9	237	267						
42 days	6	12.00	26.5	257	297	379	1.45	1.25	22.0	14.5	0.55
49 days		16.00	35.3	302	366						
56 days	8	21.00	46.3	353	435	580	1.55	1.35			0.9
63 days		25.00	55.1	377	458				21.0	14.2	
70 days	10	31.00	68.3	425	515	694	1.8	1.45			1.25
77 days		35.00	77.2	438	522						
84 days	12	41.00	90.4	473	559	857	2.1	1.6			1.8
91 days		48.00	105.8	514	603						
98 days	14	54.00	119.0	538	626	933	2.25	1.9	19.0	14.1	2.1
105 days		61.00	134.5	569	657						
112 days	16	66.00	145.5	578	662	1106	2.35	2.1			2.6
119 days		73.00	160.9	603	686						
126 days	18	79.00	174.2	617	697	1120	2.5	2.25			2.9
133 days		85.00	187.4	630	707				18.0	14.0	
140 days	20	91.00	200.6	641	716	1132	2.65	2.3			3.0
147 days		98.00	216.1	658	732						
154 days	22	105.00	231.5	674	746	1071	2.8	2.45			3.0
161 days		111.00	244.7	681	751		3.0	2.5			

DLWG = daily liveweight gain **FCE** - Feed conversion efficiency = amount of feed consumed/gain in weight

(Fig.9-12)

Such figures can then be compared to targets set for the farm, as suggested in Fig.9-12 and the quick reference in Fig.9-13. The density of the diet fed and its effects on feed intake and feed efficiency may vary these figures slightly.

The feed intake in some genotypes will be higher with a slight worse feed efficiency but increased gain.

Computerised pig models are also now available that will respond to theoretical changes in feed, the environment, the genetics of the pig and the cost of feed. They are not yet used widely because their results are sometimes variable and there are problems of obtaining accurate input information from the farm. However as they become more sophisticated they will provide valuable information to help identify inadequacies, look at "what if" scenarios and help to make better decisions.

Nutrition

The way the pig utilises its feed is dependent upon its genotype, the level of available energy, the protein quality and quantity and the limiting effects of essential amino acids. Equally important however is the temperature, ventilation and humidity of the environment in the house.

PIG PERFORMANCE TARGETS					
Age		Liveweight Target			
		Moderate		Good	
Week	Days	kg	lbs	kg	lbs
3	21	6	13	6	13
4	28	7	15	7.5	17
5	35	8.5	19	9.5	21
6	42	10.5	23	13	29
7	49	13.5	30	17	37
8	56	16.5	36	21.5	47
9	63	20.5	45	26	57
10	70	24.5	54	31	68
11	77	29	64	36	79
12	84	34	75	42	93
13	91	39	86	48	106
14	98	44.5	98	54	119
15	105	50	110	61	134
16	112	56	123	66	146
17	119	62	137	73	161
18	126	68	150	79	174
19	133	74.5	164	85	187
20	140	80	176	91	201
21	147	86	190	98	216
22	154	92	203	105	231
23	161	98	216	111	245
24	168	104	229	117	258

(Fig.9-13)

It is important to provide adequate trough space to maximise growth and reduce any predisposition to disease (Fig.9-14)

Once the rates of growth in the herd have been established assess whether target levels have been achieved and if not try to determine the reasons why. Use the checklists in chapter 3 to provide additional information.

Observation
The pig

Observations by the experienced stockperson should identify healthy and diseased pigs and those with variable growth rates.
The following should be considered when carrying out the assessment.

- Were the pigs moved into the pen as an even batch and if so is growth rate throughout the whole batch still even? This is important in relation to the presence of disease.
- Do the pigs exhibit any abnormal signs such as higher than usual levels of coughing, sneezing or skin irritation.
- Is there a history of disease or are there signs of disease?
- Do they appear settled in the pen or are there any signs of vice?
- Is the floor clean? Feed wastage can account for up to 0.4 of loss of feed conversion efficiency on some farms, particularly those that are floor feeding. Pick up a handful of feed off the floor and smell it. Has it gone rancid?
- Check the feed hoppers. It is amazing how many of them have a hole in the bottom or are of such a design that the pig scoops food out down through the slats. Waste is one of the most important factors associated with "inefficient growth".

> **Draught free pigs grow faster on less feed.**

- Is the floor wet or are the pigs wet? This will have a marked effect on the way they use energy and feed.

The environment
- Next look at the pigs on a group basis rather than individuals. Are they huddled together in a corner, or when at rest, lying on their sides not touching other pigs?
- If the latter is the case then you will know that the temperature is correct and that the airflow across the pigs is not chilling them.
- Do the skins of the animals appear shiny and pink with little hair or are they dull and dirty with excess hair growth? In the latter the pigs may be below their lower critical temperature and therefore using feed to keep warm.
- Fig.9-15 indicates the different ranges of temperatures that may be required by the pig at differing weights on

TROUGH LENGTHS, LIVEWEIGHT AND FEEDING METHODS

Weight of Pig kg	Trough Length Per Pig	
	Restricted feeding mm	Ad lib feeding mm
5	100	33(at weaning)
10	130	33
20	175	38
40	200	50
60	240	60
90	280	70
120	300	75

Single space feeder (350mm wide) 1 per 10 pigs

(Fig.9-14)

A GUIDE (ONLY) TO AIR TEMPERATURE ACCORDING TO FLOOR TYPE

Weight Pig kg (lbs)	Floor Type							
	Straw °C (°F)		Concrete °C (°F)		Perforated Metal °C (°F)		Slatted °C (°F)	
5 (11)	27-30	(81-86)	28-31	(82-88)	29-32	(84-90)	30-32	(86-90)
10 (22)	20-24	(68-75)	22-26	(72-79)	24-28	(75-82)	25-28	(77-82)
20 (44)	15-23	(59-73)	16-24	(61-75)	19-26	(66-79)	19-25	(66-77)
30 (66)	13-23	(55-73)	14-24	(57-75)	18-25	(64-77)	17-25	(63-77)
90 (198)	11-22	(52-72)	12-23	(54-73)	17-25	(63-77)	15-24	(59-75)

(Fig.9-15)

different types of floor surface. The thermo-neutral zone is the temperature range within which heat production is independent of air temperature. The limits of this range are described as the upper and lower critical temperatures (UCT, LCT). When pigs are housed below their lower critical temperature a proportion of their feed is used to maintain body heat and they are more susceptible to disease. There is a marked increase in the lower critical temperature at point of weaning, due to low feed intake and the inability of the pig to satisfy its energy requirements.

An 80kg pig with restricted feed could have a lower critical temperature of 15°C (59°F) but if it was fed ad lib the LCT could drop to 11°C (52°F). At the other extreme as pigs reach the upper critical temperature, which starts to take effect above 30°C (86°F), heat relieving procedures come into play with fouling and wetting on the floor together with soiled food, loss of palatability resulting in reduced intake and therefore reduced growth rate. A checklist of the environmental factors that can determine the upper and lower critical temperatures is shown in Fig.9-16.

If feed conversion efficiency is poor, check the factors in Fig.9-17.

Disease

During the period of observation the veterinarian and experienced stockpeople can assess the levels and presence of different diseases and their influence on growth rate and economy of production.

Use the following checklist during the clinical examinations as described in chapter 3, to identify problem

CHAPTER 9 - Managing and Treating Disease in the Weaner, Grower and Finishing Periods

areas:
- Weight for age
- Stocking densities.
- Evenness of growth.
- Effects of nutrition on growth in different environments.
- Time of feed changes and effects.
- Effects of pig movement.
- Environment changes.
- Quality of the environment, insulation, temperatures, humidity, draughts, temperature fluctuations.
- Wet pens, dirty floors.
- Spoiled feed.
- Undigested feed evident in faeces.
- Appearance of pigs skins - mange.
- Appearance of the faeces, e.g. colitis - sloppy faeces.
- Respiratory disease.
- Enteric disease.
- Records of treatments / mortalities.
- Prolapses.
- Number of pigs culled.
- Parasites.
- Examine hospital pens.

The changes in disease patterns in growing and feeding pigs in 63 intensive pig herds during a 20 year period are shown in Fig.9-18. These show the effects that changing production systems, disease and management practices may have over time and such changes may be relevant in your herd.

Diseases of the Weaned and Growing Pig

If you have a problem refer to Fig.9-19 and Fig.9-20 and then the index or relevant chapter. If you cannot identify the cause consult your veterinarian.

A pig growing at 5°C below its LCT could take 10 days longer to slaughter.

A CHECKLIST OF THE FACTORS THAT AFFECT CRITICAL TEMPERATURES

LCT	UCT
Weight of the pig. Feed intake e.g.	High levels of liveweight per m² of floor space.
Weight pig kg (lbs) / Per day feed / LCT °C 40 (88) / 1.5kg / 16 40 (88) / 2.0kg / 13	High external temperature > 30°C (86°F). High internal temperature >24°C (75°F).
Energy content of the ration. Fat depths. Group size and stocking density. Air speed - draughts. Ventilation control. Insulation of the building and floor. Floor type, slats or solid. Bedding. Wet floors. For every 1°C below LCT there can be a loss in daily gain of 12g. Monitor temperature fluctuations.	High energy intake. Fat pigs. Too high stocking density. Poor ventilation. High humidity.

LCT = Lower critical temperature
UCT = upper critical temperature

(Fig.9-16)

CHECKLIST OF FACTORS AFFECTING FEED CONVERSION EFFICIENCY

Factors	Important Criteria	Methods of Improvement
Genetics	Select from a health compatible source	Replace with genetically improved stock.
Sex	Males / females / castrates.	Split Sexes. Do not castrate.
Age	Reduce days to slaughter. Feed efficiency: 1.1 to 1 at 4 weeks. 1.5 to 1 at 8 weeks. 3 to 1 at 24 weeks.	Feed Levels. Feed quality. Maximise growth rate. Good housing. Good health.
Feeding methods	Ad lib/ waste. Wet feed is better than dry. Pellets are better than meal. Trough feeding gives better FCE than floor feeding.	Prevent waste. Change dry to wet feed. Change meal to pellets or to wet feed.
Amount fed	Check waste / carcase quality and growth.	Better management.
Feed composition	Protein. Lysine. Energy. Growth Promoters. Quality.	Assess ration types according to genotype, environment and growth. Monitor ration quality.
The environment	Too hot or cold. Too draughty or high gas levels. Too dry or too wet.	Temperature Ventilation Humidity
Levels of disease	Health control. Vaccination. SEW, SDC.	Veterinary and other advice. Management and housing control. Disease prevention.
Management efficiency	Attention to detail. Education of people. Maintenance of buildings. Purchasing good feeds.	Yourself

(Fig.9-17)

CHANGING DISEASE PATTERNS IN WEANED AND GROWING PIGS IN THE UK			
Condition	1974	1984	1996
Acute enteritis (diarrhoea)	+	++	++
Atrophic rhinitis	-	++	
Oedema disease	+++		
Exudative epidermitis (Greasy pig disease)	-	++	++
Malabsorption (villus atrophy)	-	++	++
Mulberry heart disease	-	+	++
Other viruses (influenza)	-	-	++
Pneumonia	-	-	+++
Porcine respiratory coronavirus	-	-	-
PRRS	-	-	+++
Rectal prolapse	-	+	++
Rectal stricture	-	+	++
Streptococcal meningitis	-	++	++
Vice (abnormal behaviour)	-	++	+++

CHANGING DISEASE PATTERNS IN FINISHING PIGS IN THE UK			
Condition	1974	1984	1996
Actinobacillus pleuropneumonia	-	-	+++
Ascarid infections	-	+	+
Atrophic rhinitis	-	++	-
Aujeszky's disease	-	++	-
Colitis	-	-	++
Enzootic pneumonia	+	+	+++
Lameness	-	-	++
Mange	-	+++	+
Streptococcal meningitis	-	+	+
Mycoplasma arthritis	-	-	++
PE bloody gut	-	++	+
Porcine respiratory coronavirus	-	-	+
PRRS	-	-	+++
Rectal prolapse	-	+	++
Rectal stricture	-	+	++
Salmonellosis	-	-	-
Swine dysentery	+	++	++
TGE	-	+	-

- Not significant   +++ Most significant
(Fig.9-18)

Identifying Problems in the Post-weaning Period - 5-20kg Weight

OBSERVATIONS AND CAUSES

Blown-up abdomen

Constipation
No rectum (atresia ani)
Rectal stricture *
Recto vaginal fistula
Torsion intestine *

Coughing

Actinobacillus pleuropneumonia (App) *
Ammonia *
Aujeszky's disease (AD) - pseudorabies (PR)
Bordetellosis
Dust *
Enzootic pneumonia (EP) Mycoplasma *

OBSERVATIONS AND CAUSES (Cont.)

Glässers disease (Hps) *
Parasites
Porcine reproductive and respiratory syndrome(PRRS) *
Swine influenza (SI)

Haemorrhage: Faeces

Acute enteritis
Clostridia diseases
Gastric ulcers
Haematoma
Porcine enteropathy (PE)
Swine dysentery
Warfarin poisoning

Haemorrhage: Nose

Actinobacillus pleuropneumonia (App)
Anthrax
Rhinitis
Trauma

Lameness

Actinobacillus pleuropneumonia (App)
Arthritis *
Oedema disease - bowel oedema
Erysipelas *
Foot-and-mouth disease (FMD)
Glässers disease (Hps)
Leg weakness / Osteochondrosis (OCD)*
Middle ear infection
Mycoplasma arthritis *
Streptococcal infections *
Trauma - muscles, joints, bones *

Mortality - Sudden death.

No signs and more than 1%
Determine cause by post-mortem
Actinobacillus pleuropneumonia (App) *
Acute enteritis
Anthrax
Bowel oedema - oedema disease
Clostridial disease
Glässers disease
Mulberry heart disease (MHD) *
Porcine enteropathy (PE)
Streptococcal meningitis (SM) *
Torsion intestine *
Trauma

Mortality; all causes.

More than 1.5%, including after illness
As for sudden death above
Chronic enteritis
Pericarditis *
Pleurisy

CHAPTER 9 - Managing and Treating Disease in the Weaner, Grower and Finishing Periods

OBSERVATIONS AND CAUSES (Cont.)

Pneumonia *
Porcine enteropathy (PE) *
Trauma
Vice (abnormal behaviour)
Welfare causes

Nervous signs

Abscess spine
African swine fever (ASF)
Aujeszky's disease (AD) - pseudorabies (PR)
Classical swine fever (Hog cholera)
Oedema disease - bowel oedema
Glässers disease (Hps) *
Middle ear infection *
Poisoning
Salmonella choleraesuis
Salt poisoning *
Swine fever - hog cholera (HC)
Streptococcal meningitis (SM) *
Talfan, Teschen
Tetanus

Pale pigs

Anaemia *
Actinobacillus pleuropneumonia (App)
Eperythrozoonosis (Epe)
Gastric ulcers *
Haemorrhage *
Leptospirosis
Prolapse
Shortage of iron

Pneumonia

Actinobacillus pleuropneumonia (App) *
Ascarids
Aujeszky's disease (AD) - pseudorabies (PRV)
Enzootic pneumonia (EP) *M. hyopneumoniae* *
Glässers disease (Hps)
Lungworm
Pasteurellosis
Porcine reproductive and respiratory syndrome (PRRS)*
Salmonella choleraesuis
Swine influenza (SI)

Poor pigs, wasting, hairy

Actinobacillus pleuropneumonia (App)
Chronic enteritis *
Draughts
Eperythrozoonosis
Glässers disease (Hps)
Inadequate temperature *
Poor nutrition *
Porcine reproductive and respiratory syndrome (PRRS) *

OBSERVATIONS AND CAUSES (Cont.)

Salmonellosis
Shortage of water
Swine influenza (SI)
Villus atrophy *

Diarrhoea, scour or enteritis

Campylobacter
Colitis *
Cryptosporidia
E. coli enteritis *
Poor environment *
Poor nutrition *
Porcine enteropathy (PE) *
Porcine epidemic diarrhoea (PED)
Porcine reproductive and respiratory syndrome (PRRS)
Rotavirus
Salmonellosis
Spirochaetal diarrhoea
Swine dysentery (SD)
Swine fever
Transmissible gastro-enteritis (TGE)
Villus atrophy *

Skin diseases

Erysipelas
Foot-and-mouth disease. SVD
Greasy pig disease *
Lice (visible)
Mange (red spots) *
Pityriasis rosea (ringworm like)
PRRS (small vesicles) *
Purpura
Salmonellosis (blue coloration)
Swine pox (round black lesions)
Vice (abnormal behaviour)

Sneezing

Ammonia *
Atrophic rhinitis non-progressive (AR) *
Atrophic rhinitis progressive (PAR) *
Bordetellosis
Dust *
Porcine cytomegalovirus *
Porcine reproductive and respiratory syndrome (PRRS) *

Vice - tail biting, ear biting, navel sucking

Draughts
Fluctuating temperatures
Greasy pig disease
High ammonia and carbon dioxide levels
High stocking densities
Poor environment
Uncomfortable pigs

OBSERVATIONS AND CAUSES (Cont.)

Vomiting
   E. coli gastritis
   Gastric ulcers
   Poisoning
   Porcine epidemic diarrhoea (PED)
   Transmissible gastro-enteritis (TGE)

* More likely

(Fig.9-19)

Identifying Problems in the Growing Period - 20-110kg Weight

OBSERVATIONS AND CAUSES

Blown-up abdomen
   Chronic enteritis in the large intestine
   Fermentation in large intestine
   Peritonitis
   Rectal prolapse
   Rectal stricture *
   Torsion intestine *
Coughing
   Actinobacillus pleuropneumonia (App) *
   Aujeszky's disease (AD) - pseudorabies (PRV)
   Ascarids *
   Enzootic pneumonia (EP) *
   High levels of ammonia
   Lungworm
   Pasteurellosis
   Porcine reproductive and respiratory syndrome (PRRS)
   Swine influenza (SI) *
Haemorrhage: Faeces
   Acute enteritis
   Gastric ulcers
   Porcine enteropathy (PE) *
   Salmonellosis
   Swine dysentery (SD) *
Haemorrhage: Nose
   Actinobacillus pleuropneumonia (App)
   Poisonings
   Rhinitis
Lameness
   Arthritis *
   Back muscle necrosis
   Bush foot. Claw damage *
   Erysipelas
   Foot-and-mouth disease (FMD)
   Glässers disease (Hps)
   Leg weakness, Osteochondrosis (OCD) *

OBSERVATIONS AND CAUSES

Middle ear infection
   Muscle, bone, trauma *
   Mycoplasma infections *
   Poisoning
   Poor nutrition
   Swine fever
Mortality, sudden death.
No signs and more than 1%
   Determine cause by post-mortem
   Actinobacillus pleuropneumonia (App) *
   Bloody gut (PHE)
   Clostridial diseases
   Gas poisoning slurry
   Glässers disease (Hps)
   Mulberry heart disease (MHD) *
   Pasteurellosis
   Pericarditis
   Poisons
   Porcine enteropathy (PE)
   Porcine stress syndrome (PSS)
   Torsion intestine
   Trauma
   Whey bloat
Mortality, all causes.
More than 1.5% and after illness
   Assess causes of sudden death
   Parasites
   Porcine enteropathy (PE)
   Pneumonia
   Scour
   Trauma
   Vice (abnormal behaviour)
Nervous signs
   Aujeszky's disease (AD) - pseudorabies (PR)
   Oedema disease - bowel oedema
   Glässers disease (Hps) *
   Middle ear infection *
   Poisons
   Salt poisoning *
   Streptococcal meningitis (SM) *
Pale pigs
   Anaemia *
   Actinobacillus pleuropneumonia (App) *
   Eperythrozoonosis (Epe)
   Gastric ulcers *
   Internal parasites
   Porcine enteropathy (PE)
Pneumonia
   Actinobacillus pleuropneumonia (App) *
   Aujeszky's disease (AD) - pseudorabies (PR)

CHAPTER 9 - Managing and Treating Disease in the Weaner, Grower and Finishing Periods

---

OBSERVATIONS AND CAUSES (Cont.)

Enzootic pneumonia (EP) * *M. hyopneumoniae*
Pasteurella
Porcine reproductive and respiratory syndrome (PRRS) *
Salmonella choleraesuis
Swine influenza (SI) *

Poor pigs, wasting, hairy

Enteric disease - see diarrhoea *
Poor nutrition
Poor environment *
Respiratory disease - see pneumonia sneezing *

Diarrhoea, scour or enteritis

E. coli
Campylobacter
Colitis
Porcine enteropathy (PE)
Porcine epidemic diarrhoea (PED)
Salmonellosis
Swine fever
Swine dysentery (SD)
Transmissible gastro-enteritis (TGE)

Skin diseases

As for weaners

Vice (abnormal behaviour)

As for weaners

Vomiting

Coughing
Porcine epidemic diarrhoea (PED)
Fungal toxins
Gastric ulcers
Gastritis
Transmissible gastro-enteritis (TGE)

* = more likely

(Fig.9-20)

ABSCESSES

See chapter 7 for further information.

Abscesses commonly occur as a result of secondary infection following skin damage from trauma, fighting and tail biting. Tail bitten pigs should be removed immediately from the pen and given a long-acting antibiotic penicillin or OTC injection. Such pigs should not be sent for slaughter until the abscess has been lanced and drained as described in chapter 15 and antibiotic withdrawal periods satisfied.

ACTINOBACILLUS PLEUROPNEUMONIA (APP)

The bacterium *Actinobacillus pleuropneumoniae* was previously called *Haemophilus pleuropneumoniae* and there are at least twelve different strains, some of which produce no disease and are non pathogenic, but others cause very severe disease. Strains 1, 5, 9, 11 and 12 are highly virulent and strains 3 and 6 are very mild. The organism is carried in the tonsils and respiratory tract and the incubation period is very short, from as little as 12 hours through to three days. It is transmitted by droplet infection between one pig and another and only survives outside the pig for a few days and is probably airborne for only 5 to 10 metres. Disease is dose dependent i.e. the more bacteria the pig is exposed to the more severe will be the disease. When App attacks the lungs the toxins produced cause severe damage to the tissues which turn blue to black (necrosis) with extensive pleurisy. The chest cavity rapidly fills up with fluid.

Clinical signs

Acute disease

The organism may affect the pig from weaning through to slaughter but usually the age is from 8 to 16 weeks, once maternal antibody has disappeared. Sudden death is often the only sign with blood discharged from the nose. In the live pig a short cough may be heard with signs of severe breathing difficulties and blueing of the ears. Badly affected pigs are severely depressed. Body temperature is often high. Death is due to a combination of heart failure and the toxins produced by the organisms.

Sub acute disease

This occurs at the same time as the acute disease with pneumonia characterised by abdominal breathing rather than chest breathing because the pleurisy is very painful. This abdominal breathing is used to clinically differentiate between actinobacillus pneumonia where the coughing episodes are short, perhaps one to three coughs at a time, and the prolonged non-productive ones 7 to 10 times, with EP.

Affected pigs may carry the organism for considerable lengths of time and are therefore a potential risk to younger pigs.

Diagnosis

This is based on clinical evidence, herd history, post-mortem examinations including slaughter house checks and culture of the organism in the laboratory. The lesions in the lung are very characteristic with large red-blue areas in the upper diaphragmatic lobes with an overlying pleurisy. They can be confused with lesions caused by SI. Serology can be used to identify different serotypes but in the absence of disease the interpretation can be difficult because of cross reactions between serotypes.

Similar diseases

These include enzootic pneumonia, PRRS, SI, and *Salmonella choleraesuis* pneumonia.

Treatment

☐ In view of the acute course of the disease it is important to identify clinical cases very early and treat individuals by injection. Affected pigs stop eating or drinking so that water or feed medication is usually ineffective. App usually has a wide range of antibiotic sensitivity. On the first day inject the pig twice eight hours apart and the following antibiotics are usually effective.
- Amoxycillin
- Ampicillin
- Ceftiofur. This is a very rapid acting drug and gives a good response.
- Enrofloxacin
- OTC, LA. This can be used in more chronic cases. Repeat every two days.
- Penicillin
- Penicillin/streptomycin

☐ It is important to determine when the onset of the disease is likely to occur, to assess adverse environmental factors and to apply strategic medication just prior to this time.

☐ In-feed medication during the period of risk could include:
- Phenoxymethyl penicillin 200-400g/tonne
- Chlortetracycline 500-800g/tonne
- Trimethoprim/sulpha 300-400g/tonne
- Oxytetracycline 500-800g/tonne

☐ Water medication during the period of risk can be more effective in preventing disease. Treat for 4-7 days. Similar drugs to in-feed medication can be used.

☐ Preventive feed medication is not always effective probably because of the rapid onset of disease and rapid loss of appetite.

☐ In an acute outbreak examine the at risk group three times daily to identify disease as early as possible. It may be necessary to inject or water medicate the whole group. The decision to inject is a balance between effect, and risk of more disease due to the stress of handling the pigs.

Management control and prevention

This has two aspects
a) Exclusion of virulent strains from the herd.
b) Prevention of clinical disease when virulent strains are present.

Exclusion from the herd

In breeding herds the ideal situation is to have no highly virulent strains present but only mild or avirulent strains which then naturally immunise the herd. A naive herd, (i.e. one that has never been immunised by any natural infection) is a potential time bomb. However in some countries this method of control i.e. a totally naive herd is being advocated. If a virulent strain gets in it will create havoc. Fairly effective vaccines are commercially available in most countries but they only immunise against homologous serotypes (i.e. the serotypes that are incorporated in the vaccine) and not against other serotypes. In contrast, natural infection tends to immunise against all serotypes.

In a breeding herd that is free from clinical disease (including absence of characteristic lesions in the lungs) it pays to try to keep virulent strains out. In pig disease areas where herds are close together and the level of infection is high, it may prove impossible to do so on a permanent basis. In more isolated herds it may be possible to maintain freedom from the disease for long periods (although even if extreme measures are adopted, breakdowns may occur, the sources of which are often unknown).

The following measures should be adopted:

◆ Prevent entry of virulent strains by checking that the herds which supply you with replacement breeding stock are screened on the basis of herd history, clinical inspections and absence of clinical signs and regular lung examinations at slaughter.

◆ Provide all visitors, including your veterinarian, with a hat, clean coveralls and boots and insist that they wear them.

◆ If you have a large valuable herd, install a shower and make all visitors wash their hair, hands and beard if they have one.

◆ Check that they have not come direct from another diseased herd.

◆ Build a loading bay in such a way that when lorries collect pigs the driver does not have to enter your building and you do not have to go on the lorry.

◆ Avoid loading your pigs onto lorries which already have pigs on board from other farms.
All vehicles should be empty and disinfected before arrival.

◆ Hold incoming breeding pigs in isolation, segregated from your herd for a minimum of three and optimum of six weeks and not only inspect them daily, but check that the source herd is still healthy before you bring them into your herd.

◆ Some people advocate testing the pigs in isolation serologically or micro-biologically (i.e. collecting nasal swabs and culturing for the bacterium) but these may be counterproductive because of false positive results and because the laboratory cannot always tell you whether the pigs have virulent or avirulent strains.

◆ In grower-finisher units which purchase 25 to 30kg pigs from weaner producers it is difficult to maintain freedom from virulent strains of this organism unless you are purchasing pigs from a single known source or limited number of known sources. The practice of all-in all-out by building or preferably site may also help.

◆ The organisation of a multi-site system in which the three-week-old piglets are weaned immediately

CHAPTER 9 - Managing and Treating Disease in the Weaner, Grower and Finishing Periods

from the breeding sow site into an all-in all-out nursery before coming to the grower/finisher is also likely to result in freedom from this disease.
◆ Consider adopting SEW or SDC techniques.

Prevention of clinical disease when virulent strains are present

In an infected breeding herd the most likely time to get clinical disease is in pigs over 15kg.
If it does occur consider the following:
◆ Consider routine vaccination of sows and/or incoming gilts.
◆ Operate all-in all-out, at least by room, rather than continuous throughput production.
◆ Avoid stress and overcrowding.
◆ Avoid rapid temperature fluctuations.
◆ Avoid low humidities and low temperatures.
◆ Try fogging to decrease the numbers of organisms in the air. 1% Virkon S can be of value.
◆ Increase the levels of vitamin E by 50-100g/tonne.
◆ Maintain good ventilation and a warm air flow.
◆ Keep pigs warm, dry and draught free.
◆ Provide a plentiful supply of easily obtainable water. Temporary water deprivation will trigger off disease.
◆ Consider strategic feed medication in advance of and during the likely time of onset of disease.
◆ Keep injectable antibiotics in a refrigerator ready for prompt treatment of sick pigs.

In infected grower/finisher units, consider all of the above but also do the following:
◆ Avoid introducing pigs from multiple sources.
◆ Do not mix pigs from herds with the disease and pigs from herds which are free from the disease.
◆ Practice all-in all-out and not continuous flow.
◆ Consider prophylactic medication for a period after entry.
◆ Assess the results of vaccination.

Remember that when controlling the environment:
◆ Large airborne particles >10µm are retained in nasal passages.
◆ Particles of 0.5 - 3µm penetrate deep into lung tissue. (Bacteria, App and mycoplasma)
◆ Low temperatures and high humidity produce large droplets that sediment quickly with less exposure.
◆ High temperatures and low humidity produce small droplets that sediment quickly with less exposure.
◆ Low temperatures and low humidity produce small droplets that stay airborne. A dangerous environment.

ANTHRAX

This disease is very uncommon in the growing pig unless contaminated food has been purchased. If there are sudden deaths with swollen discoloured necks or the passage of bloody faeces, anthrax must be suspected and veterinary advice sought. The disease is transmissible to the human.

ARTHRITIS

See also Lameness.

Arthritis is common in the growing pig and if a problem exists it is necessary to identify the organisms or diseases responsible, by post-mortem and bacteriological examinations. The following need to be considered as possible causes: (* common)
• Brucellosis (in countries where this exists)
• Glässers disease (*Haemophilus parasuis*) *
• Erysipelas *
• Mycoplasma arthritis *(Mycoplasma hyosynoviae infection)* *
• Leg weakness, Osteochondrosis (OCD) *
• Streptococcal infection *
• Trauma

In the weaned and growing pig erysipelas, *M. hyosynoviae* and OCD are the most common causes but in many cases the only clinical symptoms will be lameness. It is necessary therefore to consider arthritis under the general heading "lameness" and if you have a problem refer to this section to help identify the cause and then consider the specific diseases.

ATROPHIC RHINITIS (AR) - PROGRESSIVE DISEASE (PAR)

Rhinitis implies inflammation of the nose and it can be caused by a variety of bacteria and irritant substances. During the process of infection the delicate structures or turbinate bones in the nose become damaged and atrophy or disappear. Progressive atrophic rhinitis describes a specific disease where the nose tissues permanently atrophy. It is caused by specific toxin producing strains of *Pasteurella multocidia* (PMt). There are two types A and D.

Spread of disease between herds is almost invariably by the carrier pig, the organism being found in the respiratory tract and the tonsils. Spread within herds is by droplet infection between pigs or by direct pig to pig (nose to nose) contact. It can also be spread indirectly on equipment, clothes etc. When first infected pigs can carry the infection for many months. Infection is usually picked up during the second half of the sucking period or after weaning and clinical disease may be evident from three weeks of age onwards. The toxin is absorbed into the system where it damages other tissues including the liver, kidneys and lung, resulting in reduced daily gain and depressed feed efficiency. Similar organisms may also be found in the cat, dog, rabbit, poultry, goat, sheep, turkey but it is thought that these are host adapted strains and are unlikely to cause serious disease in the pig. The human may carry PMt in the tonsils for a very short period of time, although the evidence for this is limited and there are no reports of transmission by people to pigs. Experience indicates that the main and probably only method of introduction into the herd is by carrier pigs, although occasionally unexplained outbreaks of disease may occur.

Clinical signs

In sucking pigs sneezing, snuffling and a nasal discharge are the first symptoms, but in acute outbreaks where there is little maternal antibody, the rhinitis may be so severe to the extent that there is haemorrhage from the nose. By three to four weeks of age and from weaning onwards, there is evidence of tear staining and malformation of the nose associated with twisting and shortening.

Severely affected pigs may have problems eating. There is considerably reduced daily gain. In severe outbreaks pigs may not grow to market weight.

Diagnosis

This is based on clinical signs. However do not assume if sneezing is occurring in young pigs that automatically it will be progressive atrophic rhinitis. The disease is easily identified by post-mortem examinations of the nose and culture of the organism from nasal swabs. (See chapter 15 Swabbing). The snout is sectioned at slaughter at a level of the second premolar tooth and an assessment of the degree of atrophy of the turbinate bones made. The snouts are graded from 0 to 5, 0 being a perfect snout. Grade 1 would show a slight loss of symmetry of the nose, grade 2 a slight loss of turbinate tissue and grade 3 a moderate amount. It is only when grades 4 and 5 are present, when there is severe progressive loss of tissue that PAR will be suspected. (Fig.9-21).

Similar diseases

Rhinitis may be caused by the following but the distinction is less evident, less pigs are obviously affected and the turbinate bones will heal and regenerate:

Air containing high bacterial counts.
Aujeszky's disease.
Bordetella bronchiseptica infection.
Chronic respiratory disease.
Dust.
Glässers disease.

DIAGRAMATIC SECTIONS OF PIG SNOUTS

Scoring system for degrees of abnormality. Pig snouts sawn off between the 1st and 2nd premolar teeth.

(Fig.9-21)

High levels of ammonia.
Porcine cytomegalovirus infection (PCMV) (inclusion body rhinitis).
PRRS.

Treatment

- The moment PAR is diagnosed all adult stock should be vaccinated twice with a toxin derived vaccine 4 to 6 weeks apart.
- Sows should then be vaccinated four to six weeks prior to each subsequent farrowing or as per the data sheet.
- All weaned pigs should be medicated in-feed until the clinical outbreak has subsided.
- At the same time and until a good immunity has developed, antibiotic treatment should be given to the piglets. Consider using the following routines:
  Day three of age. Inject with either long-acting OTC or amoxycillin.
  Day ten. Inject with either long-acting OTC or amoxycillin.
  Inject again at weaning time with OTC or amoxycillin.
- Other antibiotics could be used depending on the bacterial sensitivity.
- The sows feed should be top-dressed with either OTC or trimethoprim/sulpha (TMS) commencing five to seven days prior to farrowing and throughout the farrowing period, or the lactating ration medicated with trimethoprim/sulpha (500g).
- At weaning time the creep feed should be medicated with OTC or CTC at dose levels of 500-800g/tonne or TMS for three weeks post-weaning.

In acute outbreaks PAR is evident clinically in up to 25% of pigs by the time they have reached 16 weeks of age. Four months after vaccination this should have dropped to around 10% and after six months down to

CHAPTER 9 - Managing and Treating Disease in the Weaner, Grower and Finishing Periods

less than 1%. Vaccination will usually prevent the establishment of infection up to approximately eight to twelve weeks of age until the pigs move into finishing houses. Here, unless the houses have been depopulated, the pigs will become infected but with few clinical signs. Infection however increases the predisposition to other respiratory diseases and depresses feed intake and performance.

Management control and prevention
- Keep disease out by purchasing pigs only from known negative sources.
- Monitor snout sections regularly.
- If the herd is infected do not breed from home bred gilts.
- Vaccinate sows.
- Maintain an old herd to produce good colostral immunity.
- Avoid continuously populated housing which may allow organisms to build up to a threshold level and initiate a disease outbreak.
- Adopt all-in all-out procedures from weaning to slaughter.
- Avoid high stocking levels.
- Avoid more than ten sows per farrowing room.
- Damp humid farrowing houses increase the risk of spread.
- Use solid divisions between farrowing crates to reduce droplet infection
- Keep weaners to less than 120 per group.
- Poor ventilation and high humidity post-weaning predispose.
- Do not re-circulate air in flat decks.
- Avoid fluctuating temperatures in flat decks.

Eradication
PAR may be eradicated from the herd after a 12 month period of sow vaccination provided all clinical evidence of disease has subsided. Piglets from vaccinated sows are weaned and segregated from disease carrying pigs until the first and second weaning accommodation has been depopulated and cleaned. The segregated pigs are then returned to the buildings. In the meantime the other finishing pigs are gradually sold to slaughter. The vaccinated "clean" pigs are not allowed contact with infected pigs and separate personnel are used between groups. PAR is only spread by close droplet contamination. An alternate and more successful method is to market all growing pigs over a 6 to 8 week period before bringing the segregated pigs back into the system. (See chapter 3 segregated disease control).

AUJESZKY'S DISEASE (AD) OR PSEUDORABIES (PR)
See chapter 12 for further information.
This is caused by a herpes virus and is a very important disease. The pig is the only natural host and the virus can maintain itself hidden in nervous tissue for long periods of time. It can affect other species including cattle, horses, dogs and cats but these always die. There are no confirmed reports of it affecting people. The outer covering of the virus contains proteins called glycol proteins which are numbered G1, G2 and G3. If one or more of these are removed by genetic engineering, the virus can no longer produce the disease but can still stimulate an immunity. Such viruses are called gene deleted and are used to produce live vaccines. Field virus can be spread between herds by sub-clinical carrier pigs, usually replacement breeding stock, and on the wind. Wind-borne infection can occur over distances of several kilometres over land and much further over water. It can also be spread by AI. Within herds it may be spread direct by nose to nose contact, or by aerosol droplets.

The virus has been eradicated or kept out of some countries (e.g. Chile, Australia, Denmark and Great Britain) and attempts to eradicate it are being carried out in other countries (e.g. USA, Ireland and the Low Countries), but in other countries it is endemic and widespread. Eradication polices range from slaughter depopulation and repopulation, to the use of gene deleted vaccines to identify by blood sampling those pigs that are carrying the disease. They can then be eliminated from the population over a period of one to two years. Because the disease is relatively slow spreading it can be eliminated.

Clinical signs
Acute disease
When first introduced into a herd AD infects the reproductive tract with high mortality in unborn piglets in utero and during sucking. In the growing period there may be fever, sneezing, coughing, pneumonia and high mortality with some nervous signs including incoordination and fits. Some strains of the virus cause severe respiratory disease and others severe rhinitis in growing and finishing pigs and complicate already existing respiratory problems.

Diagnosis
This is based on the clinical picture, serological and laboratory tests.

Treatment
- There is no specific treatment for AD, but in-feed antibiotics may help to control secondary bacterial infections during the exposure to the virus.

Management control and prevention
- In growing pigs the maintenance of a disease free breeding herd must be aimed for.
- In aujeszky free breeding herds, prevention is dependent on stopping the virus entering the herd by

- screening the sources of purchased replacement stock and blood sampling them in isolation prior to entry into the herd.
- If the breeding herd is in a country in which the infection is widespread then it may be good insurance to vaccinate the sows with gene deleted vaccine to prevent disease entering or at worst reduce the major piglet losses that can occur when the virus first enters a susceptible herd.
- The use of a gene deleted vaccine also allows the herd to be tested serologically to check that the virus has not entered.
- If the breeding herd is already endemically infected then the sows should be vaccinated routinely together with all growing pigs.

BACK MUSCLE NECROSIS
See chapter 7 for further information.

This is believed to be a manifestation of the porcine stress syndrome and is associated with severe changes in the lumbar muscles that run down each side of the spine. The onset is sudden, often after exercise and the swollen muscles are extremely painful. The condition sometimes occurs in outdoor gilts that have heavy ham muscles, when they are moved into paddocks for the first time. Within five minutes or so a number of the gilts can be very stiff and lame. The condition can take two or three weeks to resolve and the breeding capacity of the gilts may be affected.

BORDETELLOSIS

Bordetella bronchiseptica is a bacterium found in most if not all pig populations. Some strains cause a mild and non progressive rhinitis that heals spontaneously. The disease is clinically and economically of no consequence. However if toxigenic pasteurella are present in the herd then a combination of the two organisms can produce severe disease. (PAR)

Bordetella bronchiseptica can also be a secondary opportunist invader of the respiratory system.

BURSITIS

Bursitis is a common condition that arises from constant pressure and trauma to the skin overlying any bony prominence. The periosteum or covering over the bone reacts by creating bone, a swelling develops and the skin likewise responds and becomes thicker, until there is a prominent soft lump. It can commence in the farrowing houses, particularly if there are bad floors but it usually starts in the weaner accommodation on slatted floors which have large gaps. As the pig increases in weight there is increased pressure on the leg bones. Swellings develop over the lateral sides of the hocks and elbows and over the points of the hocks. Such swellings are called bursa although strictly speaking they are not. The term should apply to inflammation of bursa that cover tendons. Worn and pitted floor surfaces particularly if sharp aggregate was used in the concrete, can exaggerate the trauma to the extent that the skin is broken and secondary infection develops. If this occurs on wet dirty floors major problems can arise. Under normal circumstances if there is no secondary infection the condition commercially is not important but if breeding stock is being produced then the management system needs to be adjusted, otherwise rejection rates on breeding gilts will be high.

Wire mesh, woven metal and metal bar floors can produce high levels in weaner pigs in first and second stage housing. Identify the point at which disease first appears and alter the floor surfaces or change the environment.

Clinical signs

These can develop when piglets are 1-2 weeks old particularly where farrowing crate floors are totally slatted. Metal bars are particularly bad. Most swellings commence on the hind legs below the point of the hock or on the lateral aspects of the elbow. With repeated trauma the lesions increase in size and ultimately fluid appears. This is common in pigs 30-70kg weight. Infection with *Mycoplasma hyosynoviae* can occur and can also seen at the base of the tail over the shoulder blades and the knees.

Treatment

- There is no specific treatment that will reduce the bone reaction. Remove pigs to pens that are well bedded.
- If the swellings have become infected with bacteria inject with either oxytetracycline or ampicillin.
- If *Mycoplasma hyosynoviae* is causing infection use either lincomycin or tiamulin.
- Most lesions do not require treatment.

Management control and prevention

- Move severely affected animals onto deep bedded floors.
- Determine the point at which lesions are occurring and relate to floor surfaces.
- If the problem is arising in flat decks in breeding gilts it may be necessary to change the slats to those covered with plastic. Tri-bar or metal slats and woven mesh are bad surfaces.

BUSH FOOT / FOOT ROT

Bush foot results from infection of the claw which becomes swollen and extremely painful around the coronary band. It arises through penetration of the sole of the foot, cracks at the sole-hoof junction, or splitting of the hoof itself. It usually occurs in one foot only and is more commonly seen in the hind feet especially the outer claws, which are the larger ones carrying proportionately more weight. Infection sometimes penetrates the soft tissues between the claws and this is referred to as foot rot.

As the infection progresses inside the hoof, the claw becomes enlarged and infection and inflammation of the joint (arthritis) often develops. The condition is important because of the effect on reproductive performance of the breeding female. Foot rot involves both superficial and deep infection of the soft tissues between the claws often caused by fusiformis bacteria.

Foot pain in the boar at mating causes poor ejaculation and a shorter mating time.

Clinical signs

The pig is very lame with a painful swollen claw. Always try and examine the feet when the animal is lying down. In most cases a swelling will be visible around the coronary band which may form an abscess and burst to the surface. Invariably only one claw is involved. With foot rot the infection will be confined to the tissues between the claws.

Diagnosis

This is based on the clinical signs described above. Bush foot has to be differentiated from other forms of trauma and infection but the painful swollen claw is obvious.

Similar diseases

These include:
Erysipelas.
Glässers disease.
Leg weakness or osteochondrosis (OCD).
Mycoplasma arthritis.
Trauma

Treatment

There is a poor blood supply to the infected tissues and therefore higher dose levels of antibiotics are required for longer periods of time.
- ☐ Antibiotics which can be used, depending on the advice of your veterinarian, include:
  - Lincocin   11mg/kg liveweight.
  - Oxytetracycline 25 mg/kg liveweight.
  - Amoxycillin   15mg/kg liveweight.
- ☐ Inject daily for 5 to 7 days.
  If there is no improvement in three days change the antibiotic. Complete recovery may take 3-4 weeks.
- ☐ Anti-inflammatory injections of cortisone may be given provided the sow is not pregnant.
- ☐ An anti-inflammatory drug such as phenylbutazone may be administered either by mouth or injection.
- ☐ If there is a herd problem a foot bath containing either 1% formalin (only use in the open air) or 5% copper sulphate will help. Walk the sows through once each week on 2-3 occasions. However if there are dry cracked claws in the herd, this treatment might make them worse.

Management control and prevention

- ◆ Badly worn floor surfaces predispose.
- ◆ Sharp flint aggregates in concrete predispose.
- ◆ Pay particular attention to floors in boar pens, mating pens and loose sow housing.

> **Lame sows are less likely to conceive, have poor litters and are more likely to abort.**

- ◆ Check the quality of the floor surface around drinkers and feeders - particularly concrete slats.
- ◆ Use straw or shavings as bedding if practicable.
- ◆ Check the biotin levels in the diet.
- ◆ Wash and disinfect concrete surfaces regularly.

> **Lame boars often have poor fertility and produce small litters.**

CLASSICAL SWINE FEVER (HOG CHOLERA), AFRICAN SWINE FEVER

See chapter 12 for further information.

CLOSTRIDIAL DISEASES

See chapter 7 for further information.

Clostridial infections are relatively uncommon in growers and finishers but occur on some farms infrequently in the breeding herd. They are usually manifest either by gas gangrene of musculature or sudden death and the pig decomposes very quickly showing a distended abdomen. If an outbreak of sudden death occurs in good pigs, post mortem examinations should be carried out as soon as possible after death. Anthrax must also be considered as a possibility and veterinary advice sought.

COCCIDIOSIS

See chapter 11 for further information.

This is a disease seen in sucking pigs, occasionally growing pigs and it is rare in adults. However occasionally where finishing pigs are moved into continually populated pens to be retained as breeding animals high levels of coccidia can persist and cause disease. This may be characterised by poor growth and sloppy faeces which may occasionally be tinged with blood. An examination of a faeces sample would help in diagnosis.

Control is effected by depopulating and washing out the pen to remove the coccidial oocysts and using a disinfection such as OO-CIDE. Treatment is either by injections of sulphonamides every other day for three applications or medication of the drinking water for seven days.

COLIFORM INFECTIONS AND POST-WEANING DIARRHOEA

The bacterium *E. coli* is a common inhabitant of the intestine of the pig. There are two types, non haemolytic and haemolytic, which describe whether or not the organism breaks down blood (haemolysis) on a culture plate. In some countries haemolytic types invariably cause disease due to the toxins that they produce but in others non haemolytic strains predominate. At weaning time the loss of sows milk and IgA allow the *E. coli* to attach to the villi of the small intestines, the toxins cause acute enteritis and diarrhoea. Post-weaning diarrhoea is a common cause of mortality and morbidity.

Clinical signs

These are usually seen within five days of weaning. In severe cases a pig is found dead with sunken eyes and slight blueing of the extremities. Diarrhoea will not necessarily be seen but in less acute cases the first signs are often slight loss of condition, dehydration and a watery diarrhoea. To identify the latter press the abdomen of a suspect pig and see whether diarrhoea is evident. Dehydration results in rapid loss of weight. The changes in the intestine can be so severe as to cause haemorrhage and blood or black tarry faeces may be seen, but usually the pig dies. The diarrhoea varies in consistency from very watery to a paste with a wide range of colour from grey white, yellow and green. Colour is not of any significance. Fresh blood or mucus would normally be absent.

Diagnosis

This is based on the history of disease in the first week post-weaning although diarrhoea can develop 10 to 14 days post-weaning. Other causes e.g. rotavirus, can give similar symptoms and it is necessary to submit a live or recently dead untreated pig to the laboratory for bacteriological and virological tests to distinguish between them. Determine the antibiotic sensitivity to the *E. coli*.

Similar diseases

These include porcine epidemic diarrhoea, rotavirus, TGE and salmonella infections. A useful and simple test to differentiate between virus causes and *E. coli* diarrhoea involves the use of litmus paper to determine whether the scour is an alkaline or an acid consistency. Soak the paper in the scour, *E. coli* diarrhoea is alkaline (blue colour change) whereas viral infections are acid (red colour change).

SUITABLE ANTIBIOTICS AND MEDICAMENTS FOR THE TREATMENT OF *E. COLI* SCOUR (POST-WEANING).		
Injections	Water	In-Feed
Amoxycillin	Amoxycillin	Amoxycillin 300g/tonne
Enrofloxacin	Apramycin	Apramycin 100g/tonne
Framycetin		Combined CTC, penicillin sulphadimidine
Gentamycin	Neomycin	Furazolidone 400g/tonne
Tiamulin	Sulphonamides	Lincomycin 44g / spectinomycin 44g/tonne
Trimethoprim/sulpha (TMS)	Tiamulin	Neomycin 163g/tonne
	TMS	Tiamulin 100g/tonne
		TMS - variable levels
		Sulphonamides 200-400g/tonne
		Zinc oxide 3.1kg/tonne (Prevention only)

(Fig.9-22)

Treatment

☐ It is important to know the history of the disease on the farm and antibiotic sensitivities to the bacteria present. Sick pigs should always be treated individually and group treatment applied to the pigs at risk. Ideally by water medication. (Fig.9-22).

☐ Add zinc oxide at a level of 2,500ppm of zinc per tonne. Feed for 2-3 weeks. This is highly effective in controlling *E. coli* infection.

☐ If pigs become dehydrated, electrolytes should be provided in a separate drinker.

Management control and prevention

The principles of controlling this disease are common to the general management of the post-weaned pig. These are discussed at the beginning of the chapter and you are advised to review these and adjust your control systems as indicated. If there is a problem on the farm use the following checklist:

Pre-weaning
- Assess health and body condition of the lactating sow.
- Are there respiratory or enteric problems during sucking? Adopt control measures.
- Are the weaning problems mainly in gilt litters? If so consider *E. coli* vaccination.
- Are gilts and sows vaccinated against *E. coli*?
- Consider aspects of farrowing house environment and hygiene as discussed in chapter 7.
- Creep feeding. Consider the type, frequency and age of introduction.
- Stop creep feeding before weaning and assess the effects.

On the day of weaning - consider the significance of:
- Stress.
- Stocking density - group sizes.
- House temperatures and fluctuations.
- House hygiene.
- Water availability.
- Nutrition -
    Type - Meal or pellets, wet or dry.
        Feeding practices.
        Quality of nutrition.

After weaning consider:
- Air flow.
- Temperature fluctuations.
- Ventilation, humidity.
- Creep feed management.
- Response to different creep diets.
- Disease.
- Age and weight at weaning.
- Floor surfaces - comfort boards.
- Rate and evenness of growth.

COLITIS

"Colitis" means inflammation of the large bowel and it is very common in some countries in growing pigs. It is characterised by sloppy "cow pat" type faeces, with no blood and little if any mucus but the condition may progress to severe diarrhoea. Affected pigs are usually 6 to 12 weeks of age and in any one group, up to 50% of the population may be affected. It is not seen in adult or sucking pigs. A number of organisms have been implicated but spirochetes and in particular *Serpulina pilosicoli*, an organism distinct from a similar one that causes swine dysentery, is thought to be important. However dietary factors also precipitate disease and pelleted feed is much more likely to be associated with the disease than meal. If the incriminating pellets are ground back to meal colitis still results, demonstrating an effect of the pelleting process. Certain components in the feed are also implicated including poor quality oils and carbohydrates but specific ones have not been identified.

Clinical signs

These usually appear in rapidly growing pigs from 8 to 14 weeks old, fed ad lib on high density diets. The early signs are sloppy faeces but with pigs appearing clinically normal. As the disease and its severity progress, a very watery diarrhoea, with dehydration, loss of condition and poor growth become evident in the pigs. During the affected period daily gain and food conversion can be severely affected, with feed conversion worsening by up to 0.2.

Diagnosis

This is based on clinical signs and the elimination of other causes of diarrhoea, in particular swine dysentery. Faeces examinations in the laboratory are necessary to assist with diagnosis together with post-mortem examinations and laboratory tests on a typical untreated pig. It is possible that porcine enteropathy may be involved in the clinical syndrome and if the herd has a severe problem examination of the terminal parts of the small intestine in pigs at slaughter would be advised.

Treatment

- Antibiotic therapy is not always successful because it depends on the presence of primary or secondary bacteria, but the following drugs have given responses on problem farms, using in-feed medication.

  Dimetridazole - 200 g / tonne
  Lincomycin - 110 g/ tonne
  Monensin - 100 g / tonne
  Oxytetracycline - 400 g / tonne
  Salinomycin - 60 g / tonne
  Tiamulin - 100 g / tonne
  Tylosin - 100 g / tonne
- For the individual pig daily injections of either tiamulin, lincomycin, tylosin or oxytetracycline may be beneficial
- Weaned pigs are fed zinc for the first two weeks post-weaning to prevent *E. coli* enteritis. Colitis may develop in the 2 to 3 weeks following its removal from the diet. The response to continuing zinc oxide in the feed at 2 to 3kg per tonne should be considered.

Management control and prevention

- Disease is seen in pigs that are growing well on ad lib feeding and often it is associated with a change of diet.
- It is more common with diets high in energy and protein (14.5MJ DE/kg 21% protein). It is experienced using all types of diets but particularly those that have been pelleted rather than fed as a meal. It is thought that the pelleting process may have an effect on fats in the diet and thereby initiate digestive disturbances in the large bowel.
- It is common when fat sprayed diets are fed, try diets without.
- Mortality is low but morbidity can be high, ranging from 5 to 50%. Adopt all-in all-out management of pens.
- The same diet can be used on two separate farms and disease only appear on one, suggesting inherent causes.
- The presence of certain types of bacteria in the large bowel such as *Serpulina pilosicoli* obviously play a part in the disease. Use preventive medication in feed to control *Serpulina pilosicoli*
- It is uncommon on home milled cereal based diets.
- The response to treatment can be variable.
- Control consists of assessing the above key factors, which would include changing the diet formulation (less added fats), changing the source of feed, acidifying the diet and improving pen hygiene. A change from pellets to meal feeding is usually effective.

The following anti colitis diet fed as a meal has been effective.

Wheat 50%
Barley 11%
Full fat soya 15%
Fish meal 7.5%

Hypro soya 6.5%
Sharps (wheat by-product) 5%
Skim milk 2.5%
Vitamin lysine mineral supplement 2.5%
Analysis
    Protein 24%
    DE 14.6
    Lysine1.35

ENTERIC DISEASES

A scour or diarrhoea problem in growing pigs is likely to be associated with one or more of the following diseases. (Common ones *).
- Anthrax (rare).
- Classical swine fever (in those countries where it is still endemic).
- Coliform infections and post-weaning diarrhoea *
- Colitis (non specific) *.
- Oedema disease (diarrhoea uncommon).
- Parasites.
- Porcine epidemic diarrhoea PED *.
- Porcine enteropathy including PHE, PIA, NE and RI *.
- Rotavirus.
- Salmonellosis *.
- Spirochaetal diarrhoea.
- Swine dysentery *.
- TGE (rare in Europe now but still common in some other countries).

Refer to the above specific diseases after a diagnosis has been made in a laboratory. Use the following flow diagram to assist in interpreting the clinical picture.

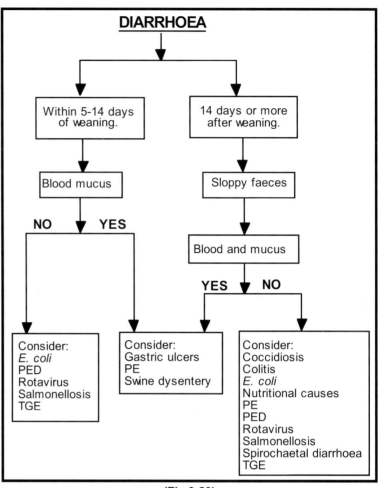

(Fig.9-23)

ENZOOTIC PNEUMONIA (EP) OR *MYCOPLASMA HYOPNEUMONIAE* INFECTION

Enzootic pneumonia is caused by a tiny organism *Mycoplasma hyopneumoniae*. It is widespread in pig populations and endemic in most herds throughout the world. It is transmitted either through the movement of the carrier pigs or by wind-borne infection for up to $2^{1}/_{2}$ - 3km ($1^{1}/_{2}$ - 2 miles) if the climatic conditions are right. The organism dies out quickly outside the pig, particularly when dried. It can however be maintained in moist cool conditions for two to three days. It has a long incubation period of two to eight weeks before clinical symptoms are seen. As an uncomplicated infection in well-housed and managed pigs it is a relatively unimportant disease and has only mild effects on the pig. However if there are other infections present particularly App, Hps, Pasteurella, PRRS or SI, the pneumonia can become more complex with serious effects on the pig.

Fig.9-24 shows the basic structure of the lobes of the lungs. EP always attacks the lower shaded areas of each of these lobes (anterior, cardiac, intermediate and anterior diaphramatic) causing consolidation of the tissues. The extent of this consolidation in each lobe is scored out of either 5 or 10 depending upon the lobe affected. Thus a severely affected pig with all lobes involved would score 55. Occasionally, particularly in disease breakdowns the diaphramatic lobes will be involved as well. If more than 15% of lungs are affected it is highly probable that EP is present in the population. Herds that do not carry *M. hyopneumoniae* rarely show consolidated lesions of more than 1 to 2% and even then they are very small.

This scoring system can be used to assess the severity of disease and its effects on the pig. (Fig.9-25).

If EP is not present in the growing population then the effects of the other respiratory pathogens are very greatly reduced. It is therefore considered a prime organism that opens up the lung to other infections.

Clinical signs

Acute disease

This is normally only seen when EP is introduced

CHAPTER 9 - Managing and Treating Disease in the Weaner, Grower and Finishing Periods

into the herd for the first time. For a period of six to eight weeks after entry there may be severe acute pneumonia, coughing, respiratory distress, fever and high mortality across all ages of stock. This picture however is extremely variable and breakdowns are experienced when disease is mild or inapparent.

Chronic disease

This is the normal picture where the organism has been present in the herd for some considerable time. Maternal antibody is passed via colostrum to the piglets and it disappears from seven to twelve weeks of age after which clinical signs start to appear. A prolonged non-productive cough, at least seven to eight coughs per episode, is a common sign around this time, with some pigs breathing heavily ("thumps") and showing signs of pneumonia. 30 to 70% of pigs will have lung lesions at slaughter.

Diagnosis

In most cases this is based on the clinical picture and examination of the lungs of pigs at post-mortem or at slaughter, combined possibly with histology of the lesions. However, these do not provide a specific diagnosis and in the herds supplying breeding stock or in special cases (e.g. litigation) it may be necessary to confirm the diagnosis by carrying out one or more of the following tests: ELISA tests, serum tests for specific antibodies, microscopic examination of stained touch preparations (TPs) of the cut surface of the lungs, fluorescent antibody tests (FATs), polymerase chain reaction (PCRs) tests and finally culture and identification of *Mycoplasmal hyopneumoniae*.

These tests are not widely available and many diagnostic laboratories cannot do them. The PCR is probably the most sensitive. FAT, serology and cultures are used in Denmark, but only FATs are available in some countries.

Similar diseases

Consolidation of the anterior lobes of the lungs at a low level can be caused by other respiratory pathogens including SI, PRRS, Hps certain viruses and other mycoplasma. Laboratory tests are required to differentiate them. Furthermore, all or some of these may occur as mixed infections together with *Mycoplasma hyopneumoniae*.

Treatment

In the herds in which the disease has become endemic a decision to medicate feed should be based on the following:
- variable growth in pigs from 10 to 20 weeks of age.

PNEUMONIA DIAGRAM OF THE LUNGS
Areas of Infection and a Scoring System

(Fig.9-24)

A GUIDE TO THE EFFECTS OF EP LESIONS ON DAILY GAIN

Total Score Max. 55	% loss in daily gain
Zero	0
1 - 10	0
11 - 20	6
21 - 30	18
31 - 40	26
41 - 55	50

(Fig.9-25)

- ongoing pneumonia treatment of individuals at more than 2.5% of the pig population.
- of lungs scoring more than 15.
- active lesions - raised above the level of the lung surface and moist or wet.

Methods of medication have been extensively dealt with in chapter 4 page.

Acute disease (Herd breakdown)

Consider the following:
☐ Medicate pigs between weaning and 16 weeks of age for 4 to 8 weeks with 500g/tonne of CTC or OTC and then reduce this to 200-300g/tonne.
☐ Inject severely affected individual pigs with either long-acting OTC, tiamulin, lincomycin or penicillin/streptomycin.

- If pigs become affected soon after weaning inject with OTC LA at weaning time or one week prior to the onset of disease.

Chronic disease
- Identify the point at which disease is occurring and apply strategic medication, either in feed, in water or by injection using the drugs outlined above.
- For strategic medication use tetracyclines 500-800g/tonne, 220g/tonne of lincomycin or 100g/tonne of tiamulin and feed for 7 to 10 days commencing one to three weeks prior to the anticipated time of the disease starting.

Management control and prevention

The EP free breeding herd
- Most breeding organisations can supply breeding stock that is deemed to be EP free and so a new pig farm can be set up or an old one repopulated EP free. The question is whether it will remain so. One rule of thumb is that if you have an uninterrupted view of an infected EP herd, particularly if it is less than 3km (2miles) away, there is a definite chance that sooner or later your herd will become contaminated by wind-borne infection. If the herd you can see is a grower/finisher as distinct from a weaner producer than the risk is greater. The risk also increases the larger the infected herd. In a pig dense regions such as in the pig rearing areas of Eastern England, Germany, the Netherlands, Belgium, Eastern Spain, Quebec or Japan, it is impossible to remain free.

  You are likely to remain EP free indefinitely if your EP free herd is in a region of low pig density, such as parts of North or Southwest France, Northern Spain or the West USA.

  Likewise if the land is hilly or mountainous or on a sea coast.

To maintain an EP free breeding herd
- Keep it closed. Introduce genes only by AI, embryo transfer, or hysterectomy and fostering.
- Purchase only EP free stock from a reputable seed stock supplier, if possible from the same source herd every time, or at least from the same breeding pyramid. (It would be sensible to check whether the source herd is also free from lesions of App).
- Isolate incoming pigs for eight weeks and check that the EP free status of the donor herd has been maintained before moving them into your herd. (This is good practice whether your herd is EP free or not).
- To be ultra careful, mix sentinel pigs from your herd in with the new pigs in isolation, one to two weeks after their delivery. The sentinels can be slaughtered and their lungs examined before the pigs move in or they can be blood tested on entry to the isolation and again five weeks later. (Whatever the health status of your herd, EP free or not, it is a good practice to put pigs from your herd alongside the isolated gilts. This helps them to gradually adapt to the health status of your herd).

To maintain an EP free grower/finisher herd
- Purchase only from an EP free source but instead of an isolation period implement an all-in all-out policy, by site if possible, or if not by building.
- Again the location is paramount.

The herd with endemic EP
- Purchase stock with EP but, depending on the health status of the herd, make sure the pigs are free from swine dysentery, mange, App and PRRS.
- Carry out isolation and monitoring procedures as above. Six weeks instead of eight weeks is probably enough. If your herd has a low health status and is intensively housed it may be helpful to medicate the feed for the incoming stock if they are EP free.

  Use tetracyclines at 300-500g/tonne for the last two weeks in isolation and the first four weeks in your herd. This allows them to become immune without becoming ill.
- Keep a broad parity spread in your sows. Sows of second parity onwards are more immune than first litter gilts and pass a better immunity to their piglets.
- Check the faeces of the growing pigs for ascarids and if present keep them under control by routine worming and all-in all-out housing procedures.
- If you are having clinical problems and poor growth later in growing pigs vaccinate young piglets against EP as per manufacturers instructions.

Increased disease is associated with the following; (consider changes)
- Overcrowding and group sizes in any one environment of more than 200.
- Variable temperatures and poor insulation.
- Variable wind speeds and chilling.
- Low temperature, low humidity environments.
- Houses with poor hygiene and high levels of carbon dioxide and ammonia.
- High dust/bacteria levels in the air.
- Pig movement, stress and mixing.
- A shortage of trough space.
- Housing with a continuous throughput of pigs.
- Other concurrent diseases.
- Poor nutrition.
- Dietary changes at susceptible times.
- Slatted floors and liquid waste.
- Less than $3m^3$ air space/pig and $0.7m^2$ floor space/pig.
- Houses that are too wide for good air flow control.
- Presence of PRRS.
- Presence of aujeszky's disease.
- Presence of App.
- Presence of swine influenza.
- Purchasing from different sources.

CHAPTER 9 - Managing and Treating Disease in the Weaner, Grower and Finishing Periods

Therefore to keep EP and respiratory disease under control:

- Optimise stocking levels by pen and house. This will not only reduce clinical signs but the energy that had been required for immunity will be available for growth and result in faster throughput. Thus the number of pigs sold per year can remain the same as at higher stocking levels.
- Optimise the ventilation and improve the hygiene to reduce noxious gases.
- Improve the insulation if necessary and maintain constant temperature control.
- Reduce the dust and bacteria in the air by changing to wet feed or to less dusty dry feed. (Note increasing ventilation does not decrease dust and may increase it).
- Check the nutrition and time of feed changes.
- Organise the grower/finisher stages so that moving and mixing is minimal.
- Operate an all-in all-out system wherever possible.
- **Vaccination**. Highly efficient EP vaccines have recently come to the market that reduce lung lesions by up to 95%. Some can be applied at one and three weeks of age and this provides excellent control during the growing and susceptible period. Vaccine could also be applied to EP negative herds if considered at risk.

Experiences of the use of enzootic pneumonia vaccines in herds with complex respiratory problems are giving very encouraging results particularly if used in conjunction with segregated weaning and segregated disease control techniques - the latter on combined breeding/finishing operations.

If you have a problem on your farm consider the following simple criteria in making the decision to vaccinate:
- The presence of *Mycoplasma hyopneumoniae*.
- A continual level of respiratory disease.
- Primary or secondary infections associated with PRRS, influenza, pseudorabies and *Actinobacillus pleuropneumoniae*.
- Heavy bacterial challenge.
- The necessity for continual in-feed medication.
- Variable and poor growth associated with respiratory disease.
- Weaning to slaughter mortalities of more than 4%.
- Finally, the cost of vaccination should be equal to or less than costs of the potential reduction in mortality and in-feed medication. Improvements in daily gain and feed efficiency become the bonus. In severely affected herds a cost benefit ratio of up to 5:1 has been achieved.

EPERYTHROZOONOSIS (EPE)

Eperythrozoonosis is caused by a small ricketsial bacterium called *Eperythrozoon suis* (Epe) which attaches itself to the red cells in the blood, damaging them and causing them to break apart. This causes an anaemia associated with a reduction in the number of red blood cells and haemoglobin the substance by which oxygen is transported around the body. When large numbers of red cells are damaged, jaundice may result.

The disease is somewhat of an enigma because the organism can be identified both in normal animals and in those severely affected with disease. It is likely that Epe is very widespread and most sources of pigs examined (varying health status) have shown evidence of the bacteria.

In the majority herds where it has been identified there have been no clinical problems and the significance therefore of the organism in relation to infection in these cases must be in doubt. However, in the past two years a positive diagnosis associated with disease has become more common. Epe can cross the placenta and be responsible for poor pale pigs at birth and high pre-weaning mortality.

Clinical signs

Epe affects all classes of pigs from sows and piglets through to weaners and growers. Clinical pictures vary, particularly if there are secondary infections involved. It is useful however, to look at the clinical symptoms in acute and chronic disease. In piglets and weaners the acute disease is manifest by primary anaemia and secondary infections, whilst the more chronic picture appears related to slow growth, variable growth rate and poor-doing pigs. The chronic symptoms in sows are associated with reproductive failure and if there is stress at farrowing, fevers and agalactia may be experienced.

If pale anaemic pigs are evident during sucking or in the immediate post-weaning period and an injection of iron has been given, the possibility of Epe should be considered.

Diagnosis

The presence of the organism does not necessarily confirm disease. The following need to be considered to clarify the relationship between Epe and disease.
- The presence of pale and anaemic pigs.
- The identification of the organism in blood smears stained with Wright's stain. Fifty microscopic fields should be examined before a negative diagnosis is arrived at.
- The clinical picture on the farm should include lowered reproductive performance.

EPERYTHROZOON SUIS - CLINICAL SIGNS		
Sows	Piglets	Weaners/Growers
Abortion	Jaundiced	Anaemia
Agalactia	Increased scour	Ear necrosis
Anaemia, jaundice	Pale pigs	Enteritis
Fever	Pneumonia	Fever
Increased repeats	Weak at birth	Pneumonia
Reduced conception		Poor doers
Reproductive failure		Pot-bellied pigs
		Scour

- Jaundice, particularly in young growing pigs from 7 to 21 days of age.
- Serological tests are being developed including an ELISA but at the time of writing they are still unreliable.
- Eliminate other causes of anaemia.
- Blood samples should be examined for packed cell volume (PCV) and haemoglobin levels. In normal pigs the mean PCV would be around 35% and in clinically affected pigs 24%. Haemoglobin levels would normally range from 9 to 14g per 100ml but in anaemic pigs they would be as low as 3 to 7g per 100ml.

Similar diseases

Actinobacillus pleuropneumonia.
Chronic respiratory disease complexed with PRRS and influenza.
Glässer's disease - *Haemophilus parasuis*.
Iron / copper anaemia.
Leptospirosis (*L.. icterohaemorrhagiae* and *L.. canicola*).
Malabsorption and chronic enteritis.
Pale piglet syndrome - haemorrhages.
Porcine enteropathy (PE, NE, PHE and PIA).

Treatment

Consider the following and discuss with your veterinarian:

☐ The response to treatment is not very good.
☐ Inject piglets with oxytetracycline at 10mg/kg daily for 4 days or use long-acting preparations, three injections each two days apart.
☐ In-feed medicate sows at 800gms/tonne of OTC for 4 weeks and repeat again 4 weeks later.
☐ Arsanilic acid in-feed at 85gms/tonne is reported to have an effect but in many countries there is no licensed product in food producing animals. Where it is available it is probably the drug of choice.
☐ The response to other drugs is poor.

Management control and prevention

Epe suis is spread by inoculation (including inoculation by insects). In a problem herd it is important to eliminate possible methods of spread including:-

Sows
◆ Vaccinating sows with the same needle - Wipe the needle between inoculation with cotton wool well dampened with surgical spirit and change every third sow.
◆ Tagging gilts - Wash the applicators between animals or hold three pairs in an antiseptic solution and rotate.
◆ Eliminate lice or mange mites.
◆ Prevent or control fighting, vulval and tail biting etc.
◆ Do not feed back placenta or farrowing house material.
◆ Control biting insects.
◆ Control internal parasites.
◆ Wear plastic arm sleeves when attending a farrowing.

Piglets
◆ Spread occurs during tailing, teething and iron injections.
◆ Control as for sows.

Weaners and growers
◆ Prevent fighting at weaning. Reduce mixing.
◆ Prevent tail biting and vice.
◆ Reduce mixing and use Stresnil to prevent fighting.
◆ Prevent spread through vaccination and inoculations between pigs.
◆ Control biting insects.
◆ Control respiratory diseases.

Do not let the infection get out of control and cause disease.

ERYSIPELAS

See chapter 7 for further information.

This is an important disease both in the young growing pig and the sow, caused by the bacterium *Erysipelothrix insidiosa*. This organism is a common inhabitant of normal healthy swine and it can be found in the tonsils in up to 50% of the population. It is passed out in faeces or via the mouth and in dirty conditions high levels of the organism can build up in the environment to present pigs with a heavy challenge. Wet feeding systems, particularly if whey or milk products are used may allow bacterial growth. The bacteria invade the blood stream through a variety of routes including a break in the skin or via the wall of the digestive tract and a septicaemia develops. Infection can also occur without clinical disease. The incubation period is 24 to 48 hours.

Clinical signs

Acute disease

This occurs as sudden death or animals acutely ill running a very high temperature. Skin lesions may also be evident as large raised diamond shaped areas over the body that turn from red to black. They may be easier to feel than to see in the early stages.

Sub acute disease

This is the more common picture with mild or few symptoms. Skin lesions are common and the pigs need not necessarily appear to be ill in spite of a temperature of up to 40°C (104°F). From the blood stream the organism may settle in the joints causing chronic arthritis and lameness. Joint problems can be responsible for condemnations at slaughter.

Diagnosis

An individual pig or a small number of pigs will show a high temperature and few other signs. Skin lesions are 10 to 50mm diamond shaped, raised and red to blue to black in colour. They are diagnostic.

The organism is easily cultured and tissue samples (e.g. spleen or liver) submitted to the laboratory provide confirmation.

The bacterium alone can cause the disease but concurrent virus infections, such as PRRS or influenza, may trigger off large outbreaks and this should be borne in mind in making a diagnosis.

Treatment

- ☐ The drug of choice is penicillin and for ease of convenience a long-acting one should be used to reduce the necessity for daily injections. If the pig is acutely ill, twice daily injections of short-acting penicillin should be used initially for the first day. Continue antibiotic cover for four days.
- ☐ Where large numbers of pigs are involved it may be necessary to inject all the pigs in the groups at risk.
- ☐ Amoxycillin, phenoxymethyl penicillin or tetracyclines in the drinking water are also effective.
- ☐ Outbreaks involving pens or complete houses of pigs sometimes occur, particularly during summer months. If the disease is acute, treatment should commence immediately via the water and be continued with in-feed medication using phenoxymethyl penicillin (penicillin V) 200g/tonne or tetracyclines 500g/tonne. Pen. V can also be used for prevention in the face of an outbreak.
- ☐ In individual outbreaks finishing pens should be washed and disinfected between batches. If wet feeding is implicated the system must be cleaned out and disinfected.

Management control and prevention

The following may predispose to disease:
- ◆ The movement of pigs involving mixing and stress, particularly when maternal antibody from the sow is disappearing.
- ◆ Diets that contain fungal toxins (mycotoxins) particularly aflatoxin.
- ◆ Sudden changes in temperature.
- ◆ Wet dirty pens particularly if they are heavily contaminated with faeces that contain high numbers of organisms.
- ◆ Water systems that have become contaminated with the organism
- ◆ During warm summer weather when pigs foul their pens.
- ◆ Sudden changes in diet.
- ◆ Heavy parasite burdens or low levels of coccidia that allow the bacteria to enter through the damaged wall of the intestine.
- ◆ Straw based systems.
- ◆ The purchase of non vaccinated boars or gilts.
- ◆ Continually populated houses with no all-in all-out procedures and disinfection.
- ◆ Virus infections particularly PRRS and SI.

Prevention - This is easily carried out by vaccination. In continual outbreaks in growing pigs it may be necessary to vaccinate pigs at 8 weeks and possibly again at 10 weeks of age. If disease is occurring earlier than this, the age of vaccination needs to be reduced. Normally however pigs are not vaccinated before 8 weeks because colostrum antibodies reduce the vaccine response.

FOOT-AND-MOUTH DISEASE (FMD)

See chapter 12 for further information.

This disease should always be considered if sudden widespread lameness appears. In all countries it is notifiable and must be reported to the authorities with all speed. As well as lameness, affected pigs salivate and blisters or vesicles are evident on the skin at the coronet at the top of the claws, the heels, nose and tongue.

FRACTURES

Bone fractures are not uncommon in sows and gilts and are usually the end result of trauma and fighting, although spontaneous ones occur in bone disease such as osteomalacia, associated with calcium phosphorus and vitamins A and D, and osteochondrosis.

Clinical signs

The onset is invariably sudden, the animal being unable to rise on its own without difficulty. A significant feature is the reluctance to place any weight on the affected leg. The muscles and tissues over the fracture site are often swollen and painful and the pig is very reluctant to move unless on three legs. An examination is best carried out when the pig is lying down. Crepitus or the rubbing together of the two broken ends of the bone can often be felt. Fractures of the spinal vertebra are common in the first litter female particularly during lactation and in the immediate post weaning period. The pig usually adopts a dog sitting position and exhibits severe pain on movement. Such animals should be destroyed.

Diagnosis

This is based upon the history, symptoms and palpation to detect crepitus.

Similar diseases

These include acute laminitis, arthritis, muscle tearing, bush foot and mycoplasma arthritis.

Treatment

- ☐ The affected animal should be slaughtered on the farm.

Management control and prevention

◆ If fractures are a recurring problem it is necessary to check that there are no diseases such as osteomalacia, osteoporosis or leg weakness (OCD).
◆ Check the calcium phosphorus and vitamin D levels.
◆ Check management procedures during the period of effect.

GASTRIC ULCERS

Erosion and ulceration of the lining of the stomach is a common condition in all pigs. It occurs around the area where the oesophagus enters the stomach (called the pars oesophagea). In the early stages of the disease the pars becomes roughened and gradually changes as the surface becomes eroded until it is actively ulcerated. Intermittent haemorrhage may then take place leading to anaemia, or massive haemorrhage may occur resulting in death. The incidence in sows is usually less than 5% but in growing pigs up to 60% may show lesions at slaughter.

The causes of gastric ulceration are multifactorial. These can be categorised as nutritional and related to the physical properties of the feed, managemental, infectious causes and miscellaneous factors.
The following need to be considered as causal or contributory:

Nutritional factors:
- Low protein diets.
- Low fibre diets. (The introduction of straw reduces the incidence).
- High energy diets.
- High levels of wheat in excess of 55%.
- Deficiencies of vitamin E or selenium.
- Diets containing high levels of iron, copper or calcium.
- Diets low in zinc.
- Diets with high levels of unsaturated fats.
- Diets based on whey and skimmed milk.

Physical aspects of the diet that increase the incidence:
- Size of feed particle - the more finely ground the meal the smaller becomes the particle size and the higher the incidence of ulcers. This is still the case if the feed is then pelleted.
- Pelleting feeds in itself increases the incidence. Feed meal.
- Particle size. Where there is a problem on the farm have the feed examined to assess the varying percentages of particle sizes. This is carried out by sifting the meal through a series of 12 to 14 tiller screens and weighing the residual amounts remaining in each screen. Particle size is also affected by the type and moisture content of the cereals that are being used, the condition of the hammer mills and the screen and the rate of flow through the grinding system. The smaller the particle size the greater the incidence.
- Sometimes there can be problems in changing from pellets to meal and a compromise is to feed alternatively.
- If the feed is home-produced and is meal, then it is necessary to check the size and quality of the screen that is being used.
- Using cereals with a high moisture content.
- Rolling cereals as distinct from grinding them will often produce a dramatic drop in the incidence but the penalties of feed use have to be taken into consideration.

Managemental factors that increase the incidence:
- Irregular feeding patterns and shortage of feeder space.
- Periods of starvation.
- Increased stocking densities and movement of pigs. Look carefully at the environment in the pens and in finishing houses. Are there undue stresses or aggressions.
- Poor management of sows in stalls and tethers.
- Transportation.
- Poor availability of food or water.

> *If ulcers are a problem then increase the screen size to 3.5mm.*

Miscellaneous factors:
- Stress associated with fluctuating environmental temperatures.
- Adverse environmental conditions that create an unhappy environment.
- Psychological stress resulting from bad or harsh stockmanship.
- The condition is more common in castrates and boars than in gilts but the reason for this is unknown. Difference in feeding patterns may be a factor.
- Split sexing may help.
- Breed. More common in certain genotypes particularly those that have low back fat measurements and a capacity for rapid lean tissue growth.

> *Consider changing from pellets to course ground meal.*

Infectious causes:
- There is a clear relationship between outbreaks of pneumonia and the incidence of gastric ulceration.
- Ulceration may occur following bacterial septicaemias such as those associated with erysipelas and swine fever.
- In the breeding sow gastric ulceration is usually confined to the individual animal and is often secondary to a specific disease.

Clinical signs

These depend on the severity of the condition. In its

most acute form previously healthy animals are found dead. The most striking sign in these cases is the paleness of the carcase due to internal haemorrhage. In the less acute form the affected pig is pale, and weak, and may show breathlessness, grinding of the teeth due to stomach pain and vomiting. The passing of dark faeces containing digested blood is often a persistent symptom. Usually the temperature is normal. When the condition becomes chronic the pig has an intermittent appetite and may lose weight. The faeces vary from normal to dark coloured depending on the presence or absence of blood. Feed intake, feed efficiency and daily gain can be affected.

Diagnosis

Ulceration should always be considered in sows or pigs which are pale, lose body condition and develop a variable appetite particularly if the faeces are black and tarry. A sample of faeces should be examined for the presence of blood and to eliminate parasites. Although the disease is usually confined to individuals or less than 5% of sows, occasionally it can become a herd problem. In such cases poor body condition is widespread through the breeding herd.

Whenever black tarry faeces are seen gastric ulceration should be suspected and in the feeding herd an examination of stomachs at slaughter should be carried out.

Similar diseases

Haemorrhage from the bowel can also arise from the intestine in cases of bloody gut (PHE) but usually this is confined to young gilts and growing pigs.

Anaemia in pigs can also be associated with eperythrozoonosis, the stomach worm *Hyostrongylus rubidus*, chronic mange and porcine enteropathy. Nutritional deficiencies particularly of minerals and vitamins can increase the incidence.

Treatment

- ☐ Move the affected animal from its existing housing into a loose bedded peaceful environment.
- ☐ Feed a weaner type diet containing highly digestible materials.
- ☐ Inject multi vitamins and in particular vitamin E together with 0.5 to 1g of iron intramuscularly and repeat on a weekly basis.
- ☐ Add an extra 100g vitamin E / tonne to the diet for two months and assess the results.
- ☐ Cull affected pigs.

Management control and prevention

- ◆ Consider the above factors and their relevance to your situation. Make alterations and adjustments accordingly.

GLÄSSERS DISEASE (*HAEMOPHILUS PARASUIS* HPS)

This is caused by the bacterium *Haemophilus parasuis*, a small organism, of which there are at least fifteen different types. It is ubiquitous, found throughout the world and is present even in high health herds. If such herds are set up using SPF or MEW techniques and are free from Hps it can be devastating when they first become contaminated, producing an anthrax-like disease with high mortality in sows.

In the majority of herds in which the bacterium is endemic, sows produce a strong maternal immunity which normally persists in their offspring until 8 to 12 weeks of age and as a result, the effects of the infection in weaners are usually nil or very minimal. The pigs become sub-clinically infected when still protected and then stimulate their own immune response. If however the maternal immunity wears off before they become infected they may develop severe disease. It can however become a secondary organism where there are other major pathogens and in particular enzootic pneumonia. Outbreaks of disease are sometimes experienced in sucking pigs, particularly in gilt herds.

Clinical signs

Acute disease

Pigs with glässers disease become rapidly depressed, with an elevated temperature, stop eating and are reluctant to rise. Hps attacks the smooth surfaces of the joints, coverings of the intestine, lungs, heart and brain. In young growing pigs meningitis or middle ear infections are common together with pneumonia, heart sac infection, peritonitis and pleurisy.

Hps also causes individual cases of arthritis and lameness with acute pain, fever and inappetance. It is respiratory spread and a characteristic feature is a short cough of only 2-3 episodes. Sudden death in good sucking piglets is not uncommon in herds with a problem and in particular when immunity in gilt litters is low.

Chronic disease

Sucking piglets are often pale and poor growing and 10-15% may be affected in a litter. Such pigs then continue into the growing period with poor growth. When long standing pericarditis is a feature sudden deaths occur.

Diagnosis

This is confirmed by clinical observations, post-mortem examinations and isolation of the organism in the laboratory but it is not an easy one to grow.

Similar diseases

These would include:
Actinobacillus suis.
App.
Mulberry heart disease.
Streptococcal meningitis.
Streptococcal septicaemias.

Post-mortem and bacteriological examinations are required to differentiate.

Treatment

- Hps has a wide antibiotic sensitivity including amoxycillin, ampicillin, OTC, sulphonamides, penicillin and ceftiofur.
- Look for the very early signs of huddling and shivering and identify clinical cases.
- Treatment must be given early, particularly if cases of meningitis are occurring. It is important to differentiate this disease from streptococcal meningitis and this can only be done by isolating the respective organisms from the brain.
- Identify the onset of disease in sucking pigs and inject 3 to 4 days prior to this to prevent disease, with long-acting penicillin.
- Treatments are best, using injections of either penicillin/streptomycin, trimethoprim/sulpha or synthetic penicillins.
- Treat for 2 to 3 days.
- Medicate the water with amoxycillin or phenoxymethyl penicillin for 4-5 days over the period of risk.

Management control and prevention

- Where the disease is a problem in sucking pigs the sows feed can be top dressed daily 7 days before and 7 days after farrowing with phenoxymethyl penicillin.
- Alternatively sows can be injected with long-acting penicillin at point of farrowing.
- Autogenous vaccines can be produced and given to the sow to stimulate an immunity but the response is serotype specific and in any one herd there may be a number of different serotypes. The vaccines need to be multivalent.
- The lactating and creep rations can be medicated with 200-300g of phenoxymethyl penicillin.
- Apply the relevant general principles discussed for the control of respiratory disease in chapter 9.

GREASY PIG DISEASE - (EXUDATIVE EPIDERMITIS)

This is caused by the bacterium *Staphylococcus hyicus* which invades abraded skin causing infection. The *Staphylococcus* produces toxins which are absorbed into the system and damage the liver and kidneys. The disease is also called exudative epidermitis which describes the oozing of fluid from the inflamed skin. In the sucking piglet disease is usually confined to individual animals, but it can be a major problem in new gilt herds and weaned pigs.

It has been shown recently that during the days immediately preceding farrowing the bacterium multiples profusely in the sows vagina. Piglets are frequently infected during the birth process or soon after. The sharp eye teeth often damage the cheeks during competition for a teat, or the knees are traumatised when seeking to suck milk. These may trigger the disease. In severe cases where the liver becomes damaged the piglet will die. Often only 50% of piglets affected during suckling will survive.

Clinical signs

These usually commence with small, dark, localised areas of infection around the face or on the legs, where the skin has been damaged. The skin along the flanks the belly and between the legs changes to a brown colour gradually involving the whole of the body. The skin becomes wrinkled with flaking of large areas and it has a greasy feel. A more localised picture is seen if the sow has passed some immunity to the piglet, with small circumscribed lesions approximately 5-10mm in diameter that do not spread.

In weaned pigs disease may appear 2-3 days after weaning with a slight browning of the skin that progresses to a dark greasy texture and in severe cases the skin turns black. Such cases usually die due to the toxins produce by the staphylococci organisms. In nurseries up to 15% of the population may be involved.

Diagnosis

This is based on the characteristic skin lesions. (See chapter 10). In an outbreak it is important to culture the organism and carry out an antibiotic sensitivity test. A moist wet area should be identified, the overlying scab removed and a swab rubbed well into the infected area. This should be returned to the laboratory in transport medium to arrive as soon as possible, certainly within 24 hours.

Treatment

- Determine the antibiotic sensitivity and inject affected piglets daily for 5 days, or on alternate days with a long-acting antibiotic to which the organism is sensitive to.
- Antibiotics include; amoxycillin, OTC, ceftiofur, cephalexin, gentamycin, lincomycin or penicillin.
- Topical application of antibiotics can also be of use. Novobiocin, an antibiotic used for treating mastitis in dairy cows, can be mixed with mineral oil and sprayed onto the skin or the piglets dipped into a solution of it.
- Piglets become very dehydrated and should be offered electrolytes by mouth.
- Ensure there are no mange problems in the herd. The mange mites damage the skin and allow *Staphylococcus hyicus* to enter.
- Long-acting injections can be given 2 to 3 days before the first signs are likely to appear as a method of prevention. Use either long-acting amoxycillin or OTC if indicated.
- In severe outbreaks an autogenous vaccine can be prepared from the organism and sows injected twice

CHAPTER 9 - Managing and Treating Disease in the Weaner, Grower and Finishing Periods

4 and 2 weeks prior to farrowing to raise immunity in the colostrum. This has proved successful on a number of farms where disease has appeared in both the sucking and weaned pigs.

☐ If the problem is occurring in gilt litters, cross suckling these piglets using older sows at birth for 4 or 5 hours can be of value.

Management control and prevention

◆ Examine the pigs to see where abrasions are taking place. For example, these may be arising from new concrete surfaces or rough metal floors.
◆ If concrete surfaces are poor, brush these over after cleaning with hydrated lime that contains a phenol disinfectant.
◆ Check the procedures for removing tails and teeth. Jagged edges of teeth can damage the gums leading to infection around the cheeks particularly when piglets fight for teat access and during mixing after weaning.
◆ The skin of the udder is one reservoir of infection. This should be sprayed daily 3 days before and after farrowing with a iodine based skin antiseptic (cow teat dip is ideal).
◆ Disinfect floors well between farrowings.
◆ Make sure that sharp needles are used for iron injections and change these regularly between litters.
◆ If mange is present in the herd treat the sow prior to entering the farrowing house.
◆ Extremes of humidity and wet pens can encourage the multiplication of the bacteria.
◆ Metal floors and side panels, in particular woven metal flooring, can cause severe abrasions particularly around the feet and legs. In such cases the first signs of greasy pig will be in these areas. Damage to the face by metal feeding troughs can precipitate disease.
◆ Check the humidity of the weaning accommodation. High levels above 70% and high temperatures provide an ideal environment for the multiplication of the bacteria on the skin.
◆ Adopt an all-in all-out policy in the weaning accommodation. Have the pens bacteriologically checked after they have been washed out and disinfected.

HAEMATOMA

A haematoma is a pocket of blood beneath the skin. They are often seen in the growing period and the most common site is the ear, where large swellings may develop following fighting or trauma. In most cases these will resolve over two to three weeks once the blood has formed a clot and the serum is reabsorbed. The clot is then slowly removed. Large haematomas on the ears cause considerable discomfort and in such cases the pig should be suitably restrained and a needle entered into the swelling. The removed fluid shows if the blood has clotted. In the growing pig it may be advisable to lance the ear at the tip leaving a 20mm open incision to allow drainage.

LAMENESS

This is prevalent in growing pigs with levels ranging from 1 to 5%. It may be caused by any of the following: (Common *)
- Arthritis caused by bacteria *
- Back muscle necrosis - a stress related disease.
- Bursitis. *
- Bush foot. *
- Erysipelas. *
- Foot-and-mouth disease.
- Fractures. *
- Glässers disease(*Haemophilus parasuis*). *
- Leg weakness or osteochondrosis (OCD). *
- Mycoplasma arthritis (*Mycoplasma hyosynoviae*). *
- Nutritional deficiencies.
- Porcine stress syndrome associated with the halothane gene.
- Streptococcal infections.
- Tail biting (see vice - abnormal behaviour)
- Trauma. *
- Foot-and-mouth disease and swine vesicular disease in those countries where they occur.

Tissue changes that cause lameness

Apophyseolysis (OCD) - Separation of the muscle mass from the growth plate on the pelvis.
Arthritis - inflammation of one or more joint.
Damage to nervous tissue - Clinical signs vary (e.g. partial or complete paralysis of one or more limbs) depending on the site of the damage.
Epiphyseolysis (OCD) - Separation of the head of the femur.
Fractured bones - Common in the hip, hock and elbow joints.
Haematoma - Haemorrhage into the tissues.
Laminitis - Inflammation of the tissues connecting the hoof to the bone. It is not common.
Myositis - Inflammation of muscles.
Penetrated sole - Damage due to trauma.
Periostitis - Inflammation of the membrane (periosteum) which covers the bone.
Osteitis - Inflammation of bone.
Osteochondrosis (leg weakness) - Growth plate and joint cartilage degeneration.
Osteomalacia - Softening of the bones due to calcium/phosphorus deficiency.
Osteomyelitis - Inflammation of all bone tissue including the spongy centre and bone marrow.
Osteoporosis - Week bones due to an imbalance of calcium and phosphorous in the diet.
Split horn - Poor hoof quality. Overgrown claws.

318 Managing Pig Health and the Treatment of Disease

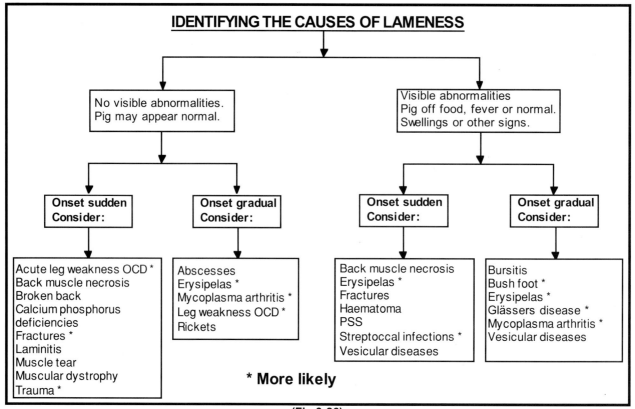

(Fig.9-26)

Torn ligaments or muscles - A common cause of lameness particularly where muscles are attached to bones.

Lameness can account for significant losses in growing pigs either because the pigs are unfit to travel on welfare grounds and require to be destroyed, or they are part or totally condemned at slaughter. Early identification of lame animals and their removal to hospital pens for treatment is a vital part of the control and healing process. Stocking density and mixing are the two major factors that precipitate traumatic disease.

Infections can also account for considerable losses particularly from tail biting and septicaemias that arise during immuno-suppressive diseases such as PRRS, EP and SI.

If there is a lameness problem on the farm it is necessary to identify the common problem and then refer to the relevant disease or diseases. Consider the following and also Fig.9-26 for identification purposes.
- If more than 2% of pigs are recorded lame per month further investigations are necessary.
- Keep records of the time lameness occurs, which house the pig is in and if possible the visual appearance of the lameness.
- If lameness involves the foot look closely at floor surfaces.
- Look for marks or scarring on the skin that might indicate external damage due to fighting.
- Look for cuts or breaks in the skin related to sharp projections from the environment. The position of these on the body of the pig will indicate the height at which these are occurring. Typical examples are worn metal feeding troughs, worn metal pen divisions and bad slats.
- If there is a high incidence of leg sores associated with fractures assess the conditions precipitating leg weakness.
- Identify the most common recurring condition and refer to it using the index in this chapter.
- Consider specific diseases.

LEG WEAKNESS - OSTEOCHONDROSIS (OCD)
See chapter 7 for further information.

This term is also referred to as osteochondrosis. Leg deformities are common in the rapidly growing pig but are usually of no commercial consequence because they do not affect the daily gain or food conversion efficiency. However the conformation defects of leg weakness can restrict the sale of breeding boars and gilts. Separation of the head of the femur at the growth plate does occur as a problem in younger growing pigs on some farms. It is characterised by the sudden onset of acute lameness with the pig refusing to put the foot to the floor. Gentle examination of the leg will determine a fracture in the hip or knee joint. Similar fractures also occur in the elbow joint and at the attachment of the hind muscle mass to the pelvis. In the growing pig heavy stocking density, rapid weight gain and environmental factors that cause the foot to slip on the floor will predispose. See chapter 7 Management control and prevention if you have problems.

LEPTOSPIROSIS
See chapter 6 for further information.

Growing pigs are often exposed to different strains of leptospira from the urine of rats, mice or other animals and they respond with positive titres in the blood. Disease however is uncommon. When it does occur it usually takes the form of acute jaundice, haemorrhage and rapid death and is caused by *Leptospira icterohaemorrhagiae*. Remember this disease can be transmitted to people.

MANGE MITES (*SARCOPTES SCABIEI*)
See chapter 11 for further information.

This is caused by the tiny mite *Sarcoptes scabiei* which burrows into the skin. It completes its life cycle from egg to adult in this tissue. Its presence affects food conversion and daily gain, particularly if the weights of infection are heavy. The disease is characterised initially by tiny red pimples over the skin particularly the back and the flanks. In the chronic condition there are thick asbestos like scabs, mainly within the ears, often with slight bleeding evident. Irritation and rubbing are constant findings together with ear shaking. If the herd is known to be infected pay particular attention to the severity of the disease at the daily clinical examinations. It is a major loss of production and growth rate in growing pigs.

MIDDLE EAR INFECTION

This is caused by a variety of bacteria, but mainly streptococci, that gain access to the middle part of the ear, the part responsible for balance. Infection probably arises from the tonsils at the back of the throat and travels down the eustachian tube to the middle part of the ear. The condition is sporadic but common and in some farms up to 5% of weaner pigs may be affected. It must be recognised early and if treatment is prompt there is usually a good response. If treatment is delayed there is the risk that infection will spread from the middle ear into the inner ear and directly to the brain, setting up a meningitis or encephalitis (inflammation of the brain). Actinobacillus pleuropneumonia has also been identified in outbreaks of the disease and bacteriological examinations should always be carried out if abnormal numbers of pigs are involved.

Clinical signs

The pig stands with its head to one side often shaking with evidence of pain. As the disease progresses there is a gradual loss of co-ordination until ultimately the pig walks around in a circle eventually falling over. Disease in the sow is often severe and such animals are best culled if the response to treatment is poor.

Treatment

☐ The response to treatment in the weaner is usually good using either penicillin/streptomycin or amoxycillin. In acute cases it is necessary to inject the pig twice daily for the first two days and then follow up with long-acting injections. Long acting OTC can also be used.
☐ Cortisone injections are also of value as advised by your veterinarian.
☐ Treatment must continue for 7-10 days and complete recovery may take up to 3 weeks.

Management control and prevention

◆ If there is a problem in your herd identify the time of onset of the disease and study the environment and other diseases for predisposing factors. These could include mange, skin trauma, vice (abnormal behaviour), mixing and fighting, greasy pig disease, joint infections and PRRS.
◆ PRRS can initiate outbreaks in some herds.
◆ Consider preventative medication using amoxycillin long-acting injections given at the time just prior to disease onset.

MORTALITY

Excessive mortality in the weaning and finishing herd is a significant economic loss. It can be assessed realistically by assuming that the overheads on the unit, excluding feed, are going to remain constant and therefore the calculation of loss for each pig can be considered as follows:
(The cost of producing a piglet to the point of weaning) + (the cost of the feed used by the pig to the point of death) + (the margin over feed that would have been made had the pig reached slaughter weight).

If the levels in the herd are above acceptable targets (Fig.9-27) then the reasons for the excess should be iden-

TARGET MORTALITY FIGURES	
Weaning to 3 weeks post-weaning	1.0%
3 weeks to 12 weeks post-weaning	0.5%
12 weeks to slaughter	1.0 to 1.5%
Culls destroyed on welfare grounds	1.0 to 2.0%
Total	3.5% to 5%

(Fig.9-27)

tified. For each pig that is found dead or destroyed note the date, age and weight, the house in which it died, the believed cause of death (Fig-9-28) and any comments. Such a system can easily be recorded on cards by house. See chapter 3. This is a simple method that is strongly recommend. The quality of nursing care given to sick pigs can significantly affect the target levels at the upper limit.

The movement to and reasons for sick pigs entering hospital pens should also be recorded.

Are you making the correct decisions in the sick pen?

RECORDED CAUSES OF DEATH.	
(i.e. those that may be readily diagnosed by an experienced pig person)	
The Weaner	The Grower Pig
Acute enteritis	Abscess
Fighting	Bloody diarrhoea
Glässers disease	Enteric problems
Meningitis	Erysipelas
Miscellaneous causes	Fighting
Oedema disease	Gastric ulcers
Post-weaning diarrhoea	Miscellaneous causes
Prolapse	Pale pig
Sudden death / stress	Rectal prolapse
Respiratory disease	Rectal stricture
Vice (abnormal behaviour)	Respiratory disease
Welfare culls (culled on welfare grounds)	Salt poisoning/water deprivation
Unknown	Sudden death/stress/torsion
	Vice (abnormal behaviour)
	Welfare culls (culled on welfare grounds)
	Unknown

(Fig.9-28)

MULBERRY HEART DISEASE (VITAMIN E / SELENIUM)

During the past few years problems associated with either the lack of availability of vitamin E and selenium, or absolute deficiencies have become major problems on some farms. These have arisen with the practice of using polyunsaturated fats in diets as sources of energy. The actual principles of vitamin E are called tocopherols and they are widespread in feed stuffs including vegetable oils, cereals and green plants.

Tocopherols are used in pig rations as dl-alpha-tocopherol acetate and measured in international units. The international unit (iu)1iu of vitamin E is defined as 1mg of a standard preparation of a specific tocopherol acetate.

Vitamin E is necessary for the optimum function and metabolism of the nervous, muscular, circulatory and immune systems, and the latter highlights its importance in maintaining the health of the pig.

Its function is basically to prevent the breakdown of oxygen at a cellular level (oxidation) when toxic products including hydrogen peroxide and hydroxyl radicals are produced. These oxidising agents are powerful tissue poisons.

The function of vitamin E in the pig
- To increase the efficiency of the immune system. Adequate levels must be available at critical times particularly as maternal antibody is dropping and pigs are being challenged by infectious agents. This highlights the importance of both diet quality and levels of energy lysine and vitamin E at these times.
- It acts as a tissue antioxidant. Heart muscle is particularly sensitive to oxidising agents, the reason why mulberry heart disease is so common.
- It helps to maintain the integral structure of muscles in the digestive and reproductive systems.
- It is involved in the synthesis of certain amino acids and vitamin C.
- It has a close relationship with selenium metabolism.

Selenium is an essential nutrient in its own right and part of an enzyme called glutathione peroxidase which also acts as a antioxidant and thus has a complementary role to vitamin E. The less selenium in the diet the greater is the requirement for vitamin E.

The recommended requirements to give a maximum boost to the immune system range from 75-220iu/kg. According to age of the pig and diet; this is in the first stage creep 220, the second stage 150, the grower 100, the finisher 60 and sow 50 iu/kg. These levels are probably higher than those necessary for maximum growth, which may be 50% less.

Polyunsaturated fatty acids PUFA's cause considerable oxidation at tissue levels and when added to diets 3iu of vitamin E should be added for each g of PUFA.

Vitamin E and selenium related diseases
Gastric ulcers - These are often stress oriented and the incidence increases where vitamin E levels are low.
Hepatosis dietetica (HD) - A condition where there is necrosis or death of liver cells.
Muscular or nutritional dystrophy (MD) (also called a myopathy) - This results from a degeneration of muscle fibres whether they be skeletal smooth or cardiac. Oedema or fluid is often produced around the tissues and muscles (PSE) as a result.
Mulberry heart disease (MHD) (also called a myopathy)- A specific disease of heart muscle and a common cause of sudden death.
Reproduction disorders - Vitamin E is involved in sperm production and ovarian function. The actual role of vitamin E on the farm is difficult to clarify.

Clinical signs

These vary according to the system affected. HD, MD and MHD are usually associated with sudden deaths in rapid growing pigs without any prior clinical signs,

usually the best pigs in the pen are affected and they range from 15-30kg in weight. Diets being fed often contain high levels of fats and yet in many cases vitamin E levels appear within normal ranges. Post-mortem symptoms are characteristic and include:
- Large amounts of fluid around the heart and lungs.
- Haemorrhagic and pale areas in heart muscle.
- Fluid in the abdomen with pieces of fibrin.
- Pale muscle areas (necrosis) particularly in the lumber muscles and hind muscles of the leg which contain excesses amounts of fluid.
- If the liver is involved it is enlarged and mottled with areas of haemorrhage interspersed with pale areas.

Diagnosis

Histological examinations of the liver, heart or skeletal muscle will confirm diagnosis and this is the most accurate method. Serum samples should be taken from pigs at risk and tested for levels of vitamin E. Normal levels are variable from pig to pig however they should be more than 1.8mg/litre. The availability of selenium can be assessed by measuring the levels of glutathione peroxidase in the serum. If levels are less than 0.025µg/ml or 0.1mg/kg in liver a deficiency should be suspected and rations checked.

If MD is the major change stiffness and muscle trembling may be seen. If back muscle necrosis is involved sudden acute lameness occurs, particularly in gilts, especially outdoors, when they are moved into paddocks for the first time. This sudden exercise precipitates disease in association with the porcine stress syndrome (PSS). Stress related problems include gastric ulcers and where lesions occur in more than 20% of pigs at slaughter, the addition of 50iu/kg of vitamin E should be assessed.

The role of vitamin E and selenium in reproductive performance is more difficult to quantify. Improvements have been noted in herds with persistent cases of agalactia and udder oedema by raising the levels in the lactating diet to 100iu/kg.

Similar diseases

These include:
    Actinobacillus pleuropneumonia.
    Glässers disease.
    Oedema disease.
    Streptococcal septicaemias.

Specific diseases associated with deficiencies of, or lack of availability include:
    Actinobacillus pleuropneumonia.
    E. coli diarrhoea.
    Oedema disease.
    Post-weaning respiratory syndrome.
    PRRS.
    Swine dysentery.
    Those diseases that occur during periods of immunosuppression.

Treatment

- Where a population is at risk inject all the pigs with vitamin E/selenium e.g. dystocel, 70iu vitamin E and 1.5mg per 50kg is adequate, but seek veterinary advice.
- Sudden death in piglets following iron injection. Inject sows 14 days prior to farrowing with vitamin E/selenium.
- Water soluble preparations are sometimes available as alternatives.
- Multi-vitamins that include vitamin E and or selenium may be used. Refer to the recommended treatment levels on the bottle label.
- Move individual pigs to hospital pens for treatment.
- Increase vitamin E levels in creep and growing rations by 100-150iu/kg.

Management control and prevention

- If problems persist change to another diet with less added fats.
- Check the levels of PUFA's in the diet.
- Check the levels of vitamin E and selenium.
- Check the levels of vitamin A. If more than 10,000iu/kg this may be increasing the requirement for vitamin E.
- Rapid growth may be a contributing factor.
- Reduce stocking densities if pigs are over crowded.
- Check there are no parasite burdens.
- Grains stored with high moisture content in high temperatures and with fungal growth may have low levels of vitamin E.
- Do not breed from animals that carry the stress gene.

MYCOPLASMA ARTHRITIS (*MYCOPLASMA HYOSYNOVIAE* INFECTION)

This is caused by the tiny organism *Mycoplasma hyosynoviae* which is ubiquitous and most, if not all herds are infected with it. It is a respiratory spread disease the organism being found in the upper respiratory tract nose and tonsils. It may be present in some herds and cause no clinical signs and yet in others cause severe disease. Infection with or without disease takes place in the young growing pig from approximately 8 to 30 weeks of age and particularly so in the gilt when first introduced onto a farm, or in the early stages of pregnancy. It is very uncommon in older sows because they develop a strong immunity resulting from repeated exposure to the organism. They pass this immunity to their offspring in the colostrum. This maternally derived immunity gradually disappears over a period of weeks. Infection then takes place as these pigs become exposed to older ones. *Mycoplasma hyosynoviae* infects joints and tendon sheaths rather than the respiratory system.

Clinical signs

Disease in the gilt is usually sudden in onset, the first signs being a reluctance to rise at feeding time. There is a considerable amount of pain and the affected pig will only stand for short periods of time. The temperature may be normal or slightly elevated. It is more common in the heavy ham straight legged animal and purchased gilts which have been reared in isolated grow out units often become diseased four to six weeks after arrival.

Diagnosis

This is based on clinical signs and the response to either lincomycin or tiamulin therapy. Joint fluid can be aspirated and examined for antibodies and isolation of the organism.

Serology is not much help because sub-clinical infection is common and so healthy animals often have antibody titres. Rising titres in blood samples taken two weeks apart together with typical symptoms strongly suggest disease.

In problem herds post-mortem examination may be necessary to reach a definitive diagnosis.

Similar diseases

These include muscle damage, leg weakness or OCD, trauma, erysipelas, glässers disease and the major vesicular diseases.

Treatment

- *Mycoplasma hyosynoviae* is susceptible to lincomycin or tiamulin injections.
- Give daily for 4 days in the early course of the disease. If the lameness is due to *Mycoplasma hyosynoviae* there should be a good response within 24 to 36 hours.
- Treatment is most effective if given early.
- Give in feed medication strategically commencing 7 days before the expected disease outbreak and continue for 14 days using 220g/tonne of lincomycin or 500-800g/tonne of OTC.
- An alternate strategy is to medicate the ration at half these levels and feed for 5-7 weeks.

Management control and prevention

Mycoplasma hyosynoviae can be a recurring problem in breeding gilts particularly during the first 6 to 10 weeks after introduction to the farm. Consider the following:
- Identify the period of onset and apply strategic preventative medication.
- In-feed medicate susceptible groups over the critical period with either 500-800g OTC or CTC per tonne, 110-220g of lincomycin per tonne or 100g of tiamulin per tonne.
- Maintain pigs on ad lib feeding during the susceptible period.
- Assess the quality of housing - in particular low temperatures and draughts which act as trigger factors.
- Remember that this is a respiratory spread disease and other factors need to be considered.
- Avoid mixing and fighting.
- Provide well bedded pens.
- In outdoor herds acclimatise gilts to cobs or large nuts before they are introduced into the outdoor herd.
- Control enzootic pneumonia and other respiratory diseases if they are a coincidental problem.

OEDEMA DISEASE (OD) - BOWEL OEDEMA

This is also called bowel disease or gut oedema. It is caused by certain serotypes of *E. coli* bacteria that produce a powerful toxin. These toxins damage the walls of small blood vessels including those in the brain and cause fluid or oedema to accumulate in the tissues of the stomach and the large bowel. Damage to the blood vessels in the brain results in some of the characteristic signs. The specific *E. coli* are described as O138, O139 and O141. Disease is generally seen 1 to 4 weeks after weaning, the peak being at 10 days. It was very common when pigs were weaned at 5 to 8 weeks of age. Since weaning ages have reduced to 17 to 26 days and starter diets have been improved the disease in its classical form is rarely seen. The *E. coli* bacteria attach themselves to the finger-like villi in the anterior small intestine and produce the toxins. This mechanism is similar to that which occurs in post-weaning diarrhoea associated with different strains of *E. coli*. During sucking the secretory IgA immunoglobulin component in milk prevents the bacteria adhering. After weaning when the IgA has disappeared the pigs becomes susceptible to disease.

Clinical signs

Acute disease

Sometimes the only sign is a good pig found dead. A typical live affected pig will show a staggering gate, puffy eyelids giving a sleepy appearance and an abnormal high pitched squeak. Pigs stop eating and in the later stages become partially paralysed and go off their legs, sometimes with nervous symptoms. Diarrhoea is not a consistent feature but breathing difficulties become evident. The damage to the brain is irreversible and most pigs die. Recovery in the few pigs that do not die takes up to 2 to 3 weeks. Certain breeds of pigs may be associated with disease suggesting a genetic predisposition.

Diagnosis

This is made from the typical clinical signs, the sudden appearance of disease after weaning, post-mortem examinations showing oedema of the greater curvature of the stomach wall, coiled colon, and eyelids and isolation of the haemolytic *E. coli* serotypes from the duodenum (anterior small intestine).

Treatment

By the time the clinical signs are seen it is often too late and most pigs die. Treatment routines are aimed at preventing the organism establishing itself and also reducing the weight of infection. The general principles of controlling coliform infections and post-weaning diarrhoea should be followed.

- Isolate the organism and determine the antibiotic sensitivity.
- Identify the stage (e.g. 10 days post-weaning) when disease first appears and apply either in-feed or water medication 3 to 5 days before this.
- In-feed antibiotics of value include apramycin 100g/tonne, framycetin 100g/tonne, neomycin 163g/tonne. Alternatively apramycin, neomycin or trimethoprim/sulpha can be used in the water.
- Individual treatments give a poor response but flunixin will help to reduce the effects of toxins and diuretics can be used to remove fluid.

It must be admitted however that the disease is most difficult to deal with and often preventative medication and treatment are unsuccessful.

Management control and prevention

- This can be difficult and unrewarding.
- Reduce piglet exposure to the *E. coli* during sucking. Adopt all the procedures in the farrowing house for the control of scour in the sucking pig.
- Consider the use of an autogenous vaccine in sows to raise colostral antibodies and block out infection in the sucking pig. This has been effective on a few farms.
- Assess the effects of no creep feeding pre-weaning.
- Restrict feed intake post-weaning.
- Assess the effects of different diets and feeding routines.
- Reduce the nutrient composition of the diet by increasing the fibre content by 10 to 15%.
- If the problem is a major one and it continues, consider a change of genotype. Some strains of pig are more resistant than others.
- Lower or alter the age of weaning.
- Alter the environment at weaning time.
- Asses the effects of adding 3% of milk powder to the diet.
- Assess the effects of zinc oxide to the diet.

PARASITES

See chapter 11 for further information.

In the weaned pig internal parasites are an uncommon problem unless the weaners are housed in continuously occupied straw based or bare concrete pens. In these circumstances coccidiosis could cause diarrhoea within 7 to 10 days of entry and strongyle infections (poor growth and sloppy faeces) within 3 to 4 weeks.

In the finisher pig if the housing is used on an all-in all-out basis and pens washed out, internal parasites cannot complete their life cycle. With the continual use of pens however ascarid infections, causing milk spot liver and coughing, may become established, but diarrhoea would be uncommon.

PASTEURELLOSIS

Pasteurella multocida bacteria are commonly involved in respiratory disease in pigs and they may be toxin-producing or non-toxin-producing strains. Either can cause pneumonia in their own right but the non toxin ones are common secondary opportunist invaders associated with primary EP or PRRS infections.

Clinical signs

Acute disease

This is characterised by severe sudden pneumonia affecting all the lung tissue, high temperatures and high mortality. Pigs show rapid breathing, discoloured skin particularly on the extremities of the ears and they are toxic.

Sub acute disease

In this form the pneumonia is less severe but often complicated by pericarditis (heart sac inflammation) and pleurisy. Coughing and emaciation are also common clinical features. The condition usually affects pigs between 10 and 18 weeks of age.

Diagnosis

This is carried out by post-mortem examination and isolation of the organism from the lungs.

Treatment

- Because the organism is usually secondary to a more specific disease antibiotic treatments should follow as for enzootic pneumonia.

Management control and prevention

- Carry out procedures as described under respiratory diseases and control strategies.
- Vaccines are available but not very effective.
- EP vaccination often prevents the pasteurella invading the lungs.

PORCINE EPIDEMIC DIARRHOEA (PED)

See chapter 12 for further information.

PED is a virus infection of the small intestine. It cycles sometimes in weaned pigs in herds which have become immune because the protection of the maternal IgA disappears after weaning. The process of continual infection maintains the virus on the farm. The disease is characterised by a sudden profuse watery diarrhoea that will last for 3 to 4 days and occurs when pigs are moved into environments where older pigs have succumbed to the disease, shed the virus and recovered. When the virus is first introduced on to the farm there is a rapid spread of diarrhoea across all breeding and growing pigs with almost 100% morbidity within 5 to 10 days. The incubation period is 2 to 4 days. Type 1 virus causes diarrhoea in growing pigs and adults only, but the type 2 virus causes diarrhoea in piglets as well

Clinical signs

There is an acute watery diarrhoea and no evidence of blood or mucus. In breeding finishing farms disease is usually sporadic, however PED is common where weaners are continually entering finishing only operations. Groups of pigs become infected when they reach a certain age and as they enter a building where infection is endemic. Mortality is usually low but morbidity can be high.

Diagnosis

This is based on the history, clinical symptoms and examinations of faeces samples for evidence of porcine epidemic diarrhoea virus by ELISA tests or electron microscopy.

Post-mortem examination of dead pigs and laboratory tests on the small intestine may be necessary to confirm the diagnosis.

Similar diseases

TGE could give a similar picture and live affected pigs are best submitted to a laboratory for differential tests.

Treatment

- The growing pig normally recovers without treatment unless there are secondary infections. In such cases antibiotics in the water or preventative medication in-feed maybe required.
- Use neomycin, apramycin, framycetin or trimethoprim/sulpha. Sometimes a good response is obtained with either lincomycin or tiamulin depending on the secondary bacteria present.

Specific treatment is of no value since this is a virus infection.

Management control and prevention

- The disease may occasionally become endemic in finishing units as new weaners are introduced onto the farm. Under such circumstances it is necessary to break the cycle by stopping purchasing for three weeks or utilising segregated disease control methods. (See chapter 3).
- All-in all-out procedures with disinfection will often break the cycle.
- The virus is easily killed by phenolic, chlorine or iodine based disinfectants or peroxides.

PORCINE ENTEROPATHY (PE)

This describes a group of conditions involving pathological changes in the small intestine, associated with a recently identified bacteria called *Lawsonia intracellularis*. The disease is world-wide in its distribution, the infectious organism exists on most if not all farms and lives inside the cells lining the small and large intestines. Disease occurs in four different forms; a) Porcine intestinal adenopathy (PIA) which describes an abnormal proliferation of the cells that line the intestines. b) Necrotic enteritis (NE) where the proliferated cells of the small intestine die and slough off (necrosis) with a gross thickening of the small intestine (hosepipe gut). c) Regional ileitis (RI) or inflammation of the terminal part of the small intestine, and d) proliferative haemorrhagic enteropathy (PHE). In the latter there is massive bleeding into the small intestine, hence the common name bloody gut.

The exact mechanisms of spread are not known but the organism is found in other species including rabbits. Infected faeces are the major vehicle for movement of the organism around the farm and those herds that have persistent problems are likely to have poor management of faeces, dirty pens and passages and heavily contaminated floor surfaces. Boars and adult pigs probably act as carriers with transfer of infection to piglets thus maintaining the cycle of infection.

Studies suggest that the organism can survive outside the pig for 2-3 weeks.

PIA and NE tend to occur in young growing pigs but sudden and severe outbreaks of PHE with high mortality can occur in pigs 60 to 90kg weight and maiden gilts. Gilts either already carry infection as they enter a farm and unknown factors trigger disease or they become infected on the farm for the first time. Ironically PE is more common in high health herds but the reasons for this are unknown.

Clinical signs

These are dependent on the nature of the changes that take place inside the small intestine and in many cases disease is so mild that signs are not detected. With PIA the pig appears clinically normal initially eats well but there is a chronic diarrhoea, gradual wasting and loss of condition, followed in some cases by a pot bellied appearance. Necrotic enteritis gives a similar picture but acute disease is manifest by bloody gut or PHE and the pig may die suddenly or appear very pale and anaemic and pass black bloody faeces. Secondary bacterial infections often increase the severity of the disease. PHE occurs frequently in young gilts, particularly within 4 to 6 weeks of arrival on the farm, at the point of service and up to the middle stage of pregnancy. Pigs with the chronic form of the PE recover over a period of four to six weeks, however there can be considerable losses in feed efficiency and daily gain of up to 0.3 and 80g/day respectively. As a consequence there can be marked variations in sizes of pigs.

Diagnosis

This is carried out by the clinical picture, post-mortem examinations, histology of the gut wall and demonstrating the organism in faeces by an ELISA test. A serological test is also available. At the time of writing only a few laboratories can do these tests. Tissue cultures have been recently developed.

Treatment

The following antibiotics have been shown to be effective against the organism.

- ☐ Penicillin, enrofloxacin, erythromycin and chlortetracyline.
- ☐ Virginiamycin - used as a growth promoter could be used to prevent disease.
- ☐ Tiamulin and tilmycosin (macrolides) also show good activity.
- ☐ When gilts are introduced onto the farm preventative medication using 300-500g/tonne of tetracycline over the first 4 to 6 week susceptible period is an effective means of control.
- ☐ Treat individual pigs with injections of long-acting oxytetracycline or penicillin and give 300-800mg of iron dextran.
- ☐ Offer creep for one to two weeks fed as a gruel.
- ☐ In acute outbreaks medicate the water for 2 to 3 days with OTC or CTC followed by in-feed medication.

Management control and prevention

- ◆ Strategically medicate incoming gilts if there are problems, commencing one week before signs usually appear and continue for four weeks as under treatment.
- ◆ Wash out and disinfect gilt pens between batches. The organism is excreted via the faeces and continual use of pens increases the exposure rate allowing endemic disease to develop.
- ◆ Where problems continue in growing pigs, pens should be washed out and disinfected between batches and pigs strategically medicated.
- ◆ Carry over of infection between batches appears to be a significant part of the epidemiology.
- ◆ Virginiamycin as a growth promoter will often prevent disease.
- ◆ In severe continuous outbreaks it may be necessary to medicate all feed with 200-400g CTC or OTC per tonne.
- ◆ *Lawsonia intracellularis* is susceptible to quaternary ammonium compounds but not particularly so to phenolic disinfectants.

Washing pens using a detergent is probably the best method.

PORCINE REPRODUCTIVE AND RESPIRATORY SYNDROME (PRRS)

See chapter 6 for further information.

Clinical signs

Acute disease

When introduced first into an EP and App free growing herd there is usually a period of slight inappetance and mild coughing but in some herds there are no symptoms at all. If EP and/or virulent App are present in the herd however, clinical signs may become severe with an acute extensive consolidating pneumonia with the gradual formation of multiple abscesses. Disease becomes evident within 1-3 weeks of weaning, pigs lose condition with pale skin, mild coughing, sneezing and increased respiratory rates. Mortality during this period may reach 12-15%.

Endemic disease

Once the acute period of disease has passed through the breeding and finishing herd PRRS virus normally then only becomes of significance in the early growing period, where severe endemic pneumonia can persist with periods of inappetance and wasting of pigs. Pigs become infected as maternal antibody disappears and then remain viraemic for 3 to 4 weeks continually excreting virus. Permanently populated houses maintain the virus at high levels, particularly in the first and second stage accommodation. Clinical disease is seen in pigs from 4 to 12 weeks of age and it is characterised by a fairly predictable time of onset, inappetance, malabsorption and wasting, coughing and pneumonia. In this post-weaning period mortality can rise up to 12% or more and persist inspite of antibiotic treatments. Secondary bacterial infections become evident in pigs at a later stage from 12 to 16 weeks of age from abscesses that develop in the lungs. These infections spread to other parts of the body, particularly joints with increased lameness.

Diagnosis

This is based on the history and symptoms, post mortem examinations and the known presence of the virus in the herd or by serological examinations and isolation of the virus.

Similar diseases

Chronic respiratory disease is caused by combination of respiratory pathogens including PRRS, SI, EP, App, Hps and pasteurella bacteria, particularly as they become additive. The diagnosis is then of multiple cause.

Treatment

☐ In the acute disease when PRRS first enters the

farm it is important to cover the period at risk, which is usually six to eight weeks, with in-feed antibiotics or by individual injections and water medication.

☐ The broad spectrum antibiotics, tetracyclines, trimethoprim/sulpha, or synthetic penicillins are the drugs of choice but if EP alone is involved tiamulin or lincomycin may be used. If App is active ceftiofur could be a drug of choice for individual treatments.

☐ In endemic disease preventive medication over the period at risk using 500 to 800g of tetracycline or trimethoprim/sulpha 400g/tonne in-feed may be used but it would be advisable to identify the major bacteria involved and determine their antibiotic sensitivities.

Management control and prevention

See also Respiratory disease and control strategies.

- Consider using segregated early weaning off site to break the endemic cycle of disease.
- Refer to the principles of SEW and SDC in chapter 3.
- Section all the buildings so that they can be managed on an all-in all-out basis, and clean and disinfect between each batch.

    It is most important to adopt this principle at the onset of disease to prevent endemic infection becoming established.

- Consider the directions of pig movement around the farm. Change these to reduce droplet contamination from older pigs to younger pigs.
- Consider farrowing once every two to four weeks thus giving an age break between groups and houses. This can be highly effective.
- Consider depopulation of the first and second stage flat decks where virus is active. Before considering this step however first check by serology that the virus is no longer circulating in the breeding and finishing herds. Elimination of virus has been successfully carried out using this technique on a number of farms. The first and second stage houses are depopulated washed with hot water and detergent and left empty for two weeks. Pigs are weaned away from the farm whilst this is being carried out and then newly weaned pigs are introduced back to the nursery.
- Live vaccines are available that can be administered by intramuscular injection to the pig at weaning time.

    Their use is claimed to be beneficial and pigs become resistant to field virus challenge. There is considerable debate as to the long term effects in the herd and the movement of live virus into the breeding herd with possible side effects. Discuss aspects of this with your veterinarian.

PORCINE RESPIRATORY CORONAVIRUS (PRCV)

See chapter 12 for further information.

PRCV is a relatively new virus that first appeared in pigs some ten years or more ago in Europe. It is related to but distinct from TGE virus, which is another coronavirus.

PRCV is respiratory spread and believed to travel long distances and because of this it is extremely difficult to maintain herds free from it and very few countries have not been exposed.

Clinically it is almost non-pathogenic and field experiences have shown that herds exposed for the first time have few if any signs of disease.

It has been suggested however that it may have an effect on lung tissue when other respiratory pathogens are present in chronic respiratory disease complexes.

PRCV does however cross react with the serological test for TGE and it therefore can confuse the diagnosis. A differential test is available.

PORCINE STRESS SYNDROME (PSS)

This term covers a group of conditions associated with an autosomal recessive gene. It includes acute stress and sudden death (malignant hyperthermia), pale soft exudative muscle (PSE), dark firm dry meat, and back muscle necrosis. Heavy muscle pigs are more likely to carry the gene.

The pig is either homozygous recessive (susceptible) heterozygous, or free of the gene.

The gene can be identified by the pigs response to the anaesthetic gas halothane but recent developments have produced gene probes using blood, that identify both the homozygous and heterozygous carriers.

Clinical signs

When the homozygous state is present and following a period of muscle activity, there is a change in muscle metabolism from aerobic to anaerobic and biochemical abnormalities develop. The body tissues become acid with a marked rise in temperature 42°C (107°F).

The onset is sudden with muscle tremors, twitching of the face and rapid respiration. The skin becomes red and blotched. Death usually occurs within 15-20 minutes. PSS is often precipitated by sudden movement. Back muscle necrosis is a more localised form. Whilst the gene produces a leaner carcase, growth rates are slower and the levels of sudden death increase.

Diagnosis

This is based on the sudden onset, symptoms, breed, susceptibility and the known presence or absence of the gene in the pig.

In many cases the pig is just found dead and a post-mortem examination is necessary to eliminate other disease. Rigor mortis (stiffening of the muscles after death) within 5 minutes is a striking feature.

Similar diseases

These include the other causes of sudden death, twisted bowel, internal haemorrhage, mulberry heart disease and pyelonephritis. Hypocalcaemia in the lactating sow although uncommon can give identical symptoms to PSS.

Treatment

This is usually ineffective but the following are worth adopting:
- ☐ Spray the pig with cold water to control the temperature rises.
- ☐ Inject 50-100ml of calcium gluconate (used in cows for milk fever) by intramuscular injections at two separate sites. Seek veterinary advice.
- ☐ Sedate the pig with stresnil.
- ☐ Do not move or cause undue muscle activity.
- ☐ Give an injection of vitamin E 2iu/kg.

Management control and prevention

- ◆ Remove the gene from the population.
- ◆ Use a homozygous or heterozygous male on stress gene free females if the gene is to be used to improve carcase quality.
- ◆ Maintain a gene free herd.

PROLAPSE OF THE RECTUM

This is a widespread condition occurring in good growing pigs from 8 to 20 weeks of age. The onset is sudden. The size of the prolapse varies from 10 to 80mm and if small it will often revert to the rectum spontaneously. In most cases however the prolapse remains to the exterior and is often cannibalised by other pigs in the pen as evident by blood on the noses of the offending pigs and on the flanks of others. The fundamental cause is an increase in abdominal pressure which forces the rectum to the exterior.

Clinical signs

At the onset the red coloured mucosa of the rectum protrudes from the anal sphincter and then may return on its own. After a short period however it remains to the exterior and becomes swollen and filled with fluid. It is prone to damage and haemorrhage and where pigs are loose housed cannibalism often results with evidence of blood on the skin.

Treatment

- ☐ Rectal prolapses must be recognised early and the pig removed from the pen.
- ☐ Replace the prolapse and retain it by a purse string or mattress suture. Return the pig to the pen. The technique for carrying this out is described in chapter 15. If the prolapse has been badly torn still replace it, and consider moving the pig to a hospital pen and treat with a long-acting antibiotic injection. In a proportion of pigs the damaged tissues become scarred with constriction leading to rectal strictures. The incidence of this is reduced by replacing the prolapse and suturing.
- ☐ In some cases the prolapse will be completely bitten off by other pigs. Here the pig should be left in the pen as most cases will progress to slaughter although a few will develop with rectal strictures.

Management control and prevention

The following may be considered as causal or contributory when adopting control measures.

Disease
- ◆ Diarrhoea - excessive straining.
- ◆ Respiratory disease - excessive coughing increasing abdominal pressure.
- ◆ Colitis - abnormal fermentation occurs in the large bowel with the production of excessive gas increasing abdominal pressure.

The Environment
- ◆ In cold weather the incidence of rectal prolapses increases. This is associated with low house temperatures and the tendency of pigs to huddle together, thus increasing abdominal pressure.
- ◆ Wet conditions and slippery floors, particularly those with no bedding, increase abdominal pressure.
- ◆ If stocking densities reach the level whereby pigs cannot lay out on their sides across the pen the incidence may increase.

Nutrition
- ◆ Ad lib feeding - Feeding pigs to appetite results in continual heavy gut fill and indigestion. There is then a tendency for abnormal fermentation in the large bowel because undigested components of the feed arrive in greater amounts.
- ◆ High density diets and in particular lysine levels increase growth rates and outbreaks may often subside either by a change to restricted feeding or using a lower energy / lysine diet.
- ◆ Water shortage - This can lead to constipation.
- ◆ Diets high in starch may predispose to prolapse - Try adding 2-4% grass meal to the diet.
- ◆ The presence of mycotoxins in feed - If there is a problem make sure that the bins have been well cleaned out. Examine the cereal sources.
- ◆ Change of diet - By studying the timing of the problem it is sometimes possible to identify rectal prolapses not only with a change of diet but also a change of housing.
- ◆ Field evidence does not identify breed as a causal factor.
- ◆ Increases in rectal prolapses have been reported in association with the use of tylosin but the evidence

- for this is unclear.
- ◆ Trauma
- ◆ Tail docking - docking tails too short can damage the nerve supply to the anal ring leading to a relaxation of the anal sphincter.

Identify those factors on your farm from the above list and making changes.

Consider collecting the following information about each prolapse to see if common factors emerge:
- Age of pig.
- Comments observations.
- Days in the house.
- Diet fed.
- House and pen.
- Number of pigs per pen
- Number of rectal strictures.
- Number of prolapses sutured.
- Outcome.
- State of prolapse.
- Tail biting.
- Weight of the pig.

RECTAL STRICTURE

This is a condition often considered a sequel to rectal prolapse. Approximately a fingers length inside the rectum the tissues gradually shrink, scar tissue develops and eventually the tube completely closes. Affected pigs in the early stage of the disease often show a very loose diarrhoea that becomes projectile and a gradual increase in the size of the abdomen, with loss of condition.

The area where the stricture occurs is supplied by two tiny arteries that originate from the aorta. Some studies suggest that if these arteries are blocked or thrombosed by bacteria a rectal stricture will result. Erysipelas, *Haemophilus parasuis*, streptococci and salmonella have been implicated. If rectal strictures occur in large numbers at predictable times consider infection as a cause and assess the effects of strategic medication by injection, water or in-feed.

Treatment

☐ There is no treatment for this condition and as soon as pigs are recognised they should be destroyed on welfare grounds. Attempting to open up the stricture by palpation has in the author's experience been a total failure.

Management control and prevention

- ◆ Determine if there is a recurring time period when this first appears.
- ◆ Approximately three weeks prior to this look for trigger factors.
- ◆ If more than 2% of growing pigs are affected apply in-feed medication at the predetermined time and assess the results. 500g of OTC per tonne for two weeks may prevent the condition if an infection such as *Haemophilus parasuis* is the predisposing cause.
- ◆ Consider all the factors outlined for the control of rectal prolapses.
- ◆ Ear tag rectal prolapses to see if they develop into strictures, often they do not.
- ◆ Replace all rectal prolapses immediately, suture and see whether this affects the incidence.

RESPIRATORY DISEASES AND CONTROL STRATEGIES

See chapter 3 for further information; reference segregated weaning.

Of all the diseases that affect growing and finishing pigs, chronic respiratory disease is the most economically important. It is extremely common and can be difficult to prevent and control. Growth rates and feed-intake are depressed together with poor feed efficiency and some herds there is heavy mortality. The control of respiratory disease requires an understanding of the complexities and interaction between the organisms that are present, the pig and the management of the environment. The prevalence of respiratory disease is affected by the following:

- The presence of respiratory pathogenic organisms.
- The virulence of the pathogens present.
- The level of the pathogens in the house environment.
- The immunity of the pig and the time of exposure to the organisms.
- The presence of secondary opportunistic bacteria.
- The interactions between management, environment, the diseases and the pig.

The presence of respiratory pathogenic organisms

The infectious agents that damage the respiratory system of the pig and the type of disease they cause are shown in Fig.9-29.

The severity of the disease will depend in part upon the number of infective agents present and the weights of infection that challenge the pig. PRCV is a relatively mild almost non clinical infection.

PRRS likewise on its own has little clinical effect on the respiratory systems, but if it is combined with swine influenza severe respiratory disease will be experienced.

Under good husbandry conditions enzootic pneumonia caused by *Mycoplasma hyopneumoniae* on its own is usually a relatively mild disease, but when complexed with PRRS, SI or *Pasteurella multocida* or combinations, serious chronic disease syndromes can develop.

Of the bacterial infections there are at least 12 serotypes (serovars) of *Actinobacillus pleuropneumoniae* but disease is dependent in part upon the virulence of the strains present, some causing no problems, others causing severe disease. Virulent serotypes vary from country to country. Individual strains within serotypes also

INFECTIONS THAT CAUSE RESPIRATORY DISEASE

Diseases *	Causal Agent *	Effects
Caused by viruses		
Aujeszky's disease (AD) (Pseudorabies PR)	Porcine herpes virus (Herpes suis)	Nervous symptoms Pneumonia (Reproductive failure in sows)
Inclusion body rhinitis (Porcine cytomegalovirus infection)	Cytomegalovirus	Non progressive rhinitis Sneezing in newborn piglets
Porcine reproductive and respiratory syndrome (PRRS), (Blue ear disease)	Arterivirus	Pneumonia Reproductive failure
Respiratory corona virus	Porcine respiratory corona virus (PRCV)	Pneumonia (very mild) Transient coughing
Swine influenza (SI) (Flu)	Influenza viruses	Fever Generalised illness Pneumonia
Classical swine fever (CSF) or Hog cholera (HC)	Swine fever virus (Hog cholera virus) (Pesti virus group. Flaviviridae)	Infertility Pneumonia
Caused by mycoplasma		
Enzootic pneumonia (EP) Mycoplasma pneumonia	*Mycoplasma hyopneumoniae* (EP)	Pneumonia
Mycoplasma flocculare pneumonia	*Mycoplasma flocculare*	Mild pneumonia Small lesions
Mycoplasma arthritis	*Mycoplasma hyosynoviae*	Lameness
Caused by bacteria		
Actinobacillus pleuropneumonia (App) (Necrotic pleuropneumonia) (Pleuropneumonia)	*Actinobacillus pleuropneumoniae*	Acute necrotic and haemorrhagic pneumonia Pleurisy Sudden death
Actinobacillus suis disease	*Actinobacillus suis* and equi	Lung nodules Septicaemia
Bordetellosis (Bordetella rhinitis)	*Bordetella bronchiseptica*	Non-progressive rhinitis Pneumonia
Glässer's disease	*Haemophilus parasuis*	Fever Heart sac infection Lameness Mild Pneumonia Pleurisy Polyserositis
Pasteurellosis	*Pasteurella multocida*	Pneumonia
Progressive atrophic rhinitis (PAR) Atrophic rhinitis (AR)	*Pasteurella multocida*, toxin producing strains	Pneumonia Progressive atrophic rhinitis
Streptococcal pneumonia	*Streptococcus suis* and other streptococci	Arthritis Meningitis Pneumonia
Salmonellosis	*Salmonella cholerasuis* (*Salmonella typhimurium*, and other salmonella)	Diarrhoea Pneumonia
Caused by Parasites		
Ascaris infection	Large White Worm (*Ascaris suis*) - migrating larvae	Acute pneumonia Coughing
Lungworm	Lungworm (*Metastrongylus*)	Mild pneumonia Coughing

* Several of the diseases and causal agents have more than one name listed here underneath each other

(Fig.9-29)

vary. The chronic respiratory disease syndrome is summarised in Fig.9-30. The greater the variety of virulent organisms in the population of pigs the more complex the picture. It is helpful in investigating a problem to determine which of these organisms are present.

Immunity

See chapter 3 for further information.

The piglet at birth receives antibodies and immunity via the colostrum. Not only do these antibodies provide protection against enteric diseases but also against all other infections endemic on the farm. These levels of passive or maternal immunity reach their maximum in the piglet a few hours after birth and they then gradually disappear over the next 3 to 14 weeks. (Fig.9-31). The actual time of this disappearance differs from one disease to another, a vital piece of information that is used to manipulate the management of the system and control disease.

When investigating a respiratory disease problem it is essential to identify the point at which disease first appears, because this highlights where management changes could reduce the effects of disease.

This biological fact can be used to control not only respiratory diseases but also many others because if the piglet is removed from the sow at weaning to a totally clean environment the disease cycle may be broken. This is now adopted as the principle of segregated early weaning. See chapter 3. Fig.9-32 suggest the ages at which piglets would have to be weaned from the sow into isolated accommodation to prevent them becoming infected with different respiratory diseases. However in some herds these ages may be less because of the herd size and increased numbers of gilts which might be actively excreting organisms. Fig.9-33 also illustrates the similar ages for enteric disease for sake of completeness. The ages given assume that the source herd contains only breeding females and sucking piglets.

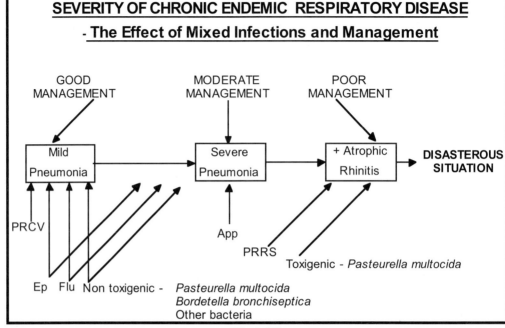

(Fig.9-30)

Management control and prevention

◆ Fig.9-34 shows the options that are available to control respiratory and other diseases. Obviously if the organism is not present on the farm there will be no disease. Disease freedom can be maintained at a national, country or at a farm level and it is therefore an important part of the control system.

◆ **Freedom from disease**
  - At a national level major diseases such as FMD, ASF, CSF, SVD, Aujeszky's (PR) and *Brucella suis*, may be eradicated either by slaughter policies or testing and slaughter. Some countries declare freedom from some diseases, for example, Ireland is free from TGE and PED. The UK and parts of the EU from aujeszky's disease and *Brucella suis*.
  - At a farm level herds can be established and maintained free of App, AD, PAR, EP and PRRS but in dense pig areas breakdowns are common.

◆ **Eradication**
  - All respiratory diseases can be successfully eradicated by total depopulation of the herd and its replacement by disease free stock. (See chapters 2 and 3). In practice the siting of the herd relative to sources of infected pigs needs careful consideration. PRCV and SI will at some stage re-infect the herd. EP and PRRS will be transmitted if infected pigs are within 2 to 3km (1 to 2 miles) and in such cases it may be advisable to restock with exposed animals and vaccinate them.
  - PRRS can be controlled by selective depopulation of first and second stage nurseries provided the disease is stabilised in the breeding and finisher herds.
  - Pseudorabies or aujeszky's disease can be successfully eradicated through the use of gene deleted vaccines and testing for field virus carrier pigs and slaughtering them.
  - By using the techniques of medicated early weaning a new disease free population can be established on another site, from an existing diseased herd.
  - Atrophic rhinitis can be eliminated by vaccination and segregated diseased control.

◆ **Control on the farm**
  - Medication and vaccination - Most if not all farms have at least one or more respiratory organisms present that require continual control procedures. The use of medication strategies for respiratory disease have been dealt with in chapter 4 and you are referred to this for further information. The use of vaccines can be limited by cost, the practical problems of administration to every pig and often two doses are required. However vaccine programmes to control AD, EP and AR have given excellent results in the field. The use of PRRS and SI vaccines are more problematical. Some vaccines are effective through the sow alone to control disease

> *Whilst the piglet is protected by maternal antibody it will not become affected with many of the infectious diseases endemic in the herd.*

CHAPTER 9 - Managing and Treating Disease in the Weaner, Grower and Finishing Periods

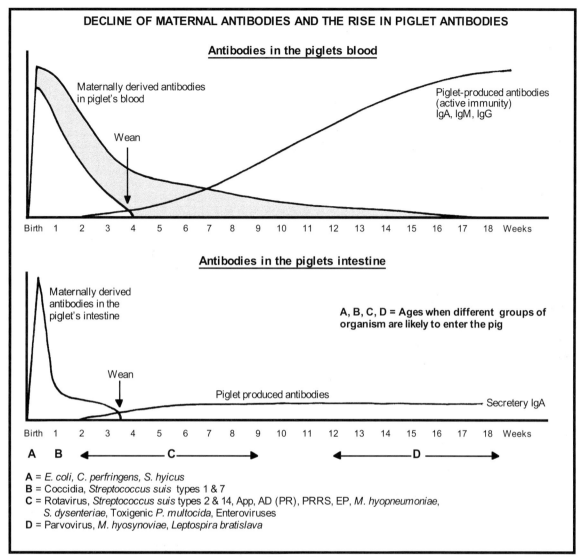

(Fig.9-31)

and the overall strategies that can be adopted are shown in Fig.9-35.

- ◆ **Management** - This involves the manipulation of the environment, the pig and nutrition, giving attention to detail and identifying the important areas and making adjustments.
- Identify the time of commencement of the disease. This is absolutely crucial to understanding the problem on the farm. If the onset of disease is identified and the incubation period calculated, then the time the pig first meets disease and the environmental factors contributing can be determined.
- Keep the pig above its lower critical temperature. Creating an environment where the pig becomes catabolic (using more energy than it is consuming) is the ideal method to trigger off respiratory disease. The LCT is commonly breached by faulty ventilation systems, a change in feed from one house to another or a change in stocking density. Draughts, shortage of water, wet floors, dirty pens, low stocking densities will have a similar effect. Look at the weight of the pig entering the house. Is it heavy enough to cope with the environment, the type of housing and floor surfaces.
- Assess the lying patterns of the pigs early in the morning and last thing at night.
- Avoid rapid changes in the environment in the house. This is particularly important where high speed ventilation systems may cause chilling. The pig will experience similar changes whenever it is moved from one house to another particularly if this is associated with a change in floor type, from a solid to a slatted floor. Contrary to popular opinion a high air flow will have little effect on the transfer of organisms between the nose of one pig and another.

Chapter 9

- A floor space < 0.5m² per pig is associated with more pneumonia. Allow 0.7m² of total area per pig.
- Pneumonia levels are less in environments that provide more than 3.6m³ of air space per pig.
- Bacterial levels above $10^4/m^3$ will predispose to pneumonia.
- Keep faeces contamination in pens at a low level because gut organisms produce endotoxins that can damage lung tissue and predispose to pneumonia.
- Avoid low temperature and low humidity environments, because the particles in the air are very small and remain suspended. Such particles are inhaled to the very bottom of the respiratory tract where the organism can attack the lung tissues.
- Maintain either a high temperature low humidity, or low temperature high humidity environment. Here the particles of water vapour are large, they attract the organisms from the air and prevent them penetrating the deep parts of the lung.
- As dust levels increase in the house so does the severity of both pneumonia and rhinitis. Dust levels of more than 4mg/m³ start to have an effect on the lungs.
- There is less pneumonia in extraction type ventilation systems than in ones that create positive pressure.
- Natural ventilation, within large cubic capacity air spaces, is ideal, because the organisms rise away from the nose of the pig by natural convection.
- Adapt all-in all-out housing systems that accommodate each week's production. This prevents the development of endemic disease.
- After houses have been washed out use a space heater to bring the temperature back to normal. This is essential for pigs from 7 to 14 weeks of age. It may be necessary in certain climates to provide heat for 7-10 days when pigs move from a solid to a slatted floor and when there is a change from dry to wet feeding.
- Keep ammonia levels at less than 25ppm, carbon monoxide at less than 30ppm, hydrogen sulphide at less than 5ppm carbon dioxide at less than 2000ppm
- Fogging - this has been used in an effort to control respiratory disease within a populated house but the results are not convincing. Fogging with water periodically will increase the humidity but it also has the disadvantage of cooling the pig by evaporation. It requires fogging at least every 5 to 10 minutes to maintain sufficient water vapour in the house.
- Make sure health control procedures are in operation that eliminate the risk of introducing new

RESPIRATORY DISEASES		
The Oldest Age at Which Pigs can be Weaned to a Segregated Site and be Free From Contamination by Pathogenic Organisms Endemic in the Herd		
Infection / Disease	Age (Days)	Medication / Vaccination * for added safety
Actinobacillus pleuropneumoniae (App)	< 28	Medication + Vaccination
Aujeszky's virus	21	Vaccination
Bordetella bronchiseptica (AR)	5	Medication + Vaccination
Influenza virus	16	None
Mycoplasma hyopneumoniae (EP)	10	Medication + Vaccination
Pasteurella multocida (toxigenic) (AR)	8 - 10	Medication + Vaccination
PRCV	? < 14	None
PRRS virus	< 16 (NR)	None
Salmonella choleraesuis	16	Medication
Other salmonella spp.	? < 21	Medication

Some of these data suggested by D.L.Harris (1996 - personal communication)
* Vaccination of the sow >2 weeks before farrowing
  Medication of the sow and/or piglets with an appropriate drug against the organism.
  Medication and vaccination are not always necessary but increase the reliability.
? Not known or guesswork
(NR) on present evidence not reliable.

(Fig.9-32)

ENTERIC DISEASES		
The Oldest Age at Which Pigs can be Weaned to a Segregated Site and be Free From Contamination by Pathogenic Organisms Endemic in the Herd		
Enteric Diseases	Age (Days)	Medication / Vaccination * of the sow for added safety
Coccidia	—	Not possible
E. coli	—	Not possible
Internal parasites	< 14	Medication
Parvovirus	< 28	Vaccination
Salmonella	? < 21	Medication
Swine dysentery	< 21	Medication
TGE	? 14	None

* Vaccination of the sow > two weeks before farrowing.
? not known or guess work

(Fig.9-33)

RESPIRATORY DISEASES. METHODS OF CONTROL	
Freedom from disease	On a national or regional basis. In integrated systems (e.g. breeding pyramid). At an individual herd level.
Eradication	Depopulate - repopulate with healthy stock (e.g. SPF or DHHS pigs). Medicate and vaccinate. Medicate and early wean. Vaccinate/test and remove.
Control on the farm	Medication. Vaccination. Management - The environment The pig Nutrition Using segregated early weaning (SEW). Using segregated disease control (SDC).

(Fig. 9-34)

CHAPTER 9 - Managing and Treating Disease in the Weaner, Grower and Finishing Periods **333**

pathogens into your herd.
- Avoid purchasing pigs from multiple sources, particularly finisher pigs.
- The larger the herd the greater is the problem.
- The more pig movement there is around the farm the more likelihood there will be of pneumonia.
- As stocking density increases there will be a greater incidence of pneumonia and this is certainly true once more than 200 pigs occupy a common air space.
- Avoid continual throughput and the mixing of different ages of pigs. The best way to maintain pneumonia on the farm is to mix pigs into a house that contains older ones that have already incubated disease and are passing out large amounts of infectious agents.
- Study the complexity of organisms on the farm in relation to the time when pneumonia occurs. This can be a sequential phenomena, that is, three or four diseases affecting the pig over a range of 4 to 12 weeks of age.
- Does the housing satisfy the environmental requirements of the pig at the different ages and weights?

◆ **Nutrition**
- Identify the time when disease first becomes evident.
- Note when nutritional changes take place. When pigs move from one house to another there is often a drop in the nutrient density of the diet. This also coincides with a drop in intake for the first 2 to 7 days.
- This reduced feed intake and change can result in catabolism and the pig dropping below the LCT.
- Maintain high energy diets at critical times. Do not change the feed for at least 5 days when pigs move from one house to another.
- Provide adequate water at all times. Look at the type of nipple drinkers, their availability and accessibility to the pig, particularly when it moves from one house to another.
- Look at the methods of feeding. Are there any features of design or feeder placement that inhibit access to the feed.
- Is there sufficient hopper space.
- Make sure there are adequate levels of vitamin E in the diet. Add an extra 50-100iu to the tonne if there is a disease problem.

◆ **Segregated weaning and segregated disease control**
- When pigs are moved from one building to another already containing pigs they are exposed to a range of viruses and bacteria many which they may not have encountered before. Some of these may produce clinical disease and others may result in subclinical infection. The end result is a large uptake of protein and energy diverted to satisfying the de-

| POTENTIAL USES FOR VACCINES ||||
Disease	Sow	Piglet	Growing pig
App		✓	✓
AR	✓		
Aujeszky's disease	✓		✓
EP		✓	✓
Porcine cytomegalovirus	not necessary		
PRCV	not necessary		
PRRS	✓	✓	✓
Salmonella choleraesuis	✓		✓
SI	✓		✓

(Fig.9-35)

mands of the immune system. This significantly depresses daily gain and food conversion efficiency. Segregated weaning to all-in all-out buildings on a week by week basis, eliminates or reduces such a challenge. The improved performance is likely to far exceed that of weaning into a continuously operated nursery containing different ages of pigs but in addition it is of great benefit in the control of respiratory disease. These procedures are discussed in detail in chapter 3.

The costs of respiratory disease are proportional to the numbers of infectious agents present on the farm, the management and environmental conditions that allow endemic disease to develop and high levels of exposure to susceptible pigs.

> *If there is a respiratory disease problem on the farm check all the key points and identify the weak ones.*

ROTAVIRUS

These viruses are widespread both in pig populations and most other mammals and there are a number of different types or groups.

Group A is probably the common pig one, but B, C and E also occur. However the frequency with which different ones occur is unknown and from a practical view point it is probably academic.

Rotaviruses are ubiquitous and they are present in most if not all pig herds with virtually a 100% seroconversion in adult stock. A further epidemiological feature is their persistence outside the pig, where they are resistant to environmental changes and many disinfectants. Maternal antibodies persist for 3-6 weeks after which pigs become susceptible to infection but exposure does not necessarily result in disease. It is estimated that only 10-15% of diarrhoeas in pigs are initiated by a primary rotavirus infection.

The fact that the virus persists in the environment accounts for widespread infection and therefore a constant risk of disease.

Clinical signs

In a mature herd disease appears after piglets are 7 to 10 days of age, with a watery profuse diarrhoea in younger animals. It becomes progressively less important with age. However if pathogenic strains of *E. coli* are present severe disease can occur with heavy mortality. Villus atrophy is a consistent feature with dehydration and malabsorption and diarrhoea usually persists for 3-4 days. Pigs look hollow in the abdomen the eyes are sunken and the skin around the rectum is wet.

The role of rotaviruses in the post-weaned pig is probably less important although they are often identified when acute *E. coli* diarrhoea occurs in the first 7-10 days after weaning.

Diagnosis

Whenever there is a diarrhoea problem in pigs from 10 to 40 days of age rotavirus infection either as primary agents or secondary must be considered. Laboratory examinations are required by electron microscopy and ELISA tests. Try the litmus test by soaking scour in litmus paper, *E. coli* infections turn blue, virus infections red.

Treatment

- ☐ There are no specific treatments for rotavirus infections.
- ☐ Provide antibiotic therapy either by injection, by mouth or in the drinking water, to control secondary infections such as *E. coli*.
- ☐ Apralan, amoxycillin, neomycin, framycetin and enrofloxacin could be used.
- ☐ Provide dextrose/glycine electrolytes to counteract dehydration.
- ☐ Provide dry warm and comfortable lying areas.

Management control and prevention

- ◆ Reduce the levels of virus in the environment by all-in all-out procedures and effective disinfection. Leave the house empty for 2 to 4 days before pigs are moved in.
- ◆ Disinfect with peroxygen based disinfectants such as Virkon S or chlorine based ones.
- ◆ Reduce the spread of virus between affected and non affected pigs. Use foot dips and clean clothing and wash hands after handling sick pigs.
- ◆ Apply control procedures outlined for coliform infections.
- ◆ If a persistent problem is diagnosed in sucking pigs expose sows to piglet scour by collecting it in wet saw dust, or mix the faeces in waters. Feed the contaminated material via the watering systems or into troughs two to three times weekly. Carry this out in weeks four and three before farrowing.
- ◆ Modified live vaccines are available in some countries.
- ◆ In the weaned pig adopt all-in all-out procedures with cleaning and disinfection in first stage flat decks. Pay particular attention to environmental stress and temperature fluctuations.

RUPTURES OR HERNIAS

Of many congenital abnormalities, ruptures at the umbilicus or the inguinal canal are most common. They are considered to be developmental defects yet have a very low heritability. Umbilical hernias can sometimes be traced back to a particular boar in which case he should be culled. Environmental factors can increase the incidence of umbilical hernias and if there is a problem (more than 2% of pigs) consider the following:

- Are prostaglandins used to synchronise farrowings. If so check that piglets are not being pulled away from the sow at farrowing and the cord stretched abnormally.
- Is navel bleeding occurring on the farm? Are naval clips being used to prevent bleeding? If so make sure they are not placed close up to the skin otherwise the tissues will be damaged and weakened.
- Identify the precise time when the ruptures appear. Do these coincide with a change of housing.
- In veranda type housing where the pigs pass through a small hole to the dunging area sudden severe abdominal pressure may cause ruptures.
- Are stocking densities high and causing increased abdominal pressure?
- In cold weather do the pigs huddle thereby increasing abdominal pressure.
- Check records to see if the boar and the sow are related.
- If the rupture is large and the pig is on a concrete floor or slats it should be moved to a soft bedded area so that the overlying skin does not become sore and ulcerated.
- Examine navels at births and two days later to see if there are any abnormalities.

Inguinal ruptures are not as important a problem unless they become very large. Where castration is the farm policy a minor surgical operation needs to be performed. This is described in chapter 15.

SALMONELLOSIS

There are many serotypes of salmonella but the ones that are most likely to cause clinical disease in pigs are *Salmonella choleraesuis*, and *Salmonella typhimurium* and to a lesser extent *Salmonella derby*. Other "exotic" salmonella serotypes may infect pigs and be shed in the faeces for limited periods but they usually remain subclinical. *S. choleraesuis* is the specific host-adapted pig serovar and can cause major generalised disease. *S. typhimurium* and *S. derby* are more likely to cause a milder disease the main sign of which is usually diarrhoea. Pigs may become long-term sub-clinical carriers of *S cholearesuis* the organism surviving in the mesenteric lymph nodes draining the intestine. Many such carriers do not shed the bacteria in faeces unless they are stressed. Some however, may become sub-clinical carriers of *S typhimurium, S. derby* and other serotypes. They may be intermittent or continuous faecal shedders but the carrier state is usually relatively short, weeks or a few months and it is self limiting.

If a pig is infected with a large dose of *S. choleraesuis* it is likely to develop severe generalised clinical disease starting with a septicaemia (blood infection) followed by severe pneumonia and enteritis. Subsequently the organism may settle out in a variety of tissues including the central nervous system, resulting in meningitis, and the joints resulting in arthritis. *S. typhimurium and S. derby* may also cause septicaemia, become generalised and involved in pneumonia but in most pigs these are transient and enteritis is the only persistent manifestation.

Salmonellosis can occur at any age but is most common in growing pigs over eight weeks of age. Severe *S. choleraesuis* infection occurs typically at around 12 to 14 week*s*.

Clinical signs

Acute septicaemia and pneumonia result in fever, inappetance, respiratory distress and depression. The skin of the extremities (i.e. tail, ears, nose and feet) becomes blue. On the ears, in *S. choleraesuis* infection, there is often a clear line of demarcation between the blue and normal skin. Foul-smelling diarrhoea which may be blood stained, is a common feature. Jaundice (yellowing) may result from liver damage and lameness from arthritis. Meningitis results in nervous signs. If untreated, mortality may be high.

Diagnosis

It is necessary to submit to the laboratory either fresh faecal samples from untreated pigs, or where available a dead or live untreated pig. This is essential to demonstrate the presence of the organism and differentiate it from other causes.

The post-mortem lesions are strongly suggestive of *S. choleraesuis*, particularly the generalised pneumonia, the appearance of the lining of the small and large intestine, the congested spleen and multiple small haemorrhages.

Similar diseases

Severe salmonellosis caused by *S. choleraesuis* can occur alone but it also commonly occurs at the same time as classical swine fever (hog cholera) in those countries in which this disease still occurs. In such countries it is important to ensure by serology and laboratory tests that swine fever is not the primary cause (NB. swine fever usually also affects sows and sucking piglets and also causes mummified litters and abortions).

Severe PRRS in herds with endemic EP may give the appearance of salmonellosis, however PRRS also causes abortions, stillbirths and precipitates scouring in piglets.

Treatment

☐ The response to the treatment of salmonella infections is often poor. It is necessary to determine the serotype, the antibiotic sensitivity and treat individual pigs at a very early stage.
☐ Preventive medication or strategic medication both in-feed or in the water are important and the drugs used are dependant on the bacterial sensitivity.

Management control and prevention

It is most important point to realise that the severity of clinical salmonellosis is dose dependant. This is true to a greater or lesser extent of all infectious diseases but is particularly so of salmonellosis. The overall aim, therefore, is to get the levels in the environment down to below the disease-producing threshold. The second aim is to reduce the spread of infection.

- Improve hygiene by frequent and thorough removal of waste.
- Optimise stocking density. Overcrowding predisposes.
- Reduce stress by reducing moving and mixing.
- Develop an all-in all-out system with cleaning and disinfection between batches.
- Avoid the movement of pig faeces between one batch and another.
- Vaccines against *S. choleraesuis* are available in some countries and can be used to help in elimination programmes if this type is present. The principle is to vaccinate the sow to produce high maternal antibody and then carry out segregated early weaning or segregated disease control programmes.
- Disinfect boots between houses.
- Control vermin and flies.
- Prevent contamination of feed by birds, rats and mice.
- Monitor raw feed ingredients and final product.

Zoonoses

It is important to remember that salmonella organisms are transmissible to people and are one of the commonest causes of food poisoning. This has two implications for you as a pig farmer.

First, you should ensure that everybody working with the pigs adopts a high standard of personal hygiene so that they do not become infected. Second, it is important that pig farmers and pig meat products have a high public image for safety and do not get linked with outbreaks of human disease. It is therefore imperative that you get salmonella under strict control by the particular use of all-in all-out procedures.

SALT POISONING - (WATER DEPRIVATION)

Salt poisoning is common in all ages of pigs and almost without exception is related to water shortage either caused by inadequate supplies or complete loss. The normal levels of salt in the diet (0.4-0.5%) become toxic in the absence of water.

Signs develop within 24 to 48 hours.

Clinical signs

The very early stages of disease are always preceded by inappetance and whenever a sow or groups of pigs are not eating always check the water supply first. The first signs are often pigs trying to drink from nipple drinkers unsuccessfully. Nervous changes are the major signs and in more advanced cases involve fits, with animals wandering around apparently blind. Often the pig walks up to a wall, stands and presses its head against it in a characteristic position. One symptom strongly suggestive of salt poisoning is nose twitching just before a convulsion starts.

Diagnosis

This is based upon the clinical signs and lack of water. Examination of the brain histologically at post-mortem confirms the disease.

Similar diseases

Aujeszky's disease, swine fever, streptococcal meningitis and glässers disease all produce nervous signs. The condition might also be confused with middle ear infection but this only affects one individual rather than a group of pigs.

Treatment

- ☐ The response to treatment is poor but involves rehydrating the animal. At a practical level this can be achieved by dripping water into the mouth of the pig through a hose pipe or alternatively via a flutter valve into the rectum where it is absorbed. (See chapter 15 Flutter valve).
- ☐ Discuss the possibility of administering sterile water into the abdomen with your veterinarian.
- ☐ Corticosteroids may also help.

Management control and prevention

- ◆ It must be a daily routine to check that all sources of water are adequate free flowing and available.

SPIROCHAETAL DIARRHOEA

This is a disease associated with spirochetes distinct from those that cause swine dysentery (*Serpulina hyodysenteriae*). It occurs mainly in young pigs appearing very similar to colitis and the possibility of *Serpulina pilosicoli* and *Lawsonia intracellularis* (PE) playing a major part cannot be discounted.

Spirochetes are common inhabitants of the large intestine and caecum and disease is often associated with changes such as the inadvertent removal of copper from the diet, withdrawal of growth promoters or a sudden change in diet.

Clinical signs

A mild to moderate diarrhoea develops two to six weeks post-weaning that persist for a few days with dehydration and loss in growth. Most cases resolve in 7 to 10 days but in some pigs chronic diarrhoea results. The disease can be difficult to differentiate from the bacterial infections, particularly colitis.

Diagnosis

This is difficult because specific organisms cannot usually be identified. If there is an on-going problem on the farm live diseased pigs showing typical signs should be submitted for post-mortem and bacteriological examinations to eliminate swine dysentery and demonstrate large populations of spirochetes associated with an enteritis.

Treatment

- ☐ In-feed medication. Lincomycin, tiamulin, monensin, dimetridazole and tylosin all have good activity against spirochetes and can be used for both prevention and treatment.
- ☐ In acute outbreaks lincomycin, tiamulin or tylosin could be used in the water.
- ☐ Inject individual pigs with either lincomycin, tiamulin or tylosin and assess the response.

Management control and prevention

- ◆ Adopt all-in all-out procedures.
- ◆ Ensure that floor surfaces are kept clean and dry.
- ◆ Provide clean sources of water.
- ◆ Use growth promoters such as tylosin or salinomycin.

STREPTOCOCCAL INFECTIONS

Streptococci are common organisms in all animals including people. They are broadly but not entirely species specific. The main species is *Streptococcus suis* which is widespread in pig populations of Europe, the Americas and Australasia and probably occurs wherever pig farming is carried out. It is associated with a variety of conditions including meningitis, septicaemia (infection of the blood), polyserisitis (inflammation of the lining of the abdominal and chest cavities), arthritis, endocarditis (infection of the heart) and pneumonia. It has also been isolated from cases of rhinitis and abortion. The pattern and relative importance of the different syndromes vary in different countries.

The situation is not as simple as it may first appear. *S. suis* is sub-divided into at least thirty-four serotypes. They vary in their pathogenicity and the diseases they cause, both between and within types. Some types appear to be non-pathogenic and have been isolated mainly from healthy pigs, some are mainly associated with lung lesions, and some have been isolated from other animal species as well as pigs. Some types, notably 2 and 14 can occasionally cause meningitis in people as well as pigs. Fortunately human cases are rare.

Different types predominate in different countries with type 2 among the commonest in most countries and the type most often associated with disease. (One exception is Denmark where type 7 is the most common). In the UK type 2 is the main cause of serious acute meningitis, along with polyserisitis and arthritis in weaned and growing pigs and it is rarely associated with pneumonia. Type 1 occurs fairly commonly in most countries and causes sporadic arthritis and occasionally meningitis in sucking piglets usually around one to two weeks of age but sometimes up to six weeks. It is a relatively unimportant condition. The syndrome that is important and worrying to the pig farmer is persistent endemic meningitis caused by type 2.

S. suis 2 is spread from one pig to another by direct nose to nose contact. It can also spread within a herd by indirect contact and in confined space by aerosol infection. Clinically healthy pigs can carry the organism in their tonsils for many months and a carrier state exists in some sows. Once a serotype has entered a herd no techniques are yet available to remove it and it becomes established in the tonsil as part of the normal flora. *S. suis* is not spread by AI or hysterectomy. The most likely source of entry into the farm is the purchase of carrier boars or gilts. There is little documented evidence to suggest that the human will transmit disease from pig farm to pig farm. *S. suis* is quickly killed by disinfectants in common use on farms, including phenolic disinfectants and chlorine and iodine based ones, detergents will also kill the organism in thirty minutes. "Savlon" is particularly effective. Outside the pig, in very cold and freezing conditions it may survive for 15 weeks or more but at normal room temperatures it dies within one to two weeks. It survives long periods in rotting carcasses. The sow passes on antibody through colostrum to the sucking pig and the disease is therefore uncommon in this group of animals unless it is introduced into the herd for the first time. It is much more common in the immediate post-weaning period often starting 2 to 3 weeks after weaning and continuing through to approximately 16 weeks of age. In flat decks or nurseries almost 100% of pigs become carriers within three weeks.

An interesting research finding is that *S. suis* type 2 is carried from the base of the tonsil to the brain, joints and serosal surfaces inside migrating white blood cells called monocytes (analogous to the "Trojan horse"). Pathogenic strains can survive and multiply in these cells whereas non-pathogenic strains cannot. There are also strains of low pathogenicity which may be activated by PRRS virus infection. PRRS may also raise the incidence of meningitis caused by pathogenic strains when it first enters a herd. Although PRRS alone does not affect the brain, it has been shown experimentally that many more pigs are affected with meningitis when they are infected with both *S. suis* type 2 and PRRS viruses than when they are infected with *S. suis* alone. *S. suis* type 14 is emerging as a new disease with the appearance of acute severe outbreaks of arthritis in both sucking and weaned pigs.

Species of streptococci other than *S. suis* may sometimes cause disease in pigs. For example, *Streptococcus equisimilis* causes sporadic cases of septicaemia and arthritis in sucking pigs, infection of the heart valves in growing pigs and ascending infection of the womb in sows. In the USA *Streptococcus porcinus* causes throat abscesses and septicaemia and is sometimes isolated from pneumonia.

Clinical signs

Acute disease

Weaners may just be found dead. In very early stages of meningitis the pig is laid on its belly, hair standing on end and shivering. Within two to three hours there are lateral jerky movements of the eye (nystagmus). The animal then lies on its side paddling and frothing at the mouth. The organism invades the blood stream and is carried around the body where it may cause arthritis and pneumonia.

Diagnosis

A history of the presence of recurring meningitis in weaned pigs is highly suggestive and is confirmed by the isolation of the organism from the brain and its specific identification, which not all diagnostic laboratories are capable of.

Because of the existence of strains that are non-pathogenic or only mildly pathogenic the isolation of *S. suis* type 2 from the tonsils of a pig is difficult to interpret. Isolation from the brain of a pig showing signs of meningitis is more conclusive.

Treatment

This must be carried out as soon as disease is recognised.
- Remove the affected pig from the group to a hospital pen. Meningitis is extremely painful and the recovery rate is increased substantially through good nursing.
- Provide warmth and bedding and trickle water into the pigs mouth from a hosepipe every 4 to 6 hours. Alternatively, water can be given by inserting a narrow hosepipe gently into the pigs rectum or using a flutter valve. (See chapter 15).
- Give intra-muscular injections of penicillin 2 to 3

- times daily for the first 24 hours.
- ☐ Use a quick acting penicillin for the first 24 hours followed by long-acting penicillin. Time is of the essence with this disease. Trimethoprim/sulpha would be an alternative drug to use.
- ☐ **Strategic medication** - This is a method to adopt on farms where disease levels remain high. The following options are available:
- ☐ Identify the onset of disease and apply strategic medication 2 to 3 days before that time.
- ☐ Strategic medication can be applied in the drinking water using phenoxymethyl penicillin, tetracyclines, synthetic penicillin particularly amoxycillin, or trimethoprim/sulpha.
- ☐ In-feed medicate continuously from day of weaning through to six weeks post-weaning. Phenoxymethyl penicillin at a level of 300g/tonne is the drug of choice. TMS could also be used.
- ☐ Inject all pigs with long-acting penicillin at weaning time.
- ☐ Assess the response to injecting pigs with long-acting penicillin five days before weaning.

Similar diseases

Similar nervous signs may occur in aujeszky's disease, glässers disease or salt poisoning (water deprivation).

Management control and prevention

- ◆ If your herd is free from this disease, try to keep it free.
- ◆ Check out your sources of replacement stock before purchase.
- ◆ Do not purchase pigs from herds with clinical cases of meningitis.
- ◆ If you have the disease endemic in your herd the incidence increases with :-
  - High stocking density in flat decks.
  - Continuous production systems which perpetuate infection.
  - PRRS infections may activate *S. suis* already in the herd.
  - Mixing of pigs post-weaning.
  - A small cubic capacity air space per pig. Provide at least $0.8m^3$ per pig at weaning.
  - Poor ventilation and high humidity.
  - High dust levels.
  - Stress.
  - Damp pens.
  - High slurry levels under perforated metal floors and the damaging effects of gases to the respiratory system.
  - Weighing pigs.
  - Tattooing, ear notching and extra stress at weaning.
  - Changes in nutritional status at critical times.
  - Low vitamin E in the diet. Assess the response to adding 50-100iu/kg

SWINE DYSENTERY (SD)

Swine dysentery (SD), which is caused by a small snake-like bacteria called *Serpulina hyodysenteriae* can be one of the most expensive diseases of the growing pig. There are two other similar bacteria, one called *S. innocens* which is non pathogenic and the other *S. pilosicoli,* associated with colitis. Disease is common in pigs from 12 to 75kg weight and occasionally in sows and piglets. It is spread entirely by the ingestion of infected faeces or from carrier pigs that shed the organism in faeces for long periods. It may enter the farm through the introduction of carrier pigs or mechanically from infected faeces via equipment, boots or birds. The disease has a marked depressant effect on feed conversion and daily gain with symptoms appearing intermittently often associated with stress, such as the movement of pigs which increases the output of organisms. The organism survives in slurry for up to eight weeks. Continual exposure to infected faeces is a major factor in the maintenance of disease in a herd

The costs of disease are associated with mortality (low), morbidity (high), inefficient production and continual in-feed medication. Disease often appears in cycles and previously affected pigs will still transmit infection to susceptible ones for at least 10 to 12 weeks. SD can be spread by flies, mice, birds (starlings) and dogs, all these species shedding the organism for up to 21 days. SD will survive outside the pig for up to eight weeks in moist conditions particularly in cold slurry but it dies out in two to three days when allowed to dry.

Clinical signs

The incubation period is normally 2 to 14 days but can be much longer. The pig may develop a sub-clinical carrier state first and then break down with clinical disease when put under stress or when there is a change of feed.

The early symptom is a sloppy diarrhoea, which stains the skin of the perineum under the anus, and a rapid hollowing of the flanks. Initially the diarrhoea is light brown and contains jelly-like mucus. As the disease progresses, blood may appear in increasing amounts turning the faeces black and tarry. The pig's appetite is decreased, it rapidly loses condition, becomes dehydrated and takes on a gaunt appearance. Spread through the herd is slow, building up in numbers as the dose rate of the causal agent builds up in the environment. Sudden death sometimes occurs mainly in heavy finishers.

Post-mortem examinations show the lesions are confined to the large bowel and sometimes the greater curvature of the stomach.

Diagnosis

This is based on the history, the clinical picture,

post-mortem examinations, gram-stained faecal or colonic smears, fluorescent antibody tests on faecal smears and the isolation and identification of *S. hyodysenteriae*. Specific identification of *S. hyodysenteriae* to distinguish it from other similar colonic spirochetes requires specialised procedures which are not available in every laboratory.

Similar diseases

These include non-specific colitis, bloody gut (PHE) and acute salmonella infection particularly by *S. choleraesuis*. Heavy infections of the whip worm, trichuris can also simulate swine dysentery.

Treatment

❒ The following drugs have an activity against *S. hyodysenteriae*: (very active *)

Carbadox *.	Ronidazole *.
Chlortetracycline.	Salinomycin.
Dimetridazole *.	Tiamulin *.
Lincomycin *.	Tylosin *.
Monensin *.	Virginiamycin.

Some strains of *S. hyodysenteriae* have become resistant to some of these drugs.
❒ With the first signs of disease medicate the drinking water with either lincomycin, tiamulin or tylosin for at least 7 days.
❒ Inject badly affected individual pigs daily for 4 days with either lincomycin, tiamulin or tylosin.
❒ In-feed medication is only of value as a prevention to suppress clinical disease.

Management control and prevention

◆ If the herd is not infected with swine dysentery carry out all the biosecurity measures discussed in chapter 2 to prevent its entry. Transmission usually requires a moderate dose of infected faeces so it can usually be kept out successfully even in pig dense areas.
◆ In infected herds control is aimed at preventing the movement of the organism between groups of pigs. Management procedures should therefore be directed towards all-in all-out systems with cleansing and disinfection between each batch. The organism is sensitive to most disinfectants and in particular phenol based ones.

The following specific management procedures should be adopted:
◆ Develop an all-in all-out housing system with disinfection. Slurry channels should be separate.
◆ Where solid dung passages are used it may be necessary to depopulate the whole house, clean and disinfect and bring in new pigs at weaning time that have not been contaminated.
◆ Control flies, they can transmit the organism from one group of pigs to another

◆ Carry out strategic medication, for example post-weaning using either lincomycin (110g/tonne) or tiamulin (100g/tonne) for a period of three weeks. This should produce a dysentery-free pig and provided this pig moves into further accommodation which as not been exposed to the organism it becomes possible to break the cycle. Segregate the herd into believed clean and infected areas and prevent transmission of faeces between them as much as possible.
◆ Use liberal disinfectant foot baths dispersed around the farm particularly when personnel move from one batch of pigs to another.
◆ Reduce the movement and handling of pigs to as little as possible particularly at weighing time when transfer of faeces is likely to take place and stress is likely to cause clinical flare ups.
◆ Do not overcrowd pigs and endeavour to keep a dry environment, the organism will die out quickly on drying. Poor sanitation and wet pens enhance the disease.
◆ One of the greatest risks is the introduction of the disease into a finishing system. This is likely when pigs have been brought in from unknown sources. Isolate incoming pigs for a period of three weeks and strategically medicate with dimetridazole 800g/tonne, lincomycin 220g/tonne or tiamulin at 100g/tonne for a period of two weeks. Water medication could also be used. This should eliminate the organism if it is present or at least lower it to a manageable level.
◆ A common source of infection is from infected pigs that are present on the vehicle which calls at your farm to collect your pigs. Infected faeces are carried back into the buildings on boots.

Eradication

Swine dysentery is a disease that no producer can afford to live with. There are therefore two options in the medium to long term: either to depopulate and repopulate the herd or attempt to eradicate the disease without depopulation. Eradication has been carried out on a number of farms successfully, although depending on farm circumstances, the success rate may only be as high as 80%. In the breeding finishing herd eradication commences with the treatment of the sow herd to eliminate the organism and produce and wean a dysentery-free pig. Such pigs must not be allowed to come into contact with any other infected pigs or their faeces on the farm. There are a number of programmes that can be adopted from this principle (Fig.9-36).
There are however some rules that need to be noted:
1. Do not start an eradication programme until clinical disease is reduced to an absolute minimum by management control and continuous preventative in-feed medication; 60g/tonne tiamulin, 55-100g lincomycin or 100g monensin could be used.

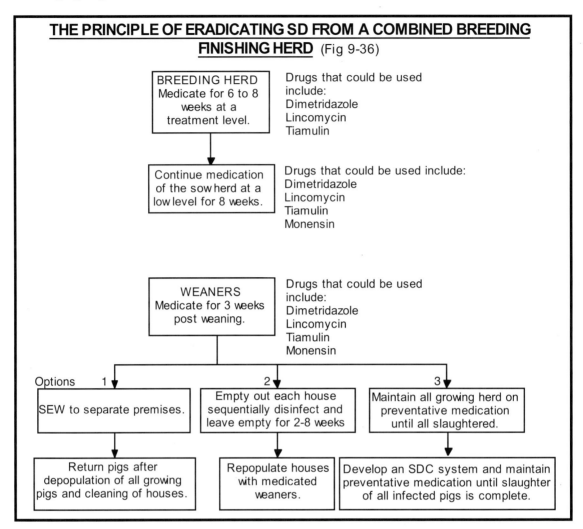

THE PRINCIPLE OF ERADICATING SD FROM A COMBINED BREEDING FINISHING HERD (Fig 9-36)

2. Maintain the preventive medication throughout the whole period of the eradication and for two months afterwards.
3. The numbers of growing pigs on the farm should be reduced to a minimum thereby reducing the susceptible population. Ideally this should start at weaner weight with all the grower pigs being sold off the farm.
4. An alternative would be to carry out segregated weaning for a period of weeks depending upon the availability of accommodation. Whilst this is going on the pigs from weaning through to slaughter can be marketed at their suitable weights.
5. One or more weaner houses should be totally emptied washed, disinfected and left empty for four weeks to give a break between clean and dirty pigs. This gap is maintained throughout the programme. Strict isolation procedures must be adopted between cleaned and infected houses.
6. As each house is emptied it should be completely cleaned down, all evidence of faeces removed and faeces channels totally emptied. Slurry channels become the most dangerous area because the organism can survive for up to eight weeks. However in practice disinfection can be carried out with individual buildings left emptied for a period of four weeks only, but this is a less reliable method.
7. Always attempt eradication during the warm summer months since the organism dies out in a matter of hours under dry conditions, whereas it can survive for weeks in cold wet conditions.
8. Prior to the commencement of the eradication programme the sow herd should be medicated for at least six weeks to remove any possible carrier state.
9. As the elimination procedures continue mice, rats and flies should be dealt with accordingly. The organism can persist for long periods of time in mice.

Drugs that have been used successfully for the eradication of swine dysentery.

Sows: Period of medication up to 8 weeks:
   Dimetridazole 500 to 800g/tonne feed.
   Tiamulin 100g/tonne feed.

Lincomycin 110g/tonne feed.
Monensin 100g/tonne feed.
Weaners: Period of in-feed medication three weeks.
Lincomycin 110-220g/tonne of creep feed.
Tiamulin 100g/tonne of creep feed.
Growers:
Lincomycin 55 to 110 g/tonne.
Tiamulin 60 to 100 g/tonne.
Monensin 100 g/tonne.

One note of warning, eradication is not always successful but it can be more cost effective than total herd depopulation and repopulation. Discuss this with your veterinarian.

SWINE INFLUENZA (SI)

Swine influenza is similar in most respects to human flu. In the pig there are at least four different serotypes each stimulating immunity to itself but not to the other serotypes. It is thus possible for the pigs to be infected by one virus and develop disease and then some two to three months later be infected by a different serotype and develop disease yet again. In large herds of over 300 sows the virus may circulate in young growing pigs, disease becoming more active in the winter time associated with reduced ventilation rates. In the growing and finishing pig disease is not seen until maternal antibody has disappeared at sometime between 7 and 12 weeks of age. SI viruses can interchange between man, pig and birds and the carrier state can exist in the pig for some two to four weeks. They are also spread by birds, particularly ducks, and for distances of 1 to 3km (1-2 miles) on the wind. Thus it is virtually impossible to guarantee or maintain a population of pigs that is free of this disease.

Clinical signs
Acute disease

The incubation period is short, less than 48 hours. The onset can be extremely rapid and dramatic. The classical picture is a house full of pigs that are normal on one day and most of them are prostrate and breathing heavily by the following morning. Severe coughing and laboured breathing will be observed. You may think most of the pigs are going to die but rest assured most of them survive, and provided the herd does not have a history of ongoing pneumonia the pigs will recover on their own, but it is always difficult to predict the outcome. Severely affected individuals or groups of pigs are therefore best given antibiotic cover.

Endemic disease

This is where the virus continually circulates through the herd infecting individual pigs within groups. SI causes severe pneumonia on its own but when it is combined with other infections such as App, EP and PRRS a chronic respiratory disease syndrome can develop.

Diagnosis

In acute disease the rapidity of development and spread, together with typical clinical signs, are diagnostic. No other disease will affect so many pigs so quickly.

In the chronic respiratory disease syndrome it is necessary to carry out serological tests and virus isolation to determine the presence and significance of the virus.

Treatment

☐ There is no treatment specifically for flu viruses. However secondary bacterial pneumonia may be involved and in such cases antibiotic treatments by injection or in the drinking water, would be advised.

☐ In-feed medication in acute disease is a waste of time because pigs do not eat. Although labour intensive, it is far more efficient to treat individual pigs that have secondary pneumonia with long-acting antibiotics, such as oxytetracycline or amoxycillin.

Management control and prevention

- Use the management procedures already outlined for the other respiratory diseases.
- Reduce the weights of exposure to other organisms.
- Vaccination is used in some countries with mixed results.
- Avoid buying pigs from sources where SI is active.

TORSION OF THE STOMACH AND INTESTINES

Clinical signs

There are usually none because the pig is found dead but the abdomen is grossly distended.

Diagnosis

This is the most common cause of sudden death in the growing pig and it is usually one of the best pigs in the group. The carcase is fresh the pig is very pale and the abdomen is very distended. Post-mortem examination shows the small and large intestines heavily congested and full of blood. The intestinal tract in the pig is suspended from a common point and this makes it liable to rotate and finally twist.

Management control and prevention

- Deaths are usually sporadic although they can be of significance where, for example, whey is being fed and bloat occurs.
- Over-feeding and abnormal fermentation of the contents of both the small and large intestine result in gas formation, increased pressure and a twist.
- Mortality in weaned and growing pigs should normally be less than 3% and up to a third of this may

be caused by torsion. If it reaches 1% or more the dietary components should be examined closely to see if there are starch based ingredients that might cause excessive fermentation. In such cases increasing the level of the growth promoter (if allowed) or adding 100g/tonne of penicillin, OTC or tylosin will reduce the bacterial multiplication.

◆ If torsion is a consistent cause of death collect information about each one including weight, age, sex, house, stocking density, environmental temperatures and feed changes. A study of this may give guidance as to contributing causes.

TRANSMISSIBLE GASTRO-ENTERITIS (TGE)
See chapter 8 for further information.

This is a highly infectious disease which in the weaning and the growing pig is clinically indistinguishable from porcine epidemic diarrhoea. If the virus is introduced into the finishing herd for the first time there is a rapid spreading illness with vomiting and a watery diarrhoea affecting almost 100% of animals. Disease disappears spontaneously over a 3 to 5 week period. Mortality is usually low but morbidity can be very high. The virus usually then dies out of the population unless there are large numbers of pigs on-site. Also if susceptible pigs are being brought in for growing and finishing, the virus is maintained in the population by continual infection. The disease then becomes endemic. The main effect on the individual pig is dehydration which is resolved in about a week. Nevertheless the disease may increase the slaughter age by 5 to 10 days.

The virus is sensitive to ultra violet radiation and in warm temperatures will only survive outside the pig for a few days. If an endemic situation therefore develops on a breeding farm a break of 2 to 3 weeks by segregated disease control is necessary, together with management and hygiene, to break the cycle of infection. Alternatively if pigs are being brought in to a finishing unit it is necessary to have a break for 3 for 4 weeks. TGE can become a major problem in SEW systems.

TUBERCULOSIS

Tuberculosis is a disease affecting human beings, mammals and birds. The causal organism *Mycobacterium tuberculosis* is sub-classified into types based on the species of host usually affected: the human type generally referred to as *M. tuberculosis* affects people and primates, the bovine type *M. bovis*, affects cattle, badgers and other wild herbivores and sometimes people; and the avian type, the *M. avian/M. intracellulare* complex, affects mainly birds. Pigs are susceptible to all three but in practice are rarely infected by the first two. Most TB in pigs is caused by the avian/intracellulare complex which causes small nodules in the lymph nodes of the neck and those that drain the small intestine. In the great majority of cases the lesions are non-progressive, they do not spread through the body, do not make the pigs ill and the organisms are not shed. The disease does not therefore spread between pigs and is rarely diagnosed in living pigs. Similarly, the *M. avium/intracellulare* complex causes non-progressive infection in normal healthy people. The main concern is that the *M. avium/intracellulare* could cause more serious disease in immuno-suppressed people and people with AIDS and the lesions in the pigs carcase at slaughter cannot be distinguished from human and bovine TB which would cause progressive disease in otherwise normal people. Therefore, in most countries if lesions are found in the neck at slaughter the whole head is condemned and if they are found in the mesenteric lymph nodes which drain the intestines the offals are condemned. If they are more widespread the whole carcase may be condemned or require cooking. If small lesions are missed by the meat inspector cooking will normally destroy the organism. The sources of infection to the pig include:

- Outdoor pigs - grazing land that has been treated with poultry manure even up to one year previously, or that which has been grazed by infected cattle or badgers infected with *M. bovis*.
- Avian TB as the name implies is found in wild birds and in particular starlings. The organism is shed in large numbers via droppings and therefore food or grain contaminated by birds becomes a potent source.
- Sawdust/shavings can be a major source of infection.
- Peat often contains *M. intracellulare* and is capable of causing lesions at slaughter. Peat is used both for bedding and gut stimulation in the young piglets. It should only be used if it as been pasteurised.
- Water contaminated by *M. avium/intracellulare* is often a source.

Clinical signs

M. avian infection has no clinical effect and there is no difference in performance between infected and non-infected pigs.

Diagnosis

TB in living pigs can be diagnosed using the skin tuberculin test but usually detected in the cervical and intestinal lymph glands at meat inspection. Normal levels are less than 1%.

Management control and prevention

If disease is evident at slaughter, consider the above potential sources and eliminate them. Remember that avian/intracellulare is an environmental contaminant - the environment is the source.

VICE - ABNORMAL BEHAVIOUR (TAIL BITING, FLANK CHEWING, EAR BITING).

Vice (abnormal behaviour Fig.9-37) in both weaned

CHAPTER 9 - Managing and Treating Disease in the Weaner, Grower and Finishing Periods **343**

and growing pigs can be a major problem on some farms with considerable economic loss.

Why do pigs mutilate each other? From our own experiences poor environmental conditions and human interactions cause varying degrees of aggravation and this is no different in the pig. If there is a problem on the farm, consider the three major contributing factors; management, nutrition and disease.

Management

Stand for a few minutes and observe pigs that are either tail biting or ear chewing and you will see that there is one overriding feature, the pigs give the impression of being very unhappy. The pig is indicating that the environment provided is far from ideal. The management factors that contribute to this are listed in Fig.9-38. Study these, identify important ones and make changes until there is a response. Remove offending pigs from the group because once the vice has become an established habit it can be difficult to stop.

Nutrition

Where there is competition for food or poor access, this tends to create aggression in the pen. Observations have shown that there is a greater tendency to tail biting when automatic feeders are used compared to manual systems. With automatic systems there is little empathy between pig and person. Increasing the salt level in the diet to 0.9% can often produce an improvement. Make sure there is ad lib water available. (Fig.9-39).

Disease

Greasy pig disease or exudative epidermitis is a little realised but important factor in the development of both tail biting, ear and flank chewing. A skin infection or wet eczema starts on the tip of the tail or ears with small areas of serum oozing to the surface. This is often initiated by a combination of feed contaminating the skin and splitting of the skin caused by trauma. *Staphylococcus hyicus* then invades and causes infection. The pig is attracted to the lesion and eventually this leads to vice. This situation is particularly apparent when pigs are first weaned into flat decks or nurseries or when they are moved into second stage accommodation particularly if mixing takes place. New concrete has an alkaline surface and the high pH and prolonged pressure to the skin, particularly when the pig is lying on slats, causes sores to develop over the ham or flanks. This can lead to infection and then vice. Greasy pig lesions on the tail are an irritant causing considerable tail movement which becomes attractive to other pigs. Other diseases such as pneumonia can result in disadvantaged pigs being traumatised by others. (Fig.9-40).

TYPES OF VICE	
The Weaned Pig	Growers
Navel sucking	Tail biting
Prepuce sucking	Ear necrosis
Ear sucking	Chewing feet
Tail biting	Flank biting

(Fig.9-37)

VICE - PREDISPOSING MANAGEMENT FACTORS	
A change in the diet	High hydrogen sulphide levels > 10ppm
A very humid environment	Long tails
Aggressive breeds	New concrete
Automatic feeding and little human/pig empathy	No bedding
Bad pen designs - badly sited feeders	Pigs too small for the environment
High carbon dioxide levels > 3000ppm	Shortage of trough space
Draughts	Trauma
Fluctuating temperatures	Uncomfortable conditions
High air speed	Unhappy pigs
High ammonia levels > 20ppm	Water shortage
High stocking densities	Wet pens

(Fig.9-38)

VICE - PREDISPOSING NUTRITIONAL FACTORS
Low salt in the diet.
Inadequate nutrition.
Rations with small particle sizes.
Diet changes.
Poor feed availability.
Feeding pellets.

(Fig.9-39)

VICE - RELATED DISEASE FACTORS
Greasy pig disease.
Wet eczema.
New concrete and skin trauma.
PRRS skin lesions.
Colitis.
Pig pox.
Skin trauma.
Pneumonia.
Parasites.

(Fig.9-40)

Treatment

☐ Determine the antibiotic sensitivity of the *Staphylococcus hyicus* if this is part of the problem and medicate feed for 7 to 10 days. Assess the results of strategic medication.

☐ Inject traumatised pigs with long-acting preparations of penicillin or OTC, or amoxycillin.

Management control and prevention

◆ Identify and correct the causal factors outlined above.

◆ Spray pigs with a 1% skin antiseptic, such as savlon, when housing is changed and continue this daily for two days.

◆ Spraying with a heavy industrial scent will help to reduce fighting when pigs are mixed.

◆ If *Staphylococcus hyicus* infection is part of the

problem there will usually be a very good response to in-feed medication with tetracyclines.
- ◆ Remove traumatised pigs from the pen to straw based accommodation immediately.
- ◆ Isolate offending pigs.

YERSINIA INFECTION

This bacterium of which two species occur in the pig, *Y. pseudotuberculosis* and *Y. enterocolitica,* is found in the intestine. It normally causes little or no disease but it has been associated, with outbreaks of diarrhoea in weaned pigs. *Y. enterocolitica* causes inflammation of the small and large intestines and *Y. pseudotuberculosis* causes small tiny abscesses throughout the carcase. The main significance of the organism relates to cross reactions that occur in agglutination tests for brucellosis. Pigs that are carrying the organism are likely to react positively. If this is the case it is necessary to determine the point in the rearing system when exposure takes place and break the cycle by management control. There is no treatment.

Medicines and Other Drugs for use in weaned and finishing pigs

Common generic medicines that are used in weaned and finishing pigs are shown in Fig.9-41. Because trade names for these medicines can vary from one country to another the right hand column can be used to categorise these for comparison of price and availability.

CHAPTER 9 - Managing and Treating Disease in the Weaner, Grower and Finishing Periods

ANTIBIOTICS AND OTHER DRUGS FOR USE IN WEANED AND FINISHING PIGS
* A Guide to Doses and Availability.

Actual Drug (Strength mg/ml)	Some Trade Names	Short Acting Injections	Long Acting Injections	Available Orally	Available In Feed g/tonne	Trade Names of Your Available Drugs
Amoxycillin (150)	Clamoxyl	1ml / 20kg	1ml / 10kg	✓	300 - 500	
Ampicillin (150)	Penbritin	1ml / 20kg				
Apramycin	Apralan			✓	100	
Baquiloprim (33) Sulpha (175)	Zaquilan	1ml / 20kg				
Ceftiofur (50)	Excenel	1ml / 25kg	1ml / 16kg			
Chlortetracycline	Aureomycin			✓	300 - 900	
Cephalexin (180)	Ceporex	1ml / 25kg				
Chloramphenicol (100)	Same	1ml / 25kg				
Cortisone (2) (anti inflammatory)	Various	1ml / 25kg				
Doramectin	Dectomax	1ml / 33kg				
Electrolytes for scour, numerous available				✓		
Erythromycin	Erythrocin			✓		
Flunixin (50) (anti toxic effects)	Finadyne	1ml / 45kg				
Framycetin (150)	Framomycin	1ml / 30kg				
Gentamycin (50)	Pangram	1ml / 10kg				
Ivermectin 1% (Parasites)	Ivomec	1m / 33kg		✓	2-6	
Lincomycin (100)	Lincocin	1ml / 10kg		✓	110-220	
Monensin	Romensin				100	
Neomycin	Neobiotic			✓	163	
Oxytetracycline (100)	Terramycin	1ml / 10kg	1ml / 10kg	✓	300-900	
Phenoxymethyl penicillin	Potencil			✓	200-300	
Phosmet 20% (mange)	Porect	Topical 1ml/10kg				
Procaine Penicillin (300)	Depocillin	1ml / 20kg				
Procaine(150) + Benzathine Penicillin (150)	Duphapen LA	1ml / 30kg	1ml / 30kg			
Penicillin(250) Streptomycin(250)	Duphapen strep	1ml / 25kg				
Phenylbutazone (200)	Phenyzene	1ml / 50kg		✓		
Spectinomycin (100)	Spectam	1ml / 5kg		✓		
Streptomycin (250)	Devomycin	1ml / 10kg				
Sulphadimidine (333) Sulphamezathine	Same	1ml / 3kg		✓	100-300	
Tiamulin (200)	Tiamutin	1ml / 20kg		✓	40-100	
Tilmicosin	Pulmotil			✓	200 - 400	
Trimethoprim (40) /sulpha (200)	Trivetrin	1ml / 16kg		✓	✓	
Tylosin (200)	Tylan	1ml / 50kg		✓	100	

* Consult your veterinarian.

(Fig.9-41)

Managing Pig Health and the Treatment of Disease

Chapter 9

10 Skin Conditions

Structure and appearance of the skin..349
How to recognise skin conditions 349
Identifying the causes of skin conditions...351
    Abscesses 352
    Anaemia..353
    Aujeszky's disease (AD) - pseudorabies (PR)...........................354
    Bursitis..354
    Cyanosis 354
    Epitheliogenesis imperfecta or defective skin...........................355
    Erythema 355
    Erysipelas 355
    Flank biting..355
    Granuloma..356
    Greasy pig disease (exudative epidermitis) 356
    Greasy skin...357
    Haematoma...357
    Haemorrhage..358
    Hyperkeratinization..358
    Insect bites..358
    Jaundice..358
    Lice..358
    Mange (sarcoptic)...359
    Necrosis of the skin 359
    Parakeratosis 361
    Photosensitisation...361
    Pityriasis rosea 361
    Porcine reproductive and respiratory syndrome - (PRRS).......361
    Preputial ulcers...362
    Pustular dermatitis 362
    Ringworm 362
    Shoulder sores..362
    Swine pox 363
    Sunburn 363
    Tail biting...363
    Thrombocytopaenic purpura - bleeding....................................363
    Ulcerative spirochaetosis (ulcerative granuloma).....................364
    Vesicular diseases..364
    Vulval oedema...365

10 Skin Conditions

Structure and Appearance of the Skin

At birth the skin and subcutaneous tissues account for up to 10% of body weight but by the time the animal has matured this has dropped to around 6%. The boar's skin over the shoulder blade is thickened by a mat of fibrous tissue. This protects the shoulder when fighting occurs.

The structure of the skin consists of three parts; an outer epidermis, which is the scaly surface of the skin, the dermis which is the main thick part and the subdermis which consists of fat and connective tissue.

The clinical appearance of the skin particularly in white breeds can be a useful guide to the health or disease state of the pig. When an examination is carried out the following should be noted.

Colour - In white skinned breeds, this may range from very pale, suggesting anaemia possibly from intestinal haemorrhage or iron deficiency, to red which may be generalised suggesting possible fever or sunburn, or localised or pimple sized suggesting insect bites or mange. Blue/black extremities (ears, feet, tail, snout) may suggest septicaemia e.g. salmonellosis, toxaemia, or circulatory failures.

Eczema - This describes dermatitis, where serum oozes to the surface giving rise to a wet lesion. It is often seen in traumatic lesions to the ears and flanks as a result of vice

Hair growth - If this is excessive it may be related to low environmental temperatures, poor nutrition, or general ill health resulting from diseases such as pneumonia, swine dysentery or mange.

Inflammation - Infection and inflammation of the superficial layers is called epidermitis and in the deeper parts, dermatitis. Epidermitis is seen typically in greasy pig disease and dermatitis is associated with bacterial infections such as staphylococci, streptococci and erysipelas. The areas of inflammation may coalesce into large patches or remain as discrete small areas or pimples.

Jaundice - The skin is a slight to moderate yellow colour but these changes are more easily observed in the mucous membranes in the eye. Jaundice may be associated with the blood parasite *Eperythrozoon suis*, leptospirosis, or where there is damage to the liver due to toxins such as aflatoxin, migrating ascarid larvae, or poisons such as warfarin.

Necrosis - When there is restriction of blood supply to an area of the skin the surface tissue dies (called necrosis) leaving a dark area. Such changes are often seen on the teats, tails and knees of piglets as a result of trauma and in skin lesions of erysipelas diamonds, where the causal organisms block the tiny blood vessels supplying small areas of the skin.

Pustules or papules - These are small areas of inflammation usually from 1-3mm in size that have red raised centres that may show evidence of pus, dead black tissue or initially appear as small vesicles (see below). They arise after infection with viruses, streptococci or staphylococci, or allergic reactions to the mange mite.

Vesicles - These are blisters containing clear fluid which are small (< 1mm) in the case of PRRS virus infection, or up to 10mm in pox virus infections. Large confluent vesicles occur around the skin horn junctions and the mouth and tongue in the vesicular diseases such as swine vesicular disease, foot-and-mouth disease, or vesicular exanthema in countries where these occur.

How to Recognise Skin Conditions

Skin diseases in the pig can be broadly divided into two groups. Those conditions or specific infections that only infect the skin and have minimal effect on the pig and those that are signs of more generalised disease.

Figure 10-1 lists the conditions that may be observed and the times when they are likely to occur, from birth through to the adult animal and indicates whether or not there is a generalised effect on the pig. Note that there are only five major diseases that have any economic significance; greasy pig disease, mange, necrosis, sunburn and the vesicular diseases.

Recognition commences by clinical observations across the herd. The following need to be considered:

- What proportion of pigs are affected?
- What age group is affected (refer to Fig.10-1).
- Is there a generalised illness associated with the condition and can this be related to a specific disease?
- Has the condition appeared suddenly or is it one that has been present in the herd for some time?
- Have you seen the condition before and can you recognise it? If not it may be advisable to consult your veterinarian or refer to the photographs.
- Do the pigs recover without treatment?

Use the progression pathway shown in Fig.10-2 together with Fig.10-3 which outlines diseases that may be responsible for the symptoms observed.

Managing Pig Health and the Treatment of Disease

SKIN CONDITIONS AND THE AGES AT WHICH THEY MAY FIRST BE SEEN

Approximate Days of Age	Sucking Pig 0 - 7	Sucking Pig 8 - 28	Growing Pig 29 - 200	Adult Pig 200 +	Generalised Effects on the Pig
Abscess	✓	✓	✓	✓	Multiple - condemnation
Anaemia	✓	✓	✓	✓	Poor growth
Aujeszky's disease	✓	✓	-	-	Illness
Bush foot	✓	✓	✓	✓	Poor growth, pain
Bursitis	-	✓	✓	✓	None
Carbon monoxide poisoning	✓	✓	✓	✓	Illness / death
Cyanosis (blueing)	✓	✓	✓	✓	Illness
Defective skin (Epitheliogenesis imperfecta)	✓	✓	-	-	None
Dermatitis/nephropathy syndrome	✓	✓	-	-	Illness
Erysipelas	-	U	✓	✓	Illness / fever
Flank biting	-	-	✓	-	None
Granuloma	-	-	✓	✓	None
Greasy pig disease *	✓	✓	✓	-	Severe to none
Haematoma	U	U	✓	✓	None
Haemorrhage	✓	✓	✓	✓	Anaemia
Hyperkeratinization	-	-	U	✓	None
Insect bites	-	✓	✓	✓	None
Jaundice	✓	✓	✓	✓	Illness
Lice	✓	✓	✓	✓	None
Mange *	-	U	✓	✓	Poor growth
Necrosis * :- Teats	✓	-	-	-	None
Mouth	✓	✓	-	-	Poor growth
Tail	✓	-	-	-	None
Ears	-	U	✓	-	None
Flanks	-	-	✓	-	None
Parakeratosis	-	-	✓	U	Poor growth
Photosensitisation	-	-	U	✓	Irritation
Pityriasis rosea	-	✓	✓	-	None
PRRS	✓	✓	✓	U	Secondary infection
Porcine stress syndrome	-	-	✓	✓	Mortality
Ringworm	-	-	U	U	None
Spirochaetosis	-	-	✓	-	None
Swine pox	-	✓	✓	✓	None
Sunburn *	-	✓	✓	✓	Irritation
Thrombocytopaenic purpura	-	✓	-	-	Mortality
Transit erythema	-	-	✓	✓	None
Trauma	✓	✓	✓	✓	Variable
Ulcer	U	U	✓	✓	Variable
Vesicular disease *	U	U	✓	✓	Poor growth

* = Economically important   U = Uncommon

(Fig.10-1)

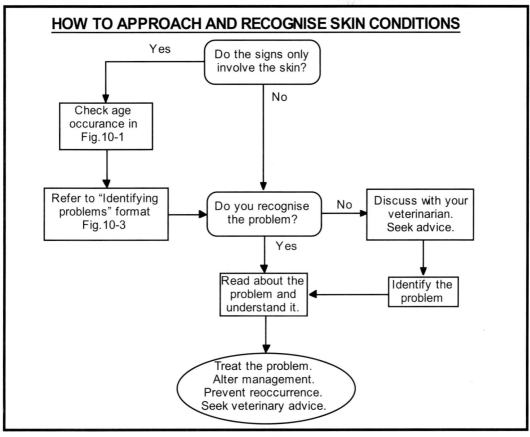

(Fig.10-2)

Identifying the Causes of Skin Conditions

If you have a problem refer to Fig.10-3 and then the index or relevant chapter. If you cannot identify the cause consult your veterinarian.

Observations and Causes

Dark greasy skin
- Greasy pig disease *
- Greasy skin
- Pityriasis rosea

Haemorrhage
- Bacterial or viral infection
- Dermatitis nephropathy syndrome
- Swine fever
- Thrombocytopaenic purpura
- Trauma *
- Warfarin poisoning

Jaundice
- Eperythrozoonosis
- Haemolytic anaemia
- Leptospirosis *
- Liver dysfunction
- Poisons - copper

Necrosis - (Black dead areas / black spots)
- Ear, tail, teat necrosis *
- Erysipelas *
- Greasy pig disease *
- Swine pox
- Vice

Open sores
- Abscesses
- Bursitis
- Flank chewing *
- Granuloma
- Shoulder sores *
- Trauma
- Vice

Reddening (Erythema) and/or blue discoloration (Cyanosis)
- Acute pneumonia
- Actinobacillus pleuropneumonia *
- Dermatitis / nephropathy syndrome
- Erysipelas
- Heart failure *
- Haemophilus parasuis
- Mastitis
- Pericarditis
- PRRS
- Porcine stress syndrome
- Purpura *
- Salmonellosis *
- Streptococcal infection
- Sunburn *
- Swine fever (Hog cholera)
- Transit erythema

Observations and Causes (Cont.)

Small red pimples
- Contact dermatitis
- Insect bites
- Mange *
- PRRS lesions
- Pustular dermatitis *
- Swine pox

Swellings (under the skin)
- Abscesses *
- Anthrax
- Back muscle necrosis
- Brucellosis (testicles)
- Bursitis *
- Fractured leg
- Haematoma *
- Mastitis
- Oedema (including bowel oedema)
- Ruptured muscles
- Tail biting *
- Tumours

Thick and roughened skin
- Callous formation *
- Chronic mange *
- Hyperkeratinization *
- Parakeratosis
- Pityriasis rosea
- Ringworm

Vesicles
- Aujeszky's disease (pseudorabies)
- Foot-and-mouth disease *
- PRRS
- Swine pox
- Swine vesicular disease *
- Vesicular exanthema

* = more likely to occur

(Fig.10-3)

ABSCESSES

Abscesses, Fig.10-4, are pockets of pus that contain dead cell material and large numbers of bacteria. The bacteria normally enter the body through damage to the skin or via the external orifices. They become walled off from the body tissues, or the bacteria are disseminated by the blood stream to develop abscesses elsewhere in the body. Near the skin surface they may become painful with an inflamed appearance.

Clinical signs

They commonly arise from fighting particularly when sows are grouped at weaning. Initially there is a break in the skin which leaves a scar followed by swellings beneath. Abscesses can also arise as secondary infection to other conditions such as swine pox, PRRS, pneumonia or tail biting and if they become widespread throughout the body, the result may be emaciation followed by death or condemnation of the carcase at slaughter.

ABSCESS ON THE NECK

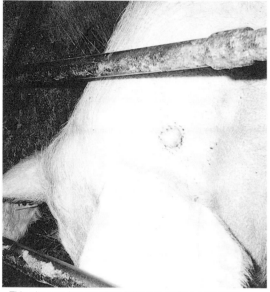

This abscess has resulted following faulty vaccination.
(Fig.10-4)

Diagnosis

This is based on the clinical signs of abnormal swellings under the skin especially with overlying scars. To confirm the diagnosis, feel and press the swelling to ascertain if the contents are fluid or solid and whether they are beneath the skin or deep seated. To examine the swelling more closely, restrain the pig by a wire noose or by heavy sedation (stresnil 1ml/10kg), and sample the contents. This is carried out using a 10ml syringe with a 18mm 16 gauge needle attached. The needle is inserted at the lowest soft point of the swelling and fluid withdrawn. If it is an abscess a white, yellow or green substance of either a watery or a cheesy consistency will appear.

Similar diseases

Haemorrhage into the tissues from a recently ruptured blood vessel or a haemorrhage of long standing is the only condition likely to be confused with an abscess. In such cases either pure blood or a very thin blood stained liquid will be withdrawn. Such pockets of blood are called haematoma and if they have been present for a long time a clot will have formed, in which case only serum or a clear liquid will be withdrawn.

Treatment

◻ This is aimed at draining the pus. Sometimes it will occur naturally after the abscess bursts but most require lancing or opening surgically. To do this make an incision approximately 15-20mm long at the lowest point particularly where it is soft and fluctuating. A sharp scalpel blade with only 15mm exposed is inserted into the abscess in a downward movement to open it up. Carry this out only when the sow is restrained. A quick controlled movement of the blade will cause little pain, far less than trying to infiltrate a local anaesthetic. The pus should be squeezed out and the interior washed using a syringe and sterile saline solution. Such a solution is made by adding 5 grams of salt to 1 litre of previously boiled water. The wound must be kept open for at least 3 or 4 days or until all the pus has drained out, otherwise the abscess may reform.

◻ See lancing an abscess or haematoma chapter 15.
◻ Most of the organisms that cause abscesses in the pig are either penicillin or oxytetracycline sensitive.
◻ If the area is badly inflamed, squeeze into the hole an antibiotic cream (a cow mastitis tube is ideal) containing penicillin/streptomycin, oxytetracycline, amoxycillin or ampicillin.
◻ Treatment should be given by intramuscular injection - if the area is inflamed or the sow is ill.
Drugs that could be used include:
- Penicillin/streptomycin daily for 3-4 days.
- Amoxycillin long-acting (LA) every other day.
- Oxytetracycline (LA) every other day.
- Penicillin (LA) every other day.

Management control and prevention

◆ Identify various projections and sharp objects in the environment. A typical example would be a neck abscess associated with worn and jagged metal on feeders. Long-acting antibiotic injections given at the time of damage will often prevent infection.
◆ Reduce fighting.
◆ Prevent tail biting. See vice chapter 9.
◆ Check injection procedures.

ANAEMIA

See chapter 8 for further information.

Anaemia arises in the sucking piglet due to iron deficiency because the sow's milk is deficient in iron and the piglet has minimal reserves. Iron forms an essential part of haemoglobin in the red blood cells and this is responsible for carrying oxygen. The piglet becomes rapidly anaemic and susceptible to other diseases such as scours, unless iron is supplied either orally or by injection. The skin is very pale particularly if there has been a severe haemorrhage both internal and external and there may also be respiratory embarrassment. Gastric ulcers with internal haemorrhages are a common cause in the growing pig. Porcine enteropathy resulting in massive loss of blood into the gut is seen in growing pigs and gilts.

AUJESZKY'S DISEASE (AD) - PSEUDORABIES (PR)
See chapter 12 for further information.

Aujeszky's disease (Fig.10-5) is not normally regarded as a cause of skin changes, but in acute outbreaks small vesicles of approximately 1mm in diameter may be seen on the skin around the nose and the mouth. Similar lesions are occasionally seen in PRRS.

AUJESZKY'S DISEASE

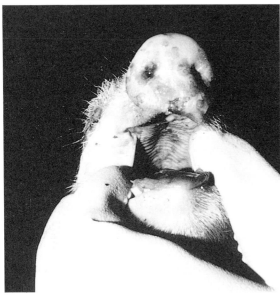

Vesicles on the nose of a 2 day old piglet
(Fig.10-5)

BURSITIS
See chapter 9 for further information.

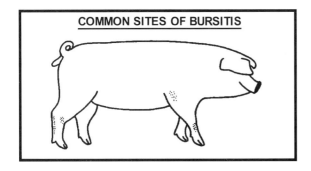

Bursitis (Fig.10-6) arises due to constant trauma of the skin particularly where it covers the bony prominences. The skin reacts, becomes thickened and small soft fluctuating swellings may be formed (false bursae).

BURSITIS

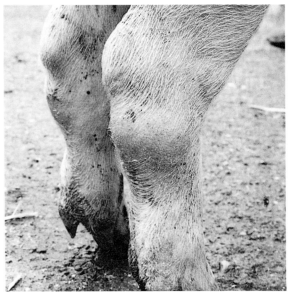

Swellings are evident on both legs below the hocks.
(Fig.10-6)

CYANOSIS

Cyanosis (Fig.10-7) is the name used to describe a blue or red discoloration of the skin which may or may not be localised to small areas, mainly the extremities. It is not a specific skin condition but a symptom of generalised disease.

CYANOSIS

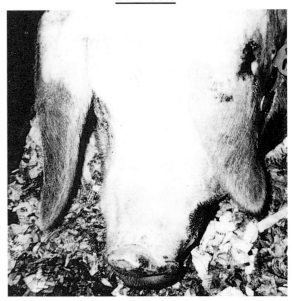

There is a clear line of demarcation on the left ear from the normal skin. This picture is typical of PRRS or blue ear disease or toxaemias.
(Fig.10-7)

The colour changes are associated either with poor circulation due to heart disease, toxic conditions, thrombosis of blood vessels or poisoning, particularly by carbon monoxide.

EPITHELIOGENESIS IMPERFECTA OR DEFECTIVE SKIN

This is a condition where the piglet is born devoid of an area of skin. (Fig.10-8). It usually occurs on the legs or flanks. Provided the area is not too large, the skin will gradually heal. If it involves an area of loose skin such as over the flank, local anaesthetic can be injected, the skin edge separated and the two edges sutured using mattress or interrupted sutures. In severe cases however the piglet should be destroyed.

EPITHELIOGENESIS IMPERFECTA

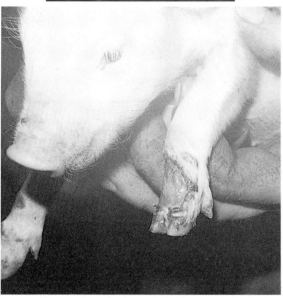

The front leg is a common site.
(Fig.10-8)

ERYTHEMA

This describes a reddening or blue discoloration of the skin, often transient, and commonly seen during transport. The pigs skin is sensitive to irritants such as urine, sawdust and disinfectants. Generalised discoloration particularly the extremities is seen in toxic conditions, bacterial septicaemias and viraemias and where there are circulatory problems. Occasionally when sows are bedded on urine soaked shavings in farrowing crates their complete body turns blue, the sow appearing quite normal. This is usually of no consequence.

ERYSIPELAS

See chapter 7 for further information.

This disease, caused by the tiny bacterium *Erysipelothrix rhusiopathiae (insidiosa)*, produces very characteristic skin lesions often described as diamond markings. The organism enters the blood stream causing a septicaemia. In the process it forms small clumps which block or thrombose tiny blood vessels supplying the skin. Affected areas appear as raised diamond shaped patches several centimetres across, scattered over the back, flanks and abdomen. Fig.10-9. They are usually pink in colour and in clean white skinned pigs are readily seen but in coloured or dirty pigs they may not be so evident. In such cases run the palm of your hand over the pig's back and sides and they can be felt as raised areas. The affected pigs may or may not be depressed and running a fever. If the thrombosis is complete and treatment is not given these areas can turn black as tissue dies and eventually slough off. The organism is very sensitive to penicillin and effective vaccines are available.

ERYSIPELAS

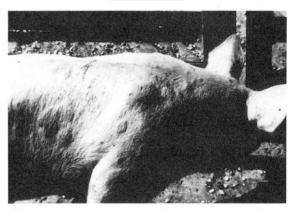

Diamond shaped skin lesions and others on the neck and flank.
(Fig.10-9)

FLANK BITING

See chapter 9; Vice for further information.

This is a relatively new condition in intensive pig producing systems but also occasionally it is seen in pigs housed in straw yards. It is often associated with ear and tail biting and usually commences as a small dark scab no more than 5-10mm in diameter. (Fig.10-10).

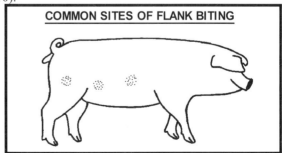

If the scab is removed a wet eczema or dermatitis is evident from which large numbers of *Staphylococcus*

hyicus can be isolated. The condition at this stage is of no consequence until the scab is removed either mechanically or by other pigs that traumatise the area. This rapidly progresses into vice and in extreme cases severe cannibalism. It is important to remove the infected pig into a hospital pen and identify the offending pigs that are responsible for the vice and isolate them too.

FLANK BITING

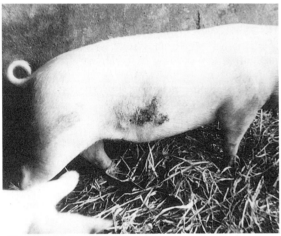

This is a developing lesion with cannibalism just commencing.
(Fig.10-10)

GRANULOMA

A granuloma (Fig.10-11) is a large mass of fibrous tissue that has been produced in response to persistent trauma and irritation to the skin and underlying tissues. Granuloma can also arise due to low grade bacterial infections. A typical example would be the large lumps seen in cases of chronic mastitis. The most common sites are over the lateral aspects of the front legs, particularly the knee, hock and elbow joints and on the hind legs over the lateral aspects of the hock and the posterior parts of the legs and feet. Occasionally the granuloma will burst to the skin surface and ulcerate. Animals showing large granuloma, particularly if they are starting to ulcerate, should be slaughtered. It is also possible to amputate large ones and you are advised to discuss this with your veterinarian.

COMMON SITES OF GRANULOMA

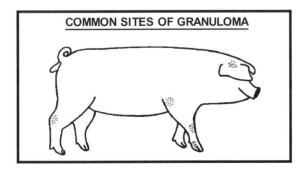

GRANULOMA

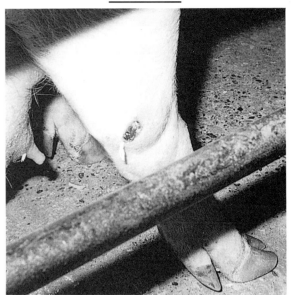

These are common on the legs. This one is starting to ulcerate.
(Fig.10-11)

GREASY PIG DISEASE (EXUDATIVE EPIDERMITIS)

See chapter 9 for further information.

Trauma and subsequent infection of the skin by the bacterium *Staphylococcus hyicus* causes a wet eczema or dermatitis. The lesions often develop to cover the whole of the piglet, the skin becomes flaky and greasy and the body turns a dark brown to black colour. (Fig.10-12).

GREASY PIG DISEASE

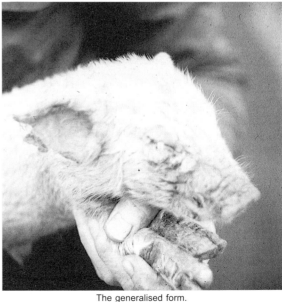

The generalised form.
(Fig.10-12)

CHAPTER 10 - Skin Conditions **357**

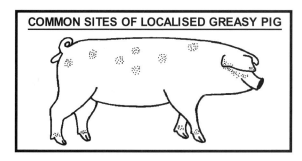

COMMON SITES OF LOCALISED GREASY PIG

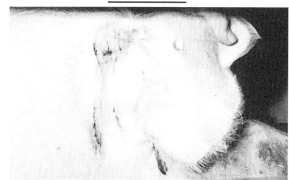

GREASY SKIN

Note the thick brown waxy deposits behind the sow's ear and beneath the eye.
(Fig.10-14)

These changes often start around the face and ears or along the abdomen. Mortality can be quite high in the generalised form due the absorption of toxins from the organism and from dehydration. A more localised form (Fig.10-13) is seen in pigs from five weeks onwards as small discrete patchy areas of wet inflammation 10-30mm in diameter, often covered over by a black scabs. The organism can also cause eczema of the tail and tips of the ears which leads to vice.

HAEMATOMA

This is a large swelling caused by haemorrhage beneath the skin into the subcutaneous tissue or muscles. (Fig.10-15). It is caused by fighting or external damage that ruptures a small blood vessel. The common sites are the ears and flanks. They can be confused with abscesses and to differentiate between them it is necessary to use a needle and syringe and sample the fluid contents. Most haematomas stop bleeding and the body defences gradually remove the serum and the blood clot. Occasionally they become infected to form an abscess, and need to be dealt with as such.

GREASY PIG DISEASE

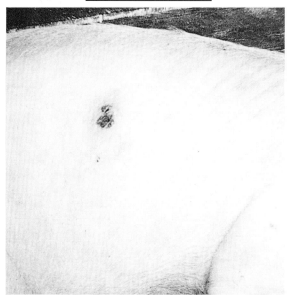

A localised lesion of greasy pig disease. This may be cannibalised.
(Fig.10-13)

GREASY SKIN

This is a condition that in the initial stages can look like greasy pig disease but is seen only in the growing pig or the sow. The skin, particularly behind the ears, eyes (Fig.10-14) between the elbow and body and the inner parts of the legs, contains a thick brown greasy material. It occasionally may involve the whole of the pig. Unlike greasy pig disease it has little if any generalised affect. It is usually of no consequence.

HAEMATOMA

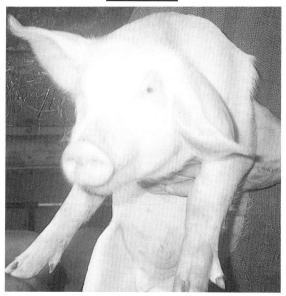

Haematoma of the ear, note the swelling.
(Fig.10-15)

Chapter 10

HAEMORRHAGE

Bleeding into the skin is not uncommon in the pig and is associated with trauma, poisons, bacterial or viral infections.

HYPERKERATINIZATION

This term describes thick layers of surface epithelial cells that become impregnated with black sebaceous material and dust from the environment. It is typically seen in confined sows, particularly over the neck and the back. (Fig.10-16). Occasionally, the condition in its extreme form will involve all the upper skin surfaces. It can be confused with mange but there is an easy and simple method of differentiation.

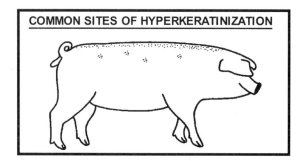

The mange mite burrows into the skin layers causing chronic inflammation and thick scabs. Hyperkeratinization on the other hand only consists of surface debris or scurf which is easily scrubbed away by the hand, leaving a clean smooth normal skin beneath. The condition is unsightly but of no consequence. It has been associated with a shortage of essential fatty acids. 4.5 litres of cod liver oil per 50 sows per week, added to the sow ration will improve the skin appearance. Alternatively essential fatty acids from other sources may be added in the diet.

HYPERKERATINIZATION

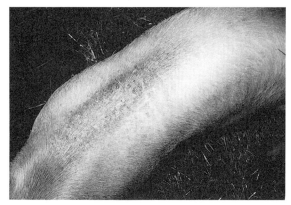

The black dead skin rubs away leaving normal healthy skin.
(Fig.10-16)

INSECT BITES

See chapter 11 (Flies) for further information.

Skin damage associated with biting insects is surprisingly common particularly in the summer months and more so where farrowing house floors are slatted. The lesions appear as small red pimples that can look very similar to the allergic form of mange but tend to be localised behind the shoulders and the flanks where biting flies gain access through slatted floors from the slurry. Sometimes it is necessary to take skin scrapings to eliminate mange particularly in herds that are monitored and believed free of the mite.

JAUNDICE

Jaundice is a yellowing of the skin and mucous membranes due to the breakdown of red cells in the blood, the accumulation of the bye-products in the liver and the production of a substance called bilirubin. The condition may be seen at any age but is usually confined to individual animals or litter mates.

In sucking pigs it is associated with a haemolytic anaemia where the piglets' red cells become sensitised by antibodies in the colostrum of the sow. (See purpura later in this chapter). Jaundice will follow the breakdown of red cells caused by the blood borne parasite *Eperythrozoon suis* and be seen in sucking and weaned pigs and occasionally in the sow. Jaundice can also occur in individual pigs under about three months of age, when the blood is infected with bacterium, *Leptospira icterohaemorrhagiae*, derived from rats' urine.

It produces a toxin that breaks down red blood cells. Jaundice can also be caused by direct damage to the liver by fungal toxins such as aflatoxin or fumonisin which may be present in feed components such as peanuts or corn. It can also be caused by coal tar toxicity from eating fragments of clay pigeons, builder's tar or by ingesting high levels of copper in feed, or by vitamin E and selenium deficiency.

In all of these there are usually other severe clinical signs such as loss of appetite, depression, and respiratory distress. It can also occur (rarely) from heavy ascarid worm infestations blocking the tube from the gall bladder to the intestine.

LICE

See chapter 11 for further information.

These insects are visible by the naked eye. Fig.10-17. They are approximately 3mm long and are commonly found behind the ears and elbows. They also congregate between the legs. They suck blood and can be responsible for anaemia and the transmission of blood borne infections.

LICE

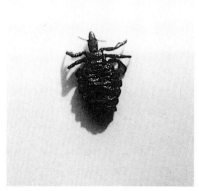

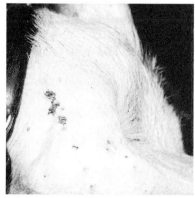

These are easily seen by the eye and are often grouped together behind the ears.
(Fig.10-17)

MANGE (SARCOPTIC)
See chapter 11 for further information.

This is caused by the tiny mite *Sarcoptes scabei* which invades the skin and causes dermatitis, proliferation of the surface cells and asbestos like lesions in chronic cases. (Fig.10-18a).

THE SITES OF CHRONIC MANGE

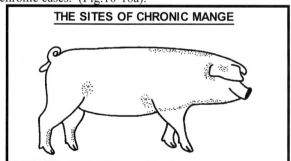

These crusts are found within the ear, behind the ears, behind the elbow and on the anterior surface of the hind legs. An allergic skin form of the disease is common when the body is sensitised to the proteins of the mite. This is shown by the appearance of very tiny red pimples throughout the body but particularly over the flanks (Fig.10-18b) that eventually turn black. Intense irritation occurs.

MANGE

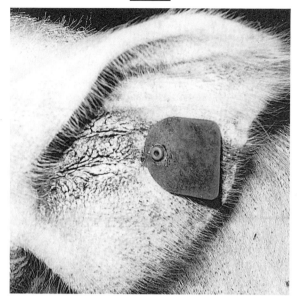

Chronic mange. Note the thick crust in the ears.
(Fig.10-18a)

MANGE

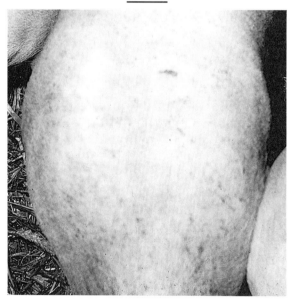

Acute mange. The skin is covered by minute red pimples.
(Fig.10-18b)

NECROSIS OF THE SKIN

Necrosis means that the cells and surrounding tissues have died. (Fig.10-19) It arises in one of three ways, from pressure on the skin from the environment, trauma causing necrosis of the teats, knees and the tail, or as a sequel to infectious diseases. It is common in the sucking pig.

360 Managing Pig Health and the Treatment of Disease

KNEE NECROSIS

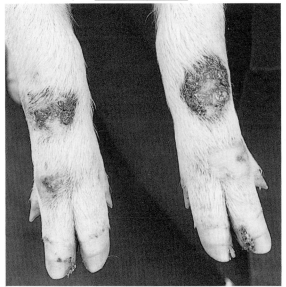

This can cause severe pain and lameness.
(Fig.10-19a)

TEAT NECROSIS

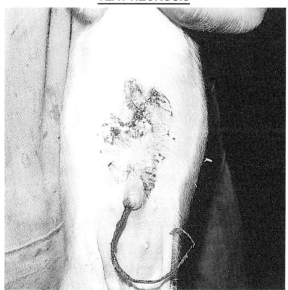

The anterior teats protected by cow gum.
(Fig.10-19c)

TEAT NECROSIS

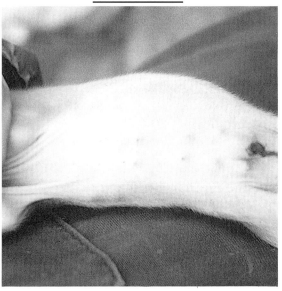

Note the small black damaged teat ends.
(Fig.10-19b)

EAR NECROSIS

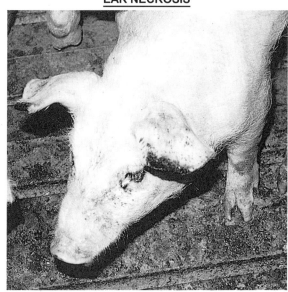

This can be so severe that most of the ear is lost.
(Fig.10-19d)

COMMON SITES OF NECROSIS OF THE SKIN

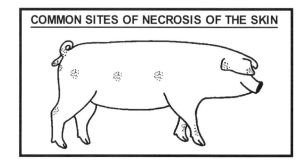

Chapter 10

PARAKERATOSIS

This is seen in pigs from 5-16 weeks of age associated with a deficiency of zinc and/or an excess of calcium which suppresses the availability of zinc in the diet. Up to 50% of pigs may be affected. The major signs are limited to the skin where gross thickening and roughening occurs over the complete body. It may start initially with small light brown spots or papules on the legs and abdomen and in young pigs it can look like greasy pig disease. Treatment and control involve analysing the levels of calcium in the diet (normal 0.6 and 0.7%). Zinc oxide or sulphate can be added to the ration at a level of 50ppm to prevent the disease. The condition is now uncommon.

PHOTOSENSITISATION

This occurs in outdoor pigs that have been in contact with substances that make the skin sensitive to ultra violet radiation. These include alfalfa, clover, rape, lucerne and a fungus that grows at the base of grass in dry weather, pythomyces charterum. Certain drugs, in particular tetracyclines and sulphonamides can also have a similar affect following prolonged use. The disease is characterised by a reddening or erythema over the white areas that are exposed to sunlight. The affected surfaces are damaged and become coagulated with serum followed by secondary bacterial infection and eventually a thick crust is formed. These changes cause a considerable amount of pain and affected animals should be moved indoors and if necessary given broad spectrum long-acting antibiotic treatment by injections. Amoxycillin could be used. Animals may abort or absorb the embryos.

PITYRIASIS ROSEA

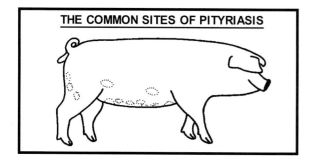

THE COMMON SITES OF PITYRIASIS

This is a sporadic condition seen in young pigs from 3 to 16 weeks of age. It is characterised by large coalescing ringworm like lesions that often start on the abdomen and spread up behind the back legs and ultimately in severe cases involve the whole of the body. (Fig.10-20). It is believed to have a hereditary background particular in the Landrace breed. The lesions are characteristic and the condition naturally resolves itself over 6 to 8 weeks. No treatment is required. It is of no consequence apart from being unsightly but may cause customer reactions if you are selling 25kg weaners to finishers.

PITYRIASIS ROSEA

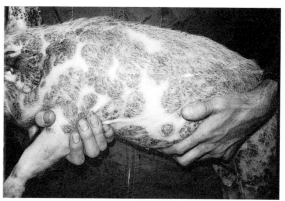

Note the raised ringworm like lesions.
(Fig.10-20)

PORCINE REPRODUCTIVE AND RESPIRATORY SYNDROME - (PRRS)

See chapter 6 for further information.

Occasionally skin lesions are seen in PRRS that are characterised by small discrete vesicles anywhere on the body but particularly around the nose and the shoulders at points of pressure. The vesicles rupture, become infected and dark coloured and ultimately heal over a three week period.

It is not uncommon where PRRS virus is active in growing pigs to see a generalised form in 1-2% of pigs. (Fig.10-21). The lesions look similar to localised greasy pig disease but close examination will show tiny vesicles covered with black scabs 1-10mm in diameter.

SKIN LESIONS ASSOCIATED WITH PRRS

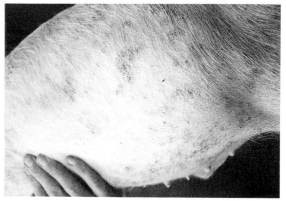

Note the tiny black lesions and the larger ones beneath the hair.
(Fig.10-21)

PREPUTIAL ULCERS

These occur as areas of wet eczema around the skin on the end of the prepuce.

Clinical signs

The ventral part of the prepuce near the opening is swollen, oedematous, red and painful. It is only shown in outdoor boars and is sporadic. The lesions are usually quite obvious and may become extensive.

Diagnosis

The cause of this condition is unknown but the possibility of a virus infection cannot be ruled out. Frost bite may be another cause. Secondary bacterial infection develops.

Treatment

- ☐ Isolate the boar until the lesions have healed.
- ☐ Apply an antiseptic antihistamine cream.
- ☐ Spray with antibiotic.
- ☐ If the prepuce is badly infected inject the pig with long-acting amoxycillin.
- ☐ Consider culling affected animals.

PUSTULAR DERMATITIS

This disease is seen in young growing pigs and occasionally in adults. The skin becomes infected with staphylococci or streptococci bacteria and small circular raised red areas appear. These are similar to acne in the human. In some cases the condition can affect large areas of skin. It is usually confined to individual animals and recovery takes place over two to three weeks. Antibiotic injections will help and lincomycin, amoxycillin or tetracyclines could be used. It can be confused with mange, localised greasy pig disease and pig pox.

RINGWORM

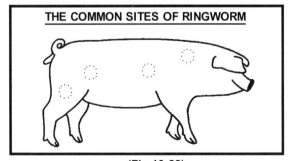

THE COMMON SITES OF RINGWORM

(Fig.10-22)

This is an uncommon condition in the pig but where it does exist it is of little economic significance. However it is a condition that can be transmitted to the human. It is caused by a dematophyte fungus. Unlike other animals there is no specific host-adapted species. Trichophyton and Microsporum species are involved. Infected skin shows gradually increasing circular areas of light to dark brown discoloration behind the ears and on the back and flanks. (Fig.10-22).

Infection can occur in all classes of stock. The fungi enter the skin through abrasions and diagnosis is made by examining scrapings from suspicious areas under the microscope to look for fungal spores. Treatment consists of washing the area with 1% savlon or hexetadene skin disinfectants or fungicides. In cases where infection is widespread, which would be rare, the pig can be treated orally with griseofulvin antibiotic at a level of 10mg/kg for a period of 7 days.

SHOULDER SORES

(Fig.10-23). They arise due to constant trauma over the bony prominences on the shoulder blade. Ultimately the skin breaks, there is an erosion and a large sore develops. It is associated with totally slatted flooring and individual sows that have a prominent spine to the shoulder blade. It is first noticed in the farrowing crates where the floors are slippery and the sow has difficulty in rising, thus constantly bruising her shoulder. Such sows should not be kept for future breeding.

SHOULDER SORES

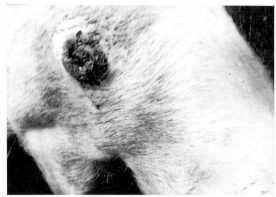

This has become a large ulcerating granuloma.
(Fig.10-23)

Clinical signs

At the highest point on the spine of the scapula or shoulder blade a reddening of the skin first appears, which gradually forms into an ulcer. In severe cases the lesion may extend to 40-70mm in diameter with the development of extensive granulation tissue. Often both sides of the shoulder are affected.

Treatment

- ☐ As soon as the condition appears move the sow into a well bedded pen. Feed ad lib for 2 to 4 weeks.

- Cut a hole slightly larger than the sore in a 70mm square piece of foam or thick carpet and place over the shoulder sore. Hold it in place with contact adhesive such as evostik. This pad will then protect the sore and allow it to heal.
- Large granuloma that sometimes develop can be surgically removed.
- Watch for cannibalism by sucking pigs. If this occurs wean the sow.

SWINE POX

This is a disease caused by the swine pox virus which can survive outside the pig for long periods of time and is resistant to environmental changes. It is a vesicular disease characterised by small circular red areas 10-20mm in diameter that commence with a vesicle containing straw-coloured fluid in the centre. After two to three days the vesicle ruptures and a scab is formed which gradually turns black. The lesions may be seen on any part of the body but are common along the flanks, abdomens and occasionally the ears. There is no treatment and the condition usually resolves itself spontaneously over a three week period.

It can be spread by lice or mange mites. It can be confused with localised greasy pig disease, pustular dermatitis and the allergic form of mange.

SUNBURN

This is common in the white non pigmented breeds, some of which can be highly susceptible to ultra violet radiation. The symptoms are similar to those in the human with rapid reddening of the skin and considerable pain.

In severe cases oedema and oozing of serum may take place with secondary bacterial infection. One major problem with sunburn in outdoor or exposed weaned sows is their refusal to stand for the boar at mating.

Ultra violet radiation can also cause embryo absorption and abortions in pure white breeds. Outdoor pigs can be protected by shades and access to good wallows throughout the year. Ensure that the breeds used have pigmented skins.

TAIL BITING

See chapter 9; Vice for further information.

Trauma to the tail and the skin is common under all conditions of management both indoors and outdoors. It is more common however in intensive conditions particularly where pigs are housed on slatted floors or solid ones without bedding.

Fig.10-24 shows a typical case, probably 2-3 days old, with considerable infection around the stump. Infection may progress into the spine or be disseminated throughout the pig causing multiple abscesses.

TAIL BITING

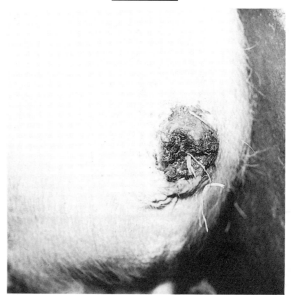

Note the swelling and infection around the tail.
(Fig.10-24)

THROMBOCYTOPAENIC PURPURA - BLEEDING

This is an uncommon condition seen only in young piglets from approximately 7 to 21 days of age. It arises when the sows colostrum contains antibodies that destroy the piglets blood platelets (thrombocytes). The immune system of the sow during the period of pregnancy recognises the platelets as foreign protein and produces antibodies against them. The formation of these antibodies is also related to the boar that is used. Disease commences 7 to 10 days after the intake of colostrum.

Clinical signs

These can be sudden and are indicated by good pigs found dead. Look closely at the skin of these and you will see haemorrhages wherever there has been bruising, teeth marks or trauma. Haemorrhages are evident throughout all body tissues (Fig. 10-25). The piglet dies through the failure of normal blood clotting mechanisms. The disease is very sporadic but up to half the litter may be affected. Invariably the pigs die.

Treatment

There is no known treatment other than good nursing. In the early stages of the disease it is worthwhile cross-fostering litters to remove exposure to any lingering antibodies in the sows milk.

Management control and prevention

- Where a sow has produced such a litter make sure she is mated with a different boar at the next pregnancy or cull her.

THROMBOCYTOPAENIC PURPURA

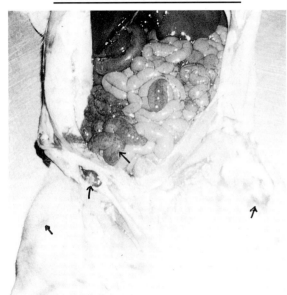

Note the haemorrhages throughout the carcase, skin and lymph nodes.
(Fig.10-25)

ULCERATIVE SPIROCHAETOSIS (ULCERATIVE GRANULOMA)

This is caused by a spirochete bacterium called *Borrelia suis*, together with secondary infections with other bacteria including streptococci and staphylococci. The disease is seen in pigs from three to ten weeks of age and skin damage is first necessary to allow the organism to enter. It causes considerable irritation in the tissues, severe inflammation and the development of fibrous tissue. Diagnosis requires laboratory examination and isolation of the organism. Control involves improving hygiene, reducing trauma and identifying the areas within the management system where infection first starts and making changes to these. Infected pigs can be treated with either penicillin, tiamulin or lincomycin. It is not a common disease.

VESICULAR DISEASES
See chapter 12 for further information.

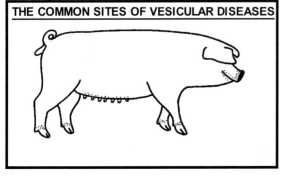

THE COMMON SITES OF VESICULAR DISEASES

These include foot-and-mouth disease, vesicular stomatitis, vesicular exanthema and swine vesicular disease. All these viral infections produce blisters or vesicles around the snout, the tongue, on the teats and at the hoof skin junctions or coronary bands. (Fig.10-26a-c). In most countries they are notifiable and if suspected must be reported to the authorities.

VESICULAR DISEASES

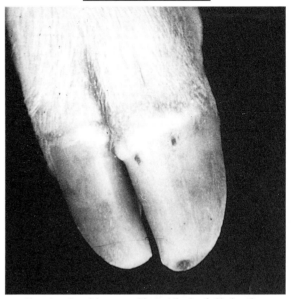

Unruptured vesicles are evident at the hoof skin junction.
(Fig.10-26a)

VESICULAR DISEASES

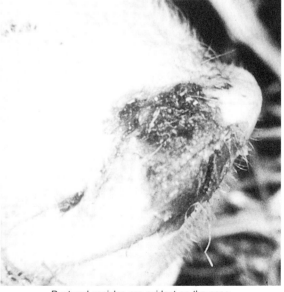

Ruptured vesicles are evident on the nose.
(Fig.10-26b)

VESICULAR DISEASES

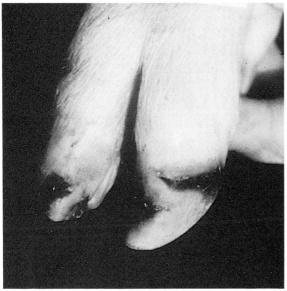

The dark areas on the hoof are due to long standing lesions of SVD.
(Fig.10-26c)

VULVAL OEDEMA

See chapter 8: Udder oedema for further information.

Fluid accumulating in the vulva at or near farrowing is a common occurrence and in mild cases is a normal physiological process and of no consequence. Fig.10-27 shows an extreme case extending into the udder, where it can interfere with milk let down and production.

VULVAL OEDEMA

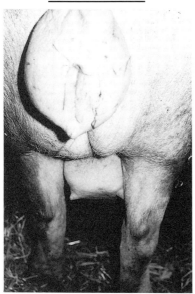

The fluid extends from the vulva between the legs and into the udder.
(Fig.10-27)

Chapter 10

11 Parasites

Internal parasites 369
    The direct life cycle 370
    The indirect life cycle 370
Recognising a worm problem 370
Management control and prevention 371
Treatment programmes for internal parasites 373
Round worms (nematodes) 373
    Kidney worms *(Stephanurus dentatus)* 373
    Large white worms or ascarids *(Ascaris suum)* 375
    Lungworms *(Metastrongylus apri)* 376
    Muscle worms *(Trichinella spiralis)* 376
    Nodular worms *(Oesophagostomum dentatum)* 376
    Red stomach worms *(Hyostrongylus rubidus)* 377
    Stomach hair worm *(Trichostrongylus axei)* 377
    Thick stomach worm *(Ascarops strongylina and Physocephalus sesalatus)* 377
    Thorny-headed worm *(Macracanthorhynchus hirudinaceus)* ... 377
    Thread worm *(Strongyloides ransomi)* 378
    Whipworm *(Trichuris suis)* 378
Tapeworms 378
    Pork bladder worm *(Cysticercus cellulosae)* 378
    Human tapeworm *(Taenia solium)* 378
Protozoan diseases 379
    Balantidium coli 379
    Coccidiosis (coccidia) 379
    Cryptosporidiosis *Cryptosporidium parvum)* 380
    Toxoplasmosis (toxoplasma) 381
Bacteria 381
    Eperythrozoonosis (Epe) 381
External parasites 382
    Flies 383
    Lice 385
    Mange - dermodectic (follicle mites) 385
    Mange (sarcoptic) 385
    Ticks 388

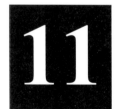

11 Parasites

A parasite is an organism that at some stage must live on or within its host to survive. The relationship is usually a disadvantage for the host but occasionally it may be beneficial in which case it is called a symbiotic relationship (symbiosis).

In its broadest sense this definition would include bacteria and viruses but the term "Parasites" as used commonly in veterinary medicine excludes these. Technically, the parasites dealt with in this chapter are all part of the animal kingdom and the cells of their bodies have true distinct nuclei whereas bacteria are members of the plant kingdom and their cells lack a true distinct nuclei. Viruses are defined differently.

Parasites in the pig are classified into two groups, internal (endoparasites) which live inside the body and external (ectoparasites) which live on or in the skin. They are generally host specific but there are exceptions.

Internal Parasites

These must all use nutrients from the host to multiply and survive. They are found in the digestive

INTERNAL PARASITES OF THE PIG	
Common Name	Scientific Name
Round Worms	**Nematodes**
Kidney worms	Stephanurus dentatus
Large white worms/ascarids	Ascaris suum
Lungworms	Metastrongylus apri
Muscle worms	Trichinella spiralis
Nodular worms	Oesophagostomum
Red stomach worms	Hyostrongylus rubidus
Stomach hair worms	Trichostrongylus axei
Thick stomach worms (2)	Ascarops strongylina and Physocephalus sexalatus
Thorny-headed worms	Macracanthorhynchus hirudinaceus
Threadworms	Strongyloides ransomi
Whipworms	Trichuris suis
Tapeworms	**Cestodes**
Pork bladder worms (Human tapeworms)	Cysticercus cellulosae (Taenia solium)
Protozoa	
Balantidium coli	Balantidium coli
Coccidia	Isospora, Eimeria species
Cryptosporidia	Cryptosporidia
Toxoplasma	Toxoplasma gondii
Bacteria	
"Epe"	Eperythrozoon suis

(Fig.11-1)

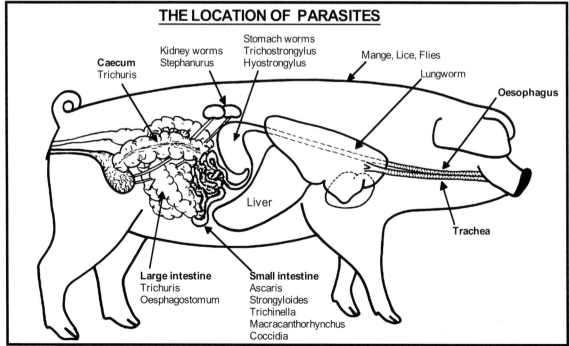

The sites where the different parasites are found

(Fig.11-2)

tract, the kidneys, liver, lungs or the blood stream. There are four groups; nematodes (roundworms), thorny-headed worms, tapeworms and protozoa. (Fig.11-1).

The location of the different worms are shown in Fig.11-2)

Controlling parasites requires an understanding of their life cycle. Procedures can then be adopted that together with anthelmintics, break this cycle and thus prevent re-infection. There are two types of life cycle, a direct one and an indirect one.

The Direct Life Cycle

This is depicted in Fig.11-3. The adult worm lays its eggs in the intestine and they are passed out in the faeces onto the ground. The eggs then develop through larval stages, but only the last stage can infect a pig and develop into an adult worm. Some larvae(ascarids and lungworm) enter the digestive tract and migrate through the liver to the lungs before they complete their cycle.

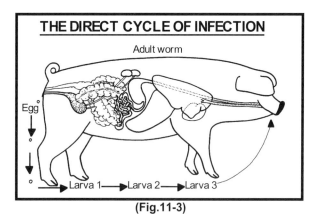
(Fig.11-3)

The Indirect Life Cycle

This requires an intermediate host as shown in Fig.11-4. It commences as a direct cycle with the eggs leaving the pig with the first stage larvae developing. The egg containing the larva is eaten by a second host such as an earth worm or a beetle, where it undergoes a further two larval stages before finally becoming infective to the pig. The pig then eats the intermediate host and thus the cycle of reinfection is completed. An indirect cycle always requires another host for development before the larva can infect the pig. Removing or preventing access to the host breaks the cycle of infection.

The length of each cycle is dependent on the temperature and humidity of the environment. Eggs and larvae do not develop in cold conditions and most die in very dry conditions. This survival time outside the pig is important in controlling continuing infections. It also takes a number of days for the larva to develop inside the egg to the infectious stage. If faeces are removed from the environment before this development has been completed then the cycle is broken. The period of time taken for the larva inside the pig to mature to an egg laying adult is called the prepatent period. Fig.11-5 shows the prepatent periods and also the time of survival of the eggs and larvae in the environment.

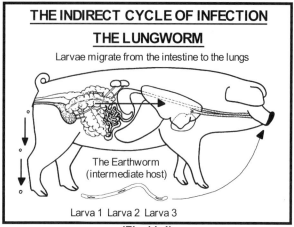
(Fig.11-4)

Recognising a Worm Problem

This is carried out by collecting faeces samples from different ages of pigs and examining them for the presence of worm eggs. 25g samples should be taken from the following animals:- 5 lean dry sows, 5 lean suckling sows, 5 separate samples from weaner faeces at 12 weeks of age and 5 separate samples from finishing pigs at 90kg. These are then submitted to a laboratory for examinations.

A 2g portion of each sample is washed through a sieve with saturated salt or zinc sulphate solution and a small amount of this liquid containing worm eggs is flooded into a glass chamber of a known size. The top of the chamber is then examined microscopically as the eggs float to the surface and the numbers of the different eggs are counted (Fig.11-6). The levels per g of faeces are then calculated.

Worms of one kind or another are almost always present in commercial pig herds. Low numbers are no problem but large numbers can cause tissue damage with malfunction of the body systems that are damaged and loss of condition. It can be difficult to assess the significance of a parasite burden but the following procedures may be adopted.

Step 1
Assess the body condition, growth rates and clinical symptoms of the group of pigs

Coughing - consider lungworm but only if the environment could give access to earth worms or beetles. Ascarid larvae as they migrate through the lungs can increase the incidence of pneumonia and coughing.

Wasting - round worms, coccidia, kidney worms or *Balantidium coli*.

Blood in the urine - kidney worms.

Blood in the faeces - coccidiosis, trichuris infection.

Anaemic pigs - stomach worms.

THE PREPATENT PERIODS OF THE COMMON INTERNAL PARASITES AND THE TIMES OF SURVIVAL OUTSIDE THE PIG				
Parasites	Development Period *	Prepatent Period	Survival Time Outside Pig	Life Cycle Type
Round Worms				
Kidney worm (*Stephanurus*)	2 - 7 days	> 9 months	1 year	Direct and indirect Earth worm
Large white worm or ascarids (*Ascaris*)	2 - 8 weeks	40 - 60 days	1 - 4 years	Direct
Lungworm (*Metastrongylus*)	1 day	21 - 28 days	1 - 2 years	Indirect. Earth worms
Muscle worm (*Trichinella*)	1 - 2 days	2 months	1 - 11 years	Indirect. Rats
Nodular worm (*Oesophagostomum*)	5 - 7 days	21 - 40 days	1 year	Direct
Red stomach worm (*Hyostrongylus*)	5 - 10 days	7 - 60 days	6 months	Direct
Stomach hair worm (*Trichostrongylus*)	5 - 7 days	3 weeks	Unknown	Direct
Thick stomach worm (*Ascarops* and *Physocephalus*)	7 - 14 days	30 - 40 days	Unknown	Indirect. Beetles
Thorny-headed worm (*Macracanthorhynchus*)	3 months	6 months	2 years	Indirect. Beetles
Threadworm (*Strongyloides*)	1 - 3 days	2 - 10 days	5 years	Direct
Whipworm (*Trichuris*)	3 - 4 weeks	35 - 45 days	6 years	Direct
Tapeworms				
Pork bladder worm (*Cysticercus*) (*Taenia*)	-	2 months - 2 years	Pig intermediate host	Indirect. People, dogs
Protozoa				
Balantidium coli	1 day	1 - 2 days	2 - 3 months	Direct
Coccidia (Isospora, Eimeria)	1 - 3 days	4 - 6 days	2 weeks - 2 months	Direct
Cryptosporidia	3 days	3 - 21 days	30 - 50 days	Direct
EPE (*Eperythrozoon*)	4 - 7 days	5 - 10 days	Unknown	Direct
Toxoplasma	1 - 2 weeks	Long. Up to 2 years	Long periods	Direct

* Period from egg to larva.

(Fig.11-5)

Step 2

Assess the type of environment and the way it could maintain parasites. Look at the ages of the pigs affected.

Step 3

Assess post-mortem and slaughter house information for evidence of parasites in the following organs:

- Liver damage / milk spot.   - ascarids
  - kidney worms
- The kidney   - kidney worms
- The stomach   - stomach worms
- The intestine   - ascarids
  - nodular worms
- The large bowel   - nodular worms
  - whipworms
  - balantidia
- Muscle   - muscle worms

Step 4

Assess the results of the faeces examinations. The egg output each day is variable and the results must be interpreted by assessing all samples, together with the types of worm eggs, their numbers (Fig.11-7) and the clinical picture. The output of eggs also varies in the sow with the stage of reproduction, with increased outputs of eggs during lactation. Never make a diagnosis on egg counts alone. Judge their significance by Steps 1, 2 and 3.

AGE OF PIG AND CLINICAL SIGNS		
Type of Animal	Common Worms	Symptoms
Sucking Piglets	Thread worms	Anaemia Bloody diarrhoea Coughing Mortality Poor growth Vomiting
Sows	Nodular worms Red stomach worms	Poor milk production Variable reproduction
Weaners Finishers	Ascarids Nodular worms Whipworms	Coughing Diarrhoea Emaciation Liver condemnation Poor daily liveweight gain Poor growth

Management Control and Prevention

"How important are worms"? This is a question often posed with the pressures and perceived necessities to routinely treat. In indoor systems where all-in all-out procedures are used, internal parasites will not build up in sufficient levels to require routine treatment.

The objective therefore is to manage the environment to prevent the pig gaining access to faeces after the larva have become infective. It can be seen from Fig.11-5 that in practical terms this is approximately 5-7 days. A routine parasite examination of faeces every six months will establish the status.

Field experiences over many years have shown that if sows are housed in stalls or tethers and they have no access to faeces, internal parasites are almost eliminated, with the exception of the ascarid or large white worm. The infective period for this larva is two to eight weeks and generally the longer period. However the egg will survive outside the pig for long periods of time. Provided good hygiene is practised on the farm and faeces and liver surfaces are monitored, it is not necessary to treat.

The danger areas for the build up of infections are the permanently populated areas such as boar, mating and gilt holding pens. Provided these are cleaned out regularly, herds can be maintained with negligible levels of parasites.

Parasite control in loose-housed sow herds is less predictable but again depends on hygiene, drainage and the regular removal of faeces. Field experiences with the foregoing provisos, also demonstrate it is not usually necessary to treat, but each herd must be assessed individually together with its history. Faeces should be examined every three months.

In finisher herds the adoption of multi-site operations or segregated systems all-in all-out have virtually negated the necessity for treatment.

In outdoor herds however parasite control is difficult. Twice yearly worming and in-between faeces examination gives good control and an insurance against the build up of infections.

Because the exposure to parasites in many commercial systems is low the corresponding immunity levels in the pig are also low. This will mean that within any given herd a number of animals will be highly susceptible and therefore the number of larvae required to produce disease is minimal.

Key Points to the Control of Roundworms

◆ Assess the husbandry system. Is there access to faeces after four days?
  - In intensive reared indoor pigs on concrete or slats treatment is unlikely to be necessary.
  - If sow stalls or tethers are used - treatment of sows is unlikely to be necessary.
  - If sows are loose-housed - how often are faeces removed?

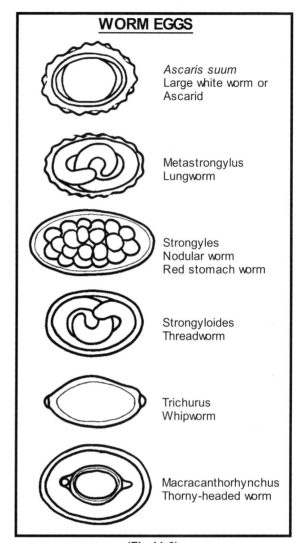

(Fig.11-6)

A GUIDE TO INTERPRETING WORM EGG COUNTS		
Worm	Eggs per Gram of Faeces	
	Low levels which are not significant (No treatment necessary)	High levels which may be significant * (If more than 50% of sample groups consider treatment)
Ascarids	< 100	> 300
Coccidia	2 - 5000	> 10,000
Kidney worms	0	any eggs
Lungworms	0	any eggs
Nodular worms	< 300	> 1000
Stomach worms	< 100	> 1000
Threadworms	< 100	> 300
Whipworms	< 100	> 300

* Treatment could be required

(Fig.11-7)

  - If sows are outdoors - worming is probably necessary.
  - If sows are housed in permanent paddocks worming is essential.

- Are there permanently populated pens on the farm? Could these create reservoirs of infection? For example - gilt pens, boar pens, or grower pens. Check faeces samples.
- Assess the history of the management system. Have parasites been a problem?
- Carry out a faecal screen every six months.
- If there is a loose-housed system with faeces remaining for two weeks or more a faeces screen should be carried out every three months. A worming programme is likely.
- If sows are outdoors use a worming programme every 4-6 months.
- Move outdoor sites regularly every one to two years.
- When pigs are weaned into arcs in the field always move to clean ground.
- Always move farrowing arcs to new ground between farrowings and burn the old bedding.
- Remember worm eggs and larva survive in warm damp wet conditions. Younger animals are more susceptible than older ones. Problems are more likely in summer than winter.
- Use farrowing, first, second and finishing accommodation on an all-in all-out basis. Wash out using a detergent between batches.
- Assess the body condition of sows.
- Examine livers regularly at the slaughter house.
- If parasites are a problem in growing pigs check the pens.
- Permanently populated grower finisher pens will help to perpetuate ascarid infections.
- When outdoor pigs are moved to fresh paddocks always worm the group of animals 14 days before hand.

All in all out systems mean no worm problems.

Treatment Programmes for Internal Parasites

- The objective of a routine programme is to maintain infection at negligible levels. It is impossible to maintain a herd completely free of all parasites because the risk of re-introduction is high and always present. The drugs used to treat parasites are called anthelmintics or parasecticides.
- Most are broad acting. Some of the common generic compounds available are shown in Fig.11-8.

Consult your veterinarian for further information and trade names.

COMMON ANTHELMINTICS		
	In-Feed	Injection
Doramectin		✓
Febantel	✓	
Fenbendazole	✓	
Flubendazole	✓	
Ivermectin	✓	✓
Levamisole		✓
Oxfendazole	✓	
Oxibendazole	✓	
Piperazine	✓	
Thiabendazole	✓	
Thiophanate	✓	

(Fig.11-8)

This list is repeated again in Fig.11-9 to show the drugs that are active against different parasites and a comparison of approximate cost ratios. If the herd is free from mange and lungworm then less costly anthelmintics can be used. The most effective time to treat outdoor sows and particularly sows remaining in permanent paddocks or yards is seven days prior to farrowing to break the cycle of infection to the piglet. However this may not be easy and the alternate is to treat the complete herd by in-feed medication every three to six months.

The following methods of treatment can be adopted:-
- Inject sows with either ivermectin or levamisole seven days prior to farrowing or two days before entering the farrowing crate.
- Mix the wormer in the feed according to the manufacturers instructions either:
  As a single dose given on one day.
  Continuously for 7 days.
  Continuously for 14 days.
- Top dress the sow or boars feed individually with the anthelmintic in pellets or use a small amount of the premix.

Alternate herd control programmes are shown in Fig.11-10.

If treatment is necessary in the herd it is likely that management control procedures are defective.
You may be spending money unnecessarily.

Round Worms (Nematodes)

KIDNEY WORMS *(STEPHANURUS DENTATUS)*

This is an important parasite commonly found in North America.

The Life cycle

The adult females form cysts in the kidney fat and pass eggs out into the urine which develop to infective larvae in 2-7 days.

SOME DRUGS AVAILABLE * TO TREAT PARASITES OF THE SKIN (ECTOPARASITES) AND INTERNAL PARASITES (ENDOPARASITES)

Active Drug	Some trade Names	Presentation / Dose Levels *	Large white worm	Eggs	Red stomach worm	Larvae	Lice	Lung worms	Mange mites	Nodular worms	Kidney worms	Thread worms	Ticks	Muscle worms	Stomach worms	Whip worms	Withdrawal period Days*	Cost comparison / spectrum of activity
Amitraz 12.4%	Taktic	Topical liquid concentrate 40ml to 10l water					✓		✓				✓				7	2.5
Amitraz 2%	Topline	Pour on to skin					✓		✓				✓				7	3.6
Doramectin	Dectomax	Injection. 1ml/33kg liveweight. (300mcg doramectin/kg liveweight)	✓		✓	✓	✓	✓	✓	✓	✓	✓	✓		✓		28	15
Febantel	Bayverm	In feed pellets	✓	✓	✓	✓		✓		✓	✓	✓				✓	35	3.6
Fenbendazole	Panacur	Pellets for top dressing. In feed for 1 day	✓	✓	✓			✓			✓	✓			✓	✓	5	1.0
Flubendazole 5%	Flubenol	Powder. Top dress or in feed for 10 days	✓	✓	✓	✓		✓		✓	✓	✓			✓	✓	7	1.6
Ivermectin 1%	Ivomec injection	1ml/33kg. (300mcg ivermectin/kg liveweight)	✓		✓	✓	✓	✓	✓	✓	✓	✓			✓	✓	28	15
Ivermectin 0.6%	Ivomec premix	Powder in feed 330g to 1kg premix/tonne	✓		✓	✓	✓	✓	✓	✓	✓	✓			✓	✓	5	10
Levamisole 7.5%	Levacide/Levadin	Injection	✓		✓					✓	✓	✓			✓	✓	28	3
Oxibendazole 2-20%	Loditac	In feed for 10 days or pellets for top dressing	✓	✓						✓		✓			✓	✓	14	3.6
Phosmet 20%	Porect	Topical liquid pour onto skin 1ml/10kg liveweight					✓		✓				✓				35	4.8
Thiophanate 22.5%	Nemafax 14	Powder in feed for 14 days	✓	✓	✓	✓						✓			✓	✓	7	2.8

* See manufacturers data sheets for further details.   Some bendazole compounds may have activity against muscle worm.

(Fig.11-9)

SUGGESTED WORMING PROGRAMMES

		Criteria	Action
1.	Indoor herd	Sows confined in stalls or tethers and the herd operates an all-in all-out system. The faecal screen is negative or low.	No treatment required. Check a faecal screen every 12 months.
2.	Indoor Sow herd	Sows loose-housed, faeces removed twice weekly. Faecal screen negative or low.	No need to treat. Monitor growing stock.
3.	Indoor Sow herd	Sows loose-housed and faeces removed periodically. The faecal screen is low.	Worm 7 days prior to entering farrowing houses. Faecal screen every 6 months.
4.	Indoor herd	Sows loose-housed, faeces removed occasionally. Faecal screen is high.	Treat sows and boars in-feed every 3-6 months. Faecal screen every 3 months.
5.	Boars	Any housing.	Treat every 3 months.
6.	Outdoor Sow herd	Carry out a faecal screen every 3 months.	Treat in-feed every 6 months. If the faecal screen is positive treat every 2 months during the summer.
7.	Feeder pigs	Milk spot livers.	Treat all the growers in the feed. Develop an all-in all-out system of pen usage. Wash pens between batches of pigs.

(Fig.11-10)

The cycle can be a direct one through the intake of infected larvae by mouth or penetration through the skin, or indirectly through infected earth worms. The larvae migrate from the intestine throughout the body over a period of 4-6 months before they finally arrive at the kidneys to mature. The cycle from egg to adult is a long one (up to a year) and the females lay very large numbers of eggs each day.

Clinical signs

Stephanurus dentatus is found only in warm wet countries because the larva dies out very quickly in cold conditions. The larvae cause severe damage, particularly in the liver, as they migrate throughout the body and they cause loss of appetite and body condition. Blood is often passed out in the urine. There is considerable wasting of muscles.

Diagnosis

This is made at post-mortem by examination of the kidneys and milk spot lesions will also be evident at slaughter. Eggs will be found in the urine.

Treatment
- See Fig.11-9.

Management control and prevention
- Prevent access to infected earth worms.
- As the worm takes so long to develop to an adult it is important to maintain a young breeding herd.
- Keep pens clean and well drained.
- See introduction.

LARGE WHITE WORMS OR ASCARIDS
(*ASCARIS SUUM*)

This is 250 to 400mm long and often seen in the faeces of sows and finishing pigs. Female worms are very prolific producing 0.5 to 1 million eggs per day and these will survive outside the pig for many years. They are resistant to drying and freezing but sunlight kills them in a few weeks. It is a common parasite found world-wide and probably the most important one economically.

The life cycle

This is direct. It takes 2-8 weeks for the larva to develop inside the egg and become infective. The eggs after ingestion hatch in the intestine, the larvae migrate through the wall and via the blood enter the liver. They then migrate through the liver to the lungs, finally reaching the trachea where they are coughed up, swallowed and returned to the small intestine to develop into adults. The cycle from egg to egg production is completed within two months.

Clinical signs

Large numbers of worms in the intestine absorb food and interfere with digestion. As the larvae migrate through the liver, liver damage (milk spot) results in condemnations at slaughter. The liver lesions heal in 5-6 weeks.

Heavy larval migration through the lungs causes coughing and pneumonia and may activate latent respiratory diseases. Both growth rate and feed efficiency may be depressed by up to 10%.

Diagnosis

This is confirmed by the presence of eggs in the faeces and evidence of liver damage (milk spot) at slaughter.

Treatment
- See Fig.11-9.

Management control and prevention
- Contaminated pens are the most common source of infection hence the adoption of all-in all-out strategies is important in control.
- See introduction.

LUNGWORMS (*METASTRONGYLUS APRI*)

This slender worm, up to 50mm in length, is found in the small bronchi (air passages) of the lungs.

The life cycle

This is indirect. The eggs are laid by the adult worm in the bronchi, they are coughed up, swallowed and passed out via the faeces. They are eaten by earth worms in which they develop through three larval stages over ten days to become infective. The cycle is completed by the pig eating the earth worm. Infection therefore only occurs where pigs have access to earth worms, for example in outdoor production. The larvae from the earth worm penetrate the intestine and migrate via the lymph nodes and blood vessels to the lungs undergoing two more larval stages in the process. The prepatent period is 3-4 weeks.

Clinical signs

These are primarily due to irritation as the larvae migrate through the lungs and the presence of the worms and their eggs in the bronchi. This produces a persistent cough and mild pneumonia. The lung damage can precipitate or enhance other respiratory diseases. Growth rates may be impaired.

Diagnosis

This is determined by the recognition of the characteristic eggs in the faeces but these are not easy to find. The worm and its eggs can be identified at post-mortem examination by cutting the posterior margins of the diaphragmatic lung lobes and extruding them by squeezing. Lungworm infection is unlikely to occur if pigs are reared on concrete.

Treatment

☐ See Fig.11-9.

Management control and prevention

- ◆ This is effected quite simply by preventing access to infected earth worms.
- ◆ If pigs are at grass then it is necessary to treat the herd and move onto clean pasture that has not had pigs on before. The larvae can survive inside the earth worm for a number of years.
- ◆ See introduction.

MUSCLE WORMS (*TRICHINELLA SPIRALIS*)

These are very tiny round worms no more than 2-4mm long. They form cysts in the muscles of the pig. When inadequately cooked pork is eaten by humans they cause disease.

The life cycle

The female worm is found in the intestine where it produces large numbers of larvae which migrate through the intestinal wall into the blood stream Some of these larvae eventually form cysts in the muscles and remain viable for many years. For the cycle to develop further the infected cyst must be eaten by another host, either people, rats or other pigs. The pig therefore can act both as an intermediate host and be involved in a direct cycle through tail and ear biting and cannibalism.

Effect on the pig

It has little effect on the pig but it is important from a public health point of view.

Effects on the human

When the larvae are eaten they migrate from the intestine and burrow into muscles particularly those of the diaphragm and jaw. In severe cases death may occur. The adult worm in the intestine can cause vomiting and diarrhoea.

Diagnosis

This is difficult but cysts containing larvae may be found in muscle at meat inspection. A blood test is also available.

Treatment

☐ There is no practical treatment for the cyst but fenbendazole has an effect.

Management control and prevention

- ◆ Control is based on ensuring that pig meat is always well cooked.
- ◆ Control of rats is important .
- ◆ Control human faeces and prevent contact with pigs.
- ◆ See introduction.

NODULAR WORMS (*OESOPHAGOSTOMUM DENTATUM*)

This species is found in the large intestine. The adult worms are 7-15mm long

The life cycle

This is direct, the egg developing to the infective larval stage in approximately one week. The larvae burrow into the wall of the large intestine where they remain for about two weeks and form nodules. They then re-enter the intestine to mature and lay eggs. The life cycle is 40-50 days and the adult worms live in the large intestine.

Clinical signs

Heavy infections cause poor growth rate. Damage to the intestine can be severe when the larvae enter and leave the mucosa. Large numbers of nodules interfere with digestion and cause enteritis and colitis with diarrhoea. Affected pigs become pot-bellied.

Diagnosis

This is by identifying the strongyle egg in the faeces and the presence of the worms at post-mortem examination.

Treatment

◻ See Fig.9-11.

Management control and prevention

◆ See introduction.

RED STOMACH WORMS (*HYOSTRONGYLUS RUBIDUS*)

This red hair like species is less than 10mm long but can just be seen by the naked eye. It is found worldwide in the stomach and is a common parasite of outdoor pigs particularly sows. It is uncommon in growing pigs.

The life cycle

This is direct. The infective larvae are taken in by the mouth and enter the stomach lining forming nodules. They take about two weeks to become adults which then return to the lumen. The complete event from egg to egg takes approximately three to four weeks. The period from egg to infective larva is from five days onwards and therefore if faeces are removed from the pigs environment more frequently than this, the cycle can be broken. Larvae are destroyed by cold and drying.

Clinical signs

The adult worms burrow into the mucous lining of the stomach where they suck blood and cause an inflammation (gastritis). Heavy infections cause anaemia, poor growth rates, loss of condition, thin sows and occasional episodes of diarrhoea.

Diagnosis

This is carried out by identifying the strongyle eggs in the faeces and/or by post-mortem examination. The eggs are similar to those of the nodular and trichostrongylus worms.

Treatment

◻ See Fig.11-9.

Management control and prevention

◆ See introduction.

STOMACH HAIR WORM (*TRICHOSTRONGYLUS AXEI*)

This is another tiny strongyle worm which as the name implies is found in the stomach. It can only just be seen by the naked eye. It is not a common worm and is considered of low significance.

The life cycle

This is direct and typical of the other strongyles. It takes 5-7 days for the larva to become infective and the prepatent period is around three weeks under ideal conditions. .

Clinical signs

On its own it would be unusual to get high enough numbers to cause problems but the worm is sometimes found in mixed infections with other worms.

Diagnosis

This is by recognising the typical strongyle egg in the faeces.

Treatment

◻ See Fig.9-11.

Management control and prevention

◆ See introduction.

THICK STOMACH WORM (*ASCAROPS STRONGYLINA AND PHYSOCEPHALUS SESALATUS*)

These worms are 10-20mm in length and are found world-wide. They are however relatively uncommon. The life cycle is indirect and involves beetles. Provided faeces are removed regularly, infection cannot occur. They must be present in large numbers to cause problems.

Treatment

◻ See Fig.9-11.

Management control and prevention

◆ See introduction.

THORNY-HEADED WORM (*MACRACANTHORHYNCHUS HIRUDINACEUS*)

These measure 100-400mm in length and are found in the intestine. The heads contain large hooks which hold the worm to the small intestinal wall and they cause nodular lesions. They are found in both temperate and tropical climates.

The life cycle

This is indirect, the larvae are eaten by the grub of the May beetle. The pig must then eat these to complete the cycle. The worms are prolific egg layers but it is an uncommon parasite.

Clinical signs

Large numbers can cause considerable damage to the small intestine and large numbers of nodules are formed.

Mild diarrhoea and loss of condition occur.

Treatment
- See Fig.9-11.

Management control and prevention
◆ See introduction.

THREAD WORM (STRONGYLOIDES RANSOMI)

These worms are very thin and hair like, 3-4mm long, and are one of the few species that can also multiply outside the host. *S. ransomi* is more important in warm climates where it is a major parasite of the sucking pig.

The life cycle

Unlike the other round worms of the intestine the threadworm larvae enter the pig by penetrating the skin or mucous membranes of the mouth and are transported by the blood to the lungs, coughed up and swallowed. They then develop to maturity in the small intestine. The infective larvae can also cross the placenta or be excreted by the colostrum and therefore infect piglets within 24 hours of birth. The prepatent period is from 3-7 days. Infection is uncommon in good dry farrowing houses.

Clinical signs

Larvae may be found in body tissues of young pigs particularly if infection has taken place via colostrum. Migration causes considerable damage and results in coughing, stiffness, pain, vomiting and bloody diarrhoea particularly from 10-14 days of age. Mortality can be high.

Diagnosis

This is carried out by recognising the eggs in fresh faeces or the presence of the worm at post-mortem examination.

Treatment
- See Fig.9-11.

Management control and prevention
◆ The eggs already contain infective larvae and infection may occur as soon as they leave the sow.
◆ Control is by good farrowing house hygiene and all-in all-out procedures to remove the free living forms.
◆ Treat the sow with broad acting anthelmintics seven days prior to farrowing before entry into the farrowing house.
◆ See introduction.

WHIPWORM (TRICHURIS SUIS)

This is about 50-80mm long and shaped like a whip. It can also affect other species including people. It is a common world-wide parasite.

The life cycle

This is direct, the eggs being passed out into the faeces where they become infective within 3-4 weeks. They can remain viable for many years outside the pig. After ingestion the larvae hatch out and penetrate the intestinal wall to develop further before moving to the large intestine and caecum where they mature into adults. In dry and hygienic environments this worm is of little significance but in poor conditions it can become a major pathogen.

Clinical signs

Large numbers can cause economic loss with depressed growth rate and feed conversion efficiency. The larvae burrow into the intestinal wall forming nodules, causing irritation, inflammation, haemorrhage and anaemia. Diarrhoea with blood and mucous occur in heavy infections.

Diagnosis

The eggs in the faeces are characteristic. *Trichuris suis* should always be considered when there is diarrhoea with blood. It is important to differentiate this from swine dysentery and colitis.

Treatment
- See Fig.9-11.

Management control and prevention
◆ See introduction.

Tapeworms

PORK BLADDER WORM (CYSTICERCUS CELLULOSAE)

HUMAN TAPEWORM (TAENIA SOLIUM)

Cysticercus is the name of the larva or cyst which forms part of the life cycle of the tapeworm *Taenia solium* found in the human. Pigs are the natural intermediate host.

The life cycle

Segments of the tapeworm in people are passed out in the faeces. They contain eggs which are eaten by the pig. The cysticercus which measures 18mm in diameter, develops in the skeletal or cardiac muscles of the pig and the cycle is completed by the human eating inadequately cooked infected pork.

Clinical signs

These are minimal but infected carcasses are condemned at meat inspection.

Diagnosis

Cysticerci are identified at meat inspection.

Treatment

☐ No highly effective compounds are available for treatment in the pig.

Management control and prevention

◆ This is achieved by preventing pig access to human faeces, by meat inspection and the burning of infected carcasses.

Protozoan Diseases

Protozoa are small single celled organisms that are found in the small and large intestine. There are four found in the pig of any significance, including coccidia, *balantidium coli*, cryptosporidia and toxoplasma. Of these, coccidia are the only one of importance and then normally only in the young pig. (Fig.11-11).

PROTOZOA AND THEIR RELATIVE IMPORTANCE				
		Infection	Disease	Signs
Balantidium coli	Piglet	Rare	Rare	None
	Weaner	Common	Common	Colitis Diarrhoea
	Grower	Common	Common	Colitis Sloppy faeces
	Adult	Common	Rare	None
Coccidia	Piglet	Common	Common	Diarrhoea
	Weaner	Common	Uncommon	Diarrhoea Poor growth
	Grower	Uncommon	Rare	Sloppy faeces
	Gilt	Common	Uncommon	Loss of weight
	Sow / Boar	Common	Rare	Loss of weight
Cryptosporidia	Piglet	Common	Uncommon	Diarrhoea
	Weaners	Uncommon	Uncommon	Diarrhoea
	Other pigs	Uncommon	Uncommon	Diarrhoea
Toxoplasma	Piglet	Common	Uncommon	Diarrhoea
	Weaners	Common	Uncommon	Diarrhoea
	Other pigs	Rare	Rare	None

(Fig.11-11)

BALANTIDIUM COLI

This single cell protozoan organism is found in the caecum and large colon as a normal inhabitant. It is debatable whether it is a primary pathogen in pigs and is more likely to be a secondary invader after bacterial or viral infections e.g. salmonella. It is thought however that if abnormal digestion takes place the parasite may multiply to large numbers, causing erosion and mild inflammation of the mucous membrane followed by colitis. Under the microscope it appears as a sphere covered with hair like structures which propel it through the liquid material in the bowel. Once outside the pig the organism rapidly forms a spherical cyst that remains infectious for long periods of time. *B. coli* uses starch from the large bowel as its source of nutrition and certain types of diet or undigested food contribute to its multiplication. The organism can also affect the human causing colitis. Soft liquid faeces, that may develop into diarrhoea, are seen in pigs from 4 to 12 weeks of age. The cycle of infection is direct.

Clinical signs

These are similar to colitis, sloppy grey faeces and in some pigs there can be considerable loss of condition.

Diagnosis

Post-mortem examinations of affected pigs should be carried out within half an hour of death. Fresh wet scrapings are taken from the lining of the large intestine and examined microscopically.

Treatment

☐ Sulphonamides and dimetridazole have a moderate effect on *B. coli*.

☐ Consider those recommended for controlling colitis.
☐ Change the components of the feed or use a different ration and assess the response.
☐ Feed meal instead of pellets.

Management control and prevention

◆ Hygiene is important in preventing a build-up of cysts in the pens.
◆ Develop all-in all-out systems.
◆ Check that other enteric diseases are not present including *E. coli* diarrhoea, salmonellosis, swine dysentery, spirochaetosis, PE and non specific colitis.
◆ Steam clean pens
◆ Use bleaches or ammonia based disinfectants to sterilise floors.

COCCIDIOSIS (COCCIDIA)

Coccidiosis is caused by small parasites called coccidia that live and multiply inside the host cells, mainly in the intestinal tract. There are three types, Eimeria, Isospora and Cryptosporidia. Disease is common and widespread in sucking piglets and occasionally in pigs up to 15 weeks of age. Diarrhoea is the main clinical sign.

The life cycle

Tiny-egg like infected structures called oocysts are passed out in the faeces into the environment where they develop (sporulate). This takes place within 12-24 hours at temperatures between 25°-35°C (77°F-95°F). Oocysts can survive outside the pig for many months and are very difficult to kill. They are resistant to most disinfectants but OO-CIDE (Antec) is effective. The oocysts are eaten and undergo three complex developments in the wall of the small intestine to complete the cycle. It is during this period that damage occurs. Sows faeces are one source of infection and it is important that they are removed daily from the farrowing house. The life cycle in the piglet takes 5-10 days and disease therefore is not seen before five days of age.

Clinical signs

Coccidiosis causes diarrhoea in piglets due to damage caused to the wall of the small intestine. This is followed by secondary bacterial infections. Dehydration is common. The faeces vary in consistency and colour from yellow to grey green, or bloody according to the severity of the condition. Secondary infection by bacteria and viruses can also result in high mortality, although mortality due to coccidiosis on its own is relatively low. Occasionally disease is seen in young boars and gilts that are housed in permanently populated pens and floor fed.

Diagnosis

Coccidiosis should be suspected if there is a diarrhoea problem in sucking pigs from 7-21 days of age that does not respond particularly well to antibiotics. Diagnosis however is not easy in some outbreaks because identifying oocysts in the faeces of infected pigs can be difficult. In other outbreaks however clear signs are evident at post-mortem examinations. The oocysts do not pass out into the faeces until approximately 3-4 days after diarrhoea is seen, by which time the pig may have recovered. Faeces samples for laboratory examination should be taken from semi-recovered pigs rather than pigs with scour.

Diagnosis is best made by submitting a live pig to the laboratory for histological examination of the intestinal wall. *Isospora suis* is the most pathogenic of the three types of coccidia.

Treatment

- For this to be effective it must be given just prior to the invasion of the intestinal wall.
  Once clinical signs have appeared the damage has been done.
- Medicate the sow feed with either amprolium premix 1kg/tonne, monensin sodium 100g/tonne or sulphadimidine 100g/tonne.
  Feed from the time the sow enters the farrowing house and throughout lactation.
- Inject each litter with a long-acting sulphonamide at six days of age.
- Medicate small amounts of milk powder with a coccidiostat such as amprolium or salinomycin and give small amounts daily to the piglets from three days of age onwards top dressed on the creep feed.
- One or two doses of toltrazuril (Baycox Bayer) at a level of 6.25mg/kg is effective in controlling disease.
  It is prepared by mixing 250ml of glycerol, 125ml water and 125ml of Baycox together. A 2ml dose may be given once at 4, 5 or 6 days of age, the exact time determined by the response, and repeated again at ten days of age. If there is no response it is unlikely that coccidiosis is the problem.
  Specifically discuss this method of treatment with your veterinarian who may prepare this for you.

Management control and prevention

- Once the oocysts have become established in an environment the sow plays only a minor role. The oocysts contaminate the environment by other means such as flies, dried faeces, dust and faeces contaminated surfaces.
  Hygiene and insect control are important.
- Remove sow and piglet faeces daily.
- Improve the hygiene in farrowing houses, in particular farrowing pen floors and prevent the movement of faeces from one pen to another.
- Ensure as far as possible that slurry channels are completely emptied between farrowings.
- Thoroughly wash and disinfect the farrowing houses with OO-CIDE (Antec) or other substances that are active against oocysts.
- If farrowing crate floor surfaces are made of concrete and pitted, brush these over with lime wash and allow it to dry before the next sow comes into farrow. See chapter 15.
- Keep pens as dry as possible and in particular those areas of the floor where the piglets defecate.
  An effective method is to cover the wet areas with shavings and remove them daily.
- If creep is fed on the floor stop creep feeding until piglets are at least 21 days old.
- Control flies. See later in this chapter
- In outdoor herds control can be difficult.
  Always move farrowing arcs to new ground between farrowings and burn bedding.
- If floor boards are used in farrowing arcs disinfect these with OO-CIDE (Antec).
- Wallows can be an ideal focus of infection particularly during lactation. Increase the amount of shade and provide sprays. Provide alternating wallows.
- Site wallows well away from the source of food.

CRYPTOSPORIDIOSIS (CRYPTOSPORIDIUM PARVUM)

This is a small single-cell organism which infects the cells at the base and top of the finger-like villi in the small intestine. The oocysts are passed out in the faeces and the cycle of infection is direct.

C. parvum can survive outside the pig for 6-10 weeks. The condition is usually unimportant unless pigs are exposed to heavy infections or they are part of a secondary infection following other primary causes of diarrhoea.

The life cycle
This is similar to *Eimeria* and *Isospora* species.

Clinical signs
These are associated with villus atrophy in piglets 7-21 days old and mild malabsorption manifest by diarrhoea. Cryptosporidia also infect humans, rats, mice and other species.

Diagnosis
Oocysts can be detected in the laboratory in stained smears of faecal scour or by histological examinations of the small intestine at post-mortem.

Treatment
- No drugs are effective against this condition and prevention therefore is important.

Management control and prevention.
- Apply the same criteria as outlined for the control of coccidiosis.

TOXOPLASMOSIS (TOXOPLASMA)
This is caused by the protozoa *Toxoplasma gondii* which affects animals and people. The life cycle is indirect. Cats are primary hosts and the only one that sheds infective oocysts in their faeces. Pigs may become infected by ingesting feed or water contaminated with cat faeces, by cannibalism of other infected dead pigs, by ear and tail biting or by eating infected rodents or other uncooked meat. Feed back of placenta is contraindicated. In the pig the organisms form cysts in muscles and other organs where they remain viable for long periods of time. These can develop then into the mature parasites when eaten. Pork therefore is a source of human infection.

Clinical signs
Clinical disease in the pig is uncommon. There are usually few signs or none at all. If infection occurs in the first 6-8 weeks of pregnancy the organism may cross the placenta and abortion may result but if it is later on piglets may die and become mummified. Occasionally increased stillbirths or premature piglets with tremor and coughing may occur. Piglets may also be born weak and lethargic. Diarrhoea may be seen.

Diagnosis
The presence of the parasite rarely results in clinical disease. In cases of abortion foetal fluids from aborted piglets can be tested for the presence of antibodies. Serology can also be carried out on blood samples from pigs.

Treatment
- Sulphonamides and trimethoprim are effective by in-feed medication but treatment is rarely indicated.

Management control and prevention
- Keep cats out of piggeries.
- Keep cats out of feed and grain stores.
- Control rodents.
- Reduce and prevent cannibalism.

Bacteria

EPERYTHROZOONOSIS (EPE)
Eperythrozoonosis is caused by a small ricketsial bacterium called *Eperythrozoon suis* (Epe) which attaches itself to the red cells in the blood, damaging them and causing them to break apart. This causes an anaemia associated with a reduction in the number of red blood cells and haemoglobin the substance by which oxygen is transported around the body. When large numbers of red cells are damaged, jaundice may result.

The disease is somewhat of an enigma because the organism can be identified both in normal animals and in those severely affected with disease. It is likely that Epe is very widespread and most sources of pigs examined (varying health status) have shown evidence of the bacteria. In the majority herds where it has been identified there have been no clinical problems and the significance therefore of the organism in relation to infection in these cases must be in doubt. However, in the past two years a positive diagnosis associated with disease has become more common. Epe can cross the placenta and be responsible for poor pale pigs at birth and high pre-weaning mortality.

Clinical signs
Epe affects all classes of pigs from sows and piglets through to weaners and growers. Clinical pictures vary, particularly if there are secondary infections involved. It is useful however, to look at the clinical symptoms in acute and chronic disease. In piglets and weaners the acute disease is manifest by primary anaemia and secondary infections, whilst the more chronic picture appears related to slow growth, variable growth rate and poor-doing pigs. The chronic symptoms in sows are associated with reproductive failure and if there is stress at farrowing, fevers and agalactia may be experienced. If pale anaemic pigs are evident during sucking or in the immediate post-weaning period and an injection of iron has been given, the possibility of Epe should be considered.

EPERYTHROZOON SUIS - CLINICAL SIGNS		
Sows	Piglets	Weaners/Growers
Abortion	Jaundiced	Anaemia
Agalactia	Increased scour	Ear necrosis
Anaemia, jaundice	Pale pigs	Enteritis
Fever	Pneumonia	Fever
Increased repeats	Weak at birth	Pneumonia
Reduced conception		Poor doers
Reproductive failure		Pot-bellied pigs
		Scour

Diagnosis

The presence of the organism does not necessarily confirm disease. The following need to be considered to clarify the relationship between Epe and disease.
- The presence of pale and anaemic pigs.
- The identification of the organism in blood smears stained with Wright's stain. Fifty microscopic fields should be examined before a negative diagnosis is arrived at.
- The clinical picture on the farm should include lowered reproductive performance.
- Jaundice, particularly in young growing pigs from 7 to 21 days of age.
- Serological tests are being developed including an ELISA but these are presently unreliable.
- Eliminate other causes of anaemia.
- Blood samples should be examined for packed cell volume (PCV) and haemoglobin levels. In normal pigs the mean PCV would be around 35% and in clinically affected pigs 24%. Haemoglobin levels would normally range from 9 to 14g per 100ml but in anaemic pigs they would be as low as 3 to 7g per 100ml.

Similar diseases

Actinobacillus pleuropneumonia.
Chronic respiratory disease complexed with PRRS and influenza.
Glässer's disease - *Haemophilus parasuis*.
Iron / copper anaemia.
Leptospirosis (*L. icterohaemorrhagiae* and *L. canicola*).
Malabsorption and chronic enteritis.
Pale piglet syndrome - haemorrhages.
Porcine enteropathy (PE, NE, PHE and PIA).

Treatment

Consider the following and discuss with your veterinarian:
- ☐ The response to treatment is not very good.
- ☐ Inject piglets with oxytetracycline at 10mg/kg daily for 4 days or use long-acting preparations, three injections each two days apart.
- ☐ In-feed medicate sows at 800g/tonne of OTC for 4 weeks and repeat again 4 weeks later.
- ☐ Arsanilic acid in-feed at 85g/tonne is reported to have an effect but in many countries there is no licensed product in food producing animals. Where it is available it is probably the drug of choice.
- ☐ The response to other drugs is poor.

Management control and prevention

Epe suis is spread by inoculation (including inoculation by insects). In a problem herd it is important to eliminate possible methods of spread including:-

Sows
- ◆ Vaccinating sows with the same needle - Wipe the needle between inoculation with cotton wool well dampened with surgical spirit and change every third sow.
- ◆ Tagging gilts - Wash the applicators between animals or hold three pairs in an antiseptic solution and rotate.
- ◆ Eliminate lice or mange mites.
- ◆ Prevent or control fighting, vulval and tail biting etc.
- ◆ Do not feed back placenta or farrowing house material.
- ◆ Control biting insects.
- ◆ Control internal parasites.
- ◆ Wear plastic arm sleeves when attending a farrowing.

Piglets
- ◆ Spread occurs during tailing, teething and iron injections.
- ◆ Control as for sows.

Weaners and growers
- ◆ Prevent fighting at weaning. Reduce mixing.
- ◆ Prevent tail biting and vice.
- ◆ Reduce mixing and use Stresnil to prevent fighting.
- ◆ Prevent spread through vaccination and inoculations between pigs.
- ◆ Control biting insects.
- ◆ Control respiratory diseases.

External Parasites

There are five groups of these (Fig.11-12): ticks, mites, lice, mosquitoes and flies. They can cause considerable skin irritation, sometimes resulting in loss of blood and poor growth.

EXTERNAL PARASITES	
Common Name	**Scientific Name**
Flies	Musca, Drosophila, Stomoxys
Follicle Mite	Demodex phylloides
Lice	Haematopinus suis
Mange Mite	Sarcoptes scabiei var. suis
Mosquitoes	Anopheles, Culex, Aedes
Ticks	Boophilus
	Amblyomma
	Ixodes

(Fig.11-12)

Some can transmit diseases. For example, the pig louse may carry swine flu viruses or swine pox. Flies can mechanically transmit bacteria and viruses from one pig to another, directly in the case of biting flies or indirectly by contaminating feed. Flies can also transmit infections from one pig farm to another if they are less than 3km (2 miles) apart. In South East Asia mosqui-

> ***Do not let the infection get out of control and cause disease.***

toes can transmit the deadly Japanese B. encephalitis virus from pigs to people. In Africa they transmit African swine fever virus from pig to pig.

Mites, lice and ticks are important (Fig.11-13) because of their effect on growth, feed efficiency and spread of disease. They are a nuisance to the pigs and pig attendants.

FLIES

As pig farms have become more intensive over the last ten years and animals have been kept in controlled environments a variety of flies, spiders, cockroaches and other insects have established themselves in these warm places. The most important of these is the house fly of which there are two types; the common house fly (*Musca domestica*) and the lesser house fly. Other flies that occasionally cause problems are the blue bottle (*Calliphora*), the stable fly (*Stomoxys calcitrans*) and the fruit fly (*Drosophila*). An understanding of the different life cycles from egg to adult is important in their control.

Life cycle

The common house fly, which is world-wide in distribution is by far the greatest problem in farrowing and weaner houses. It has a life cycle from egg to egg of 7 to 14 days. The adults lay up to 400 eggs. The fruit fly has a slightly longer life cycle, from 8-30 days and is a more prolific egg layer producing up to 900 eggs. The eggs of all species hatch into larvae which develop into pupae and finally adults. The common house fly breeds in slurry, in manure heaps and any damp moist places, particularly if food is present. The fruit fly breeds in damp feed.

Disease risks

Flies make contact with faeces, skin and discharges from all surfaces of the pig. It follows therefore, that if the number of flies in the environment reaches a high enough level they can become major transmitters of disease organisms, not only within a building, but also between buildings and sometimes between pig herds. Such infections include pathogenic strains of *E. coli*, *Serpulina hyodysenteriae* which causes swine dysentery, salmonellae, streptococci, rotavirus and TGE. In a laboratory test, a large number of flies from a farrowing house were cultured to determine the bacteria present. Bacillus bacteria, moulds, staphylococci, yeast's, streptococci and coliforms were isolated. This illustrates the potential for the dissemination of organisms. Major outbreaks of greasy pig and coccidiosis can be maintained by very high fly populations. When sows are sick with mastitis, flies are attracted to the udder and skin surfaces in great numbers and they can be responsible for enhancing severe outbreaks.

They have also been shown experimentally to trans-

EXTERNAL PARASITES: THEIR RELATIVE IMPORTANCE				
		Infection	Disease	Symptoms
Lice	Piglet	No	No	Lice visible
	Weaner	Uncommon today	Uncommon	Anaemia Irritation
	Adult	Uncommon today	Uncommon	Irritation
Sarcoptic mange	Piglet	Common	Rare	Skin lesions.
	Weaner 7-15kg	Common	Uncommon	Red papules. Thickened skin
	Grower	Common	Common	Crusts Rubbing
	Adult	Common	Common	Crusts. Rubbing Thickened skin
Ticks	Rare indoors. Can occur outdoors in certain areas.			Ticks visible

(Fig.11-13)

mit *Streptococci suis* type 2 which causes meningitis and because adult flies can live for up to four weeks and travel up to 2.4km (1.5 miles), transmission between farms becomes a possibility. They can be responsible for piglet diarrhoea persisting in farrowing houses.

If fly populations are allowed to build up, particularly in farrowing houses, they cause annoyance to pigmen and distress to sows and piglets. Fly dirt causes heavy contamination of surfaces, particularly around warm areas, lamp surfaces and lights.

Large fly populations on a pig farm can also be a nuisance to nearby communities.

Management control and prevention

- ◆ **Keep the numbers low**. This is the most important factor in the control of flies, to prevent the build-up of the population. In countries with warm summers, fly control should commence at the onset of the breeding period and be maintained throughout.
- ◆ **Break the breeding cycle**. Flies require a minimum temperature, moisture content and light in order to breed. Eggs hatch best at 35°C (90-100°F) and multiplication is reduced when the temperature is below 16°C (63°F). Moisture is a major requirement and humidity between 25-65% is ideal. It is interesting that the breeding activity is impaired when light levels are reduced.
- ◆ **Identify the breeding grounds**. This is an important part of control because if the breeding grounds can be removed, or the conditions for breeding changed, the reproductive cycle will be broken or much reduced.

Waste feed that accumulates in and around pens, particularly where there is moisture, provides an ideal environment for flies to lay eggs. Crust on top of slurry becomes a major breeding ground especially if slurry tanks are not completely emptied. Cracks and crevices in walls are an attractive area for flies to breed in, as are solid manure heaps. Farrowing houses harbour large populations that be-

come sources of infection for other houses.
- **Use all-in all-out systems** with cleaning and washing of the houses between batches of pigs.
- **Identify resting sites.** Where contact insecticides are to be used for control it is important to identify the resting sites of the flies. These are creep lids, lamp tops and walls where it is warm. For the fruit fly this can be a problem, because this species does not move around the building, but lives on roofs, walls and in cracks where there is moist feed at ground level. Residual sprays are of value.
- **Hygiene.** Having identified the breeding grounds, keep them clean by pressure washing frequently and applying a residual insecticide. Where flies have built up to large numbers it is necessary to completely empty slurry channels and remove the crust material. Bedding used in farrowing houses that contaminates slurry will exaggerate the problem and provide better breeding conditions.
Solid muck stored on the farm is a prime breeding site and should be moved well away regularly each week.
- **Creep feeding.** Creep feeds contain high levels of milk products and sugar which provide nutrition and encourage both breeding and feeding. Delay creep feeding until pigs are at least 14 days of age (they probably do not eat much anyway before that age). This will reduce breeding levels.
- **Monitoring the population.** A useful technique is to hang a white card of approximately 150x200mm in size from the roof of each house. This card should be soaked in a sugar solution and dried. Weekly, over a 48 hour period the dots of the fly faeces should be counted. This will give an indication of the build-up over a period of time and predict a population explosion so that intensive prevention and treatment routines can be carried out.

Methods of control

These include electrocution, sprays (either daily or residual), paints and baits, larvacides, fly traps and biological predators such as other flies, beetles and wasps. In-feed medication using insecticides that pass through the sow have also been reported. The main chemicals used include pyrethrins, organophosphorus compounds (OPs), lindane and BHC. Some of the products available and their uses are listed Fig.11-14. The following procedures can be used:

- **Pulse medication** - This involves use of an automatic, battery-powered spray that ejects insecticide into the environment on a periodic basis. This is carried out every 10-20 minutes and is a very good method of keeping fly populations at low levels.
- **Contact baits** - These are one of the best methods of controlling flies, because they have immediate access to the insecticide as soon as they hatch.

SOME COMMONLY USED INSECTICIDES FOR FLIES		
Chemical (Trade names)	Manufacturer	Application
Azamethipos (Alfracon OP)	Ciba-Geigy	Residual spray, bait paint, granules
Trichlorphon (OP) (Dipterex OP)	Bayer	Manure heaps
Neoprene (Neporex)	Ciba-Geigy	Larvacide
Methomyl (Muscamone)	Sanofi	Granules, paint-on baits
Golden malrin (Dichlorvon)	Ciba-Geigy	Crystals
Iodenphon (Nurvanol OP)	Ciba-Geigy	Buildings, manure heaps
Bromophon (Turbair OP)	Pan Britannica	Buildings, yard
Diazinon (Sheep dip)	Many	Slurry crusts
Deltamethrin (Spot-on)	Mallinckrodt	Sow skin
Permethrin (Stomoxyn)	Mallinckrodt	Spray, roof/walls
Fenitrothion (Durakil OP)	Antec International	Slurry, faeces heaps, residual larvacide
Pyrethrins	Many	Knockdown sprays
Cryomazine	Ciba-Geigy	Granules, liquid, larvacide

(Fig.11-14)

Such surface baits can either be sprayed on the ceiling or painted on the walls, particularly over warm areas where the flies rest. Some products contain a fly attractant. An excellent method of control is to sprinkle small crystals containing the fly attractant and the insecticide over the top of creep lids or other flat surfaces every other day. When selecting the insecticide look at the history of use on that farm and as soon as there is evidence of resistance developing change to an alternate chemical. Make sure the manufacturer's instructions are followed and in particular, that the siting of the insecticide is to best advantage.

- **Sprays** - There are many products available; but if they have to be used daily for control, the battle is lost because large numbers of flies will have built up.
- **Electrocution** - These fly traps are a promising addition to the range of controls.
- **Sheep dip** - This successfully kills maggots and small amounts can be added periodically onto slurry crusts provided there are no contraindications to the product being used as such. Waste oils will have a similar effect.
- **Larvacides** - These are substances such as neoprene which inhibit larval development and thus stop the cycle. They are sprayed or applied to the breeding grounds such as faeces heaps and slurry.
- Alternate contact baits every three days with knock down sprays.
- **Biological control** - House flies can be controlled using the predator fly, Orphyra. This fly is at-

tracted to the areas where the house fly deposits its eggs. Its larva cannibalise the house fly larva and then cannibalise themselves thus the life cycle is a limiting one. This method of control is also effective against the fruit fly. Artificially produced pupae are placed in the contaminated houses in small trays and allowed to pupate over a 10-14 day period. It takes 3-6 weeks to achieve control and the populations are maintained at a low level by periodic inputs of further pupae. The production of pupae on the farm using purpose built culture chambers and special media is the most cost effective method. For further information contact Salus QP Ltd. Predator wasps have a similar action.

LICE

These are relatively uncommon in herds today, particularly if mange treatment is carried out because this will also destroy the pig louse.

The life cycle

This is direct. The adult female lays 2-4 eggs per day over a period of 20-30 days. The eggs are attached to the hair by a cement like substance and they hatch out as nymphs 10-21 days afterwards. The cycle from adult to adult is approximately 30 days. They are blood sucking and cause a certain amount of irritation but their economic effects are probably relatively low. They are aesthetically however not acceptable and severe infestations can cause anaemia.

Diagnosis

They are easily visible on the skin.

Treatment

☐ Lice are one of the easier conditions to eliminate from the farm. It is important to treat the whole breeding herd to break the cycle from the sow to the sucking pig. The feeding herd also has to be treated if infested.
☐ Treat all the breeding herd in one operation.
☐ Use either ivermectins, diazinon, lindane or deltamethrin 1%. Deltamethrin (Coopers spot-on) has long lasting effects and is used as a pour on. Two doses given ten days apart will totally eradicate lice. All drugs are ineffective against the eggs hence the necessity to treat twice.

Management control and prevention

◆ Lice are the easiest disease to keep out of the herd. They will only enter on a pig.

MANGE - DERMODECTIC (FOLLICLE MITES)

These tiny mites *Demodex phylloides* are unimportant from a disease aspect. They live at the base of the hair follicles, around the face and on the abdomen producing small papules. Rarely do they cause clinical disease.

Treatment

The response to treatment is poor but the mite is sensitive to those drugs used for mange control.

MANGE (SARCOPTIC)

Mange is a parasitic disease of the skin caused by one of two mites either *Sarcoptes scabiei* or *Demodex phylloides*. Sarcoptic mange (sometimes called scabies) is by far the most common and important because it is irritant and uncomfortable for the pig, causing it to rub and damage the skin which becomes unsightly. It significantly depresses growth rate and feed efficiency.

The life cycle

This is direct and takes 14-15 days from adult to adult to complete. Fig.11-15.

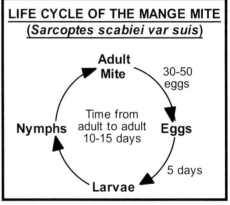

(Fig.11-15)

The mite spreads directly from pig to pig, either by close skin contact or contact with recently contaminated surfaces. The boar helps to maintain infection in the herd because he is constantly in direct skin contact with breeding females and he remains a chronic carrier. If pigs are housed in groups there is increased opportunity for spread. The mite dies out quickly away from the pig, under most farm conditions, in less than five days. This is an important factor in control. If a herd is free from mange, it is one of the easiest of diseases to keep out because it can only be introduced by carrier pigs. However, once it is introduced it tends to be come permanently endemic unless control measures are taken.

Clinical signs (See also chapter 10)

Acute disease

The common signs are ear shaking and severe rubbing of the skin against the sides of the pen. Approximately three to eight weeks after initial infection the skin becomes sensitised to the mite protein and a severe allergy may develop with very tiny red pimples covering the whole of the skin. These cause intense irritation and rubbing to the point where bleeding may occur. The incubation period to the appearance of clinical signs is approximately three weeks although it may be several months before signs are noticed in large pig populations, particularly in feeder pigs housed in pens with solid partitions.

Chronic disease

Thick asbestos-like lesions develop on the ear, along the sides of the neck, the elbows, the front parts of the hocks and along the top of the neck. (Fig.11-16).

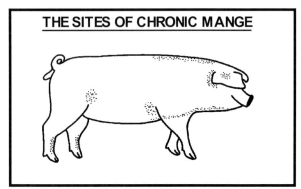
(Fig.11-16)

Diagnosis

Persistent skin irritation with small red spots on the skin developing into asbestos-like thickening suggests the presence of disease. The skins of pigs can also be examined at slaughter for evidence of the small red pimples. Herds with active disease always show a high level of grade 2 or grade 3 lesions (Fig.11-17). Average grade scores at slaughter indicate the degree of infection and its economic significances. Diagnosis is confirmed by demonstrating the presence of the mite. To do this scrapings are taken from suspicious lesions on the skin and particularly inside the ears. A teaspoon is an ideal instrument to scarify material from the interior of the ear. This material can be spread onto a piece of black paper and left for ten minutes. Mange mites which are rounded in shape and only 0.5mm in length may be just visible to the naked eye. However to positively identify the mite the scrapings should be submitted to a laboratory for microscopic examination.

Average grade score of pigs examined at slaughter
< 0.3 - Very low level, unlikely to be mange. Other factors such as fly bites can cause similar lesions.
0.5 - Disease well controlled no economic effect.
1 - 1.5 - Active disease, considerable irritation and rubbing.
2+ - Severe disease; expect losses of 0.1 in feed efficiency and 7-10 days extra to slaughter.

Similar diseases

Mange can be confused with the normal dead scurf of the skin (hyperkeratinization - see chapter 10) that is often seen over the back and the neck but this flaky material can be rubbed away leaving normal skin beneath. The mange scabs on the other hand penetrate the skin surface, are not easily removed and skin damage is evident. Other diseases that might be confused with mange include greasy pig disease, swine pox and sun burn. Occasionally in mange free herds ear scrapings may reveal mite eggs and mites but no clinical disease. Such mites are indistinguishable from porcine *Sarcoptes scabiei*. This particularly occurs in pigs bedded on old straw that has been contaminated by other animals such as rats or birds with their own host specific mites. Such mites do not survive long or cause disease in the pig.

Management control, treatment and prevention

Mange is an expensive disease not only because of its economic effects on the pig but also the costs and necessity for repeated treatment. Drugs available are shown in Fig.11-18. There are three aspects to consider:

1. Maintain a free herd

If the herd is mange free make sure purchased pigs are also free. Insist upon a veterinary declaration of the disease status. Examine incoming pigs carefully during their period of isolation. Take skin scrapings from suspicious lesions. Two injections of ivermectin, doramectin or related compounds ten days apart usually eliminates the mite but if in doubt keep the pigs out.

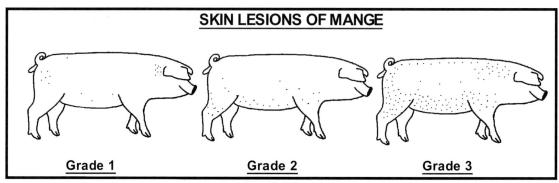
(Fig.11-17)

2. Control the parasite

This can be can be carried out either by spraying, applying a oily liquid containing phosmet 20% to the back of the pig, (the drug is absorbed through the skin) or by in-feed medication or injection. The objective of any control programme however must ultimately be to eliminate the parasite.

Control programmes - These are based on the fact that the sows and boars in the breeding herd are the permanent reservoirs of infection, the growers and finishers being constantly removed to slaughter. The aim is to prevent the suckling sow infecting her piglets thereby producing potentially mange free animals. Such grower and finisher pigs are separated from skin contact with the breeding herd.

The success of control programmes depends also on people and the following should be noted:
- Is there sufficient labour available to carry out the recommended programme?
- Is the correct equipment or methods of feeding sufficient?
- Can the correct dose levels be given?
- Carry out herd inspections to assess the level of disease particularly in sows and boars.
- Maintain the discipline of treating the sow seven days prior to farrowing. Set up a system of documentation.

Suggested programmes:
Programme A
- **Adult stock** - Examine the breeding herd for the presence of chronic lesions. Identify such animals for special treatment. These chronic lesions, found especially in the ears behind the elbow and on the legs, can be difficult to eradicate and they remain a constant source of infection.
  If they are evident in the ears dress them three times, once every 10 days with either 1ml of phosmet or spray with 1% benzyl benzoate. If they are on the skin scrub with amitraz every 10 days.
- Treat all the breeding herd (gilts, sows and boars) with phosmet 20% 1ml to 10kg weight on one day. Repeat this 10-14 days later.
- Repeat this programme every three months. Alternatively, treat sows twice yearly but give them one single dose just prior to farrowing.
- **Weaners** - Treat pigs on the day of weaning with 0.75 - 1ml of phosmet using a pump applicator or give an ivermectin injection. Alternatively either medicate the creep feed with ivermectin for 7 days or the water for the first five days of weaning. The latter is best carried out using a water tank with a water bowl attached. The total weight of weaned pigs is calculated and the required daily ivermectin dose added to sufficient water that will be consumed in 24 hours. The water in the tank is agitated three times daily. The water is freshly medicated each day. Ivermectin as a sheep drench has been used successfully for this purpose at a dose level of 12.5ml/100kg liveweight. Discuss with your veterinarian.
- Treated pigs should only be moved into **cleaned washed pens** that have been sprayed with a parasecticide such as amitraz and left empty for at least three days, preferably five to six.
- If mange is active at the onset in the growing herd medicate with ivermectin in-feed for seven days.

Programme B
- Treat all the sow herd with a single injection of ivermectin and repeat every 6 months.
- Treat sows with phosmet seven days prior to farrowing.
- Treat weaners as in A.
- Inject boars every three months.

Programme C
- **All breeding adult stock** - Medicate feed for seven days with ivermectin at a level of 100 mcg/kg liveweight.
- Repeat every six months. Round worms are also treated.
- Treat sows with phosmet seven days prior to farrowing.
- **Weaners** - Treat as in A.

Programme D
- Alternate the phosmet and ivermectin treatments on a three monthly basis.

If home bred gilts are retained for the breeding herd inject these animals twice with ivermectin ten days apart.

3. Eradicate it

If the control programmes outlined above are carried out efficiently for a period of six months it becomes possible to eradicate mange mites because there will only be a low population present in the breeding herd. At the point where there is no clinical evidence of mange in the growing pigs or sows a final eradication in the sow herd should be carried out. There are two methods:
1. Control first followed by eradication: Fig.11-19.

SOME DRUGS * USED IN THE TREATMENT OF MANGE		
Generic Substance (Trade Name)	Method of Application	Comments
Amitraz 0.1% (Taktic) (Topline)	Spray Pour on	Spray 3 times 10 days apart.
Benzyl benzoate	Liquid	Topical application to chronic lesions
Diazinon 0.05%	Spray	Spray 3 times 10 days apart
Doramectin (Dectomax)	Injection	Repeat in 14 days
Ivermectin (Ivermec)	Feed / Water / Injection	Feed for 7-10 days / Medicate for 5 days. / Repeat in 14 days
Lindane 0.06%	Spray	(60 days withdrawal) Repeat in 10-14 days
Melathion 0.5%	Spray	Repeat in 10-14 days
Phosmet 20% (Porect)	Pour on	1ml/10kg repeat in 14 days
Toxaphene 0.5%	Spray	Repeat in 10 - 14 days

* For specific uses see the relevant data sheets

(Fig.11-18)

2. Immediate whole herd eradication: Fig.11-20.

Once the programme has been completed wait at least seven months before success can be claimed. This is determined by the lack of any clinical evidence, the observations of finishing pigs at slaughter and regular scrapings of ears particularly of boars and finishing pigs.

If the eradication has failed the appearance of the allergic skin conditions can be sudden.

The economics of eradication are sound. The costs of the programmes are approximately the same as the amount of money spent on control over a 6-9 month period. The costs however are concentrated into a 4-6 week period.

Management control and prevention

- Treat regularly to prevent a build up of numbers.
- Disease is less easily spread where sows are housed in individual confinement.
- Treat boars regularly every 2-3 months. They are a constant source of infection.
- The mite will only live away from the pig for a maximum of five days.
- The mite is host specific, except that on rare occasions pig attendants develop a localised lesion, and it is easily kept out of the herd.
- Always treat animals twice 10-15 days apart.
- Leave pens empty for three days after infected pigs move out and spray the pen after washing with a mange dressing.
- Treat pigs in the hospital pens regularly.

TICKS

Ticks are found on most species of animals including humans. They are not generally host specific. They are not commonly found on pigs indoors. They differ in species and incidence from region to region so local knowledge is useful. If they do attach to pigs it is invariably to those kept outdoors. They are not usually themselves of any importance but they can spread a number of diseases, including classical swine fever and African swine fever.

The life cycle (Figs.11-21 and 22)

This is similar to the mange mite, from the egg to a larva then a nymph and finally the adult. Both the nymph and adult suck blood. Each part of the life cycle may be on one or a number of different species.

Clinical signs and diagnosis

Ticks are easily seen by the naked eye and they are often engorged with blood.

Treatment

- All the drugs used for the treatment of mange are effective.
- Spray contaminated areas in the environment if practical.

1. CONTROL FOLLOWED BY ERADICATION	
STEP 1	Only purchase breeding stock from mange free herds. Carry out a control programme for 6 months.
STEP 2	Identify chronically infected animals and cull them.
STEP 3	Examine the growing herd for mange clinically, by ear scrapings and skins at slaughter. All pigs should have been treated.
STEP 4	If Step 3 is clear proceed. If not look to the efficiency of the control programme and delay eradication.
STEP 5	Medicate the sow, boar and gilt rations with ivermectin for 10 days to give 100mcg of ivermectin per kg live wt (see manufacturers instructions). Repeat again in 14 days. Alternatively treat the herd with phosmet followed a further 14 days later with ivermectin in-feed for 10 days.
STEP 6	Make sure that the hospitalised pigs are treated. They can be a reservoir of infection.
STEP 7	Continue treatment of weaners for 4 weeks after Step 5 has been completed then remove all treatments.

(Fig.11-19)

2. IMMEDIATE WHOLE HERD ERADICATION	
This programme should only be attempted when there are few if any symptoms of disease in the herd.	
One month prior to commencement	Examine all pigs in the herd particularly sows and boars for chronic skin lesions. Cull these animals or inject with ivomec and treat topically with amitraz or other available topical dressing.
STEP 1 Day 1	Only purchase breeding stock from mange free herds. Medicate all weaners and growers 7-50kg in-feed with ivermectin using ivomec premix 330g/tonne of feed for 10 days or as per manufacturers recommendations.
STEP 2	In planning Step 1 the current recommended withdrawal period should be observed which means no slaughter pigs for the designated period.
STEP 3 Day 1	Medicate all finisher pigs 50-120kg in-feed with 400g/tonne of ivermectin premix.
STEP 4 Day 1	Medicate all sows, gilts and boars in-feed with 1.25kg of ivomec premix per tonne. Feed each animal 2.7kg of feed once per day. Feed lactating sows extra non medicated feed.
STEP 5 Day 1 to 10	Any sick animals that fail to eat during the 10 days inject with ivomec 1ml per 33kg liveweight.
STEP 6 Day 1	Inject all pigs in the sick pen with ivomec followed by in-feed medication.
STEP 7 Day 5	Spray pens sides to pig height with topical dressing.
STEP 8 Day 7	Wash and spray all boots with topical dressing. Change to new pig clothing.
STEP 9 Day 10	Stop all medication.
STEP 10 Day 20	Repeat the programme after a 10 day gap.

(Fig.11-20)

> *More mange mites*
> *- More disease*
> *- More mange mites.*

Management control and prevention

◆ Keep pigs away from the infected environments where possible.
◆ Use the same parasecticides as for mange.

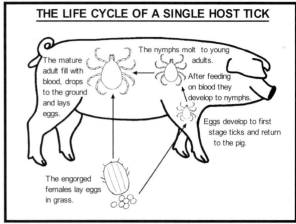
(Fig.11-21)

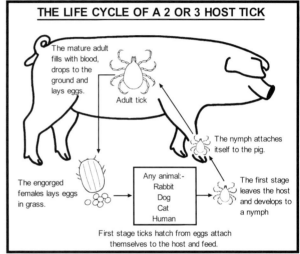
(Fig.11-22)

Chapter 11

Managing Pig Health and the Treatment of Disease

12 Exotic Diseases

Introduction 393
    What are exotic diseases? 393
    Why this chapter has been written 393
    Which countries are free from which diseases? 394
Diseases 394
    African swine fever (ASF) 394
    Aujeszky's disease (AD) - pseudorabies (PR) 396
    Blue eye disease (BE) 400
    Brucellosis 401
    Classical swine fever (CSF) - hog cholera (HC) 403
    Foot-and-mouth disease (FMD) 406
    Japanese B. Encephalitis (JBE) 408
    Leptospirosis 408
    Porcine epidemic diarrhoea (PED) 410
    Porcine respiratory coronavirus (PRCV) 411
    Swine vesicular disease (SVD) 411
    Teschen disease 412
    Transmissible gastro-enteritis (TGE) 414
    Vesicular exanthema of swine (VES) 415
    Vesicular stomatitis (VS) 415
Protecting your herd against serious infectious diseases 417
    Vaccinate 417
    Biosecurity 417

12 Exotic Diseases

Introduction

Terminology

Enzootic (= endemic) disease - This means that the disease, or at least the infection causing it, is permanently present in a population. In relation to diseases of pigs the population may be a herd or the herds in a region, a country or a continent. Strictly speaking 'endemic' should only be applied to populations of people (demos meaning people e.g. democracy) and 'enzootic' should be used for animals but in practice the two are interchangeable.

Epizootic (= epidemic) disease. - A disease which spreads, usually fairly quickly, to a large proportion of the pig population. The term 'endemic' is often used instead but strictly speaking "endemic' applies to people not animals.

Erosion - A shallow ulcer.

Exotic disease - A disease which does not occur in the region or country of your pig farm.

Pandemic disease - A disease which is widespread throughout a region or the world.

Ulcer - A localised inflamed surface or gut lesion from which the skin or surface membrane has been removed by trauma, chemicals or infection.

Vesicle - A blister containing clear or yellow-tinged liquid under the superficial layers of the skin or surface membrane of the mouth or gut.

Vesicular diseases - Viral diseases in which vesicles are a prominent feature. The vesicular diseases of pigs are foot-and-mouth disease (FMD), swine vesicular disease (SVD), vesicular exanthema of swine (VES) and vesicular stomatitis (VS)

What are Exotic Diseases?

Exotic diseases are infectious diseases that normally do not occur in the region of your pig farm either because they have never been present there or because they were eradicated and then kept out by government control measures.

A disease in your region which is under a government eradication programme is becoming an exotic disease. It will certainly be a notifiable disease. That is to say, if you suspect it you must report it to the authorities. Since the presence or absence of different diseases vary from region to region and country to country, what may be an exotic disease to some pig farmers may be enzootic (endemic) to others. For example, if you farm

> *If you farm in a free area forget the disease*
> *If not, take care. Learn to recognise it*

in the UK or Denmark, aujeszky's disease (pseudorabies) is an exotic disease because it has been eradicated, but if you farm in Ireland it is still an enzootic disease although the Irish are trying to get rid of it. Fig.12-1 should help determine the exotic diseases in your region. Beware, though, that situations change both for the better and the worse.

Why this Chapter has been Written

Free, fringe and enzootic areas

Pig producing regions of the world can be classified as free, fringe or enzootic.

"Free" describes those regions, countries or continents which are free from the causal agent of a particular disease.

"Fringe" refers to areas which are generally free but which are always under threat of re-infection from outside (for example through the importation of disease-carrying animals or animal products). Fringe areas may suffer sporadic outbreaks which then have to be controlled and stamped out. Such outbreaks may occur several times a year, or several years apart.

"Enzootic" refers to those areas that are permanently infected. The infection is endemic (enzootic) in them.

The risk of disease to your herd

If, in relation to a disease described in this chapter, you farm in a free area, it poses no risk to your herd and you need not concern yourself further about it. If, however, your farm is in a fringe area then it is of concern because there is a risk to your herd. Your herd or your neighbours' herd might be where an outbreak starts or spreads to. Since it is likely that a serious exotic disease is under government control, it is probably mandatory for you to report it if you suspect it. It follows that you should have some idea what it looks like if only to know when to seek help. If you farm in a fringe area you should also have some idea of what precautions you should take to prevent it entering your herd. You should also be aware of what the authorities are likely to do if the disease is confirmed in your herd. Finally, if a disease described in this chapter is enzootic in the region in which you farm it is not, from your viewpoint, an exotic disease but is a constant threat to the herd. You had better be aware of it and take action to keep it out.

Which countries are Free From Which Diseases?

Fig.12-1 highlights the important diseases. You can then read more about the disease situation in your country. Bear in mind though that this is thought to be the situation at the time of writing. It may have changed by the time you read this. Also, whereas the information in some countries is fairly reliable, in others it is not and in some there is very little information. The most reliable information is that in the countries listed in North and South America, the Antipodes and the EU.

Diseases

AFRICAN SWINE FEVER (ASF)

African swine fever (ASF) resembles classical swine fever (CSF) (hog cholera) so closely that laboratory tests are required to differentiate them. The clinical signs and post-mortem lesions of the two diseases are almost indistinguishable. ASF is caused by a unique virus which is distinct from that of CSF and which infects only domestic and wild pigs and a variety of soft bodied ticks. The virus is endemic in Africa south of the equator, in warthogs and bush pigs, but the infection in them produces no clinical disease. It circulates between warthogs and the soft bodied ticks which inhabit their burrows. The ticks transmit it through all stages of their life cycle and perpetuate it. It is also endemic in the domestic pigs of some African countries.

ASF virus is relatively tough and can survive in the environment and in pig carcasses for a long time. Curing and smoking pork products does not destroy it. Its main method of spread from country to country is via waste uncooked pork products fed to pigs. Mostly, the waste products have come off aeroplanes or ships but in one case at least it was waste food given to a boar by a returning tourist which resulted in twelve herds being infected and slaughtered. Its spread between herds within a country is by direct and, to a lesser extent, indirect contact between pigs. Indirect contact usually involves contamination from dead pig tissues and secretions.

Importance of ASF

- When virulent strains cross into domestic pigs they cause very serious disease. Virtually all the pigs in the infected herd become ill and the majority die. It is not surprising that all countries regard it as important. There is no vaccine for it and those European, South American and Caribbean countries which have been infected have adopted a slaughter policy to eradicate it. Mild strains of the virus also occur which cause a milder but still serious disease in domestic pig herds.
- It was carried from Africa to Portugal in 1957 and again in 1960. It spread through Portugal and into Spain. Outbreaks then appeared in France, Italy, Belgium, the Netherlands, Malta, Cuba, Brazil, Haiti and the Dominican Republic. It has been eradicated by slaughter from all of these except the Italian island of Sardinia where pigs are kept free-ranging to forage for food. There are no ticks that transmit it there and although it is a virulent strain which causes severe disease in wild boars on the island they are not a major factor in its spread. At the time of writing there are a few cases still occurring in Sardinia and by the time you read this it may have been eradicated.

Should you be concerned about ASF?

Outbreaks occur from time to time in domestic pig herds in Africa even in the large control areas in South Africa where a slaughter policy exists. Herds usually become infected by eating warthog flesh and blood or from tick infestations or from other infected domestic pigs. If your pig farm is in an infected region of Africa it is clearly at risk. To keep it out you should adopt biosecurity measures described. The central aim of your biosecurity must be to keep your herd well away from live and dead warthogs, their ticks and other domestic pigs. If the disease is still present in Sardinia and your farm is in Sardinia or to a lesser degree mainland Italy there is some risk. It spread from Sardinia to the mainland in 1983 in boar meat and could do so again. Pig farms in Sardinia could be infected from direct or indirect contact with infected pigs.

In indoor herds reasonable biosecurity should prevent contamination. If your pigs run outside the herd should be double ring fenced. Soft bodied ticks are not a risk in Italy. While the disease is still present in Sardinia, there is a small chance of it appearing in pigs in Western Europe which have been illegally given infected uncooked pork products from Sardinia. Such products would most likely be brought back by holiday-makers ignorant of the risks to domestic pigs and be fed to back-yard pigs or pet pigs. You have a duty to warn anyone you know with back-yard pigs or pet pigs against feeding any household waste

The main threat to pig herds outside Africa is the introduction of infected pork products in waste food from aeroplanes and ships arriving from the southern half of Africa. This is unlikely to occur in the EU, North America or the Antipodes because of the strict rules governing the disposal of such waste but the rules may not be so strict in some other countries. There is a small theoretical risk of seagulls carrying scraps of such waste from ships to coastal pig farms. Alert your veterinarian promptly if several of your pigs become ill with a high fever, and if he suspects ASF or CSF, (he would not be able to distinguish between them) he will have to notify the veterinary authorities who will close your herd and carry out laboratory tests. If the diagnosis of ASF is confirmed the herd will be slaughtered.

CHAPTER 12 - Exotic Diseases

DISTRIBUTION OF EXOTIC DISEASES IN DIFFERENT PIG REARING REGIONS MAY 1997

	FMD	SVD	CSF	ASF	PR	TGE	PED	JBE	PRRS	B. suis	PRCV	B. eye
N. America												
Canada	-	-	-	-	-	+	? -	-	+	-	-	-
Mexico	-	-	- +	-	- +	+	? -	-	? -	+	? -	- +
USA	-	-	-	-	- +	+	? -	-	+	+	+	-
S. America												-
Argentina	-	-	+	-	+	-	-	-	+	-	-	-
Brazil	- +	- +	- +	-	+	-	-	-	-	- +	-	-
Chile	-	-	? -	-	-	-	-	-	-	? -	-	-
Europe - EU												
Austria	-so	-	+	-	+	+	+	-	+		+	-
Benelux *	-so	-so	-so	-	+	+	+	-	+		+	-
Denmark	-so	-	-	-	-	-	-	-	+	+ so	+	-
Finland	-so	-	? -	-					+		+	
France	-so	-	-	-	- +	+	+	-	+	-so	+	-
Germany	-so	-	+	-	- +	+	+	-	+		+	-
Iberia *	-so	-	-	-	+	+	+	-	+		+	-
Ireland	-	-	-	-	+	-	-	-	+	-	-	-
Italy *	-so	so	- so	- +	+	+	+	-	+		+	-
Sweden	-	-	-	-	-	-	-	-	+		+	-
UK	-so	-	-	-	-	+	+	-	+	-	-	-
Europe - Non EU												
Bulgaria	-so		+	-	+	+		-			? +	
Byelorussia	-so		+	-	+	+					? +	
Czech / Slovakia	-so		+	-	+	+					? +	
Hungary	-so		+	-	+	+		-			? +	
Latvia	-		+	-	+	+					? +	
Lithuania	-		+	-	+	+					? +	
Poland	-so		+	-	+	+				+	? +	
Russia	- +		+	-	+	+					? +	
Ukraine	-so		+	-	+	+		-			?+	
Antipodes												
Australia	-	-	-	-	- +	-	-	-	- +	-	-	-
New Zealand	-	-	-	-	- +	-	-	-	-	-	-	-
S. E. Asia												
China	? +	+	+	-	+	+		+		+		
Japan	-	-	+	-	+	+	+	+	+	? -		-
Korea	-	-	+	-	+	? +	+	+	+	? +		-
Philippines	+	? +	+	-	+	+		+	+	+		-
Thailand	+	? +	+	-	+	+		+	+	+		-

FMD - Foot-and-mouth disease
SVD - Swine vesicular disease
CSF - Classical swine fever (Hog cholera)
ASF - African swine fever
PR - Pseudorabies (Aujeszky's disease)
TGE - Transmissible gastro-enteritis
PED - Porcine epidemic diarrhoea
JBE - Japanese B. encephalitis
PRRS - Porcine reproductive and respiratory syndrome
B. suis - *Brucella suis* which causes brucellosis
PRCV - Porcine respiratory coronavirus
B. eye - Blue eye disease

Blank square: no information   - Disease absent   + Disease present
- + Disease absent from regions but present in others.
? - Disease thought to be absent but may be present at a low level.
?+ Disease thought to be present but insufficient information.
so Sporadic outbreaks: May be several each year or one now and again or a real risk of one occurring. Countries in Europe are officially regarded as free of FMD.

* Benelux: Belgium, Netherlands, Luxembourg
* Iberia: Spain and Portugal
* Italy includes Sardinia and Corsica

(Fig.12-1)

Clinical signs

In the acute form of the disease caused by highly virulent strains, several pigs develop a high fever 40-42°C but may not show any other very noticeable signs for a couple of days. They then gradually lose their appetites and become depressed. If they are white skinned pigs their extremities (nose, ears, tail and lower legs) become cyanotic (blue-purple colour) and discrete haemorrhages appear in the skin particularly on the ears and flanks. They lie down huddled together shivering, breathing abnormally and perhaps coughing and they do not want to get up. If you make them get up they are unsteady on their legs. Within a few days they become comatosed and die. Pregnant sows abort. The disease spreads through the herd over several days or sometimes more slowly over several weeks and many pigs die. Some may die very soon after they become ill.

In Sardinia the virus has remained fairly virulent, but elsewhere less virulent strains have become evident. Some outbreaks of the disease in African countries, in which the virus is endemic in the domestic pig population, are milder, run a longer course and spread more slowly through a herd with fewer deaths. Some affected pigs become very thin and stop growing and develop signs of pneumonia, skin ulcers, and swollen joints.

Milder strains may also be introduced accidentally into pig herds in countries outside Africa in waste food from ships, aeroplanes or returning travellers. The disease may then go unrecognised for some time.

Diagnosis

Pigs that die early in an outbreak may have no very noticeable lesions but as the disease progresses the lesions then are striking. Bright red haemorrhages in the lymph nodes, kidneys, heart and linings of the body cavities are common findings. There may also be excess haemorrhagic fluid in the body cavities and gelatinous fluid in the lungs. The spleen may be enlarged, darkened and crumble on slight pressure.

The veterinarian will have to send samples to a laboratory which specialises in CSF and ASF diagnosis. The best samples to send are blood, lymph nodes, spleen and in chronic cases, serum for serology. In case it is CSF and not ASF the tonsils might also be sent. The veterinarian should consult the appropriate veterinary authorities on how best to send these.

The tonsils of the pig are very easy to find. Laying the dead pig on its back, cut away the skin and flesh under and between its lower jaw bone and also tongue. The pair of tonsils are two large red patches each about the size of the end half of your thumb or perhaps slightly bigger. Their surfaces are covered with small pits or depressions.

In South Africa and countries outside Africa it is essential to isolate and identify the virus. Only about six laboratories in the world can do this. In African countries in which the disease is endemic in the domestic pig population the veterinarian may only send serum samples for antibody detection.

Virus may be isolated in primary cultures of pig bone marrow or peripheral blood leucocytes. Infected cells haemadsorb i.e. pig red cells will adhere to them. Virus can also be detected in infected cells by fluorescent antibody tests. ELISA tests are also used to detect antibodies. In doubtful cases samples can be injected into experimental pigs.

Serum antibody titres may be tested in a number of ways. The indirect immunofluorescence (IIF) and the ELISA tests seem to be the most favoured.

> **Rapid accurate laboratory diagnosis is essential.**

Treatment

There is no treatment.

Management control and prevention

- No effective attenuated or inactivated vaccines have been developed and so none are available.
- Prevention in countries outside Africa has to be on a national basis by restrictions on incoming pigs and pork products, compulsory boiling of waste animal products under licence before feeding to pigs and the application of a slaughter policy when the disease is diagnosed.
- Prevention in Africa is based on measures to keep warthogs and materials contaminated by warthogs away from the herd.

AUJESZKY'S DISEASE (AD) - PSEUDORABIES (PR)

In Europe the name 'aujeszky's disease' (AD), after the Hungarian who helped identify the causal agent, is preferred to pseudorabies. This is to avoid confusion with rabies, a name which tends to alarm people. It is totally unrelated to rabies. Nevertheless, pseudorabies (PR) is the name most commonly used in North America and other parts of the world.

The two names, aujeszky's and pseudorabies, are therefore synonymous. Pseudorabies describes the clinical signs of aujeszky's in dogs. Another early name was 'mad itch' reflecting the most striking clinical sign in cattle.

Aujeszky's disease (AD) virus is primarily an infection of pigs which represent its only known reservoir host. It is sometimes transmitted naturally from pigs to individual cattle, horses, dogs and cats which develop nervous signs and rapidly die. These animals are end hosts and do not usually spread it. It has never been known to cause disease in people.

Should you be concerned about AD

There is a wide spectrum of risk and concern.

At one end of the spectrum, if you are involved with pig farming in Australia or Chile, which are remote from infected regions, your herd is perfectly safe. Australia and Chile are free from the virus and with careful import controls, unlikely to become contaminated. You can ignore this section.

In Canada, the UK or Denmark your herd is relatively safe from this disease because it has been eradicated from all three countries. However, if you are farming in Canada you should be aware that you could become infected from the USA. Also, if you are a British pig farmer you should not be complacent; it could get back into the UK from other EU countries with the movement of pigs, possibly for slaughter, now that there are no barriers to trade. If you are a Danish pig farmer you can feel a little more reassured in that your Slaughterers Association is likely to have more sense than to import pigs for slaughter from countries which have this virus. The virus could blow over the sea again from Germany to some of the Danish islands as it did before the vaccination of neighbouring German pig herds was financed.

The AD virus was also reported to have been eradicated from Eastern Germany before it came to be reunited with Western Germany in which the AD virus is enzootic. Since reunification, there has been movement of pigs from the West of Germany into farms in the East so if you are involved with pig farms in the East you should be aware that your herd may be vulnerable. Several countries of the EU (other than the UK and Denmark) are variously taking steps towards eradication of AD but most are still a long way from achieving it. If you live in these countries your herd is at risk.

Major attempts are being made to eliminate it from the USA. (See Fig.12-2). There are 5 main stages in the eradication programme. The 24 states in stage V are now regarded as free from AD and the 8 in stage IV are pretty close to being free. You will see that Iowa is only in stage II. This is because of the concentration of pigs there, 25% of the national herd. It is a daunting task but it is hoped that Iowa will be approaching stage V by the year 2000. If you are a pig farmer in the USA it is still a risky time for you. Eradication is underway in New Zealand.

At the other end of the spectrum, AD is widespread throughout most regions of Italy, Spain and Portugal, Central and Eastern Europe, South East Asia including China and Central and South America. It is considered to have been eradicated from one state, Sonora. in Mexico but it is still enzootic in the others.

For many readers of this book, therefore, it is not an exotic disease and is a constant threat to your herds. You should vaccinate routinely

Importance of AD

- AD is an economically-damaging viral disease of pigs although not anything like as damaging as swine fever. Some governments (e.g. the UK, Norway, Denmark, N & S Ireland, the Netherlands, Canada, the USA, and Chile) take it seriously and adopt control policies, which may include compulsory vaccination or in the case of the UK and Denmark, slaughter and eradication policies.
- In a susceptible (unvaccinated) herd large numbers of pigs may be clinically affected and some sows may abort. Mortality in suckled piglets is high but much lower in growing pigs. Unfortunately, it can spread on the wind so standard precautions of farm biosecurity cannot be entirely relied on to keep it out. On the credit side, there is only one serotype of the virus and attenuated vaccines are highly effective.

Clinical signs

The susceptible breeding herd

The earliest sign is usually a few pregnant sows aborting. If there is a farm dog in close contact with the

PSEUDORABIES ERADICATION FROM THE USA					
Situation on 1st December 1996					
Stage II	Stage II/III	Stage III	Stage III/IV	Stage IV	Stage V
Iowa	Indiana Michigan Minnesota Nebraska N. Carolina	California Florida Georgia Hawaii Illinois Kansas Louisiana Massachusetts US Missouri New Jersey Ohio Pennsylvania Texas	Wisconsin	Alabama Arizona Arkansas Kentucky Oklahoma S. Dakota Tennessee Virgin islands	Alaska Colorado Connecticut Delaware Idaho Maine Maryland Mississippi Montana Nevada New Hampshire New Mexico New York N. Dakota Oregon Puerto Rico Rhode Island S. Carolina Utah Vermont Virginia Washington W. Virginia Wyoming
(1)	(5)	(13)	(1)	(8)	(24)

Data courtesy of USDA-APHIS-VS

(Fig.12-2)

pigs, it may develop a severe acute nervous disease which is distressing to see and which always progresses to death. The farms cats disappear presumed dead. In newborn piglets an acute severe fatal nervous disease develops. This is first evident by rough haired listless appearances. They stop sucking and within 24 hours, tremble, become incoordinated, salivate excessively and go into convulsions, rolling their eyes forward and backward. They often emit a high pitched squeal.

Affected suckled piglets may show a variety of clinical signs such as walking in circles, sitting like a dog, or lying on their sides paddling their legs. Some may vomit and others may develop diarrhoea. They die within 24-36 hours of the onset of nervous signs. Mortality in piglets may be very high, approaching 100%. Subsequent litters may be born weak and/or start showing clinical signs as soon as they are born.

> *If sows abort, the farm dog goes into convulsions, and piglets become dull, hairy and start shaking, call your veterinarian urgently.*
>
> *Early vaccination can reduce the losses.*

If there are weaned pigs on the farm, the younger most recently weaned ones develop early signs similar to, but milder than, the suckled piglets and fewer of them develop nervous signs and die. Vomiting and diarrhoea are sometimes a feature. If the virus is a pneumotropic strain, causing pneumonia as well as nervous signs, older weaned pigs start sneezing, develop a nasal discharge, breath heavily and start coughing. The virus infection tends to cause flare-ups of enzootic pneumonia caused by *Mycoplasma hyopneumoniae* and may trigger off secondary bacterial infections such as *Pasteurella multocida* and *Actinobacillus pleuropneumoniae*.

Affected weaned pigs run a high fever 41-42°C (106-107°F). Many of those that develop nervous signs and/or severe pneumonia die but the death rate is usually less then 10%. Most of the rest recover fully in 5-10 days but some may be left stunted and grow poorly.

The susceptible grower-finisher herd

The earliest signs here are usually depression, lack of appetite, staring coat and fever 41-42°C (106-107°F) and respiratory diseases similar to those described above for older weaners are common. Relatively few pigs develop nervous signs or they may be mild (e.g. muscle tremors). Although all, or nearly all of the growers and finishers may be affected, most recover in 5-6 days and start to grow well again when they have recovered their appetites. The mortality is usually less than 2%.

Variations on the above clinical picture

These are common partly because of variations in the virulence of different strains of the virus and partly because of the differing immune status of pigs. If the virus is a mild one a herd may seroconvert to become positive in routine serological tests without the pig attendants being aware of anything seriously wrong. All strains of the virus have an affinity for nerves. Some also tend to have a strong affinity for the respiratory tract causing severe pneumonia while others do not.

In modern pig production cattle are not usually reared in close proximity to pigs but on those farms where they are some of the cattle may become sick, develop a relentless itching and die. Farm cats may also develop nervous signs and die.

Diagnosis

In acute severe outbreaks a strong presumptive diagnosis can be made on the typical clinical signs, particularly those in newborn piglets. The diagnosis is strengthened further if dogs, cats, cattle or horses are affected. On the other hand, in milder outbreaks and in grower-finisher herds where there are no sucking piglets, diagnosis may be difficult or impossible. Furthermore, even when sucking piglets are involved this disease can easily be confused with porcine reproductive and respiratory syndrome (PRRS) which is caused by an entirely different type of virus. Both diseases cause abortions, the birth of weak and premature litters and a high piglet mortality but in PRRS there are no nervous signs in piglets and weaners. The disease in grower/finisher pigs can also be confused with influenza which results in similar clinical signs and takes a somewhat similar course.

To confirm the diagnosis you will have to resort to laboratory tests. Whole dead young piglets should be submitted if possible. If not, tonsils and smears made from the pharyngeal region on microscope slides can be submitted. See chapter 15 (Swabbing). The laboratory should be able to do a rapid fluorescent antibody test (FAT) and have the results in a matter of hours. This test is fairly reliable in sucking piglets but much less so in grower/finisher pigs and so a negative result may be false and unreliable.

In grower/finisher pigs virus isolation has to be attempted and this delays the result considerably. The best tissues to submit for this are brain, spleen and lung which should be kept chilled on ice during transport. If no dead pigs are available nasal swabs can be submitted and should be sent in transport medium containing antibiotics. Blood samples from pigs in the early stage of the disease and from recovered pigs can be tested for rising antibodies but this delays the result about two weeks.

Virus isolation is carried out in cell cultures. The virus produces changes in the cells (cytopathic effects) and can be demonstrated by fluorescent antibody tests.

A variety of serological tests have been developed for aujeszky's virus including serum neutralisation tests, ELISAs, and latex agglutination tests. The ELISA is usually the test of choice and yields results fairly quickly. ELISA kits are commercially available and some of them are able to differentiate antibodies produced by gene deleted vaccine virus from those produced by natural infection from a wild virus.

Post-mortem lesions

AD damages the pig's nervous system but this damage (i.e. lesions) can only be seen through a microscope, not with the naked eye.

The only gross lesions that can be seen by the naked eye are those in the lungs and respiratory tubes and areas of necrosis on the tonsils and abdominal organs. An untrained pig person would not be able to distinguish AD lesions from those caused by influenza, PRRS, *Mycoplasma hyopneumoniae*, *Actinobacillus pleuropneumoniae*, or *Pasteurella multocida* so, unless you are veterinary trained it is probably a waste of time to open up pigs suspected of having died of AD.

Treatment

- There is no treatment available specifically against the virus.
- No treatment is effective in sucking pigs.
- Antibiotics will prevent secondary infections particularly of the respiratory system and also reduce bacterial damage.

Management control and prevention

◆ **Vaccination of the herd**

In countries which are free of the AD virus, vaccination is not practised and generally is not allowed.

In enzootic and high risk areas routine vaccination is practised and may be compulsory as part of an eradication scheme.

The great break-through in vaccination was the development of gene-deleted attenuated-virus marker vaccines. In these a small part of the genetic code of the viral DNA has been removed so that not only is the virus non-pathogenic when it multiplies in the pigs (thus producing immunity but no disease) but also it fails to stimulate a full complement of antibodies. This is because the missing piece of genetic code is not coding for one antigen. This is therefore absent from the vaccine virus.

Special commercially available serological test kits can distinguish antibodies which have been stimulated by the marker vaccine from those that have been stimulated by natural infection with a gene-complete wild virus. Pig herds in a control and eradication area can thus be vaccinated to protect them from the worst ravages of virulent AD virus and at the same time serologically screened for natural infection. The widespread use of gene-deleted marker vaccines in a controlled region has the added advantage of suppressing the spread of wild virus and thus reducing its level in the region. There is only one main serotype of AD virus which produces a strong long-lasting immunity. Vaccinated pigs can become infected but multiplication of the virus in the pigs' tissues is limited and so less is shed into the environment. Vaccination also prevents the virus from crossing the placenta of pregnant sows to infect the unborn piglets.

Piglets which are suckled by vaccinated sows receive colostral protection which lasts about 6-8 weeks. This is the age when the virulent AD virus would do most damage. During this time the pigs cannot be vaccinated successfully because the maternal antibodies neutralise the vaccine virus before it has had time to stimulate an immunity.

◆ **National or regional control and eradication programmes**

Individual countries and regions within countries are variously trying to suppress or eliminate the AD virus (e.g. Ireland, Norway, the Netherlands, France, the USA, and Mexico). The approach used is blanket vaccination of all 8-12 week old commercial slaughter pigs with a relatively cheap inactivated vaccine. Breeding stock is vaccinated with a longer lasting gene-deleted vaccine over a limited period to reduce the level of virus in the pig population. This is combined with routine testing of sow sera using the differential ELISA to monitor for natural infection. Tests have also been developed for use on colostrum which is easier to collect than blood. The disease may also be made notifiable (i.e. when a veterinarian diagnoses it he has to report it to the authorities who take the appropriate action).

> *If your pig farm is in a region where AD is enzootic vaccinate the herd routinely.*

◆ **On-farm eradication**

First try and identify how it arrived before deciding which is the best option.

If your herd is infected and the disease is in a stable state there are various methods of eradicating it.

1. Slaughter the herd, clean and disinfect the premises and repopulate with negative breeding stock. This is expensive and is unlikely to be cost effective in most commercial herds.
2. In a weaner production unit, vaccinate all the breeding stock with gene-deleted vaccine. Later test all the sows with the differential ELISA and remove those that are positive for wild virus.

Follow this by one of two options:
   a) Depopulate the weaner accommodation and rear the pigs elsewhere. Then, after all the grower/finishers have been slaughtered and/or the youngest of them reared elsewhere, gradually restock the weaner, grower and finisher accommodation as subsequent sows are weaned or
   b) Change to a three-site or multi-site system with all-in all out rooms or buildings.

On-farm precautions

If your herd is free of AD virus you should of course endeavour to keep it free but it is not always easy to do so particularly in a pig-dense area.

Unfortunately, the AD virus can spread on the wind several km over land and much further over water, so standard precautions of farm biosecurity such as those described earlier in chapter 2 cannot be entirely relied on to keep it out of your herd. Also, semen from infected boars is thought to spread it so the use of artificial insemination with bought in semen could in theory contaminate the herd.

> *AD virus can spread from farm to farm on the wind*

Rats, which are normally thought of as dead end hosts, also become infected and are said to spread it from farm to farm. This possibility is disputed by some authorities.

Infected pigs can become long-term sub-clinical carriers. Any replacement pigs coming on to the premises should come from known safe sources and be quarantined. These should as a minimum be physically separated from your pigs, for at least a month, preferably six weeks and blood tested prior to integration. AD virus can be carried on the tonsils of the wild boar and be excreted intermittently. Make sure the farm is pig-proof.

> *If there is a risk of AD in the area check on the health status of your replacement stock and segregate them for a month after arrival*

The causal agent is a herpes virus and like the herpes viruses of humans (e.g. the causes of cold sores and chicken pox) the AD virus can lie latent in the pig's nerve cells. Stress (e.g. the stress of transport) can reactivate it and the pig starts to shed virus again. The main spread between pigs is aerosol and nose to nose contact. It is not spread in faeces or urine.

The AD virus is not thought to survive long in pig meat and if this is true the illegal feeding of pig meat scraps to neighbouring "back-yard" pigs is unlikely to trigger off an outbreak which could then spread to your herd. However, mink farms have been reported to become infected from feeding pig meat waste products. Unwashed pig lorries which have carried infected pigs do not seem to be such a major factor in the spread of AD as, say, SVD. Nevertheless, it would be unwise not to adopt safe methods of loading your slaughter pigs.

BLUE EYE DISEASE (BE)

(So-called because the whole eye develops a bluish tinge as a result of corneal opacity).

Blue eye disease (BE) is characterised by clinical signs of nervous derangement, reproductive problems and opacity of the surface of the eyes (corneal opacity). It is thought to be caused by a paramyxovirus.

Should you be concerned about blue eye disease (BE)?

BE was first recognised in central Mexico in 1980 and was later diagnosed in many other regions of Mexico. If you are involved in pig farming in Mexico, you should be concerned about it.

It has never been diagnosed in any other countries and is unlikely to spread to them.

In Japan, a paramyxovirus (the Sendai virus) can cause nervous disorders and reproductive problems but it is probably a different virus.

If you are involved with pig farming outside Mexico and your country has strict controls over imports of live pigs, particularly from Mexico, do not be concerned.

But beware! You could confuse ontario encephalitis (the nervous form of vomiting and wasting disease) which occurs in Europe and North America with it.

> *If you farm in Mexico, and piglets suddenly develop convulsions, consider blue eye, ontario encephalitis or pseudorabies.*

Clinical signs

When the disease first breaks out in a susceptible breeding herd the first clinical signs are usually seen in the farrowing house. Piglets are hunched with rough coats for a short time and then suddenly develop acute nervous signs. They have difficulty walking, start to shiver, and sit in abnormal postures. Some lie on their sides, paddle their legs and roll their eyeballs back and forth. The eyes of some piglets water and the eyelids swell and get stuck together. Worst affected are piglets under 2 weeks of age. Up to 90% die. Older weaned piglets may develop blueing of the pupils (black centres) of the eyes. Up to 65% of litters may be affected. The disease disappears slowly and spontaneously after several weeks.

Older pigs of a month or more in age show milder transient signs of loss of appetite, fever, sneezing and coughing. Nervous signs, such as an unsteady walk, are less common.

Some adult pigs also show clinical signs including blueing of the eyes. There is an increased return rate in sows lasting about 6 months. Abortions and stillbirths may occur. Up to 40% of boars have testicular enlargement, which is usually one-sided, followed by shrinking

> *BE will not be of concern unless you farm in Mexico.*

with a concurrent loss of fertility.

Diagnosis

In acute severe outbreaks a strong presumptive diagnosis can be made based on the nervous signs, corneal opacity, infertility and testicle changes.

For confirmation of the presumptive diagnosis serological tests have to be done in the laboratory. Virus isolation from brain tissue can also be demonstrated.

Post-mortem

There are no lesions indicative of BE that can be seen with the naked eye.

Similar diseases

Diseases with similar clinical signs include aujeszky's disease (AD), PRRS, ontario encephalitis (vomiting and wasting disease), and brucellosis. However, none of them have all the clinical signs of BE.

Treatment

☐ There is no effective treatment.

Management control and prevention

◆ **Vaccination**
This should be a useful method if and when an effective vaccine is developed.

◆ **Biosecurity**
This should reduce the chances of your herd being infected. Read the final section of this chapter.

◆ **On-farm eradication**
Once a herd has been infected and clinical signs have disappeared the virus may disappear. To help this do not introduce replacement stock into the herd for 1 - 2 months.

BRUCELLOSIS

Brucellosis in pigs is caused by a bacterium called *Brucella suis*. There are five different types, called biotypes, which behave in slightly different ways outside the pig.

In most parts of the world where *B. suis* infects pigs, the most common biotypes causing disease are 1 and 3 with biotype 2 in Europe. Biotype 2 is enzootic in wild hare populations in Northern and Central Europe. Hares transmit it to pigs.

Biotype 4 is enzootic in reindeer and caribou in Siberia, Alaska, and Canada. Pigs are not generally kept where reindeer and caribou are plentiful and type 4 is thought not to be very pathogenic to pigs. Human cases of type 4 infection are not caught from pigs.

Should you be concerned about Brucellosis?

B. suis is not present in the UK or Ireland and if you work in these countries you need not be concerned about it.

It was thought to have disappeared from France and Denmark because no clinical cases had been diagnosed for a number of years. Then over recent years outdoor breeding herds were established which, of course, were exposed to hares. At least one of these in each country caught brucellosis from infected hares. The hares associated with the French (Normandy) outbreak had been recently introduced from Poland by hunters, because the hare population of Northern France had dropped so low.

It is assumed that *B. suis* is still enzootic in the hare population of Scandinavia and Central Europe but there is insufficient evidence to define the precise area where infected hares exist. It is present in the USA, South America parts of Asia and Australia.

Importance of Brucellosis

- *Brucella suis* is not a highly epizootic infectious organism like, say, TGE or FMD. It spreads slowly between and within herds and you should be able to keep it out of your herd if you take sensible precautions. But it is a serious disease and you must always think of it as such.

> *If brucellosis is suspected in your herd, take great care that you and other pig attendants do not get infected. Call in your veterinarian.*

- If it gets into your herd, it is difficult to eliminate. It causes long term reproductive losses and some biotypes (1 and 3 particularly) also cause a very nasty disease in people. Fortunately, the hare biotype-type 2- is less pathogenic to people.

Clinical signs

In a susceptible breeding herd

The earliest sign is usually a few pregnant sows aborting. No other pigs may appear to be affected. If the early abortions are few in number they may be missed particularly in loose-housed sows and in outdoor herds.

> *If sows abort at all stages of pregnancy, and the farm is in a swine brucellosis region call in your veterinarian and request an accurate diagnosis.*

The first sign noted then may be a high return to service and vaginal discharges. These returns are 30-50 days after mating if the disease has been introduced to the herd by an infected boar. The females are infected by him at mating. If sows are already pregnant abortions may occur at any stage. The infection arising from contaminated rooting materials or vaginal discharges.

In the boar, *B. suis* tends to multiply in the testicles and/or the male accessory reproductive glands and is then shed in the semen for prolonged periods. The reproductive tracts of sows and gilts become infected when served by the boar or inseminated artificially. This results in a large proportion of very early abortions. The infection in the sows' reproductive tracts is not permanent and eventually clears up spontaneously. In contrast, the infection in the boars' reproductive tract is usually permanent, the damage that it does is irreversible.

It may then be noticed that some of the boars' testicles are becoming enlarged. A few growing pigs and adults, and a slightly greater number of sucking piglets and weaners start to develop partial or total paralysis in their hind quarters. This is the result of infection and damage to the spine. Some pigs may become lame with swollen joints.

Mortality is likely to be low and the disease may spread slowly but the long term damage to production can be serious.

Diagnosis

The combination of abortions, returns to service, vaginal discharges swollen boar testicles, lame pigs and young pigs with posterior paralysis is strongly suggestive but laboratory tests have to be done to make a definitive diagnosis. Best samples to submit are aborted piglets, swabs of vaginal discharges, dead pigs, and blood samples from at least 10 sows, preferably from those which have aborted or returned to service.

The most sensitive and accurate laboratory method is to culture and identify the organism on selective medium which is not difficult. The products of abortion are teeming with organisms. The organism can also be cultured from semen, testicles and accessory organs, lymph nodes, fluid from swollen joints, and in the early stages, from blood.

A variety of serological tests can be done on blood samples, including agglutination and complement fixation tests, ELISAs, and card and plate tests. Both false positive and false negative results occur which is why you need to blood test at least 10 sows and boars, preferably more. Serological tests are unreliable for diagnosis in an individual pig and should be done only as herd tests.

Post-mortem

It would be risky to open a dead pig to look for lesions. In the early stages of the disease the organism is spread throughout the pig's body. Even in the later stages it is fairly widespread. It can infect you through tiny cuts and abrasions on your hands or by being splashed or rubbed into your eye or mouth.

> ***Do not open up a dead pig for post mortem examination. The risk of catching brucellosis is too great.***

Treatment

- Treatment with antibiotics is not very effective and generally should not be attempted. Affected pigs should be destroyed.
- If your herd becomes infected the most reliable method of control is to slaughter the herd, clean up the premises and restock with brucella-free pigs. This is also the safest procedure from the pig attendants' and public's stand-point and in the long term is usually the least costly. Depending upon the country in which you work, it may mandatory to do so.

> ***If your herd becomes infected the best course of action is to slaughter the herd, clean up the premises and restock with brucella-free pigs.***

- Other approaches include repeated herd blood tests with removal of positive reactors. This may be effective if only a few pigs are infected but is likely to be unsuccessful if many pigs are positive.

Management control and prevention

◆ **Vaccination**

The brucella vaccines which have had widespread use for brucellosis in cattle are not effective in pigs. The low incidence of the disease has not made it cost-effective to develop vaccines for pigs and none are available

◆ **National or regional control and eradication programmes**

There is a move in a number of countries, including the USA, to gradually eliminate this disease mainly by compulsory slaughter of herds in which the organism is diagnosed combined with various other procedures depending on the particular programme.

◆ **Farm precautions**

If your herd is free of *Brucella suis* you should endeavour to keep it free by adopting the methods of biosecurity described in the last section of this chapter.

The main method of spread is by pig-to-pig contact, through venereal transmission during mating and on-farm do-it-yourself artificial insemination. Other materials include the eating or rooting of aborted piglets, dead piglets, aborted afterbirths or materials contaminated by vaginal discharges from aborted sows. Exposure of cut or abraded skin to infected materials may also result in transmission. Sows shed the organism from the vagina for at least 30 days after aborting, sometimes much longer. Suckling sows also shed the organism in milk which then infects their piglets. The organism does not spread on wind and rarely on other vectors so the main defence of your herd depends on preventing exposure to infected pigs and the introduction of brucella-free replacement pigs.

- ◆ **Protection of personnel**
Brucellosis in people, also called undulant fever, is a serious long-lasting disease which does not respond well to treatment. Infected people get recurrent attacks of clinical disease over many years. It causes a variety of symptoms including severe headaches, meningitis and bad dreams, severe backache, depression and lack of energy and interest, damaged testicles and changes of personality. It is therefore essential that if the organism infects your herd, you take every precaution against people becoming infected.

If the herd becomes infected take every precaution against people catching it.

Main precautions to take
- ◆ Wear protective clothing and take it off and wash your hands before eating.
- ◆ Wear rubber gloves when handling affected pigs or infected materials.
- ◆ Protect your eyes against splashing infected materials into them.
- ◆ Do not touch your eyes or put your fingers or any instruments on or in your mouth when working with affected pigs.
- ◆ Protect any bare skin on your arms or face that might have cuts and abrasions.
- ◆ Get rid of the disease as soon as possible.

CLASSICAL SWINE FEVER (CSF) - HOG CHOLERA (HC)

Classical swine fever (CSF), otherwise known as hog cholera (HC) or just swine fever, is a specific viral disease of pigs. It affects no other species. It is a notifiable disease in most countries of the world.

Importance of CSF
- CSF is one of the most economically-damaging pandemic viral diseases of pigs in the world. Many governments take it very seriously and adopt strict control policies, which include compulsory vaccination or slaughter and eradication policies.
- In a susceptible (unvaccinated) herd almost all the pigs are affected. It causes generalised disease, including fever, malaise, lack of appetite, diarrhoea, paralysis, abortion, mummification and the birth of shaking piglets. Mortality is high.
- Fortunately, there is only one serotype of the virus and attenuated vaccines are highly effective. Also, it does not spread on the wind or on insects or birds so standard precautions of farm biosecurity should keep it out. However it persists in uncooked and cured meat and these should not be fed to pigs.

Should you be concerned about CSF?

If your pig farm is in the United States, Canada, Chile, Australia, New Zealand or Ireland, which can be regarded as free countries and which are most unlikely to be recontaminated, you need not be concerned about it.

If your pig farm is in Western Europe, most of which can be regarded as a fringe region, (i.e. free from the virus but at risk of re-entry) you should be concerned because although your country is probably free from the virus, there is a real risk that it might get back in from Germany, Austria, Central Europe or Eastern Europe.

If your pig farm is in Germany, Austria or Poland, although the domestic pig population is free from the virus, it is endemic in the wild boar population which poses a threat to your herd. This might also be true of Italy.

If your pig farm is in the South of Brazil, although your area may be free from the virus there is a risk of it getting back in from the North.

The virus is thought to be endemic (enzootic) throughout the rest of Central and Eastern Europe, S.E. Asia and Africa so if you are involved in pig production in any of these areas you may need to vaccinate your pigs routinely.

Clinical signs

If you are involved in pig farming in one of the fringe regions identified above you should be able to recognise the early clinical signs so that you can alert you veterinarian. If the disease is suspected he/she will report it to the authorities. They will carry out laboratory tests and depending on your country's policy, will probably slaughter your herd, a very distressing experience even if you are paid compensation.

The virus that causes CSF varies in virulence. Some strains are highly virulent and cause acute (i.e. rapid) serious disease. Some strains are of low virulence and cause chronic (i.e. long-lasting) disease, others are intermediate causing sub-acute disease.

Acute disease

Clinical signs usually appear first in a small number of growing pigs which show non-specific signs of depression, sleepiness, and reluctance to get up or to eat. If you get them up they may wander to the feeder but eat very little or nothing and wander away again to lie down. They walk and stand with their heads down and tails limp. Over the following few days these signs get worse and more pigs become affected.

Younger piglets may appear chilled, shiver and huddle together.

Initially affected pigs may appear to be constipated but this generally changes to a yellow-grey diarrhoea as the disease progresses. Early on some of the pigs may develop conjunctivitis (inflammation of the eye surface) with thin discharges. This gets worse, the discharge getting thicker with time until some of the eyelids are completely closed and adhered.

A constant early sign, which persists throughout the disease until just before death, is a high fever, over 42°C (107°F). Check the sick pigs' rectal temperatures. If they are all high suspect CSF.

> *If a number of your pigs become drowsy, reluctant to get up or to eat, and hang their heads and tails, take their temperatures. If most are above 42°C (107°F), call your veterinarian urgently*

As the disease progresses the affected pigs become very thin and weak and develop a staggering walk. Initially this is probably through weakness but later it is due to infection of and damage to the spinal nerves. Partial paralysis of the hind end results in a drunken walk and a tendency to fall to a sitting or lying position. Diarrhoea worsens and some pigs vomit a yellowish bile. The pigs' skins go purple, first over the ears and tail, followed by the snout, lower legs, belly and back. Affected pigs die in 10-20 days. Some pigs go into convulsions before death.

Sub-acute disease

The early signs in growing pigs are similar but they progress more slowly and are less severe. Affected pigs may be ill for up to 30 days before they die.

Chronic and aberrant disease and persistent infection

The virus can cross the placenta and infect the piglets in the sow's uterus. Sows that have been inadequately vaccinated that become infected, or sows which become infected with a virus of low virulence, may appear normal but give birth to shaking piglets many of which die. (Note: there are also other causes of shaking or trembling piglets).

If the virus crosses the placenta before the piglets' immune systems have developed they may be born apparently healthy although possibly weak and may grow on to be persistent carriers without at first showing clinical signs. They shed virus so they are a menace to other pigs. At several weeks or months of age they may develop typical clinical signs but these are likely to be milder, last longer and without the high temperatures.

Virus that infects the piglets in the uterus may cause other effects, namely, death, mummification, abortion or the birth of weak piglets some of which may be deformed. Vaccination of sows during pregnancy with some of the original attenuated virus vaccines resulted in trans-placental infection of unborn piglets with similar adverse results. The newer attenuated vaccines are claimed to be safer.

Low virulence strains of the virus may also multiply in the reproductive tracts of unvaccinated boars or boars which have been inadequately vaccinated. The vaccine virus itself in some of the older attenuated vaccines was thought to do this, resulting in returns to service and abortions.

Diagnosis

In acute or sub-acute outbreaks a presumptive diagnosis can be made on the typical clinical signs and post-mortem lesions but African swine fever and *Salmonella choleraesuis* infection produce some similar signs and lesions. *Salmonella choleraesuis* is frequently a concurrent pathological infection with CSF virus, triggered off from its latent state by the CSF virus infection.

In chronic or aberrant cases the clinical signs and lesions are less diagnostic and may only raise a suspicion of CSF.

In all suspected cases laboratory tests should be done to confirm the diagnosis. Investigations are usually carried out by the authorities.

> *Rapid accurate laboratory diagnosis is essential.*

It is best to send whole dead pigs to the diagnostic laboratory so the pathologists can sample what they want. If only samples can be sent the tonsils are best.

The tonsils of the pig are very easy to find. Cut away the skin and flesh under and between the lower jaw bone including the tongue. The pair of tonsils are two large red patches each about the size of the end half of your thumb or perhaps slightly bigger. See chapter 15 (Swabbing). Do not freeze them but send them packed with ice.

Virus is present throughout the body. In addition to the tonsils the next best organs to send are the spleen, kidneys and last few inches of the small intestine (before it meets the large intestine).

The laboratory should be able to carry out rapid tests and let you know the diagnosis on the same day they receive the samples.

A quick and fairly accurate test, which has been used for a number of years, is the direct fluorescent antibody test (FAT) carried out on frozen sections of the tonsils or other organs. It can sometimes give false negative results but this can be avoided if a sufficient number of pigs' tonsils are sampled. The CSF virus also cross reacts in the FAT test with bovine virus diarrhoea virus (BVDV) of cattle and the border disease virus (BDV) of sheep, either of which may sometimes infect pigs. These viruses can cause trans-placental infection of unborn piglets in the sow's uterus resulting in infertility and piglet problems similar to those of CSF. Such congenital infection may also result in newborn piglets which are shedding virus and thus infecting other pigs. The false positive results obtained in an FAT may cause awkward problems if there is a control or eradication policy in force. Specific antibodies against specific antigens of the CSF virus differentiate it from BVDV and BDV. Fortunately, BVDV and BDV are relatively rare infections in pigs kept separately from cattle and sheep. One source of infection with BVDV, however, may be the feeding of raw milk by-products to pigs. Another source may be the accidental presence of BVDV in live attenuated aujeszky's disease (pseudorabies) or other vaccines. Recent vaccination (i.e. a few days) of pigs with attenuated CSF vaccine may also cause positive FAT results.

Post-mortem

Normally it requires a trained person to interpret post-mortem examination findings but in the case of CSF an untrained pig person should be able to recognise some of the more marked lesions

If pigs are laid on their backs after death and opened up for examination the picture is striking. There are usually many small haemorrhages throughout the body and larger haemorrhages in some organs such as lymph nodes. Some of these may be bright red and filled with blood. Larger haemorrhages may also be present in the lungs and under the skin.

The kidney surfaces are often described as looking like mottled ducks' eggs in that they are covered with variable sized bloody spots.

The spleen may have dark raised areas of dead tissue. Similar areas of dead tissue occur in other organs (e.g. the tonsils) but are more difficult to find.

The lungs may show severe pneumonia, haemorrhage and pleurisy usually resulting from secondary bacterial infection.

The stomach and gut are usually empty except for scant liquid which may be brightly coloured. Fairly unique lesions to look for are raised so-called 'button ulcers' on the inner lining of the large intestine near its junction with the small intestine.

Management control and prevention

◆ **Vaccination**

In most national CSF eradication programmes and in countries which are free of the CSF virus, vaccination against CSF is not practised and generally is not allowed.

In enzootic and high risk areas routine vaccination is practised and may be compulsory.

Inactivated vaccines were in common use but they sometimes contained live virus which resulted in infection. Inactivated vaccines have now largely been replaced by live attenuated vaccines, the most recent of which are relatively safe and effective. Pigs develop protective immunity one week to ten days after vaccination and the immunity lasts two to three years (i.e. the lifetime of many sows and boars). Piglets which are suckled by vaccinated sows receive colostral protection which lasts about 6-8 weeks. During this time they cannot be vaccinated successfully because the maternal antibodies neutralise the vaccine virus before it has had time to stimulate an immunity.

There is only one mutationally-stable serotype of CSF virus which produces a strong long-lasting immunity. The virus in CSF vaccines was attenuated by frequent passage in rabbits (so-called 'lapinised vaccines' or 'Chinese strain vaccines'). These are still available in some parts of the world but many vaccines now contain viruses that have been attenuated by continual growth in cell cultures.

In a circumscribed region in which the CSF virus is endemic it is usual to blanket vaccinate all pigs over two weeks of age initially. Piglets born to vaccinated sows would be vaccinated over 8 weeks age. This policy usually results in elimination of the virus from that region.

◆ **National eradication programmes**

A number of countries in which CSF was enzootic have successfully eradicated it, most notably Canada and the USA, the UK and most EU countries on mainland Europe.

Generally, an eradication policy starts with compulsory large scale vaccination over a limited period to reduce the level of virus in the pig population. Vaccination is then stopped and the disease is made notifiable. When CSF is then diagnosed the whole herd and other in contact animals are slaughtered. Theoretically, it would be useful to carry out national serological testing at the same time (as has been done in eradicating aujeszky's disease), but vaccination results in almost life-long positive tests. Also, BVDV and BDV infections cause false positive results.

> *If CSF is enzootic in your area vaccinate your herd routinely*

◆ **National preventative programmes**

Countries which are free of the CSF virus prevent re-infection from outside by controlling the importation of pigs and pig meat products, unless they have been well processed, from regions in which the CSF virus is still present. In addition, swill (waste human food) containing meat products must be sterilised by heating in licensed premises.

The disease is also legally notifiable. If a case does occur the herd is slaughtered, all in-contact pigs are traced and monitored or killed and a standstill order is placed on pig movements in the area around which the case occurred. Attempts are made to find out the source of the infection. This is likely to be illegally imported pig meat scraps which have been given to pigs without first thoroughly cooking them. Other possibilities are the illegal importa-

Managing Pig Health and the Treatment of Disease

tion of infected semen, the return of unwashed pig lorries from an infected region and contact with wild boar or unprocessed meat.

◆ **On-farm precautions**

If you farm in a country where CSF is endemic or where there is a risk of CSF occurring consider routinely vaccinating your herd if vaccination is allowed. This will greatly reduce the possibility of contamination.

CSF virus does not spread as readily as some other viral infections (e.g. TGE and FMD). Unlike FMD it is not windborne. Thus the conscientious application of simple biosecurity measures should keep it out of the herd.

If CSF is in your country important precautions include reducing visitors to a minimum, taking precautions against contamination from vehicles, and not allowing pig meat products near any pigs. Any replacement pigs coming on to the premises should come from known safe sources and should be quarantined. In some areas the disease has become very mild and spread can go unrecognised.

Pig buildings should be protected from stray animals, particularly wild pigs.

FOOT-AND-MOUTH DISEASE (FMD)

See chapter 10.

FMD is called a porcine vesicular disease because one of its most prominent clinical signs is the appearance of vesicles (blisters containing a clear fluid) in the mouth, on the lips and nose, on the teats and around the coronets of the feet just above the hooves. There are four vesicular diseases of pigs which are difficult or impossible to differentiate clinically: FMD, swine vesicular disease (SVD), vesicular exanthema (VES), and vesicular stomatitis (VS). Of these, FMD is the most widespread and important with SVD being of secondary importance in some regions (e.g. the EU). The other two have very limited distribution and VES has disappeared. Because of the importance of FMD and the difficulty of distinguishing it from the others, all four have to be considered in this chapter.

Importance of FMD

- FMD is the most important restraint to international trade in animals and animal products. Consequently, large sums of money have been invested in control and eradication programmes and also into research. As a result more is known about the FMD virus than about almost any other animal infection.
- It generally produces severe disease in pigs and cattle.
- FMD is so important because it is highly infectious, spreads rapidly throughout animal populations and over long distances on the wind and hence it is difficult and costly to control. Also because of its damaging and debilitating effect on cattle, a great deal of effort and tax-payers money has been spent keeping it out of large areas of the world. It would be highly irresponsible to let it back in.
- If you live in an FMD-fringe area that is also free of swine vesicular disease (SVD) you should be aware of what early clinical signs would make you suspicious and what you should do if you suspected them in your herd. If you farm in an endemic area or a fringe area in which SVD is present then you should know a bit more, particularly about the clinical signs in pigs and vaccination regimes.
- If you farm in an FMD-free country that takes sound precautions against its entry, the risk to your herd is negligible unless you farm in California where vesicular exanthema may pose a very small risk.

Early clinical signs

In cattle the early clinical signs are much more definitive or suggestive than in pigs. For example in a dairy herd several cows may suddenly show depressed milk yield, go off their feed, run a fever, have a dramatic drop in milk yield, and a little later start salivating profusely, the saliva running from their mouths (slavering). If you see such signs, jump into action, ring the vet. Veterinarians who have to deal with FMD say that if a farmer telephones to say that several cows are salivating profusely they think first "FMD?".

If after cows have started salivating and smacking lips, vesicles are noticed on the lips, on the teats and around the coronets, the areas above hooves - your worst fears are probably true. The probability is that your pig herd has been infected too.

> **If you keep cattle as well as pigs and some of the cattle go off their food and start salivating profusely think "FMD?"**

In pigs early signs are lameness a drop in food consumption and some pigs appear depressed and have fevers of about 40.5°C,(105°F). In piglets sudden death due to cardiac failure is common. What should make you strongly suspicious is the appearance a little later of vesicles up to 30mm. diameter, similar to those described above for cattle. They are most plentiful around the coronets but are less plentiful on the nose and lips although this is where you are likely to see them first. They often appear on the teats of recently farrowed sows. By then the sows and some of the other pigs may be dribbling saliva and chomping their jaws. If they are on bedding they may not appear lame but if they are on concrete they probably will be.

The early signs of swine vesicular disease (SVD) when it is severe, are indistinguishable from FMD so you should suspect it too.

If you farm near the coast of California where FMD and SVD are extremely unlikely, vesicular exanthema could be a possibility. If you farm in Georgia, the Carolinas or Central or South America and it is summer/autumn time perhaps you should think of vesicular stomatitis. The clinical signs of all four diseases are almost indistinguishable.

Within 24 hours many of the vesicles will have burst. On the lips and teats they may leave shallow erosions but on the coronets of the feet secondary infection and trauma may convert them into raw jagged-edged ulcers.

If the pigs are not killed some may lose their complete hooves (so-called "Thimbling"), sows may abort, as a result of fever, and in severe outbreaks some may die. Boars may go lame and stop serving sows, so there is an infertility side effect. There may also be an increase in mortality among suckled piglets. This is often the first sign.

In endemic areas where vaccination is carried out routinely the disease is not a serious economic problem in pig herds. In fringe areas, particularly where vaccination is not allowed (e.g. in the EU) it is a serious problem because the herd will almost certainly be slaughtered out and although compensation is likely to be paid, the farm cannot be restocked for at least six weeks, it is therefore out of production and in a negative cash flow for a long time.

Diagnosis

Rapid accurate diagnosis is essential.

FMD cannot be distinguished from SVD on clinical grounds, or from VES in California, although SVD is often much milder. To differentiate these diseases and confirm the presumptive diagnosis, samples have to be sent to a laboratory capable of making a diagnosis.

There are not many of these. The main one is the World Reference Laboratory at Pirbright near London in England. There is also one on Plum Island off the coast of NY in the USA and one near Melbourne in Australia.

The samples sent are blood and pieces of the skin that overlay the blisters plus vesicular fluid if this is available. Once the samples have been received by the laboratory diagnosis is fairly rapid.

> **Diagnosis of suspected FMD must be rapid and accurate.**

Tests called ELISAs are used for virus identification and if it is FMD they also indicate what serotype it is. The virus may also be grown in cell culture and the identification confirmed by other tests. A molecular genetic test called a PCR (polymerase chain reaction) may also be used to 'fingerprint" the virus. The gene (genome or RNA) of FMD repeatedly undergoes minor changes as the virus spreads through animal populations so by identifying the precise sequence in the gene the laboratory staff are able to make an assumption where it may have come from by the most recent isolate with a similar sequence.

> **If a group of pigs go off their feed and have blisters on their nose and lips and go a bit lame suspect FMD or SVD. Contact your veterinarian urgently**

Treatment

☐ There is no treatment. Animals should be destroyed.

Management control and prevention

◆ **Vaccination**

In endemic and high risk areas routine vaccination may be practised mainly to protect the breeding stock.

Most FMD vaccines are produced in cell suspension cultures and inactivated by ethylenamine derivatives. An adjuvant is added to make them more potent. Oily adjuvants are used in swine.

Vaccination in pigs is problematical. This is because protection is short-lived lasting only about six months. It is also partly because there are seven serotypes of FMD and protection against one leaves animals susceptible to the others. Vaccines must be multivalent (several serotypes) in most endemic regions. Since FMD is largely a winter disease, vaccination should be carried out in the autumn.

Serotypes - There are 7 main serotypes: A, O, C, SAT 1, SAT 2, SAT 3 and Asia 1. There are also many strains within serotypes. Careful selection of the strains for incorporation in vaccines is essential to ensure they are effective.

◆ **Precautions**

Countries in free and fringe areas apply strictly enforced national preventative measures against the introduction of infection. The main features of these measures are control over the importation of cloven-hoofed animals and of meat from such animals from counties in which FMD occurs. The virus does not survive rigor mortis but it can persist in bone marrow and lymph nodes of infected carcasses for several weeks.

If the disease does enter a free or fringe area, a slaughter policy is implemented, all diseased and in-contact animals being slaughtered. A standstill on animal movement is imposed and tracings are carried out to check possible spread of the disease through previous contacts. Ring vaccination may be used around the affected region.

If you farm in an FMD-risk region you should take strict precautions against the contamination of your herd. If you have a cattle or goat herd or a flock of sheep as well as a pig herd you should also adopt preventative measures for them and keep a wary eye for the appearance of typical clinical signs.

Unfortunately, none of the measures described prevent the windborne spread of FMD. Infected pigs can produce huge quantities of infective virus as aerosols. They produce far more aerosol virus than cattle, goats or sheep. In dry weather when there are strong thermals the aerosol virus is rapidly inactivated so the wind does not carry infective aerosols very far. Strong winds, hills and objects such as high buildings and trees create turbulence and disperse the plume of airborne virus as they would a plume of smoke from a bonfire. In humid overcast weather with a steady light wind blowing over flat countryside infective virus may survive long enough to infect other herds up to 60km (36 miles) distant. Over water, given the same climatic conditions, infective virus has been shown to travel up to 300km (180 miles) so siting your pig herd on an island in a lake is not going to stop it.

Windborne infection is impossible to guard against. Even if your pig herd is in closed buildings, the aerosol virus can get in through the ventilation system and you may carry it in from outside on your boots or clothes.

If vaccination is permitted and the pig herd is in a high-risk area you should consider routine vaccination to reduce the susceptibility of your herd.

JAPANESE B. ENCEPHALITIS (JBE)

Japanese B. encephalitis (JBE) is caused by a virus (a member of the flavivirus group) which is spread by mosquitoes. The pig is the natural amplifier and reservoir host. In other words it serves to multiply up the virus and keep it going. Many other species can be infected including most domestic animals and many wild animals such as rabbits, mice, birds, bats, snakes and lizards.

Should you be concerned about JBE?

You should be if you work in South Asia or visit pig farms there.

JBE is confined to a large area of South Asia, about 6500 x 6500km (4000 x 4000 miles), centred on the China Sea and stretching from Ceylon to Japan and from New Guinea to Mongolia and Eastern Russia. This includes such major pig producing countries as China, Taiwan, Korea, Thailand, the Philippines and Japan.

> *If you intend to visit pig farms in South Asia get yourself vaccinated*

If you live outside this area of South Asia, there is no risk to your herd and no risk to you unless you decide to visit pig farms in the area, in which case get yourself vaccinated twice, preferably three times, before you go.

Importance of JBE

- JBE is not a very important disease of pigs causing only sporadic reproductive problems.
- Its main importance is its threat to public health.

> *Japanese B. encephalitis is transmitted by mosquitoes and causes a serious disease in people*

Clinical signs

The main clinical signs are degeneration of the boar's testicles and infertility and the birth of abnormal piglets. These include mummified foetuses, dead piglets with subcutaneous oedema (excess clear bodily fluid under the skin), hydrocephalus (water on the brain), and weak piglets sometimes with nervous signs.

> *If sows give birth to piglets with a variety of abnormalities, and one or more boars become infertile, and you work in S. Asia, suspect JBE.*

Diagnosis

This requires laboratory examination of dead stillborn piglets and affected boars' testicles.

Definitive diagnosis depends on the isolation of the virus in tissue culture and demonstration of antibodies in stillborn piglets serum, usually by an ELISA.

Similar reproductive problems are caused commonly by parvovirus, aujeszky's disease, PRRS, certain strains of influenza, CSF(hog cholera), and some enteroviruses.

Post-mortem

There are no specific lesions visible to the naked eye.

Treatment

- There is no effective treatment.

Management control and prevention

- Vaccination - In countries in which this disease is endemic young breeding gilts and boars are vaccinated twice before the mosquito season starts commonly with an attenuated vaccine but inactivated vaccines are also available.
- Trying to control mosquitoes in pig herds is a waste of time.

LEPTOSPIROSIS

See chapter 6 for further information.

It can take several forms depending on the serotype or serovars involved. The main serotypes that cause disease in pigs are:

- *Leptospira pomona*

- *Leptospira tarassovi*
- *Leptospira bratislava/muenchen*
- *Leptospira icterohaemorrhagiae*

Leptospira hardjo is widespread in the cattle populations of the world and causes bovine abortion. It causes transient infections and antibody responses in pigs but no disease.

L. pomona and *L. tarassovi* are the only serovars that can be regarded as exotic.

L. POMONA INFECTION

The risk to your herd

This is enzootic in many pig rearing parts of the world including North, Central and South America, Australia, New Zealand, South East Asia and Eastern and Central Europe. If you are involved in pig farming in any of these areas it is not an exotic organism and your herd is at risk.

L. pomona is definitely not present in the UK or Ireland and is thought not to be present in other countries of Western Europe with the possible exception of Italy. So if you are involved in pig farming in Western Europe (except Italy) you can regard it as an exotic organism. The risk to your herd is probably negligible.

If you are involved in exporting pigs from countries of Western Europe, the pigs for export will probably have to be blood-tested for antibodies to *L. pomona*. You will probably be frustrated to find that a small number will be positive. This is because they have encountered the mosdok serovar, which is present in some species of wildlife, which sometimes cross-infects pigs causing little or no clinical disease. This is so closely related to *L. pomona* of pigs that it stimulates a positive immune response. It never develops into a herd problem. The pig can be thought of as an end host.

Importance of *L. pomona*

- Once it establishes itself in a herd it is difficult to eliminate.
- It causes reproductive failure with consequent loss in production and income.
- It also infects people with a disease sometimes called "swine herds' disease", a severe flu-like condition sometimes with meningitis. There is another disease in the human called Weil's disease and this is caused by *L. icterohaemorrhagiae*.
- If you are involved in the supply of breeding stock from a farm that has just become infected you would be wise to stop sales.
- If you are involved in the export of breeding stock the importing country will usually require you to either test serologically for *L. pomona* or to put all the pigs for export on a course of streptomycin to eliminate the carrier state. The problem with the former is that some other leptospira serovars that circulate in rodents and hedge-hogs can cross-infect pigs causing no disease but causing cross reactions with *L. pomona* and false positive results. The problem with the latter is that in some countries (e.g. the USA) streptomycin is not allowed to be used in pigs.

> *If you are working in a herd with L. pomona take care not to contaminate your skin, lips or eyes with pigs' urine.*
> *L. pomona causes a nasty disease.*

Clinical signs

The disease spreads slowly through the herd causing infertility, abortions and the birth of weak premature piglets. The sows which abort are not otherwise clinically ill. If pregnant cattle are in close contact with the pigs, some of them may also abort.

If any of the pig workers on the farm go down with flu-like symptoms and develop a bad headache call the doctor immediately. Fortunately the disease in people responds to antibiotics if caught soon enough.

> *If sows are aborting and giving birth to weak litters, consider L. pomona, call your veterinarian and tell your pig people to take great care of their hygiene.*

Diagnosis

This requires the help of a diagnostic laboratory. Send paired blood samples (i.e. sows sampled on the day they abort and two weeks later) and freshly aborted piglets. The piglets may yield a rapid diagnosis if certain tests are done. Serology on the paired samples inevitably results in at least a two week delay.

The laboratory is likely to carry out micro-agglutination/lysis tests to demonstrate rising antibody titres in the sows and the presence of antibodies in the piglets' serum. The latter is conclusively diagnostic. The laboratory may also try to demonstrate the leptospiras in aborted piglets' tissues using fluorescent antibody tests (FATs) and sections stained with aniline dyes.

Management control and prevention

- ◆ Vaccination - Routine vaccination of breeding stock is practised commonly in countries in which the organism is enzootic but not so much in fringe and free areas. The vaccine, like all bacterial vaccines (bacterins) does not provide a solid immunity but usually raises the resistance sufficiently to prevent clinical signs.

  Vaccines used are inactivated and contain an adjuvant.

- ◆ Take care in the sources of your replacement stock to ensure that they are not carrying the organism.

- The organism is spread in urine from carrier animals. It can live fairly long periods in water contaminated by infected urine. Do not provide water from questionable streams and keep your water supplies and tanks clean and free from contamination.
- Contamination from pig lorries are a minor risk as compared to other infections unless the lorry has other pigs present.
- Also read the last section of this chapter.

L. TARASSOVI

This appears to be a pig adapted strain that causes reproductive problems similar to but milder than *L. pomona*.

There are very few recent reports of this in pigs. It seemed to be confined to Central and Eastern Europe, Australia and New Zealand and presumably is still there. It is believed to be still present in Hungary and Western Russia so if you live in these countries your pigs may be at risk.

PORCINE EPIDEMIC DIARRHOEA (PED)

This is an acute rapidly spreading diarrhoea similar to transmissible gastro-enteritis (TGE) but less severe. It is caused by a member of the corona virus group but is distinct from that of the TGE virus.

Should you be concerned about PED?

PED is thought to be widespread throughout most regions of Western and Central Europe except Denmark, Sweden, Ireland and possibly Austria. If you are a pig farmer in Denmark, Sweden, Ireland or Austria be aware of PED because it could get into your country and put the herd at risk.

If you are a pig farmer in the rest of Western or Central Europe, your herd is at risk. It has also been reported in China and Taiwan. Its not known whether it exists in other countries of SE Asia. If you are involved with pigs in China and Taiwan or possibly other countries of SE Asia then you might encounter it.

It has not been reported in North, Central or South America, Australia or New Zealand. If you live in any of these do not worry about it unless a specific alarm is raised, which seems most unlikely.

Importance of PED

- PED is not a very important disease economically. Mortality is low, clinical disease lasts about a week or so and then disappears spontaneously and the majority of affected pigs recover fully.
- It is important because it can be mistaken for TGE, which it is not.

Clinical signs

There are two strains of the PED virus. Type 1 causes diarrhoea in growing pigs and adults but not in sucking pigs. Type 2 causes diarrhoea in all age groups.

> *If growing and adult pigs develop an acute watery scour, (whether the piglets do or not) consider PED and TGE and call the veterinarian urgently.*

When the virus enters a susceptible herd it spreads fairly rapidly though it. The diarrhoea is watery and tends to squirt out like a hose-pipe but it has no blood in it. Very few piglets die. Each affected pig scours for about 3-5 days and then stops spontaneously. Depending on the size of the herd the clinical disease disappears in 1-2 weeks and the herd develops a strong immunity. The disease is unlikely to recur in less than two years and usually much longer.

Diagnosis

The clinical signs often give a strong indication. Confirmation and differentiation from TGE has to be done in a laboratory. Submit freshly dead piglets and blood samples from sows taken at the beginning of the outbreak and 10 days later.

Post-mortem

Very few piglets usually die so there are not many to examine. The stomach and gut contain watery and gassy fluids.

Treatment

☐ Antibiotics have little effect. Supportive measures such as the provision of electrolyte solutions and warmth are helpful with piglets and weaners. It is sensible to try to spread infected faeces from scouring pigs around the whole herd to develop a rapid immunity.

Management control and prevention

- **Vaccination**
  Vaccines are not available and would probably not be cost-effective.
- **National control programmes**
  Individual countries such as Ireland, and Denmark would not admit sero-positive pigs.
- **On-farm eradication**
  The virus seems to disappear from the herd spontaneously. If your herd is selling breeding stock it should stop doing so for about six weeks and then it may start selling again. You may want to put some pigs from a susceptible herd in first to act as sentinels but, unlike TGE, this is rarely necessary.
- **On-Farm precautions**
  - Its not known whether this virus is carried by birds (like TGE).
  - It does not seem to be windborne.
  - Nevertheless it is difficult to keep it out.
  - Refer to the final section of this chapter.

PORCINE RESPIRATORY CORONAVIRUS (PRCV)

Around 1986 several laboratory workers in Belgium and France and later in other countries who were carrying out routine testing of blood samples for TGE began to realise that an epidemic of antibodies, (i.e. positive tests) for TGE was rapidly spreading but no clinical TGE was occurring.

The cause was found to be a highly infectious virus, identical to TGE except that it had lost its ability to multiply in the intestines and therefore did not cause diarrhoea. It multiplied mainly in the lungs and appeared to be windborne by the rapidity of its spread.

It spread right across Western Europe and to the UK but not to Ireland which remains free. Very few herds escaped.

Should you be concerned about PRCV?

No!

If your pig farm is in Western Europe (except Ireland), the chances are that you already have it and probably do not know it.

If you live elsewhere you are unlikely to get it.

Importance of PRCV

There are two points of importance.
1. It cross reacts with TGE on most tests which is why countries that do not have it do not want it. (There is a special test which can differentiate between the two). If you are involved in the export of breeding pigs from Western Europe you will find difficulty in finding sero-negative breeding herds.
2. Since it spread through Western Europe TGE has almost disappeared. It is assumed that it has naturally vaccinated the national herds.

Clinical signs

A transient coughing, lasting only a few hours, which is generally not noticed by the pig people.

No other clinical signs!

It is often found in pneumonia in mixed infections with PRRS, influenza and mycoplasma but whether or not it is playing any role is not known.

Diagnosis

Blood tests done in a diagnostic laboratory capable of carrying out the differential test.

Management control and prevention

◆ **National importation programmes**
Individual countries which are free from this infection and TGE will only import pigs that are sero-negative for TGE and PRCV
◆ **On-farm precautions**
None!

SWINE VESICULAR DISEASE (SVD)

Although the virus which causes swine vesicular disease (SVD) virus is different from that causing foot-and-mouth disease (FMD) it produces a disease in pigs that is clinically indistinguishable from FMD. So if you are concerned about SVD in your pigs read also the FMD section.

Should you be concerned about SVD?

If your pig farm is in the UK, mainland Europe or S.E. Asia you should be aware of the possibility of it becoming infected with SVD, however low the risk might be. The herd will probably be slaughtered if it gets infected.

If your pig herd is in Ireland, where SVD has never occurred and which does not import pig meat products, the risk is extremely low. It is just conceivable that it could be brought in on an inadequately disinfected pig lorry returning from mainland Europe where the virus periodically circulates.

If you farm in North or South America, or Australia or New Zealand, the risk of your pig farm becoming infected with SVD or FMD is virtually nil.

Importance of SVD

- Although clinically SVD is similar to FMD it causes little impact on productivity. Often it can be so mild that the pigs do not appear lame particularly if they are on straw bedding. What is more, it is strictly a disease of pigs and does not infect cattle, goats, sheep or other species. Why then is it regarded as so important that governments, such as those in the EU, bring in costly slaughter and eradication policies? It is for the very reason first stated, namely, that it is clinically indistinguishable from FMD. They are afraid that if SVD became widespread in the pig populations of FMD free and fringe areas that pig farmers and pig veterinarians may become accustomed to seeing vesicles on pigs noses and feet and not report them or even consider FMD.
- One could argue that an expensive slaughter policy is unnecessary, that SVD could be made notifiable (i.e. any pigs with vesicles would have to be reported to the authorities) and that accurate rapid tests (e.g. ELISAs and PCRs) could be available in all diagnostic laboratories, but such an argument would be academic. The fact is that most governments in free and fringe areas would adopt a slaughter and eradication policy if there were a risk of contamination. If you farm in such an area you have to live with such a policy.

Unless you farm in Italy or S. Asia your herd will be slaughtered if it gets SVD

Clinical signs

SVD does not infect or affect cattle, sheep, goats or any species other than the pigs. So, unlike FMD, if you keep other livestock they will not be affected.

Clinical signs of SVD are much the same as FMD so read that section.

If there is no slaughter policy and pigs are not killed some may lose the claws off some of their toes. SVD does not usually cause abortion and boars are not sufficiently lame to stop serving sows. Mortality among all age groups is low.

The pigs recover completely in 2-3 weeks but you may see bruises under the claws which gradually move down under the horn as it grows (about 2mm per week). See chapter 10.

In fringe areas (e.g. in the EU) it is a serious problem because the herd will almost certainly be compulsorily slaughtered and although compensation is likely to be paid, the farm cannot be restocked for at least three months. This is twice as long as for FMD because the SVD virus is much tougher and survives longer. Furthermore, after that time small numbers of susceptible pigs may have to be introduced onto the farm to act as sentinels. If there is still residual virus in the premises these sentinels are likely to come down with disease and the farm will have to be emptied and disinfected again.

> **Cattle, sheep and goats are not affected by SVD**

The pig farm is a long time out of production even if the sentinels do not develop disease but if they do it is even longer with all the financial hardship that this will cause. So-called recrudescences on farms which had been slaughtered out, disinfected and later restocked, were a major problem in the early days of the SVD eradication programmes in Europe.

Diagnosis

This is the same as for suspected FMD. Read the FMD section. SVD cannot be distinguished from FMD on clinical grounds so to confirm the presumptive diagnosis, samples have to be sent without delay to an appropriate laboratory.

Management control and prevention

- ◆ Vaccination
  There is only one main serotype of SVD and theoretically it should be possible to produce an effective vaccine but in endemic areas the disease is too mild to warrant it. Vaccination is not allowed in fringe areas because it might mask the disease and go undiagnosed.
- ◆ Other precautions
  Countries in free and fringe areas apply strictly-enforced national preventative measures against the introduction of SVD. The main features of these measures are control over the importation of pigs and of pig meat products from counties in which SVD occurs. Pig meat products are particularly dangerous because, unlike the FMD virus, SVD virus is tough and survives rigor mortis. If infected pig meat gets into the food chain there is a risk of uncooked waste being eaten by pigs which could trigger off an outbreak. To prevent this many countries have brought in cooked waste feed policies which forbid the feeding of animal products to pigs unless they have been processed through a licensed processing plant.

> **Do not let pig-meat products contaminate your pigs or those of your neighbours**

If the disease does enter a free or fringe area, a slaughter policy is implemented similar to that described for FMD. All diseased and in-contact pigs are slaughtered. A standstill on animal movement is usually imposed and tracings are carried out to check possible spread of the disease through previous contacts.

If you farm in the EU which is an SVD-risk region you should keep in mind the possibility (small though it may be) of contamination of your herd and you should take simple appropriate precautions.

The greatest risk is from contaminated pig lorries returning from Italy where the disease is still present. The virus survives well in lorries and pigs can become infected by mouth or via skin abrasions. The lorry collecting your pigs for slaughter is the obvious danger.

> **Prevent pig lorries that carry slaughter pigs from contaminating your herd**

You should not feed pig meat products.

Windborne spread does not occur in SVD so the simple precautions outlined later in this chapter should be effective.

TESCHEN DISEASE

Also called Talfan disease, benign enzootic paresis or poliomyelitis suum.

Teschen disease is caused by a porcine enterovirus, serotype 1, of which there are highly virulent and mildly virulent variants. Teschen disease is not really an exotic disease although it may be widely regarded as such which is why it is included in this chapter. The virus probably exists throughout the world wherever pigs are kept but most infections are sub-clinical and outbreaks of clinical disease are rare.

The name Teschen disease is traditionally used for the most severe form of the disease, large outbreaks of which were reported many years ago near the borders of Germany and Poland and in Madagascar. Since then smaller, generally milder, outbreaks have occurred from time to time in other regions of the world. These milder outbreaks have usually been called by other names such as Talfan disease (Talfan is a hill in Wales where an outbreak occurred) to evade the application of a slaughter policy. Most countries in the western world had erroneously made Teschen disease notifiable very early on before it was realised that the virus was so widespread. Teschen disease was quietly removed from the EU lists of notifiable diseases several years ago.

Importance of Teschen/Talfan disease

The severe outbreaks that occurred in central Europe and Madagascar were regarded with some trepidation by other countries which is why slaughter policies were brought in. The introduction of such policies made the disease officially important. In reality the disease is now rare and unimportant.

Should you be concerned about Teschen/Talfan?

No, not unless your farm is in a country in which it's still notifiable because then, if your pigs develop the disease, overzealous officials may want to slaughter your herd.

The virus multiplies in the intestines and is shed in large quantities in the faeces. It is relatively tough, can survive outside the body, and is highly infectious requiring only a small dose of infected faeces to be ingested to establish infection in the intestines. It is therefore easily transmitted between herds on clothes, boots, lorries, machinery and equipment. It can also spread between herds through the movement of young sub-clinical carrier pigs.

Within a herd the virus cycles in the weaner and follow-on accommodation. It is prevented from multiplying in the intestines of suckled piglets by the sow's lactogenic immunity, i.e. the secretory antibodies present in her milk. After the pig has been weaned the lactogenic immunity ceases to be supplied and the virus is able to multiply in the intestines but it cannot get to the nervous system (CNS) because whenever it escapes from the gut it is neutralised by the sow's colostral antibodies which are still circulating in the pig's blood stream. The virus multiplies in the intestines harmlessly for several weeks until the pig has developed an active immunity which stops it from multiplying. The pig is then immune and virus free. If its a young gilt which is retained later for breeding it will in turn pass on its antibodies to its piglets.

The virus can only reach the central nervous system (CNS), multiply in the nerves and cause damage when there are no circulating specific antibodies or when they are at too low a level. It can then be carried in the blood stream to the CNS. This situation may arise if the mother has never been infected with the virus, if the newborn piglet didn't get enough colostrum, or if the virus enters a naive herd for the first time.

Clinical signs

The disease is directly analogous to human poliomyelitis which is caused by three serotypes of human enterovirus. The Teschen virus cannot infect people or other animals and the human polioviruses can not infect pigs.

Affected pigs develop an ascending paralysis of muscles which may progress to a complete hind end paralysis. In other words the pig partially loses the use of its lower back legs, and then its thighs and then the rear end of its body. The partial loss may progress to a total paralysis. It is an infection of the motor nerves only and not the sensory nerves. The pig still has sensation and can feel pin pricks. Initially the pig may be slightly off its feed and a little depressed for a day but after that it is otherwise fine with a good appetite and normal temperature. Its only problem is that it can't walk around very well to eat and drink and in severe cases can't rise from a dog-sitting position. Since in the severe form of the disease the motor nerves are totally destroyed the disease is irreversible. The pig never recovers, which if a lot of pigs are affected, is serious.

> *If a number of weaned pigs develop a swaying walk in their hind legs but no other clinical signs, think of Teschen/Talfan disease.*

When cases occur these days they are usually in weaned and young growing pigs. The disease does not often progress to full paralysis probably because the pigs have a level of immunity or because it is a milder strain of the virus. The pigs develop a drunken swaying gait from which many may recover spontaneously. It was anticipated that the disease might be a problem in herds set up by medicated early weaning or segregated weaning or in the development of all-in all-out multi-site production systems but this does not seem to have happened.

Diagnosis

The clinical signs are suggestive but not conclusive. Other conditions can cause a swaying gait in weaned pigs including injuries to the feet or back, bone weakness, poisonings such as arsanilic acid poisoning, the early stages of bowel oedema, or bacterial meningitis after treatment. Lack of a fever or any other signs of illness rule out classical swine fever (hog cholera), African swine fever and aujeszky's disease (pseudorabies).

Serum samples can be taken to demonstrate rising antibodies in paired blood samples taken from a group of pigs at the start of the disease and 10-14 days later. Single blood samples are no good because sub-clinical infection is fairly common and so positive blood samples are also common even when no disease has been observed.

Microscopic examination of the brains and spinal cord of pigs which have been killed will show changes typical of any virus disease but they are not specific for Teschen disease.

Treatment

There is no effective treatment.

Management control and prevention

- Effective attenuated or inactivated vaccines could be made fairly readily but there are none available commercially because the disease is so uncommon that they would not be cost effective.
- The only preventative measure is to ensure that all piglets receive a good drink of colostrum

TRANSMISSIBLE GASTRO-ENTERITIS (TGE)

See chapter 8 for further information.

TGE is an economically-damaging highly-infectious disease of pigs that is enzootic in most pig rearing countries of the world. Thus, for the majority of readers it is not an exotic disease but is enzootic and a serious risk to your herd.

Should you be concerned about TGE?

A few countries are thought to be free of it, which is why it is mentioned briefly here. They are Australia, New Zealand, Ireland and Denmark.

Australia and New Zealand are so remote from sources of infection and have such strict import controls that they are most unlikely to be contaminated.

Ireland and Denmark are more at risk. If you are involved in pig farming in either you should be aware of TGE because it is enzootic in the UK and mainland Europe. Both Ireland and Denmark have strong pig industry (producers and slaughterers) associations which take every legitimate precaution to keep TGE out but since it is commonly spread by flocks of starlings and on pig lorries and their drivers' feet, it might get in. (It did get into Ireland once several years ago but fortunately did not spread). The proximity of Denmark to Germany suggests that Denmark is at most risk but the prevalence of antibodies to porcine respiratory coronavirus (PRCV), which is antigenically closely similar to TGE, in Denmark probably reduces this risk. PRCV is not present in Ireland.

Importance of TGE

- If your herd is fully susceptible to TGE and it becomes infected up to 100% of piglets under 2 weeks of age will die. Many older sucking pigs and some weaned pigs will also die. A proportion of recently bred sows will return to service. As a rule of thumb you can predict that the number of young pigs that die will be >1.5 times the number of breeding females in the herd. The precise number depends on the actions you take and the concurrent diseases present in your herd.
- If the herd is farrow to finish you will suffer a substantial loss of revenue and negative cash flow for 4-5 weeks about 4-5 months after the outbreak and another one 4-5 months later.

Clinical signs

When TGE first enters the herd it causes acute diarrhoea in all age groups including sows. In piglets and young weaned pigs the faeces are very liquid, brightly coloured (grey, yellow, green and faun), gassy, shooting out as if from a hose-pipe and smelling strongly (typical of this disease).

Young piglets also vomit bright green or yellow vomitus. Baby piglets die in a few days.

Diagnosis

In an acute severe outbreak in a breeding herd or a farrow-to-finish herd the clinical picture provides a strong presumptive diagnosis. A main feature, which differentiates it from other diarrhoeas is that all age groups are affected. Mild outbreaks of TGE may be difficult to distinguish from PED on clinical grounds. Also TGE in grower-finisher herds may be confused with other conditions. To confirm the diagnosis, samples have to be sent without delay to a laboratory. The best samples are freshly dead or dying piglets. In grower/finishers send the youngest. Also send paired blood samples from early in the outbreak and again ten days later.

The best test, which will give an answer in a matter of hours, is to freeze the ileum (last part of the small intestine), section it for histology and carry out fluorescent antibody tests (FATs) on the sections. ELISAs may also be available in some more sophisticated laboratories. Polymerase chain reaction (PCR) tests would be possible but are probably not available. The blood samples can be subjected to serum neutralisation tests to detect rising antibody titres. Unfortunately these results take at least 2 weeks.

Treatment

- See chapter 8.

Management control and prevention

- The most important precautions are careful loading of pig lorries and keeping out visitors, starlings and other birds such as seagulls.
- Vaccination - There is only one main serotype of TGE and theoretically it should be possible to produce an effective vaccine but because of the type of

immunity involved most commercially available vaccines are not very effective

VESICULAR EXANTHEMA OF SWINE (VES)

The virus of vesicular exanthema of swine (VES) is different from those causing foot-and-mouth disease (FMD) and swine vesicular disease (SVD) but it produces a disease in pigs that is clinically indistinguishable from FMD and SVD both of which are described in detail above. Unlike FMD it only effects pigs.

You only need be concerned about VES if you have a pig farm in California, near the West coast. To everyone else it is no more than an historical curiosity. This account is therefore brief.

Importance of VES

- Infact it has not occurred since 1959 but the virus is still present in sea mammals and fish so it could occur again and you should not dismiss it completely.
- The main importance of VES is that clinically it resembles FMD and if it occurred again a slaughter policy would be applied.

Where is it?

Viruses that are virtually identical to VES virus are present in marine mammals and fish along the Pacific coast of the USA. It is therefore assumed that the source of VES was waste sea food fed to pigs as garbage or finding its way to pigs from farmed-mink fed sea-food.

History

The story of VES is unusual. It was first diagnosed in pigs in Southern California in 1932. Because of its close similarity to FMD all the pigs were destroyed. It kept reappearing in California from time to time, the pigs being slaughtered each time. Then in 1952 the virus escaped from California in a train-load of infected pork. Garbage fed pig herds came down with the disease and it spread from them to neighbouring herds until herds in 43 states were affected. It was eventually stamped out in 1956 by a major slaughter policy combined with a ban on feeding uncooked garbage to pigs. It was declared an exotic disease in the USA in 1959

The only cases outside the USA were in slaughter pigs on ship from the USA bound for Hawaii in 1947 and in pigs fed uncooked pork scraps from an American military base in Iceland in 1955.

The source of the virus remained a mystery until 1972 when an essentially similar virus was isolated from San Miguel sea lions. When inoculated experimentally into pigs it caused typical signs of VES.

Clinical signs

VES does not affect cattle, sheep, goats or any species other than the pigs and sea mammals. So, unlike FMD, if you keep other livestock they will not be affected.

Clinical signs of VES are much the same as FMD so read the section on FMD. Mortality is low but there may be some deaths in sucking piglets. Growing pigs may become debilitated.

Diagnosis

This is the same as for suspected FMD and SVD and requires laboratory tests to identify it.

Management control and prevention

- ◆ No vaccines are available.
- ◆ The cooked garbage policy in the USA should prevent its reappearance but its conceivable that an ignorant or careless person may break the rules.
- ◆ If you farm in California do not feed waste sea food to your pigs. Also, do not allow anyone working in your herd to take sandwiches or other food into the pig buildings. Provide a designated eating place for them away from the pigs. This is a good policy anyway.

VESICULAR STOMATITIS (VS)

This disease occurs mainly in South and Central America, occasionally in the USA and rarely as epidemics extending as far North as Canada and as far South as Argentina. If you farm in any of these areas you should be aware of it. The infection is more widespread involving wild life including sea mammals.

It does not occur outside the Americas. The only confirmed reports outside the Americas were France during World War 1 and South Africa during the Boer war - both associated with horses.

Importance of VS

- The VS virus produces a disease in pigs that is clinically indistinguishable FMD, SVD and VES. Most often however infection of pigs is subclinical.
- In itself it is not very important in pigs. In severe outbreaks the foot lesions may be painful and make pigs lame and there may be a reduction in growth rate. On the other hand it can be so mild that the pigs do not appear lame or ill.
- If you are concerned about VS read also the sections above on FMD and SVD (and if you work in California VES).

Species affected

In domesticated animals, VS is primarily a disease of horses and cattle only occasionally causing clinical disease in pigs. A range of wild animals including wild pigs, deer, racoons and sea mammals. People can also be infected developing flu-like symptoms.

> *VS is primarily a disease of horses and cattle only occasionally occurring in pigs.*

Clinical signs

The initial signs in affected swine are drooling saliva and a rise in body temperature to 40-41°C (106-107°F). Thereafter the clinical signs are so closely similar to those of FMD, that they need not be repeated in detail here. Like FMD, the most striking feature is the appearance of vesicles (blisters) up to 30mm diameter on the nose, lips, and teats and around the coronets of the feet which may make the pigs lame. These burst leaving erosions and ulcers. Those on the nose and mouth then heal rapidly but those on the feet may become secondarily infected and permanent damage may result. Mortality is usually low and most pigs recover in one to two weeks.

One difference from FMD is the relatively small proportion of pigs in a herd outbreak that show vesicles. Most may not although many may seroconvert as a result of sub-clinical infection. Another difference from FMD is that usually when an outbreak occurs in a pig herd it rarely if ever spreads to cattle and horses on the same farm and vice versa.

Occurrence and spread

The Americas can be divided into enzootic and epizootic regions. In the enzootic region the virus is present and cycling among animals and insects all the time. The enzootic region covers Central America, Mexico, the coastal plains of South Eastern USA and the North West of South America. The rest of the USA, Canada and South America constitute epizootic regions.

The virus is not present in these all the time but outbreaks occur seasonally and intermittently, several years often passing between epizootics. Epizootics usually start in the USA in late spring or early summer often after heavy rain, presumably reflecting the rise in the insect population. They usually end with the first frost although the 1982-83 outbreak in the USA persisted into winter.

The virus is spread mechanically by a variety of insects and has been isolated from face flies, black flies, eye gnats, sand flies, leaf hoppers and mosquitoes. The virus may multiply in some of these insects and can pass vertically through the ovaries to the offspring. Insects are therefore thought to act as reservoirs, perpetuating the virus in the enzootic regions.

It is thought that in the spread between pigs in epizootic regions insects get the virus on their mouth parts from feeding on the lesions left after the vesicles have burst and carry it mechanically to other pigs in the same herd or in neighbouring herds. It is unlikely that they get infected from sucking the pigs' blood. The erosions and ulcers are initially teeming with virus and although the virus is assumed to be carried around the body in the blood stream it is at very low undetectable levels.

The virus can also spread between pigs by direct contact particularly when pigs are tightly packed together, for example, during transport or when pigs fight after mixing. The virus is thought to be spread in these circumstances by getting into cuts and abrasions.

The virus can also be carried from herd to herd through the movement of pigs but pigs do not appear to become long term sub-clinical carriers.

Diagnosis

VS is notifiable in most epizootic areas, i.e. if you suspect it in the herd you or your veterinarian have to report it to the authorities.

The clinical signs of VS are similar to those of FMD and SVD both of which are subject to government slaughter and eradication policy in Canada, the USA, Mexico, Chile, South Brazil, and Argentina. It is therefore crucial to reach a fast accurate diagnosis. This can only be done by delivering samples to a laboratory equipped and capable of doing the appropriate tests. The aim is to eliminate the possibility of the disease being FMD or SVD (or in California VES).

The best samples to submit are vesicular fluid, if available, which has high concentrations of virus and/or vesicular tissue (e.g. the thin superficial skin layer over the vesicle) which also contains virus. If these samples are from pigs or cattle the authorities will probably only allow you to send them to a designated FMD laboratory in case the disease is FMD. If they are from a horse then they cannot be FMD (horses do not get FMD, SVD, or VES) and you may be allowed send them to other laboratories (e.g. in the USA, the USDA-NVSL at Ames or other State laboratories).

The possibility of the disease being FMD or SVD (or in California VES) should be eliminated and an accurate identification of the VS virus made. The first of these, namely, elimination of FMD, SVD and VES can probably only be done in the designated FMD laboratories. Other diagnostic laboratories may be able to do the second, namely, identification of the VS virus in samples from horses. This is done by demonstrating the presence of the VS virus in the vesicular fluid or tissue first by ELISA which is rapid giving an answer in a few hours time.

Paired blood samples (i.e. one sample taken during the early stage of the disease and one 10-14 days later) may also be taken. The authorities will probably allow these to be tested in non FMD-designated laboratories (e.g. in the USA, State laboratories). The tests used are generally ELISAs with back-up neutralisation and complement fixation tests. In horses, rising antibody levels to the VS virus have to be demonstrated in the blood samples to be sure that an active VS infection has taken place. This is because in epizootic regions some old horses may have positive antibodies from the last outbreak. Pigs generally do not live so long so single positive samples would be strongly indicative of active infection.

Unfortunately blood sampling and serology may mean a delay of at least two weeks which is too long.

Management control, prevention and Treatment

◆ **Vaccination**

It is possible to produce an effective live attenuated vaccine or an inactivated vaccine but in practice the low incidence of the disease in swine, even in the face of big outbreaks in cattle and horses makes vaccination uneconomical. Furthermore, in the USA vaccination of pigs against VS is not allowed. There are numerous serotypes of VS virus but only two (Indiana 1 and New Jersey 1) are known to affect pigs.

◆ **National precautions**

If your pig farm is in an epizootic area, which most states in the USA are for example, and VS is confirmed, the herd will not be slaughtered out to get rid of the virus because the disease is self limiting and disappears spontaneously. It is likely, however, that the authorities will quarantine your farm until they deem that the virus has gone.

In the USA, animals in any state in which outbreaks of VS are occurring cannot be legally moved to any other state or to the EU without testing and quarantine.

Countries which are completely free from VS (e.g. countries in Europe) apply national preventative measures against the introduction of VS. The main feature is control over the importation of cattle and pigs from countries in which VS occurs.

In practice it is most unlikely that VS would get into such countries, spread and become established. Pig farmers in these countries should not worry about this disease

If the disease did enter such a country, which could be through the movement of horses, a standstill on animal movement would probably be imposed and the affected animals would be isolated and might be slaughtered. Infact, it has only been identified once in Europe and that was in American military horses in France in the first world war. It did not spread or persist.

◆ **On-farm prevention and disease management**

As with other infectious diseases, if you are a pig farmer in an epizootic region be careful about the source of newly introduced pigs into your herd. Isolate them for a month to six weeks to ensure that they, or the source from which they have come, are not incubating this disease or any other.

VS is not as contagious as, say, FMD or TGE, but if the disease breaks out in neighbouring pig herds you should tighten the biosecurity of your own farm.

In the case of VS, the gap in the protective measures is that the virus is spread by insects and, of course, it is difficult to stop their movement.

If the disease breaks out in your herd the most urgent thing for you to do is to get an accurate diagnosis. Call your veterinarian immediately.

If possible, make the affected pigs comfortable by providing clean bedding. Also, give them soft food. Put them in clean pens to reduce the likelihood of secondary infections. If secondary infections occur, treat with antibiotics.

Use insect sprays and repellents to reduce the spread in your herd and to your neighbours' herds. If you supply other herds with stock, stop the movement of pigs from your herd for 30 days. (The authorities will probably insist on this anyway).

Protecting Your Herd against Serious Infectious Diseases

See chapter 2 for further information.

Vaccinate

If you farm in a country where one or more serious infectious diseases are enzootic or where there is a risk of them occurring, and if vaccines are available and vaccination is allowed, you should vaccinate your herd routinely. This does not completely prevent your herd becoming infected but it greatly reduces the chances as well as reducing the damage. Of the diseases described in this chapter effective vaccines are available in enzootic countries against classical swine fever (hog cholera) and aujeszky's disease (pseudorabies). Less effective or shorter lasting ones are available in some countries against foot-and-mouth disease, porcine reproductive and respiratory syndrome and transmissible gastro-enteritis.

Biosecurity

Whether you can vaccinate or not you should protect your investment by applying appropriate biosecurity measures. This is not just to keep out the infectious diseases covered in this chapter, although of course if you are in a high risk area this is crucial, but to keep out some of the more serious diseases covered in other chapters too.

Some viruses, such as transmissible gastro-enteritis (TGE) virus and foot-and-mouth disease (FMD) virus spread very readily and if they are spreading in your neighbourhood they are difficult to keep out of the herd no matter what precautions you take. This is partly because they are highly infectious so that it only takes the entry of a few viable virus particles to set off a major outbreak. It is also because they are carried on the wind, or on birds or flies which are difficult or impossible to guard against. Fortunately not all infectious agents are like that. Some viruses and bacteria spread less readily. Examples in this chapter are swine vesicular disease (SVD) and classical swine fever (hog cholera). You can keep them out fairly reliably if you take appropriate biosecurity precautions.

Vehicles

You should take precautions against contamination from vehicles. The lorry picking up pigs for slaughter is a particular danger. Always insist that it has been well washed out before visiting the herd and that it also always visits your herd first. You should also take precautions against contamination from such lorries by building a safe pig-loading bay and by not allowing the driver into your pig buildings.

> **Do not let slaughter-pig lorries or their drivers contaminate your herd**

Pig meat products

You should not feed pig meat products unless they have been thoroughly cooked. You may not be permitted to feed them in your country and it is safer not to feed meat products at all. Do not allow anyone to take sandwiches or food into the pig buildings. Provide a designated eating place for them away from the pigs. Also, if you know of any 'back-yard' type pigs or pet pigs in your neighbourhood stress to the owners the importance of not feeding human waste food or scraps from the table. Maintenance people and builders may keep pigs at home.

> **Do not let pig-meat products contaminate your pigs or those of your neighbours**

Incoming pigs

Any replacement pigs coming on to the premises should come from known safe sources and should be quarantined, or at least physically separated from your own pigs, for at least a month, preferably six weeks. You can use the second half of this time to apply acclimatisation procedures to adapt them to the microbial flora of your herd, and to your feed and management procedures. The pigs can also be vaccinated if necessary.

Physical barriers

If some or all of your pig buildings are open sided or easy to access, they should be ring-fenced or walled off to protect your herd from stray animals, (particularly wild pigs), or human intruders entering your pig buildings. If your buildings are fully walled with limited access (e.g. like many in Denmark, Canada and in the mid-western states of the USA), and if the doors are strong and lockable, then a fence may not be necessary.

The necessity for strong physical barriers depends on the country in which you farm.

The most dangerous animals are wild pigs, particularly where they may be infected with classical swine fever (hog cholera) virus as in Germany, Poland and possibly Italy.

Stray dogs can spread transmissible gastro-enteritis (TGE) and probably other diseases. Whether you should keep a guard dog in the compound depends on the level of crime (pig rustling and equipment thefts). Some pig farms in countries such as Portugal have them patrolling between two parallel perimeter fences. Cats can be an asset if they are contained within the pig buildings all the time as they are in Denmark. They help to keep down the mice and rats. But if dogs and cats are kept in the pig compound or buildings, do not feed them pig meat products.

> **Erect stout barriers to keep intruders and stray animals away from your pigs**

Foxes can be a problem, particularly in outdoor breeding herds but it is not known what pig diseases they may spread.

Badgers in the UK can spread bovine TB and hares in Denmark, Poland and possibly neighbouring countries under some circumstances spread *Brucella suis* and have infected outdoor breeding herds.

Birds, mainly starlings, spread diseases in their droppings including avian TB, erysipelas and most seriously, TGE.

Thieves are a menace, not just because they steal your pigs or equipment but also because they are probably dirty and unhygienic and may well infect your herd.

Visitors

Reduce visitors to a minimum and make any that have to enter your pig building change into clothes and boots that are kept on the farm. One way of ensuring that they change all their clothes before entry is to insist on them taking a shower. If they wash their hair while showering it adds to the farm biosecurity. Compulsory showering helps to deter visitors and raises biosecurity attitudes. You might also insist that visitors stay away from other pigs for a period of time before visiting. A minimum period would be one night. Some pig farmers with large herds insist on two nights down-time. If you do not insist on down-time, check whether your visitors have come from contaminated places like pig farms, slaughter houses, animal renderers, or post-mortem rooms. If they have, do not let them in. Make them sign a visitors' book stating that they have not been in such places.

> **Reduce visitors to a minimum. Check on where they have come from. Make them change into your clothes and boots.**

You and the other pig attendants should follow the same rules and keep away from contact with other pigs and contaminated places too.

Control of rodents and flies

Rats can carry a variety of diseases from one pig farm to another. Mice do not travel much between pig farms but they do perpetuate infections such as salmonella and swine dysentery. Flies can carry infections such as streptococci that cause pig meningitis and can travel up to about 3km (2 miles) between pig herds.

Water, feed and bedding sources

Check on the source and cleanliness of the water you provide to your pigs. Water can bring a number of infections such as leptospira and salmonella. If in doubt, chlorinate it. Check also the water storage tanks and pipes.

Scrutinise feed sources and constituents. Avoid meat and bone meal. In the USA where there is a very rapid turn round of grains through the compounders it is thought that feed may spread TGE. If you are worried about this store it for a few days before feeding it.

Bedding, if used, should come from a pig-free source and not become contaminated by birds, rats or mice during storage.

> **Consider bird-proofing your buildings. It will pay for itself in saved feed as well as protecting your herd**

"Keep out notices"

Provide large notices and a siren/klaxon type door bell so visitors can contact farm workers without need for entering the farm. Alternatively provide a mobile phone number as many mangers now carry these.

Chapter 12

13 Poisons: Recognition, Treatment and Control

Dose effect 423
Intake of poisons..423
Detoxification and excretion 423
Factors in the pig that influence the effects of a poison...........................423
How to recognise poisoning..423
Clinical signs of different poisons...425
Potential poisons 426
    Algae..426
    Arsenic...427
    Coal tars..427
    Copper 427
    Ethylene glycol...428
    Fluorine 428
    Herbicides...428
    Iron dextran..428
    Insecticides 429
        Carbamates 429
        Chlorinated hydrocarbons 429
        Pyrethrins 429
        Organophosphorus compounds (OPs)..429
    Lead 430
    Manganese 430
    Medicines..430
        Carbadox 430
        Furazolidone 430
        Monensin 430
        Olaquindox 431
        Penicillin...431
        Salinomycin..431
        Sulphonamides 431
        Tiamulin 431
    Mercury...431
    Metaldehyde...431
    Mycotoxins..431
        Aflatoxins..432
        Ergot toxins 433
        Fumonisins..433
        Ochratoxin and citrinin...433
        Trichothecenes..434
        Zearalenone 434
    Nitrates and nitrites 434
    Plants...435
        Bracken *(Pteridium aquilinum)*...435
        Cocklebur *(Xanthium)*..435
        Deadly nightshade *(Solanum)* 435
        Oak leaves and acorns 435
        Pigweed *(Amaranthus)*..435
        Pokeweed *Phytolacca)*..435
        Sorghum *(Sorghum)* 435
        Yellow jasmine *(Gelsemium)*..435

Water hemlock (*Conium maculatum*) 435
Salt (water deprivation) 435
Selenium 436
Toxic (slurry) gases 436
    Ammonia 436
    Carbon dioxide 437
    Carbon monoxide 437
    Hydrogen sulphide 437
    Methane 437
Warfarin 438

13 Poisons: Recognition, Treatment and Control

Dose Effect

Most poisons and medicinal products are dependant upon the size of dose for their clinical effects. These progress from:
- No clinical signs.
- A therapeutic effect.
- A toxic effect.
- A lethal effect.

The degree of toxicity is measured by a term LD_{50} which is the dose that will kill 50% of the exposed population.

Intake of Poisons

A toxic compound may gain entry by mouth and the intestinal tract, the respiratory tract, the eye, the womb, through the skin or by injection. It is transported via the blood stream and deposited in various tissues throughout the body. It is important to know which of these are involved so that relevant tests can be carried out.

Detoxification and Excretion

Water soluble poisons are excreted by the kidney in the urine. Other poisons are first detoxified in the liver into water soluble compounds and then excreted in the urine. Some poisons are detoxified in to non-water soluble substances which may then be combined with other substances to neutralise them further. Fat soluble poisons are likely to accumulate in the liver. Poisons may also be excreted through the skin or through the milk with possible adverse effects on sucking piglets. Some may be absorbed across the placenta of the pregnant sow and affect the foetus. Tissues used for testing include liver, kidney, blood and stomach contents.

Factors in the Pig that Influence the Effects of a Poison

- The age of the pig.
- Its weight and size. Generally the younger the pig the more severe the effect.
- The nutritional status and feed intake.
- The health status.
- The droplet size of the toxin. The smaller the size the greater the absorption.
- Sex. Gilts and sows for example are more susceptible to organophosphorus poisoning.

How to Recognise Poisoning

This is never easy because of the myriad of potentially toxic substances likely to be present on a farm, however always look for the most common and obvious first.

A poison may only affect an individual animal within a group because it was the only one inadvertently exposed to it. For example a toxic dose of medicine was administered by mistake.

> *If litigation is a possibility, document in detail all your observations and the time they were made.*

Similarly most or all the pigs in a pen, a number of pens or a complete building may be affected, indicating a much wider exposure. Finally a complete herd may be affected - invariably associated with a common feed, water source or airborne pollution.

Step 1 - Study the history carefully

Consult with your veterinarian
- Is the onset rapid - usually within 48 hours? If so, are a number of pigs affected?
- Is only a particular age group affected, for example gilts, sows, sucking piglets? If so, what is common to the group?
- What routines, medicines, management procedures have been applied to the group recently?
- Is a particular area of the farm or a number of pens affected? If so are there any common factors?
- Does the appearance of the condition coincide with the introduction of a new batch of feed or feed ingredients, a change in water or other local change?

Step 2 - Clinical signs

- List the clinical signs. (See Fig.13-1 and Fig.13-2).
- Common features of poisoning include:
- Rapid onset - (There are however exceptions depending on the dose level and period of exposure).
- A defined group of pigs affected.
- A number of pigs with identical clinical signs.
- Not a recognisable disease.
- Rectal temperatures are usually normal.

Managing Pig Health and the Treatment of Disease

Poison	General	Nervous	Digestive	Circulatory	Reproductive	Urinary	Skin	Sudden Death	Liver	Respiratory	Lameness
Algae		✓		✓				✓	✓	✓	
Arsenic: Inorganic			✓	✓							
Organic		✓	✓					✓			✓
Coal Tars		✓			✓		✓	✓			✓
Copper	✓		✓	✓				✓	✓	✓	
Ethylene glycol	✓	✓				✓		✓		✓	
Fluorine		✓	✓								✓
Herbicides		✓		✓			✓	✓		✓	
Iron dextran								✓		✓	✓
Insecticides (except OPs)	✓	✓									
Aldrin	✓	✓						✓			
Benzene hexachloride	✓	✓						✓			
Chlorinated	✓	✓						✓			
Organo-phosphorus	✓	✓	✓	✓				✓		✓	
Lead		✓	✓							✓	
Manganese			✓								✓
Medicines - General	✓	✓		✓	✓	✓		✓		✓	
Medicines - Specific											
Carbadox	✓	✓	✓					✓	✓		✓
Furazolidone		✓							✓		
Monensin	✓	✓	✓	✓						✓	✓
Olaquinidox	✓	✓									
Penicillin		✓	✓	✓					✓		
Salinomycin	✓								✓		
Sulphonamides						✓					
Tiamulin	✓							✓	✓		
Mercury		✓	✓				✓			✓	
Metaldehyde		✓									
Mycotoxins:	✓	✓							✓		
Aflatoxin			✓	✓		✓			✓		
Ergot				✓				✓			
Fumonisins					✓					✓	
Ochratoxin and			✓			✓			✓		
Trichothecenes		✓	✓								
Zearalenone			✓		✓						✓
Nitrates / Nitrites			✓	✓				✓		✓	
Plants - General	✓	✓	✓	✓		✓				✓	
Bracken								✓		✓	
Salt (water deprivation)		✓						✓			
Selenium	✓							✓		✓	✓
Toxic gases											
Ammonia	✓									✓	
Carbon dioxide		✓									
Carbon monoxide				✓			✓	✓		✓	
Hydrogen sulphide		✓		✓				✓		✓	
Methane		✓									
Warfarin				✓			✓	✓		✓	

(Fig.13-1)

Clinical Signs of Different Poisons

A broad outline of how different poisons affect different systems of the pig is given in Fig.13-1. This can be used to help identify possible causes, particularly if used in conjunction with Fig.13-2. Specific systems of the body may be affected and develop the following signs:

Circulatory system
Anaemia.
Cyanosis (blue discoloration of skin).
Increased respiration.
Jaundice.
Haemorrhage.

Digestive system
Abdominal pain.
Diarrhoea - with or without haemorrhage.
Rectal prolapse.
Salivation.
Vomiting.

General effects
Generalised malaise.
Reduced feed intake or complete inappetance.
Reduced growth.

Locomotor system
Abnormal gait.
Ataxia.
Incoordination.
Lameness.

Nervous system
Blindness.
Excitation.
Fits.
Incoordination.
Spasmodic movements.

Reproductive system
Abnormal oestrus.
Swollen vulva.
Abortion.
Embryo absorption.
Failure of fertilisation.

Respiratory system
Coughing.
Difficulty breathing.
Pneumonia (found at post-mortem examination).
Sneezing, nasal discharge.

Skin
Colour.
Haemorrhage.
Irritation.
Vesicles.

Urinary system
Blood in the urine.
Cystitis / pyelonephritis (found at post-mortem examination).
Excess mineral deposits (found at post-mortem examination or in the urine).
Pus.

CLINICAL SIGNS AND POSSIBLE POISONS		
Signs Observed	Possible Poisons	
Individual or Grouped Sows/Boars		
Blindness Incoordination Lameness Nervous fits Trembling	Algae Arsenic Chlorinated hydrocarbons Lead Mercury	Organophosphorus compounds Medicine overdose * Plants Water deprivation * Vitamin E / selenium
Diarrhoea Inappetance Vomiting	Arsenic Bad food * Mercury Monensin * Moulds	Nitrates / nitrites Organophosphorus compounds Plants
Breathing difficulty Circulation problems Skin discoloration	Algae Carbadox Carbon monoxide	Ergot Monensin Warfarin
Sudden Death	Algae Bracken Coal tars	Nitrites Toxic gases *
Abortion Reproductive failure	Carbon monoxide Ergot toxin	Medicines * Mycotoxins *
Blood, mucus, pus in the urine	Ethylene glycol Mercury Mycotoxins	Oak leaves and acorns Plants
Sucking Pigs		
Fits Incoordination Lameness Nervous Trembling	BHC Furazolidone * Iron dextran	Medicine overdose * Organophosphorus compounds Penicillin *
Diarrhoea Inappetance Vomiting	Bacterial toxins Medicine overdose Penicillin	
Breathing difficulty Skin discoloration	Ammonia Bacterial toxins Carbon monoxide Iron dextran	Medicine overdose Nitrates / nitrites Vitamin E / selenium
Sudden death	Coal tars Furazolidone Iron dextran Medicinal anaphylaxis (shock)	Nitrates / nitrites BHC Toxic gases
Weaned and Growing Pigs		
Blindness Coma Fits Incoordination Lameness Trembling	Arsenic (arsanilic acid) Coal tars Hydrocarbons Medicines Monensin	Olaquindox Organophosphorus compounds Plants Water deprivation Toxic gases
Diarrhoea Inappetance Vomiting	Arsenic Carbadox Copper Lead Mercury	Monensin Mycotoxins Oak leaves and acorns Plants
Breathing difficulties Circulatory problems Skin discoloration	Bacterial toxins Carbadox Monensin	Nitrates / nitrites Toxic gases Vitamin E / selenium
Sudden death	Bracken Organophosphorus compounds	Salt Toxic gases Vitamin E/selenium

* More likely to occur

(Fig 13-2)

Step 3 - Post-mortem examinations and records of mortality

Post mortem examinations may assist in differentiating between a specific disease and toxic conditions. Samples from tissues are probably required for further laboratory tests. The number of deaths and whether they are sudden or after a short or prolonged illness may characterise certain poisons.

The information assessed from steps 1 to 3 will raise a suspicion of poisoning.

Step 4 - Identify the possible sources of the poison

- List the chemicals on the farm - sprays, pesticides etc.
- List the medicines on the farm.
- What injections have been given?
- Are rodenticides used and available?
- Are parasecticides used?
- Could any sources of feed be suspected?
- Is there evidence of spoiled or mouldy feed or mould in the feed delivery system?
- Consider water, bedding and other environmental contaminants.
- Are sprays / disinfectants used?
- In out-door herds consider plants, water and environmental contaminants.
- Do any of the signs fit into Fig.13-1 or Fig.13-2?

Step 5 - Identify the toxin

Use Fig.13-1 to identify the potential toxin or toxins, together with the history and symptoms.

Step 6 - Read about the poison

Refer to the poison in the text and administer treatments in conjunction with veterinarian advice.

Step 7 - Confirm the poison

Refer samples to a lab for confirmation. (Fig.13-3).

Potential Poisons

ALGAE

If drinking water becomes heavily contaminated with green and blue toxin producing algae, acute disease and high mortality can take place. Poisoning is only likely to be seen in pigs outdoors where there is access to ponds used as drinking water (unless of course indoor pigs derive their water from such sources). Large numbers of algae appear in the water during periods of warm sunny weather. Wind blows the organisms to the waters edge where they are ingested by the pig. The algae produce highly toxic substances that cause massive damage to the liver and haemorrhage and / or affect the nervous system causing coma and respiratory failure. Post mortem examinations show a grossly enlarged liver with haemorrhages.

TOXIC LEVELS OF POISONS		
Poison	Non Toxic Levels. Less Than	Reported Toxic Levels from Mild to Severe Effect
Ammonia	25ppm	50 - 150ppm
Arsenic - Inorganic	50 mg/kg livew't Liver, 1 ppm kidney 1ppm	10 - 200 mg/kg in feed Liver, kidney 10ppm
Organic	100ppm in feed	1000ppm for 2-3 days in feed 400ppm for 14 days in feed 300ppm, 21-28 days in feed
Carbadox	50ppm in feed	100 - 300ppm in feed
Carbon monoxide	30ppm	60 - 250ppm
Clay-pigeons	-	10 - 15g ingested
Copper	200ppm in feed	200 - 600ppm in feed Liver > 250ppm Kidney > 60ppm 20 mg/kg liveweight
Ergot	0.2% sclerotia	0.3% sclerotia
Furazolidone	400ppm in feed	500 - 1000ppm in feed
Hydrogen sulphide	50ppm	80 - 900ppm
Lead		600 mg/kg in feed Liver or kidney 3ppm
Mercury	Kidney <2ppm Liver 0.3ppm Feed 1ppm	Liver 40 - 70ppm Kidney 40 - 100ppm 2 - 13 mg/kg liveweight 1.5 - 10ppm in feed Single dose of 5 - 15mg/kg
Metaldehyde		V. small amounts of pellets
Monensin	100 ppm in feed 10 mg/kg livew't	200 - 400ppm in feed 20 mg/kg liveweight
Nitrates	150 - 400ppm	1500ppm
Nitrites	10mg/kg livew't	15 - 20mg/kg liveweight 40ppm in water
Nutritional poisons	See Chapter 14	
Olaquindox	100 ppm in feed	300 - 500ppm in feed
Salt	2% ad lib water	0.5% in feed - no water
Selenium	0.1 - 0.3ppm	3 - 10ppm in feed, >12ppm in liver
Tiamulin	150ppm in feed	200ppm in feed
Warfarin		Low levels

ppm = g/tonne = mg/kg

(Fig.13-3)

Clinical signs

The onset of symptoms is usually sudden and within one to two hours. Death within 24 hours. Pigs show sudden collapse, muscle tremors, convulsions, discoloured skin and bloody diarrhoea.

Diagnosis

A history of pigs having access to water showing evidence of algae blooms suggests poisoning. Clinical signs and post mortem examinations provide strong diagnostic evidence. A sample of the algae should be sent to a laboratory for identification and information sought on how to control it.

Treatment

There is no specific treatment.

Give gastrointestinal absorbents such as charcoal and kaolin as a drench in water or in feed if practicable.

Pigs should be removed immediately from the source

of water and housed away from sunlight in warm surroundings.

Management control and prevention

Provide an alternative source of water or if this is not possible install a fence to allow access to only a small area of the waterline. Protect this by a muslin barrier to hold back large numbers of the algae.

Multi-vitamin injections particularly the B complex may help.

ARSENIC

Arsenic exists as both inorganic and organic compounds. Inorganic arsenicals are little used today except in a few rodenticides, insecticides and weed killers.

Organic arsenicals are less toxic than the inorganic ones and are used in some countries to control swine dysentery, to treat eperythrozoonosis or as growth promoters. The common chemicals are arsanilic acid, sodium arsanilate, roxarsone (3-nitro - 4-hydroxyphenyl arsonic acid) and carbasone.

Clinical signs

Poisoning with inorganic compounds results in acute illness with severe damage to the intestinal tract. Clinical signs include vomiting, acute diarrhoea and colic, dehydration, convulsions, collapse and death.

The onset of clinical signs in organic arsenical poisoning vary according to the level of intake. At low levels nothing may be seen for two to three weeks, when mild signs of incoordination and possibly blindness occur. With high doses clinical signs may be seen within two to three days, as incoordination, paralysis of the hind legs and blindness. The blindness is often irreversible. Affected animals continue to grow if they can get to feed and water. Very high doses of organic arsenicals may cause gastro-enteritis.

Diagnosis

This is determined by the history, availability of arsenical compounds and analysis of feed or suspect substances.

Treatment

There is no effective antidote but if the compounds are removed immediately most pigs recover.

COAL TARS

The distillation of coal tar and crude petroleum products produces a variety of substances including creosols or phenolic compounds, crude creosote and pitch. These substances are used as disinfectants and preservatives and may be eaten by pigs. Pitch is used as a binder in clay pigeons and it only requires 10-15g ingested over a seven day period to produce mortalities. Tar papers, bitumen on floors and creosote treated wood are further sources of poisoning. Coal tar preparations are also irritant to the skin.

> *If you suspect poisoning always seek veterinary advice.*

Clinical signs

The first signs of clay pigeon poisoning are prostration or coma leading rapidly to sudden death. Pigs may be found dead.

Low levels of intake interfere with the absorption of vitamin A and produce signs of deficiency including piglet malformation and stillbirths. If the skin of a newborn piglet comes into contact with phenolic disinfectants, contact areas, particularly the teats and soles of the feet may be burnt.

Diagnosis

This includes a history of access to phenolic and other coal tar preparations. Look for evidence of contamination particularly in outdoor pigs.

Treatment and control

There is no effective treatment.

The environment should always be examined for evidence of exposure particularly where sows are outdoors.

Injections of vitamin A using multi-vitamin preparations may be of value.

COPPER

Copper sulphate is added routinely in some countries to grower rations as a growth promoter at levels between 50-175ppm. Levels above 250ppm may interfere with normal growth rate particularly if the levels of zinc and iron in the ration are low. If the levels of zinc and iron are normal a level of 500ppm becomes toxic. Plants such as subterranean clover may also produce a mineral imbalance in outdoor pigs by increasing the retention of copper.

Clinical signs

These are usually gradual in onset unless there has been a massive intake of copper. In acute poisoning there is severe gastro-enteritis, abdominal pain, diarrhoea and jaundice, an enlarged liver and blood in the urine. In less acute cases there is anaemia and reduced growth rate.

Diagnosis

This is based on history, clinical signs and post-mortem findings. Laboratory tests for copper levels of more than 250ppm in the liver and 60ppm in the kidney confirm the diagnosis.

Treatment

The response to treatment is poor.
Calcium versonate by injection can be of help.
Seek veterinary advice.

ETHYLENE GLYCOL

This is a substance commonly used in antifreeze liquids in engine coolants. Ethylene glycol is very toxic and only 4-5ml per kg body weight are required to produce signs.

Clinical signs

In acute poisoning pigs vomit, become depressed, lose locomotor function, develop kidney failure and die. Death may occur within 12 to 24 hours and is often the only sign observed.

The tissues throughout the body become acid. In less acute cases pigs suffer depression, gastro-enteritis, abdominal distension, difficult breathing and nervous symptoms.

Diagnosis

This is based on history of access to antifreeze, clinical signs and post-mortem lesions.

Treatment and control

There is no treatment although some success has been reported using 5% sodium bicarbonate intravenously to reduce the acid state of the blood. Seek veterinary advice.

FLUORINE

Fluorine poisoning is uncommon in swine but may occur on heavily contaminated pastures. In acute cases of poisoning, diarrhoea, lameness and nervous signs may be seen. In chronic cases however lameness may be the only symptom.

Diagnosis

This is carried out by assessing fluorine levels in bone which should be less than 600ppm.

HERBICIDES

Poisonings associated with herbicides are much more common in cattle and sheep than in pigs. The important ones however include arsenic, borax and pentachlorphenols (PCPs). The latter can be absorbed through intact skin or mucous membranes to which they are highly irritant.

PCP's are used widely as preservatives, insecticides, fungicides and molluscicides but generally they are inactivated in soils when used correctly. Contact with treated wood used in feeding troughs can cause salivation and severe irritation to the mouth.

Clinical signs

These include nervous changes, respiratory distress, tremors, muscle weakness, convulsions and death.

Diagnosis

This can be difficult but a careful examination of the products on the farm and their access will often assist.

Treatment

If nervous signs are severe use a sedative such as stresnil. Give electrolytes.

IRON DEXTRAN

Iron injections as iron dextran are given by intramuscular or subcutaneous injections to piglets between one and seven days of age. This is to correct the development of iron deficiency that leads to anaemia. A dose level of 100-200mg per piglet is required. If sows or gilts become deficient in vitamin E and / or selenium during pregnancy, piglets are also born deficient. Under such circumstances the enzymes which metabolise the iron cannot function and the iron then becomes toxic.

Clinical signs

The piglet becomes acutely lame, a dark swelling occurs at the site of the injection (usually the thigh) and about 50% of the litter or more die within hours.

Diagnosis

The association between injections and symptoms is usually clear and the clinical signs are typical. The cut muscle surface where the iron has been injected loses all its structure and appears almost like wet fish muscle. This is due to necrosis (death) of the tissues.

Treatment

The initial reaction often is to blame the iron. It is true that inferior quality iron dextrans (usually the cheap ones) are more likely to be associated with severe disease than better quality ones but the primary problem is selenium/vitamin E deficiency.

As soon as the condition is recognised all the piglets that have had iron within the last two days should be injected with vitamin E/selenium according to the manufacturers recommendations.

All females due to farrow within seven days should be injected with vitamin E/selenium.

Sows within the last month of pregnancy should be injected with vitamin E, two weeks before farrowing.

Management control and prevention

Excessive oxidation of fats in the sow feed is the most common cause of low vitamin E status. Oxidation results from poor storage of cereals or corn and particularly in situations where the bottoms of feeds bins are not cleaned out and moisture has gained access.

As a precaution add an extra 150iu/tonne of vitamin E to the sow feed for the next two months.

Check the sources and storage facilities of all feed grains.

INSECTICIDES

Insecticides by virtue of their actions are toxic or lethal poisons and it is important that the manufacturers instructions are followed when using them. Furthermore most of these chemicals are absorbed through the skin and therefore become potentially hazardous to the operator. Take note of the detailed recommendations for use, particularly when handling the concentrate. Poisoning in pigs from insecticides may arise from incorrect application, pigs eating contaminated feed or accidental exposure. Insecticides are available as four different chemical types; carbamate, chlorinated hydrocarbons, pyrethrins and organophosphorus compounds (OPs).

All insecticides act on the nervous system and the general symptoms are similar. These include muscle tremors, hyperactivity and ultimately convulsions and death.

CARBAMATES

The most common of these are carbaril and methomyl which are often used to destroy worms and other insects. They act by blocking the transmission of nervous impulses at nerve muscle junctions and act in a similar manner to organophosphorus compounds. The antidote is atropine sulphate by injection and veterinary advice should be sought.

CHLORINATED HYDROCARBONS

These include aldrin, benzene hexachloride (BHC), lindane, chlordane, dieldrin, methoxychlor and toxaphene. They are highly effective against insects, but due to their side effects and toxicity to humans a number of them are now prohibited. BHC is still used in large animals and dogs and lindane is the best known proprietary name used in pigs. Most hydrocarbons are restricted to use on crops.

Clinical signs

All chlorinated hydrocarbons stimulate the central nervous system and signs include twitching of the muscles of the face, generalised muscle trembling and shivering, followed by fits coma and death. Some pigs may stand with heads pressed against the wall continually licking and chewing, others show loss of leg function (ataxia). Symptoms appear within 24 hours. The chlorinated hydrocarbons are absorbed by the body fat.

Diagnosis

Whilst the history assists in indicating the type of poison, a laboratory analysis of the brain, kidney, liver and fat tissues is required for confirmation. Pseudorabies and salt poisoning (water deprivation) can give similar signs.

Treatment and control

There are no known antidotes but severe nervous signs can be controlled by barbiturates.

Chlorinated hydrocarbons are excreted slowly from the body over a long period of time and suspected carcasses should be destroyed and not used as food.

PYRETHRINS

Pyrethrins are naturally occurring substances found in the chrysanthemum plant and have a powerful knock down effect on insects. Synthetic compounds are manufactured that have similar effects. Toxicity is relatively low and it is unlikely to be seen unless massive doses are either absorbed through the skin or taken in by mouth. All compounds have an effect on the central nervous system causing excitation, convulsions, coma and death. Marked muscle trembling and paralysis may also be seen. Most pigs die from respiratory failure.

Treatment

Pigs usually recover naturally and none is required. Activated charcoal or attapulgite given by stomach tube will reduce absorption.

ORGANOPHOSPHORUS COMPOUNDS (OPS)

These groups of drugs are widely used as insecticides and pesticides. OPs and similar carbamate insecticides affect the chemical transmitters that control the nerve endings in muscles. The result is over activity causing muscles to go into a continual spasm.

Clinical signs

The continual and excessive stimulation of the muscles in acute poisoning causes excessive salivation, the passing of faeces and urine and a very stiff awkward gait. This may be followed by vomiting, diarrhoea and muscle tremors of the face and body. Death can be fairly rapid, within 1 to 4 hours and is caused by respiratory failure.

Diagnosis

A history of exposure to OPs gives rise to a suspicion and together with the clinical signs point to a diagnosis. The insecticides will be identified in the stomach or in the suspect material such as feed, but detection is unlikely in body tissues.

Treatment and control

The antidote is atropine sulphate at 0.5mg/kg bodyweight by intramuscular injection. The response is usually seen within 3 to 5 minutes. Consult your veterinarian immediately.

Move affected pigs to well bedded hospital pens.
Give activated charcoal or attapulgite by mouth if possi-

ble to absorb the insecticide.

LEAD

Compared to ruminants swine are not easily poisoned by lead and lead poisoning is rare. A level of at least 30mg per day is required before any signs are seen. Lead acts on the central nervous system causing pain, grinding of the teeth, blindness, severe muscle twitching and incoordination. Kidney tissue is a good source for sampling and levels of more than 4ppm indicate poisoning.

Treatment

Calcium EDTA 1% solutions are used for treatments at a level of 110mg/kg.

MANGANESE

Normal levels in the diet range from 3 to 10ppm. At 60ppm feed intake and daily gain are affected. Levels above 3000ppm may produce clinical signs including a slight stiffness and abnormal gait. Poisoning would be rare.

MEDICINES

Sometimes reputable medicinal products, which normally at correct dosages may be highly beneficial, cause a toxic or allergic reaction. This may be because they are given to the wrong species by accident, e.g. cross contamination of feed, administration of too high a dose, or are given with another drug with which they are incompatible. They may cause a hypersensitivity reaction in an individual. If the medicament causing the problem is in the feed, analysis of feed samples should confirm the tentative diagnosis. If the feed is suspected random samples should be retained in case a liability dispute arises. (See chapter 15 Sampling Feeds)

CARBADOX

This drug (Mecadox, Pfizer), is used as a growth promoter at a level of 10-20ppm (10-20g/tonne) and also in the treatment and prevention of swine dysentery at 50ppm. Poisoning may commence at 200ppm in a mild form and acute disease at 300ppm or more, usually because mistakes have been made in mixing it in feed. At the lower level of 200ppm there is reduced feed intake and growth rate, hard faeces and excessive hair growth. Incoordination, posterior paralysis and death occur after 5 to 10 days of continuous consumption. There is no antidote. At post-mortem examination lesions may be found in the kidneys and adrenal glands.

FURAZOLIDONE

Furazolidone is a member of a group of drugs called the nitrofurans that have been used over many years for treating enteric and respiratory diseases.

The drug is used orally for treating piglet diarrhoea and by in-feed medication to control post-weaning enteric disease. Levels of up to 400ppm cause no problems. At levels above 500ppm inappetance and mild nervous signs are seen, progressing to ataxia, fits, coma and death. The drug is fairly quickly excreted from the system and pigs return to normal 4 to 5 days after withdrawal. Newborn piglets become depressed, hypothermic and lay on their sides, paddling and frothing at the mouth. These effects are most likely to occur if the drug is given immediately at birth rather than 6 to 7 hours after colostrum intake.

It is common to dose piglets at birth to prevent diarrhoea. Those with low birth weight (< 800g) are susceptible to poisoning.

MONENSIN

This substance is used as a growth promoter and marketed under the trade name Rumensin (Elanco). It is also an effective drug in the treatment and prevention of swine dysentery. There is a narrow gap between therapeutic and toxic levels. The therapeutic level in swine is 10mg/kg or 100g to the tonne. Clinical signs are seen when levels are twice this and heavy mortality occurs when they reach 400g/tonne. Most poisonings occur in pigs either through the accidental addition of rumensin or where the calculated inclusion level has been incorrect.

Clinical signs

Clinical signs of poisoning usually occur within 12 hours of intake and include heavy and difficult breathing, frothing around the mouth, loss of use of the hind legs and generalised muscle weakness. Diarrhoea may also be seen. The toxic effects of monensin are exaggerated if either of the antibiotics salinomycin at 60ppm or tiamulin at 100ppm are also contained in the feed. Some affected pigs, particularly those that have lost the use of their hind legs may take two to three weeks to recover but many of these die.

Diagnosis

This is based on the clinical signs and post-mortem lesions, both of which are characteristic, together with the history of the use of monensin. The lesions observed at post-mortem examination include pale areas in the muscles of the diaphragm, thighs, lower shoulders, back, ribs and heart necrosis (with equal distribution on each side). The bladder may contain red-brown urine. Feed samples should be examined for the presence of monensin. A test for this is fairly quick and straight forward. Contamination of pig feed is not uncommon because the drug is used widely as a growth promoter in cattle and if it occurs in the presence of tiamulin or salinomycin can become toxic.

Treatment

There is no antidote for monensin poisoning.

OLAQUINDOX

This is used as a growth promoter and to control post-weaning diarrhoea. The margins between therapeutic and toxic dose are narrow. The normal level is up to 100ppm but 300ppm or more will give rise to inappetance and incoordination with progressive loss of limb function as the dose rate is increased.

PENICILLIN

Penicillin and in particular the combination of procaine penicillin and benzathine penicillin occasionally causes vomiting in individuals or small groups of pigs when given by intramuscular injection. This is particularly marked in piglets less than ten days of age where an acute sensitivity reaction sometimes occurs. Within 3 to 4 minutes of injection piglets collapse lay on their side paddling and frothing at the mouth. Fortunately this episode passes off within thirty minutes with most pigs returning to normal. Long-acting injections of penicillin given to weaners will also cause a proportion of pigs to vomit but this is of no consequence.

SALINOMYCIN

Salinomycin is used as a growth promoter in pigs at levels of between 30-60ppm. It should not be used simultaneously with tiamulin and there must be seven days between the last exposure to salinomycin and the commencement of treatment with tiamulin (see monensin). Poisoning is associated with a marked drop in feed intake and growth rate and sudden death.

There is no antidote.

SULPHONAMIDES

High levels of sulphonamides form crystals in the kidneys and cause damage but poisoning is uncommon because when high levels are inadvertently mixed in feed the pigs will often reject it. Some sulphonamides and in particular sulphadimidine are excreted in the faeces and urine and are recycled back into the pigs again. If recycling occurs during the withdrawal period tissue residues will appear at slaughter. In consequence some countries have either banned or restricted its use. Other sulphonamides used for treatment do not recycle to the same extent.

TIAMULIN

This antibiotic is used extensively to treat swine dysentery and enzootic pneumonia. Levels of up to 120ppm have no toxic effects on the pig but above 200ppm the skin reacts to contact with contaminated faeces or urine, with marked red discoloration. After prolonged use bleeding into the muscles may occur along with increased mortality.

Tiamulin should not be used in conjunction with monensin because it enhances the toxicity of the monensin or salinomycin. (See monensin and salinomycin). There is no antidote.

MERCURY

Mercury exists in two forms, organic and inorganic. Organic compounds are used as fungicides to treat seed grains prior to sowing. Poisoning occurs if swine are fed corn or cereals that have been treated or contaminated with such a fungicide. Inorganic mercury as mercury chloride is used as a disinfectant and in some paints, batteries and thermometers.

Clinical signs

Mercury is a cumulative poison so clinical signs vary depending upon the duration of intake as well as the dose and the type of mercury. As a poison mercury acts primarily on the gastro-intestinal tract causing vomiting and bloody diarrhoea. Dead (necrotic) pieces of tissue may be seen in the faeces. Damage to the kidney also occurs leading to signs of uraemia. Pigs stop eating and lose body condition. White crystalline deposits may be seen in the urine. Nervous signs maybe seen including ataxia, blindness, wandering, partial paralysis, coma and death.

Diagnosis

The clinical signs and post-mortem lesions may suggest mercury poisoning which may be confirmed by finding the source of poisoning and by laboratory analysis of mercury levels in the kidney and liver (normally less than 1ppm).

Treatment

This is carried out by a combination of sodium thiosulphate 20% solutions given intravenously at 1ml/5kg body weight together with dimercaprol by intramuscular injection at a level of 3mg/kg body weight. Seek veterinary advice.

Feed pigs with either milk or egg protein which act as an absorbent.

METALDEHYDE

Metaldehyde is widely used to kill slugs and other garden pests and it is presented either as a meal with bran or pelleted. Clinical signs start within one hour of ingestion and effect the nervous system, with severe tremors, incoordination, convulsions, high temperatures and death due to respiratory failure. If pigs eat large amounts, it is necessary to anaesthetise them using barbiturates for a period of 6 to 12 hours whilst the drug is excreted. There is no specific antidote.

MYCOTOXINS

Under certain conditions fungi multiply on cereals, corn, cotton seed and other food materials sometimes producing chemicals called mycotoxins (Fig.13-4). They require adequate moisture, oxygen and carbohydrates to multiply and temperatures from 10°C to 25°C (50°F to 77°F). Multiplication may still take place however outside these ranges and crops that are already diseased are more likely to succumb to fungal infection. The presence of fungi including recognised toxic species however does not necessarily mean that the toxins are present. Each requires precisely the right substrate and environmental conditions to produce toxins. The common fungi causing disease (mycotoxicosis) in the pig include species of *Fusarium, Aspergillus* and *Penicillium,* but because of the variable requirements for growth and toxin production particular species tend to predominate in certain geographical areas. Toxins are not destroyed by heating but modern treatments used in the processing of animal feeds such as temperature and pressure may reduce the actual fungal load.

Factors that may increase the likelihood of mycotoxins in feed
- Cereals left over after screening.
- Damaged or broken grains.
- Storage of moist grain.
- Storage in warm damp conditions.
- Damaged leaking feed bins.
- Fluctuating environmental temperatures.
- Fungal growth in liquid feeding systems.

Diagnosis of mycotoxicosis

This can often be frustrating because although the clinical signs may be suggestive they are rarely diagnostic. It may be impossible to detect the toxin in the feed because of patchy distribution and/or the samples taken are toxin free. Also the effect of the toxin may have been delayed and the feed containing the toxin has been consumed. Alternatively the laboratory may be testing for the wrong toxin.

Effects of mycotoxins

The specific effects of the various toxins on the pig are shown in Fig.13-4. *Fusarium* species require high levels of moisture and relative humidity (>88%) for multiplication and toxin production whereas *Aspergillus* and *Penicillium* multiply at lower levels.

Aflatoxins and some of the ochratoxins are immunosuppressive and can enhance effects of generalised disease.

Methods of preventing mycotoxicosis

Wherever a fungal toxin is suspected consider the following actions:
- Immediately replace the feed or cereal sources by alternate ones.
- Examine carefully the meal or pellets for evidence of fungi.
- Empty all feed bins out and examine for bridging of feed or presence of mouldy feeds. If feed bins are contaminated, empty them and treat with a non toxic fungicide.
- Examine all automatic equipment and in particular feed hoppers and automatic dispensers for evidence of mouldy feed.
- If wet moist grain is stored, mould inhibitors such as propionic acid, calcium propionate or sorbic acid will prevent growth.
- Once mycotoxins have developed in feed there are no methods that can destroy them. However their effects can be mitigated by regrinding the feed and mixing with an alternate source at a ratio of 1:10 and feeding to growing stock on a test basis first.
- A feed sample should be sent to a laboratory for examination (see chapter 15 Sampling Feeds).
- Check other sources of poisoning, including straw and wet bedding materials.

AFLATOXINS

These are produced from the fungus aspergillus and are probably the most common and important of the mycotoxins in pigs. The aspergillus species commonly concerned grows in maize, soya beans and peanuts. The main species involved are *A. flavus* and *A. parasiticus* and countries where maize and peanuts are not fed aflatoxicosis is uncommon. The effect of the toxins are dependent upon the dose and the age of the pig, the

A GUIDE TO MYCOTOXIN LEVELS IN FEED: MILD TO SEVERE DISEASE				
Fungus	Toxins	No Clinical Effect	Toxic Level	Clinical Signs
Aspergillus sp	Aflatoxins	< 100ppb	300 - 2000ppb	Poor growth Liver damage Jaundice Immunosuppression
Aspergillus sp and Penicillium sp	Ochratoxin and Citrinin	< 100ppb	200 - 4000ppb	Reduced growth Thirst Kidney damage
Fusarium sp	T2 DAS DON (Vomitoxin)	< 2ppm	4 - 20ppm	Reduced feed intake Immuno-suppression Vomiting
Fusarium sp	Zearalenone (F2 toxin)	< 0.05ppm	1 - 30ppm	Infertility Anoestrus Rectal prolapse Pseudo pregnancy
			< 30ppm	Early embryo mortality Delayed repeat matings
Fusarium sp	Fumonisin	< 10ppm	20 - 175	Reduced feed intake Respiratory symptoms Fluid in lungs Abortion
Ergot	Ergotoxin	< 0.05%	0.1-1.0% Ergot bodies by weight (sclerotium)	Reduced feed intake. Gangrene of the extremities. Agalactia due to mammary gland failure.

ppm - parts per million ppb - parts per billion.
sp - species - each of these fungi have several species only some of which are toxic

(Fig.13-4)

younger the animal and the larger the dose the greater the effect. It is more common for pigs to be exposed to low levels of aflatoxins for long periods of time and the effects therefore tend to be sub-acute rather than acute. Feed levels up to 200ppb produce clinical signs and levels above 300ppb may be fatal.

Clinical signs

These include reduced growth and feed efficiency and at the upper levels the effects of liver damage and failure include jaundice. Aflatoxins do not have a direct effect on reproductive efficiency but abortion and agalactia may occur. They are immuno-suppressive and therefore increase the severity of concurrent diseases, such as PRRS, flu viruses and mycoplasma pneumonia. There are different types of aflatoxins designated B_1, B_2 and G_1, G_2 and the effects of the toxins are enhanced where poor quality, low protein diets are fed. If levels in the feed are low it can take four to six weeks for symptoms to appear.

Diagnosis

Wherever there is poor growth in a herd associated with poor nutrition and chronic infectious diseases the possibility of toxins in the feed should be considered and tested for. Post-mortem lesions include jaundice, anaemia, fluid in the abdomen, poor clotting of the blood and liver haemorrhage. Histological examinations of the liver may help to confirm the diagnosis. Follow the steps outlined at the beginning of the chapter and also see "Diagnosis of mycotoxicosis".

Treatment

There is no specific treatment. Remove the suspect source until it has been tested.

Raising the vitamin and protein levels in the feed by 10% for two to three weeks, could be beneficial, as could raising the lysine content of the diet to growing pigs by 0.2% for four weeks.

ERGOT TOXINS

These are produced from the fungus ergot (*Claviceps purpurea*) that affects wheat, oats, ryegrass and other grasses by entering the seed and developing into a dark elongated body called a sclerotium. This contains toxic alkaloids, one of which is ergometrine which has the effect of contracting small blood vessel walls, thus restricting the blood supply particularly to the mammary gland and the body extremities.

Clinical signs

Levels of more than 0.1% of the sclerotium in the ration will produce clinical signs. These usually occur over a period of weeks and are associated with poor growth rates, increased respiration and general depression. The most sensitive blood vessels are those found in the mammary glands of maturing pregnant gilts. The restricted blood supply then causes agalactia in lactating animals and gives rise to increased piglet mortality. Lameness is also common due to necrosis and sloughing of the hooves. Tail and ear necrosis are also common.

Diagnosis

There are two methods, the examination of food to identify black/brown sclerotium which can be seen with the naked eye and the laboratory identification of the alkaloids.

Treatment

There is no specific antidote.
Remove the affected feed.
Treat areas of gangrene with antibiotics.
Some pigs may have to be destroyed on humane grounds.

FUMONISINS

These are produced by the fungus *Fusarium moniliforme* growing in corn (maize) and the toxins cause excess fluid to leak out into lung tissue (pulmonary oedema). This is a recently recognised uncommon disease called the porcine pulmonary oedema syndrome. Toxins also have a mild effect on the liver resulting in jaundice and orange-yellow coloured lesions evident at post-mortem examination. It usually takes five to ten days of continual exposure for the signs of acute respiratory distress, cyanosis (blue colour) of the skin, jaundice, high morbidity and mortality to appear.

OCHRATOXIN AND CITRININ

Other aspergillus species, *Aspergillus ochraceous* and *Penicillium viridicatum,* produce toxins called ochratoxin and citrinin. These species are ubiquitous in Northern climates and are found in oats, barley, wheat and maize. Levels of toxin of more than 1ppm in the diet cause mild clinical signs particularly if spread over long periods of time. If the levels of intake exceed 1mg/kg mortality may occur.

Clinical signs

The main signs include reduced growth and feed efficiency. Liver damage occurs but the main effect is on the kidneys resulting in increased water intake.

In young growing pigs oedema (fluid between the tissues) may occur with generalised stiffness. In acute poisoning mortality can be high. Gastric ulceration is also a consistent finding and in herds with high levels, the possibility of these toxins being present in feed should be considered.

Diagnosis

The clinical signs and post mortem findings are indicative of ochratoxin and citrinin poisoning and this may be confirmed by identifying the toxins in the feed or in kidney tissue at slaughter. The toxins can also be identified in serum.

Treatment

There is no specific antidote.
Remove the suspected sources.
Increase the vitamin levels in feed.
Recovery is slow.

TRICHOTHECENES

Trichothecenes are produced by other species of the fungus *Fusarium* mainly *F. graminearum,* and *F. sporotrichioides* growing in wheat and corn (maize) and the common toxins are called T-2, DAS and DON (vomitoxin). Their significance is that they are immuno-suppressive and also affect the production of blood cells by the bone marrow.

Clinical signs

Levels of 1ppm or more reduce feed intake and at high levels (10 to 20ppm) they cause vomiting and inappetance but at such levels pigs refuse to eat the food.

Diagnosis

This is based on clinical symptoms, a history of sudden vomiting within 10 to 15 minutes of feeding and inappetance. In such cases feed should be changed and samples tested.

Treatment

None is required - the toxins are rapidly excreted.
Change the feed source.

ZEARALENONE

This toxin called F2 is produced by a strain of *Fusarium graminearum* which appears in corn (maize). It is an oestrogenic toxin and it is produced in high moisture environments in maize growing areas well before harvest. Rectal and vagina prolapses are common symptoms in the young growing stock.

Clinical signs

The most striking clinical feature is the swollen red vulva of immature gilts. The other signs are dependent up on the levels present in the feed and the state of pregnancy. The following may be used as guidelines to the symptoms that may be observed.
Boars - Semen may be affected with feed levels above 30ppm but not fertility. At higher levels poor libido, oedema of the prepuce and loss of hair may occur.
Gilts (Pre puberty) 1 - 6 months of age - 1 to 5ppm in feed causes swelling and reddening of the vulva and enlargement of the teats and mammary glands. Rectal and vagina prolapses also occur in the young growing stock.
Gilts (mature) - 1 to 3ppm will cause variable lengths of the oestrus cycle due to retained corpora lutea and infertility.
Sows - Levels of 5 to 10ppm can cause anoestrus, which may also be associated with pseudo pregnancy due to the retention of corpus luteum. F2 toxin will not normally cause abortion however. If sows are exposed during the period of implantation litter size may be reduced. In lactation piglets may develop enlarged vulva.
Effects on pregnancy - Embryo survival to implantation does not appear to be affected at levels less than 30ppm but above this complete loss between implantation and thirty days occurs followed by pseudo pregnancies. Low levels of 3 to 5ppm do not appear to affect the mid part of pregnancy, but in the latter stages piglet growth in utero is depressed, with weak splay-legged piglets born. Some of these may have enlarged vulvas.
Effects on lactation - 3 to 5ppm has no effect on lactation but the weaning to service interval may be extended.

Diagnosis

The clinical signs are distinctive. Rations that are suspected of contamination should be examined both for the presence of zearalenone and also other oestrogen like substances. Removal of the suspect feed will be followed by the regression of symptoms within three to four weeks.

Treatment

None is required provided the toxin source is removed. Sows that are in deep anoestrus may respond to injections of prostaglandins.

NITRATES AND NITRITES

If these substances are absorbed from the small intestine in sufficient quantities, nitrite reacts with haemoglobin in the blood to form met-haemoglobin which reduces its oxygen carrying capacity. Poisoning occurs when nitrates and ammonia in slurry and straw are converted to nitrites by bacteria, or if the pig drinks drainage water that as become heavily contaminated. Nitrate itself is only slightly toxic, until it is converted to nitrite. Silage effluent is a particularly heavy source of nitrites.

Clinical signs

These are related to a shortage of oxygen in the blood stream. There is a marked increase in the respiratory rate with animals showing a staggering gait and general weakness. The mucous membranes become dark red, almost blue. There may be sufficient irritation of the digestive tract to cause a gastro-enteritis. Clinical signs of poisoning will develop when 10 to 20mg of nitrites per kg liveweight are eaten. Mortality becomes very high above the latter level.

Diagnosis

Sudden prostration of groups of pigs or a pen of pigs, that have had access to potential sources of nitrates and nitrites, including whey and milk bye products, must always raise a suspicion. Post-mortem examinations show that the blood and musculature are a dark brown colour due to the formation of met-haemoglobin. This is a diagnostic feature.

Treatment

Intravenous injections of 10mg/kg methylene blue. Consult your veterinarian.

PLANTS

Poisoning from plants eaten by pigs kept outdoors is rare but the following species may cause problems from time to time.

BRACKEN (Pteridium aquilinum)

Bracken produces a toxin that destroys the vitamin thiamine. Pigs are normally resistant to bracken poisoning and it needs in excess of six weeks of constant exposure particularly to fresh bracken shoots and the rhizomes.

Clinical signs

Sudden death is often the only sign, although prior to this respiratory distress may be seen associated with oedema or fluid in the lungs.

Diagnosis

This is based on history, clinical signs if seen and enzyme tests carried out on serum.

Treatment and control

If sows are likely to have access to large amounts of bracken, injections of thiamine should be given every two weeks. Where clinical signs are seen all the group at risk should be injected with thiamine.

COCKLEBUR (Xanthium)

This is found in waste places and the edges of ponds and rivers. Poisoning occurs when pigs eat the two-leaf seedling. The mature plant is unpalatable. The toxins cause depression, vomiting, weakness, rapid breathing, convulsions and lowered body temperature. Death occurs within a few hours. Lesions seen at post-mortem examination include ascites (liquid in abdominal cavity) and liver congestion and necrosis. Treat with mineral or sunflower oil by mouth.

DEADLY NIGHTSHADE (Solanum)

These plants are found in waste areas and hay fields. The berries are very poisonous and will produce an acute haemorrhagic gastro-enteritis with considerable salivation, trembling, paralysis, leading to coma and finally death. Poisoning in pigs is rare. Treatment requires the use of pilocarpine. Consult your veterinarian.

OAK LEAVES AND ACORNS

Whilst ruminants are more susceptible to acorn poisoning, outdoor pigs may be affected occasionally. Young oak leaves or green acorns are the major sources and signs are seen two to three days after ingestion. These include abdominal pain and constipation followed by haemorrhagic diarrhoea. The kidneys may also be affected.

Treatment

There is no treatment but remove the pigs from the sources immediately.

PIGWEED (Amaranthus)

This is a characteristic clearly defined disease associated with the accumulation of oedema (fluid) around the kidneys. The signs start with trembling and an uncoordinated gait and pigs characteristically lie on their bellies. Acute kidney damage occurs usually within two to three days which in severe cases is followed by coma and death. The characteristic changes of fluid around the kidneys and history of access to the plant are diagnostic. There is no treatment and pigs should be removed immediately from the source.

POKEWEED (Phytolacca)

This plant produces oxalic acid which causes acute abdominal pain, vomiting, haemorrhagic diarrhoea and haemorrhage from the kidneys. There is no treatment

SORGHUM (Sorghum)

These course grasses contain hydrocyanic acid and intake causes difficult breathing, convulsions and a very bright red coloured or chocolate brown blood associated with the formation of nitrites. Treatment is as for nitrites.

YELLOW JASMINE (Gelsemium)

This plant is found in woodlands and can cause poisoning. The onset is sudden and acute with incoordination, weakness, coma and death usually within 48 hours. There is no specific treatment. Sedate with azaperone (Stresnil) to control convulsions.

WATER HEMLOCK (Conium maculatum)

This is found in open, moist or wet ground and it is highly toxic. Death can occur within 30 to 50 minutes associated with violent muscular spasms, dilated pupils, convulsions, coma and death. There is no specific treatment. Use sedatives to control convulsions.

SALT (WATER DEPRIVATION)

Salt poisoning or water deprivation is the most common poisoning to be seen in swine. It arises where there is a shortage or complete lack of water and the normal salt in the diet then becomes toxic. The normal levels of salt in the ration vary between 0.4 and 0.6% and even at these levels water deprivation can result in toxicity after 48 hours. The higher the level of salt in the diet the shorter is the period of water deprivation before signs are seen. However in the presence of ad lib water the pig can tolerate up to 2% or more of salt in the diet. The first signs are inappetance and whenever this occurs in a pen of apparently healthy pigs or an individual always check the water supply first.

Clinical signs

These appear within 24 to 36 hours of water deprivation. Pigs become inappetent, wander aimlessly, are blind and stand with their heads pushed into the wall of the pen. Recurrent fits are common. These start with a characteristic twitching of the nose, the head then goes back and the pigs fall over. They eventually lie on their side with convulsive leg movements, froth at the mouth and become comatosed and die.

Diagnosis

This is based on clinical signs and a history of water deprivation. Diagnosis can be confirmed by histological examination of the brain in which the lesions are diagnostic.

Treatment

The response to treatment is poor particularly if pigs have developed fits. Rehydration of the pig is important and this can be achieved by dripping water through a flutter valve (see chapter 15) into the rectum or allowing water to drip onto the tongue from a hose pipe. An alternate technique is to inject sterile water at body temperature into the abdominal cavity. This technique requires veterinary advice and direction.

SELENIUM

See chapter 14; Vitamin E / Selenium for further information.

Selenium is a highly toxic mineral but it is required in very minute amounts for normal bodily functions. Selenium poisoning is rare and usually occurs when selenium supplement has been wrongly mixed into the ration. Levels above 3ppm in the diet have a clinical affect on the pig and when they reach 10ppm severe clinical signs develop. The toxic dose of selenium by injection is approximately 0.8mg/kg. Problems are more likely to occur with a deficiency producing muscle myopathies and mulberry heart disease.

Clinical signs

Pigs become anorexic with loss of hair and separation of hooves at the coronary band. Paralysis of front and hind legs is common. As the disease progresses there is liver and kidney failure and the pigs become toxic.

Diagnosis

The clinical picture of selenium toxicity is characteristic and almost diagnostic. Confirmation is by the identification of abnormal levels in feed, the liver and the kidneys of affected pigs. Levels above 3ppm are diagnostic.

Treatment

There is no specific treatment.

TOXIC (SLURRY) GASES

AMMONIA

Ammonia is the most common poison in the pig's environment. The concentrations of the various gases found in piggeries are expressed as parts per million (ppm). Generally ammonia levels are less than 5ppm in well run pig houses. The human respiratory tract can detect levels at around 10ppm. Levels of 50 to 100ppm affect performance, particularly daily gain which may be reduced by up to 10% during prolonged periods of exposure. At levels of 50ppm and above the clearance of bacteria from the lungs is also impaired and therefore the animal is more prone to respiratory disease.

Clinical signs

These include increased coughing and respiratory rates, irritation of the mucosa lining the respiratory tract and an increased incidence of pneumonia. Pigs are restless, uncomfortable and may show increased levels of vice, such as tail biting, ear biting and flank chewing.

Diagnosis

This is based on the assessment of air quality by the pig person and observed effects on the pig. Ammonia levels can be measured easily using glass sampling tubes. These are thin glass tubes containing a chemical to which syringes are attached. By drawing air through the chemical, a colour change takes place which indicates the ppm of the gas being tested for. (See chapter 15).

Treatment

Increase ventilation rates.

Management control and prevention

Where levels reach above 30-50ppm ventilation must be improved and other measures taken.

Increase the drainage of urine from the house and remove solid faeces daily. If a slurry system is used, remove slurry regularly and prevent a crust developing on the surface. Proprietary products that include an extract of the yucca plant are effective in reducing ammonia production in slurry.

When designing houses keep the surface area and depth of the slurry to a minimum.

Slurry systems that are flushed every twenty minutes reduce ammonia levels.

Do not store slurry under slats. Empty frequently to holding areas. Make alterations to the diet to reduce nitrogen excretion.

CARBON DIOXIDE

This gas is a normal component of air in levels up to 300ppm. It is only toxic in very high levels >3000ppm and rarely causes problems in piggeries. However if CO_2 levels are high then there are significant risks that the levels of other more toxic gases will be critical. Increased levels cause pigs discomfort and restlessness which may lead to vice and cannibalism.

CARBON MONOXIDE

Carbon monoxide poisoning in swine occurs where faulty gas heaters are used in farrowing houses and ventilation is poor resulting in an increase in stillbirths. Also, the decomposition of faeces, particularly in slatted floored finishing houses produces high levels. 50ppm are not uncommon and suggest inadequate ventilation. Levels of 250ppm however interfere with the uptake of oxygen by the haemoglobin in the pig's blood and similarly in people. Instead of oxyhaemoglobin, carboxyhaemoglobin is formed and the oxygen carrying capacity of the blood is reduced. This markedly increases the number of stillborn piglets. Levels may rise to 50%. Carbon monoxide affects the blood of unborn piglets more quickly than the sow.

Clinical signs

Sows may show dark coloration of the mucous membranes and stillborn piglets are often bright red due to the formation of the carboxyhaemoglobin in the blood. Such levels of carbon monoxide can have a similar effect on people so care should be taken in investigating the housing area.

Diagnosis

If gas heaters are used in farrowing houses and a sudden rise in stillbirths occurs, inadequate combustion must immediately be suspected together with poor ventilation. Carbon monoxide levels can be measured using glass sampling tubes.

Treatment

Improve the ventilation immediately, and identify and remove the source of production.
Administer oxygen but this may be impractical.

HYDROGEN SULPHIDE (H_2S)

This is one of the important toxic gases found in piggeries and it is potentially lethal. The gas is produced by anaerobic bacterial decomposition of organic matter, particularly that found in faeces and slurry. The greatest source of H_2S and indeed the greatest potential for disasters comes from slurry that is held in pits beneath slatted finishing houses. Pockets of gas may become trapped and when the slurry is agitated and removed from the house there is a risk of acute and fatal poisoning not only to pigs but also to people. There is a low concentration of H_2S in most pig houses, usually less than 100 ppm. H_2S concentrations can be detected by the human nose within the range of 0.05 to 200 ppm. When levels get above the upper limit the sensitivity of the nose to detect the gas decreases significantly and the situation becomes potentially dangerous.

Clinical signs

These are dependent on the levels in the air and the following sequence of events can be considered in both pigs and humans:

Less than 50 ppm:	little effect but detected by people.
200 to 250 ppm:	slight breathing difficulties, distress and irritation of the eyes, nose and back of the throat. The environment is becoming dangerous.
250 to 400 ppm:	breathing starts to become very difficult with muscular spasms and disorientation.
400 to 600 ppm:	pigs become totally disorientated and some start to relapse into a coma.
600 to 1000 ppm:	the pig develops fits and convulsions and becomes extremely short of oxygen Its skin goes blue (cyanosed) and death ensues.

METHANE

Methane gas is highly explosive when levels reach 1% or more, this is the main risk on farms. As a poison the gas is largely inert and would only cause problems to pigs if the levels were so high as to displace oxygen. This would take place above a concentration of 80% and the signs would be acute respiratory embarrassment.

A SUMMARY OF TOXIC SLURRY GASES

Gas	Acceptable Levels in piggeries	Toxic Levels	Clinical Effects In People	Common on Farm Problems and Dangers
Ammonia	< 25ppm	> 50ppm	Difficult breathing Irritation	Agitation of the slurry pits when emptying.
Carbon dioxide	< 2000ppm	Uncommon	Difficult breathing Headaches Drowsiness	Power failure. Ventilation failure.
Carbon monoxide	< 30ppm	> 60ppm	Difficult breathing Asphyxiation Drowsiness	Faulty heaters. Deep slurry pits.
Hydrogen sulphide	< 5ppm	> 80ppm	Irritation Sickness Headaches Unconsciousness Death	Release of gas after slurry pits are agitated.
Methane	Non toxic unless 80% or more in air.	> 80%	Irritation Explosive atmosphere >1%	Rare.

(Fig.13-5)

WARFARIN

Warfarin is one of a group of chemicals (rodenticides) that are used to control rat and mice populations. Poisoning by these substances is common in pigs due to accidental exposure. A single dose of warfarin of 3mg/kg is fatal. Doses of less than 0.06mg per day for seven to ten days will produce poisoning. Warfarin acts by preventing blood clotting.

Clinical signs

Severe haemorrhage is present throughout the carcase of dead pigs and in the skin, particularly where trauma has occurred. Lameness with haemorrhage in the joints and anaemia are consistent features.

Diagnosis

This is based on the history of the use of warfarin and the typical post-mortem lesions of widespread haemorrhage throughout the carcase.

Treatment

Give injections of vitamin K, 5mg/kg on day one and then 2mg/kg daily for five days.

If you open the door of a finishing house and there are no sounds, stop and think:
TOXIC GASES or ELECTROCUTION
and
DO NOT ENTER.

14 Nutrition and Disease

The role of amino acids 446
The role of energy 446
Common diseases and conditions associated with nutrition 447
    Abortion and seasonal infertility... 448
    Anaemia.. 450
    Colitis 450
    Diarrhoea.. 451
    Fractures... 454
    Gastric ulcers... 454
    Lameness.. 456
        Calcium and phosphorous.. 456
        Osteodystrophy... 456
        Osteoporosis (OP) and osteomalacia (OM)......................... 456
        Rickets... 457
        Vitamin A 457
        Leg weakness or osteochondrosis 458
    Prolapse of the rectum.. 458
    Reproduction... 459
    Respiratory diseases.. 461
    Salt poisoning - (water deprivation)... 461
    Torsion of the stomach and intestines 462
    Udder oedema and failure of milk let down................................. 462
    Water... 463
Minerals and vitamins 465
    Biotin... 465
    Choline.. 465
    Copper... 465
    Cyanocobalamin B_{12} 465
    Folic acid 465
    Iodine 465
    Iron 466
    Magnesium... 466
    Manganese... 466
    Nicotinamide... 466
    Pantothenic acid... 466
    Potassium... 466
    Riboflavin B_2 466
    Sodium and chloride... 466
    Thiamine.. 467
    Vitamin E / selenium (mulberry heart disease).............................. 467
    Vitamin K 468
    Zinc... 468
Non nutritional supplements.. 468
    Probiotics... 469

Chapter 14

14 Nutrition and Disease

This chapter looks at the role nutrition may have on disease syndromes but for more extensive information on nutrition itself the reader is referred to specific books dealing with this (e.g. The Science and Practice of Pig Production. Whittemore CT Longman Group UK Ltd).

A major role for the stockperson on the farm is to judge the interaction between the pig, its age and/or productive cycle against the quality, content and intake of feed. The role of management in this respect has an important influence not only on the levels of disease in the herd but also whether the pig maximises its biological potential.

The essential nutrients include protein and amino acids, energy, essential fatty acids, water, vitamins and minerals. A guide to the normal requirements is shown in Fig.14-1 both by weight of pig and ration type.

If you feel you have a feed related problem study Fig.14-2. First identify the problem by symptoms and this will suggest potential nutrient deficiencies or problem areas. You would be advised at this time to consult with your feed supplier because a knowledge of the composition of the diet will then assist in determining more specific areas, for example insufficient energy or lysine for the particular age group of pigs in that environment. Fig.14-3 relates the clinical signs to possible causes where there are deficiencies or excesses of minerals and similarly Fig.14-4 of nutrients and vitamins, although it would be uncommon today to see many of them. Details of individual nutrients are given in subsequent pages. The most common problems on farms today however relate to the failure of the diet to satisfy the amino acid and energy requirements for the pig.

A GUIDE TO NUTRIENT REQUIREMENTS AT DIFFERENT STAGES OF LIFE FINAL DIETARY LEVELS						
	Liveweight kg Ad libitum Feeding					
Type of Ration	6-10 Creep	10-20 Weaner	20-50 Grower	50-100 Finisher	Dry Sow	Lactating Sow
Crude protein %	23 - 25	19 - 22	18 - 20	16 - 17	13.5 - 13.8	17 - 18
Crude fibre %	1 - 3	2 - 4	2 - 5	3 - 4	4 - 5	2 - 5
MJ DE/kg	15 - 16	14.5 - 15	13.8 - 14.1	13.5 - 13.8	13.3 - 13.8	14.2 - 14.8
Essential Fatty acid (linoleic) mg/kg	100	Unknown not considered necessary				300
Lysine %	1.3 - 1.5	1.25 - 1.35	1.0 - 1.1	0.85 - 0.95	0.6 - 0.7	1.0 - 1.15
Arginine (as a % of Lysine)	40					
Histidine (")	35					
Isoleucine (")	60					
Leucine (")	110					
Methionine plus cystine (")	60					
Phenylalanine plus tyrosine (")	95					
Threonine (")	60					
Tryptophan (")	18					
Valine (")	75					
Calcium g/kg *	10 - 12	8 - 10	8 - 10	8 - 10	8 - 11	9 - 12
Phosphorus g/kg *	8 - 10	6 - 8	6 - 8	6 - 8	6 - 8	7 - 9
Sodium chloride g/kg	2 - 3.5	2 - 3.5	2 - 3.5	3 - 4	5	5
Magnesium mg/kg	40	40	40	40	40	40
Iron mg/kg *	100	80	60	60	80	80
Zinc mg/kg *	100	100	90	90	75	75
Manganese mg/kg	80	60	30	20	200	200
Copper mg/kg *	175	175	100	100	5 - 15	5 - 15
Iodine mg/kg	1.0	1.0	0.5	0.14	0.4	0.4
Selenium mg/kg	0.2	0.3	0.2	0.2	0.1	0.1
Vitamin A iu/kg *	7500	7500	8000	8000	8500	8500
D_3 iu/kg *	2000	2000	2000	2000	2000	2000
E iu/kg *	100 - 250	100 - 150	100	60 - 80	- 80	- 100
K mg/kg	4.5	3.5	2.5	2.5	3.5	3.5
Riboflavin B_2 mg/kg *	15	10	7.5	7.5	10	10
Nicotinamide (niacin) mg/kg	35	25	17	17	25	25
Pantothenic acid B_5 mg/kg *	22	17	11	11	11	11
Cyanocobalamin B_{12} mg/kg	40	35	15	12	20	20
Choline mg/kg	1000	660	550	550	1350	1350
Thiamine B_1 mg/kg	4.0	2.0	1.5	1.5	1.5	1.5
Pyridoxine B_6 mg/kg	5	3	2	2	2	2
Biotin mg/kg *	1	1	0.22	0.22	1	1
Folic acid mg/kg	1	1	1	1	3.0	3.0

mg/kg = g/tonne = ppm   mg/kg x 0.0001 = %   g/kg x 0.1 = %
CP = Crude Protein   DE = Digestible Energy   MJ = Megajoules   iu = International Units
* Diets usually supplemented to these levels

(Fig.14-1)

CLINICAL PROBLEMS ASSOCIATED WITH NUTRITION

Abortion
Energy
Fungal toxins present
Iron

Anaemia haemorrhage
Aflatoxin
Anticoagulants
Coal tar poisoning
Copper
Iron
Protein
Vitamin E - Selenium (gastric ulcers)

Bone fracture, malformed bones, lameness
Calcium *
Magnesium
Manganese
Nicotinamide
Phosphorus *
Vitamins * - A, D_3, E

Diarrhoea, colitis
Excess protein, tapioca
High levels of wheat
Increased levels of potassium and magnesium
Iron
Nicotinamide
Pantothenic acid

Haemorrhage
Vitamin K

Nervous symptoms, incoordination, lameness
Biotin
Calcium
Copper
Magnesium
Manganese
Pantothenic acid
Phosphorus
Vitamins * - A, B_6, D_3, * E
Water *

Poor growth, poor appetite
All aspects of nutrition *
Amino acids * - lysine, arginine, histidine, isoleucine, methionine, cystine, threonine, tryptophan
Energy *
Feeds of poor digestibility *
Iron *

CLINICAL PROBLEMS ASSOCIATED WITH NUTRITION

Magnesium
Phosphorus
Potassium
Protein *
Sodium chloride *
Vitamins -* A, B_6, B_{12}, * D_3, choline, riboflavin, pantothenic acid niacin
Water *
Zinc

Poor litter size
Choline
Energy *
Folic acid
Lysine *
Other essential amino acids
Vitamin E *

Reproductive failure
Choline
Energy *
Folic acid
Iodine
Lysine *
Manganese
Other essential amino acids
Riboflavin
Vitamins - B_{12}, * E

Respiratory diseases
Energy
Protein
Vitamin E

Skin changes
Iron *
Essential fatty acids * - linoleic acid
Nicotinamide
Potassium
Riboflavin
Salt
Zinc

Sudden death
Selenium *
Thiamine
Vitamin E *
Water - salt poisoning

* Likely to occur. Others uncommon or rare

(Fig.14-2)

MINERALS. CLINICAL SIGNS OF DEFICIENCIES AND EXCESSES

Mineral	Signs of Deficiency	Signs of Excess
Calcium	Agalactia Depressed milk yield * Fractures * Hypocalcaemia Osteomalacia * Osteoporosis * Posterior paralysis in sows * Rickets	Changes in bone formation If zinc is low (parakeratosis) more than 1% may cause problems. Reduced strength of bone
Copper	Leg weakness Loose faeces if suddenly withdrawn	* Jaundice 200 - 600g/tonne Haemorrhage Death
Iodine	Enlarged thyroid glands Reproductive failure Weak hairless pigs at birth	Rare > 800mg/kg
Iron	* Anaemia * Increased respiration More prone to piglet diseases Poor growth Pale skin	Death in piglets deficient in vitamin E Muscle degeneration > 5000 mg/kg
Magnesium	Infertility Rare Poor growth Weak joints	Loose faeces > 0.5% in diet.
Manganese	Infertility Rare Lameness Poor growth Weak piglets	Inappetance > 2000ppm
Phosphorus	Poor growth * Rickets See calcium also Soft bones	Changes in bone formation. Posterior paralysis in sows.
Potassium	Anorexia Rare Heart malfunction Incoordination Poor growth	Loose faeces > 1.2% in diet.
Salt (Sodium chloride)	Low water intake Poor growth and feed efficiency Unthriftiness	* Common Any level if water is short Death > 2 - 8% if water short Fits Incoordination Thirst
Selenium	* Mulberry heart disease Muscle changes Sudden mortality	Diarrhoea Feet deformity Lameness Respiratory distress Sudden death 5 - 10g/tonne
Water	* All systems affected Failure to thrive Nervous convulsions (water deprivation) Predisposition to disease	Colic
Zinc	* Dry thick skin (parakeratosis) Poor appetite	Reduced feed intake > 3000g/tonne Up to 2500g/tonne in diet none.

* Likely to occur. Others uncommon or rare

(Fig.14-3)

NUTRIENTS AND VITAMINS. CLINICAL SIGNS OF DEFICIENCIES AND EXCESSES		
Nutrient	**Signs of Deficiency**	**Signs of Excess**
Amino Acids	A predisposition to disease. Poor growth.	Digestive disturbances.
Biotin	Infertility. Anoestrus. * Lameness. * Poor hoof quality.	Unknown. Unlikely.
Choline	Poor litter size. Poor growth.	Unknown. Unlikely.
Cyanocobalamin (B_{12})	Poor growth. Infertility. Anaemia.	Unknown. Unlikely.
Energy *	* Infertility. Loss in weight. Poor fat deposition. Predisposition to: * Cystitis pyelonephritis. * Post-weaning enteritis. * Respiratory disease. * Villus atrophy and malabsorption. * Thin sow syndrome.	Deposition of excess fat.
Fat and fatty acids * (Linoleic)	Dry skins in sows and piglets. Loss of weight in lactation. Poor growth.	Colitis. Digestive disturbances. Loose faeces.
Folic Acid	Anaemia. Poor litter size. Poor growth.	Unknown. Unlikely.
Nicotinamide (Niacin)	Diarrhoea. Dermatitis. Poor growth. Paralysis.	Unknown. Unlikely.
Pantothenic Acid (B_5)	Poor appetite and growth. Goose-stepping gait. Diarrhoea.	Unknown. Unlikely.
Protein *	Lean tissue gain reduced. Poor growth. More prone to disease.	Diarrhoea.
Pyridoxine (B_6)	Poor growth.	Unknown.
Riboflavin (B_2)	Infertility. Weak piglets.	Unknown. Unlikely.
Thiamine (B_1)	Poor appetite and growth. Sudden death.	Unknown. Unlikely.
Vitamin A	Rare but reports of: Infertility. Incoordination. Poor bone growth. Poor sight. Congenital defects, born blind.	* Epiphyseal plate changes. * Increased incidence of OCD. * Increased requirements for vitamin E. Joint pain. * Leg weakness. * Mulberry heart disease.
Vitamin D_3	Fractures. Lameness. Rickets. Rubbery bones or osteomalacia. Swollen joints.	Calcification of soft tissues.
Vitamin E * (Mulberry Heart Disease)	Agalactia. Discoloration of fat. * Gastric ulcers. * Liver, heart and muscle changes. MMA syndrome. Oedema disease. Porcine stress syndrome. * Predisposition to: App. E. coli diarrhoea. Respiratory disease. Swine dysentery. * Reduced immune responses. Sudden death. Udder oedema.	
Vitamin K	Enhances warfarin poisoning. Poor blood clotting.	Unknown. Unlikely.

* Likely to occur. Others uncommon or rare.

(Fig.14-4)

THE ROLE OF AMINO ACIDS

These are substances which when linked together in different combinations form different proteins. There are approximately 22 amino acids and whilst the pig can synthesise the majority of these, there are a number it cannot and these are described as essential for normal health and metabolic processes.

The essential amino acids:
- Arginine
- Isoleucine
- Histidine
- Leucine
- Lysine
- Methionine plus cystine
- Phenylalanine plus tyrosine
- Threonine
- Tryptophan
- Valine

Field experiences constantly reinforce the importance of good quality proteins and amino acid availability particularly during periods of stress, management change and when the immune system is challenged.

Critical time periods are in the first 14 days post-weaning, and from 6 to 12 weeks of age when maternal antibodies are declining to EP, PRRS and App and when pigs are exposed to new endemically infected environments. During these periods of challenge you are advised to feed or continue feeding the higher quality diet. The advent of segregated early weaning, which removes many pathogens and environmental contaminants that are normally exposed to the pig, has increased the nutritional requirements necessary to satisfy the increased growth. This is particularly true of lysine and energy.

The quality of the protein in the pigs' diet is a reflection of the amount and the availability of these essential amino acids. High quality protein contains all of the essential amino acids at acceptable levels, poor quality protein is deficient in one or more. When proteins enter the intestinal tract they are broken down into the separate amino acids which are absorbed into the blood stream and transported around the body. These amino acids are then built into different types of proteins to satisfy the many diverse requirements of the body. It can be seen therefore, that where there is a deficiency of one or more essential amino acids in the diet, the metabolic functions of the pig are compromised leading to biological inefficiency and possibly disease. The major roles of the amino acids are in the production of muscle protein, digestive enzymes, haemoglobin in the blood, gamma globulins (antibodies), milk protein and in hormone metabolism. Since the proteins used in pig diets are of variable quality some of the essential amino acids may be deficient. These are called the limiting ones and in most cases lysine is the most likely, followed by methionine and both are often added to diets routinely. If the diet is deficient in one or more of these essential amino acids then protein synthesis will only continue to the level associated with the first limiting amino acid. The amounts of each amino acid required in the diet are expressed as a percentage of the total lysine requirement. (Fig.14-1).

Enteric diseases such as *E. coli* enteritis in the sucking pig, transmissible gastro enteritis, colitis and swine dysentery, which severely damage the lining of the intestine and its capacity to absorb nutrients can have a profound effect on the absorption of amino acids and exacerbate the effects of the disease. It is important when dealing with such diseases to ensure that the diet has a high level of amino acids during the recovery period.

THE ROLE OF ENERGY

Energy in the diet is measured either by calories (Mcal) as used in the USA and Canada or joules (MJ) as used in Europe. In some countries the kilocalorie (kcal) is used and in others the Megacalorie(Mcal) = 1000 kcal. To convert calories to joules multiply by 4.184.

Thus 1Mcal = 4.184 MJ. The most common nutritional deficiency in pigs is that of energy and the amount available in the diet is usually measured either as digestible energy (DE) or metabolisable energy (ME). (ME = 0.96DE). Digestible energy is the amount of energy which is present in the feed and readily digested and absorbed from the intestine into the body.

KEY FACTORS THAT CREATE AN ENERGY DEFICIENCY
- A low energy diet.
- A low protein diet.
- An incorrect diet for the age of the pig.
- Poor feed intake.
- Poor palatability.
- Floor feeding.
- Poor access to the feed.
- Faulty feed hoppers.
- Toxic gases affecting palatability.
- Shortage of water.
- High stocking density.
- Wet pens.
- Draughts.
- Poor insulation of floors and buildings.
- Changing / low environmental temperatures.
- Faulty heaters.
- The movement of pigs from one house to another.
- The mixing of pigs.
- Movement from a solid to a slatted floor.
- A change from dry to wet feeding or vice verse.
- The genetic make-up of the pig - the more lean the pig the more susceptible it is to the environment.
- Exposure to infection and disease.
- Excessive use by body tissues and body products.
- Parasites.
- The requirement of body tissues.
- Reproduction and pregnancy.
- Growth of the foetus.
- Lactation.

USE THIS AS A CHECK LIST IN YOUR HERD

(Fig.14-5)

The pig could not operate without adequate sources of energy because it is the fuel that supports maintenance and drives the whole of the metabolic processes resulting in the production of meat and milk. Fig.14-5 shows the key factors that contribute to an energy deficient state. If there is poor growth problem in your herd you would be advised to check this list and identify those factors that are likely to have a bearing on your problem and then refer to the index or other chapters relating to the problem area.

Energy requirements are determined by the weight of the pig, its growth rate, the amount required for maintenance and its stage in the reproductive cycle. The requirements for energy in the lactating sow should not be underestimated. Fig.14-6 shows the critical periods of energy demand in the pig through its life and diseases that may be associated if an energy deficiency arises. Daily feed intake and the energy level per kg of feed are crucial factors which help the pig to maintain a positive (anabolic) energy state instead of a negative (catabolic) one. The intake of energy is also essential to maximise reproduction performance (see chapter 5). The relationship between feed intake and energy used by the pig on the one hand and that lost to the environment is a complex one. The survival of the piglet in the first 2 to 3 days of life is highly dependent on a regular supply of energy and if the sows nutrition is inadequate leading to poor quality milk, the susceptibility to disease and piglet mortality rises. Diarrhoea in the neonatal period and up to 14 days of age is often precipitated by intermittent periods of catabolism associated with low environmental temperatures. The introduction of creep feed at an inopportune time can, through indigestion and abnormal fermentation, initiate a sequence of events leading to scour or increased susceptibility to rotavirus, PRRS, joint infections or glässers disease. If you have an intransigent scour problem on your farm and you are feeding creep to sucking piglets stop doing it. Many problems become lesser ones or disappear. See diseases of the sucking piglet in chapter 8.

In the newly weaned pig the quality and availability of carbohydrates and other energy sources are vital if a healthy rapid growing pig is to be produced. Within 12 to 24 hours after weaning most pigs become energy deficient for a short period, which affects the degree of villus atrophy and the rate of their regeneration. The immune system also does not respond efficiently and the results are more disease or a greater incidence. The important changes in management and feeding practices are considered in detail in chapter 9.

The significance of maintaining a positive energy balance in the pig and its role in the precipitation of disease is often not appreciated on the farm. Aspects of this are

Do not feed creep to piglets if you have a scour problem.

THE ENERGY CRISES	
The Critical Time Period	Diseases or Conditions to which a Deficiency of Energy may Contribute
From birth to day 3	E. coli enteritis Hypoglycaemia Joint infections
Day 3 to weaning	E. coli enteritis Glässers disease Immuno-suppression Septicaemia
The weaned pig to 7 days post-weaning	E. coli enteritis Glässers disease Malabsorption Poor growth Streptococcal meningitis Streptococcal septicaemia
Growing pig 5 - 14 weeks old	Actinobacillus pleuropneumonia Atrophic rhinitis Colitis Enzootic pneumonia Immuno-suppression Mycoplasma arthritis Pasteurella pneumonia Poor metabolism and growth Porcine reproductive and respiratory syndrome.
Finishing pig	Aujeszky's disease (pseudorabies) Enteric disease Immuno-suppression Pneumonia Poor metabolism and growth
Dry sow or gilt	Abortion in late pregnancy Anoestrus Cystitis pyelonephritis Embryo resorption Litter size Pseudo pregnancy
Lactating sow	Poor subsequent litter size and fertility

(Fig.14-6)

dealt with in the relevant chapters and specific diseases. Conditions however are highlighted here from field experiences, so that you can assess them in relation to problems on your farm.

Common Diseases and Conditions Associated with Nutrition

Figures 14-3 and 14-4 highlight signs of deficiencies and excesses documented in the literature. In practice today, using modern well formulated premixes, problems with most of the individual nutrients would be uncommon or rare. Problems usually only occur due to gross mismanagement in the preparation of the premixes, prolonged storage under adverse conditions, the failure to add nutrients over a prolonged period of time or incorrect mixing.

COMMON DISEASES AND CONDITIONS ASSOCIATED WITH FEEDING AND NUTRITION	
• Abortion.	• Torsion of the stomach / intestines.
• Colitis.	• Water deprivation.
• Fractures of bones.	• Anaemia.
• Lameness	• Diarrhoea.
- Osteochondrosis	• Gastric ulcers.
- Osteomalacia	• Mycotoxicosis.
- Osteoporosis	• Reproduction.
• Mulberry heart disease.	• Salt poisoning.
• Prolapse of the rectum.	• Udder oedema and mastitis.
• Respiratory disease.	

(Fig.14-7)

The roles of energy and protein in disease generally have already been highlighted but there are a number of specific conditions that are initiated by faulty feeding in one form or another. (Fig.14-7)

ABORTION AND SEASONAL INFERTILITY

Embryo loss and abortion

Embryo loss occurs when there is death of embryos followed by absorption, or expulsion. Healthy embryos grow into foetuses. Abortion means the premature expulsion of a dead or non-viable foetus. There is often alarm when an abortion is seen but it should be remembered that there can be loss of embryos at any time during early pregnancy, which often goes unseen.

Embryo loss or abortion can be considered in three main groups: First, during the period from fertilisation to implantation; second, during the period of implantation at around 14 days post-service to 35 days; and finally, during the period of maturation, which results in premature farrowings. It can be seen therefore that losses can take place at any stage from approximately 14 days after mating, when implantation has taken place, through to 110 days of pregnancy.

The maintenance of pregnancy

Pregnancy is maintained due to hormonal changes initiated by the implantation of embryos at day 14. These changes allow the corpus luteum (the body from which the egg is released) in the ovary to develop and produce the pregnancy hormone progesterone. The presence of the corpus luteum is necessary to maintain the pregnancy throughout the whole of the gestation period. The loss or failure of the corpus luteum through any cause initiates the farrowing process, hence an abortion, or if near to term a premature farrowing.

Methods of Investigation

It is worthwhile monitoring the levels of abortion in your herd continually and comparing them to the normal levels. The following information should be recorded with each abortion:

- Sow number.
- Parity.
- Boar used.
- Date of service.
- Date of abortion.
- Housing.
- Feed and amounts given.
- Clinical observations of the sow and any disease history.
- Condition of the aborted piglets - alive fresh, recently dead or mummified.

If you are using the farrowing rate loss analysis sheet illustrated in chapter 5 you will be doing most of this anyway.

It is important to study the herd history and environment. For example, is there a seasonal effect or an association with a particular area of the housing or management practice? You should also note the clinical state of the sow at the time of abortion. Does she show other clinical signs or is she apparently normal? You should examine the aborted foetuses too. Are they fresh with no signs of any decomposition, or are they decomposing or mummified. Such observations, particularly if recorded over a period, may be of help to your veterinarian in leading to a possible diagnosis of the cause.

There are three parts to the investigations that must be carried out. First, collect information about the individual sows, then request post mortem examinations and serological tests, and finally, assess the clinical evidence and feeding procedures in the herd.

The object of these is to identify the area of failure and by management studies, examination of records, clinical examinations, and laboratory tests the cause may be identified.

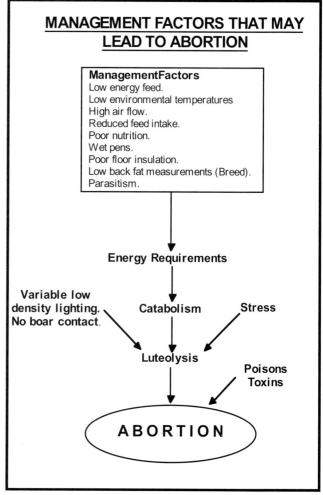

(Fig.14-8)

Non Infectious Causes

Seasonal infertility

Experiences have shown that 70% of all abortions fall into this category. Because the sow historically only produced one litter per year, with farrowings during early spring, there is an in-built tendency for the animal not to maintain a pregnancy during the summer and autumn periods. This is well recognised with summer infertility and the autumn abortion syndrome, where environmental factors are likely to cause the corpus luteum to disappear.

A catabolic state

If the metabolism of sows are allowed to progress to a negative energy or catabolic state so that they are having to use their body tissues to maintain the energy equilibrium, then individual susceptible animals may abort. Clinical examinations will identify possible changes in the environment. For example, the removal of bedding, poor quality feeds, or a drop in feed intake. The latter may simply be associated with a change in stockpeople. Outbreaks of abortion may occur when there are changes from pellet feeding to meal feeding, or where feed is presented by volume and not by weight. Wet, damp environments or high air movement cause chilling and increase demands for energy. An important feature of environmental abortions is that the sow remains normal, often eating feed in the morning, and expelling the litter in the afternoon. Some people call these "Farrowing abortions". The aborted foetuses are perfectly normal and the sow shows no signs of illness. The underlying initiating mechanism is regression of the corpus luteum.

Light

Another contributing factor is decreasing daylight length. To maintain a viable pregnancy requires constant daylight length. Ideally this should be 12-16 hours per day. Light intensity experienced by the sow can be affected by a number of environmental inadequacies, for example, poor lighting in the first place, followed by fly faeces and dust on lamps gradually reducing the availability of light. High walls surrounding animals, or automatic feeders in front of sows producing shadows. A simple tip here is to make sure that you can read a newspaper in the darkest parts of the building at sow eye level. If not, then problems may start. Painting the roofs and walls white to increase the reflection of light is one way of improving the environment and on a number of occasions abortions have ceased after such simple improvements.

Abortions, anoestrus and sows found not in pig commonly occur during the period of summer infertility when sunlight is intense and the weather is hot. This is particularly evident in outdoor sows where levels of pregnancy failure may reach 15-30%. In such cases the abortions are so early that the foetuses are either not seen or there is progressive embryo mortality and a delayed return to oestrus. Look for slight mucous discharges from the vulva and if present refer to chapter 6 "Endometritis".

The following factors are important indoors or outdoors as applicable (Fig.14-9):

- Ultra violet radiation may cause regression of the corpus luteum particularly in white breeds. The outdoor breeding female should always be derived from at least one pigmented parent.
- Provide extensive shades so that the sows can protect themselves from the sun.
- Site the arks in the wind direction so that with open ends cooling can take place.
- Provide extensive well maintained wallows suitably sited so that sows do not have too far to reach them.
- Always maintain boars within the sow groups for the first six weeks of pregnancy at least.
- Increase feed intake from days 3 to 21 after mating.

A CHECKLIST FOR ABORTIONS	
Abortion Level. Is this more than 1.5% of sows served?	- Take action
Are sows ill?	- Probably disease
Are sows otherwise normal?	- Probably non infectious - Maternal failures
Is the problem seasonal?	- Autumn abortion syndrome
Do they occur in a particular part of the farm?	- Environmental
Are the aborted pigs fresh or alive?	- Suggests the environment
Are mummified pigs present?	- Suggests infection
Is the dry sow accommodation uncomfortable?	- Suggests the environment
Are sow pens wet, draughty, poorly lit?	- Suggests the environment
Does the ventilation system chill the sows?	- Suggests the environment
Are there factors that place the sows in a negative energy state?	e.g.: High chill factors Draughts Low feed intake A change in bedding Availability
Are sows short of food	- Check feed intakes by volume and weight
Is the food mouldy?	Check for mouldy feed
Do the sows experience 14 hours of good light at eye level?	
Are the lights dirty, covered in fly dirt?	
Can you read a newspaper in the darkest corner?	
Do your sows have boar contact in pregnancy?	
Are any other diseases evident in the sows?	e.g.: lameness cystitis kidney infections
Are the abortions associated with stress?	

(Fig.14-9)

> *Empty feed bins monthly.*
> *Examine internal surfaces monthly*
> *Examine feed daily*
> *Treat Bins regularly with a mould inhibitor.*

- Increase the mating programme by 10-15% over the anticipated period of infertility.
- Because boar semen can be affected follow each natural mating 24 hours later by purchased AI.

The role of energy in abortion is detailed in Fig.14-8.

Changes in energy requirements as shown in Fig.14-8 may result in luteolysis or regression of the corpus luteum and abortion. Abortions can also be associated with specific infectious diseases or mouldy feeds. See also chapter 6.
- To prevent the latter:
- Always check your feed bins. Are they water tight?
- When were they last inspected internally?
- Do they contain bridged mouldy feed?
- Are the bins filled with warm feed?
- Do you regularly treat the bins to prevent mould growth.

ANAEMIA

Anaemia is a condition associated with either a reduction in the number of red cells in the blood, the amount of haemoglobin they contain, or the volume of the red cells themselves.

It can arise in one of three ways:
- Loss of blood through haemorrhage. Typical examples would be gastric ulceration, trauma to the vulva or a ruptured liver.
- Lack of haemoglobin due to dietary insufficiencies, particularly iron and copper.
- Reduced numbers of red cells. These are produced in the bone marrow and any disease, infection or toxic state affecting it may result in anaemia.

The common causes of anaemia are shown in Fig.14-10 but iron deficiency and anaemia in piglets are the most common and important. From a purely nutritional aspect anaemia in growing and adult animals would be uncommon but disease will often give rise to a secondary anaemia. Anaemia is also common, secondary to specific diseases such as actinobacillus pleuropneumonia or glässers disease.

Clinical signs

The pig is pale and becomes breathless on exertion. The mucous membranes of the eyes are pale. They can be compared to a normal pig if there is doubt about interpretation. Haemorrhage may be obvious to the exterior or it can occur through bleeding into the tissues or the gut. Warfarin poisoning can cause severe bleeding into the tissues.

Diagnosis

Anaemia can be diagnosed on clinical grounds and by examining a sample of blood. This is tested for the red cell volume and the haemoglobin levels. (Normal levels 9-15g/100ml), anaemia <8g/100ml). A stained blood smear will also confirm the shape and size of the red cells and whether there are any bacteria present. Specific cell types are involved in the different anaemias. Iron dextran toxicity associated with vitamin E deficiency may give rise to anaemia in piglets.

Treatment

☐ The intestine can absorb only small amounts of iron daily which may not be enough to reverse the anaemia quickly. Nevertheless iron and copper levels in the feed should be checked. It is also helpful to give an injection of iron dextran 300-500mg depending on the age of the pig.
☐ Specific treatment and prevention will depend on the cause. Refer to the specific conditions in the index.
☐ In severe cases electrolytes can be given either by injection or by mouth.

Management control and prevention

◆ Carry out regular worming programmes and/or check faeces samples for parasites every 3 to 6 months and monitor iron levels in feed.

COLITIS

"Colitis" means inflammation of the large bowel and it is very common in some countries in growing pigs. It is characterised by sloppy "cow pat" type faeces, with no blood and little if any mucus but the condition may progress to severe diarrhoea. Affected pigs are usually 6 to 12 weeks of age and in any one group, up to 50% of the population may be affected. It is not seen in adult or sucking pigs.

A number of organisms have been implicated but spirochetes and in particular *Serpulina pilosicoli*, an organism distinct from a similar one that causes swine dysentery, is thought to be important. However dietary factors also precipitate disease and pelleted feed is much more likely to be associated with the disease than meal. If the incriminating pellets are ground back to meal colitis still results, demonstrating an effect of the pelleting process. Certain components in the feed are also implicated including poor quality oils and carbohydrates but specific ones have not been identified.

THE COMMON CAUSES OF ANAEMIA	
Eperythrozoonosis in all ages.	The stomach worm (*Hyostrongylus rubidus*).
Fungal toxins.	The whip worm (*Trichuris suis*).
Gastric ulcers.	Umbilical haemorrhage
Iron deficiency in piglets.	Vaginal haematoma.
Mange (*Sarcoptes scabiei*).	Vulval biting.
Mycotoxins	Warfarin poisoning.
Porcine enteropathy - Bloody gut (PHE).	

(Fig.14-10)

Clinical signs

These usually appear in rapidly growing pigs from 8 to 14 weeks old, fed ad lib on high density diets. The early signs are sloppy faeces but with pigs appearing clinically normal. As the disease and its severity progress, a very watery diarrhoea, with dehydration, loss of condition and poor growth become evident in the pigs. During the affected period daily gain and food conversion can be severely affected, with feed conversion worsening by up to 0.2.

Diagnosis

This is based on clinical signs and the elimination of other causes of diarrhoea, in particular swine dysentery. Faeces examinations in the laboratory are necessary to assist with diagnosis together with post-mortem examinations and laboratory tests on a typical untreated pig.

It is possible that porcine enteropathy may be involved in the clinical syndrome and if the herd has a severe problem examination of the terminal parts of the small intestine in pigs at slaughter would be advised.

Treatment

☐ Antibiotic therapy is not always successful because it depends on the presence of primary or secondary bacteria, but the following drugs have given responses on problem farms, using in-feed medication.

    Dimetridazole - 200 g / tonne
    Lincomycin - 110 g/ tonne
    Monensin - 100 g / tonne
    Oxytetracycline - 400 g / tonne
    Salinomycin - 60 g / tonne
    Tiamulin - 100 g / tonne
    Tylosin - 100 g / tonne

☐ For the individual pig daily injections of either tiamulin, lincomycin, tylosin or oxytetracycline may be beneficial

☐ Weaned pigs are fed zinc for the first two weeks post-weaning to prevent *E. coli* enteritis. Colitis may develop in the 2 to 3 weeks following its removal from the diet. The response to continuing zinc oxide in the feed at 2 to 3kg per tonne should be considered.

Management control and prevention

◆ Disease is seen in pigs that are growing well on ad lib feeding and often it is associated with a change of diet.
◆ It is more common with diets high in energy and protein (14.5MJ DE/kg 21% protein). It is experienced using all types of diets but particularly those that have been pelleted rather than fed as a meal. It is thought that the pelleting process may have an effect on fats in the diet and thereby initiate digestive disturbances in the large bowel.
◆ It is common when fat sprayed diets are fed, try diets without.
◆ Mortality is low but morbidity can be high, ranging from 5 to 50%. Adopt all-in all-out management of pens.
◆ The same diet can be used on two separate farms and disease only appear on one, suggesting inherent causes.
◆ The presence of certain types of bacteria in the large bowel such as *Serpulina pilosicoli* obviously play a part in the disease. Use preventive medication in feed to control *Sepurlina pilosicoli*
◆ It is uncommon on home milled cereal based diets.
◆ The response to treatment can be variable.
◆ Control consists of assessing the above key factors, which would include changing the diet formulation (less added fats), changing the source of feed, acidifying the diet and improving pen hygiene. A change from pellets to meal feeding is usually effective.

The following anti colitis diet fed as a meal has been effective.

Wheat	50%
Barley	11%
Full fat soya	15%
Fish meal	7.5%
Hypro soya	6.5%
Sharps (wheat by-product)	5%
Skim milk	2.5%
Vitamin lysine mineral supplement	2.5%

Analysis

Protein	24%
DE	14.6
Lysine	1.35

DIARRHOEA

Whilst diarrhoea may be initiated by nutrition it is also associated with one or more of the following diseases. (Common ones *). See chapter 9.

- Anthrax (rare).
- Classical swine fever (in those countries where it is still endemic). See chapter 12
- Coliform infections and post-weaning diarrhoea *.
- Colitis (specific disease). *
- Oedema disease (diarrhoea uncommon).
- Parasites.
- Porcine epidemic diarrhoea PED. *
- Porcine enteropathy including PHE, PIA, NE & RI. *
- Rotavirus.
- Salmonellosis. *
- Spirochaetal diarrhoea.
- Swine dysentery. *

- TGE (rare in Europe now but still common in some other countries).

Refer to the above specific diseases after a diagnosis has been made in a laboratory. Use the Fig.14-11 to assist in interpreting the clinical picture.

Pre and Post-weaning

Changes in the intestine of the pig at weaning

Fig.14-12 shows the cross section of the small intestine of the weaned piglet to consist of many thousands of finger like projections called villi, which increase the absorptive capacity of the small intestine. During suckling they are continuously bathed by sows milk which contains the immunoglobulin IgA. This becomes absorbed into the mucous covering the villi surfaces and prevents *E. coli* and other organisms attaching to the fingers. If they are unable to attach they are unable to cause disease. The secretary IgA also helps to destroy bacteria. After weaning time however no more IgA is available, the levels rapidly decline and bacteria damage the villi causing them to shrink. This atrophy reduces the absorptive capacity of the gut and the ability of the pig to use its food. The enzymes produced by the cells of the villi are likewise reduced. The changes result in malabsorption of food and poor digestion with or without the development of scour. The villi normally regenerate within 5 to 7 days after weaning from cells at their base called enterocytes, which multiply and migrate upwards causing the villi to return to their normal length. The rate of multiplication and regeneration is in part an environmental temperature and energy dependent phenomena. If the pig is weaned in an environment below its lower critical temperature (LCT), the rate of regeneration of the villi is reduced and in some cases ceases. (This results in the hairy pig that doesn't grow). Feed intake is a crucial part of the equation.

Other factors also increase the demand for energy and it is critical the balance is made in the first 24 hours of weaning. Draughts must be avoided.

Before weaning the piglet receives milk as a liquid feed at regular intervals. As a result the bacterial flora of the gut, although relatively simple compared with that of a mature pig, is stabilised.

At weaning cessation of milk removes secretory IgA and there is a period of starvation, followed by irregular attempts to eat solid feed. This results in a dynamic disruption of the bacterial flora of the gut which may last for 7 to 10 days before stabilising. This bacterial disruption may also contribute to poor digestion and possibly scour, particularly when high levels of pathogenic strains

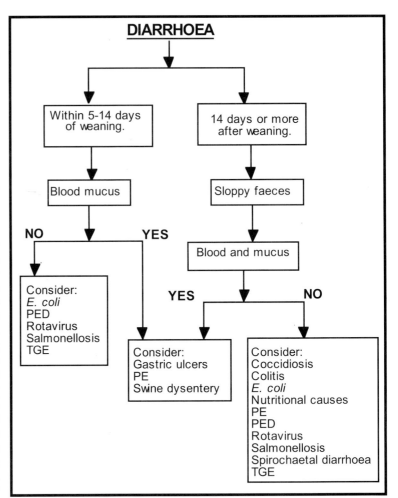

(Fig.14-11)

The greater the villus atrophy the poorer the growth rate of the pig.

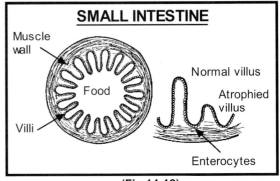

(Fig.14-12)

of *E. coli* are involved.

Before weaning the piglets led an ordered life, being "called" with their litter mates to suckle and obtain small amounts of milk at regular intervals, sleeping between meals in a warm creep. All this suddenly changes at weaning, the pigs finding themselves in strange surroundings with strange piglets, and only solid feed. Psychological trauma is inevitable and is likely to affect some pigs more than others, resulting in impaired digestibility and lowered resistance to disease. The more this psychological stress can be minimised the better

If poor growth is evident in the first seven days post-weaning the following options or variables need to be considered:

- Check that the weights of all pigs at weaning are to the target level.

> **The pig must balance its energy requirements during the first 72 hours post-weaning. If not, disease is likely to occur. Fig.14-13.**

- Check the ages of the pigs at weaning.
- Heavier but younger pigs will have a more immature digestive system.
- Group the pigs by weight or keep them in their litter groups.
- Use a highly digestible and palatable diet and mix and soak this for the first day or two with water.
- Use different diets according to body weight and age.
- Use open dishes for feeding for the first three days at least, instead of troughs.
- Feed small quantities of creep four to five times daily and remove uneaten stale feed.
- Provide easy access to fresh clean water.
- Use in-feed medication for the first ten days post-weaning.
- Check that the environmental temperature is constant and satisfies the pigs requirements particularly in the first four days post-weaning.
- Maintain a dry house without draughts.
- Reduce any form of stress.
- If pigs are housed on slatted floors provide solid comfort boards for them to lie on for the first few days.
- Remove the smallest piglets from each pen after 7 to 10 days and place them together in one pen in the same room. Their diet can then be adjusted accordingly.

Key factors that dictate the degree of villus atrophy

- Age of the pig at weaning.
- Weight of the pig at weaning.
- The environmental temperature and its fluctuations.
- Feed intake and availability of feed.
- Digestibility of the feed.
- Quality of the proteins.
- Levels of milk proteins.
- Levels of bacterial and viral challenge.

Nutrition

Only minimal amounts of solid food are eaten during the suckling period and very little before 10 days of age.

Key points to maximising feed intake

- Pigs at weaning time will eat a warm gruel better than a solid food.
- Gruel feeding reduces the degree of villus atrophy and dehydration.
- Pigs need to be encouraged to feed in the first 2 to 3 days post-weaning because the maternal discipline of suckling every 40 minutes is lost.
- Provide creep feed for the first 72 hours in open dishes 5 to 6 times a day. This will encourage the pigs to eat and avoid over eating. Piglets naturally "root" pellets from the floors rather than a trough. Recently washed metal troughs have unattractive smells.
- By experiment place the feeders in the most attractive part of the pen.
- A small pellet or crumb will increase intake. Pellet size should be 2mm or less.
- Examine the piglets mouths at weaning time to ensure there has been no damage to the gums during teeth removal. Pigs with sore infected gums will not eat.
- Use a highly palatable diet.

Creep feeding / options

The term "creep feed" here means the pre-starter diet offered to piglets before and just after weaning until they can be changed to a cheaper starter diet.

When sows were loose-housed in farrowing pens the pre-starter had to be placed in a "creep" where the sows could not get to it. Now that sows are farrowed in crates

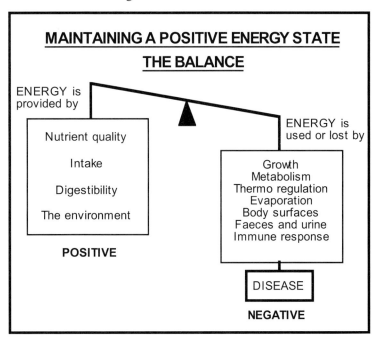

(Fig.14-13)

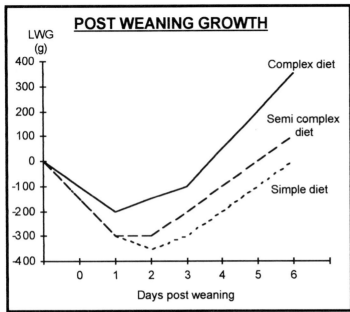

Complex diet - Cooked cereals and skim milk
Semi complex and simple diets - Wheat, barley, soya.
Courtesy of Frank Aherne

(Fig.14-14)

or tethers the creep is placed outside the warm creep area in a cooler part of the pen to keep it fresh but the term "creep feed" is still used.

There are a number of options:

- No creep given pre-weaning.
- Different creeps given pre and post-weaning.
- Mixed creeps given post-weaning.
- A high dense diet used pre-weaning and a low one post-weaning.
- A low dense diet used pre-weaning and a high one post-weaning
- Restricted feed for varying periods of time.
- Choice feeding.

By trial and error determine the best methods that produce a healthy rapid growing weaner.

On most farms the best method is to offer very small quantities of fresh creep feed several times a day for the last 7 to 10 days before weaning and to continue this for one to three days after weaning while gradually changing to starter rations.

Nutritional components of a good creep diet

Whilst it is not the purpose of this book to discuss nutrition in detail nevertheless Fig.14-14 shows the effects on growth rate of a simple diet compared to a complex one. A complex diet could consist of the following:

Cooked cereals 38 %, maze oil 11%, milk products 45%, Glucose and sugars 5% plus minerals and vitamins, MJ DE/kg 16.4, Protein 21 to 23%, lysine 1.3 to 1.4%, oil 20%.

FRACTURES

See also lameness in this chapter for further information.

Bone fractures are not uncommon in sows and gilts and are usually the end result of trauma and fighting although spontaneous ones occur in bone disease such as osteomalacia, associated with calcium phosphorus and vitamins A and D, and osteochondrosis.

Clinical signs

The onset is invariably sudden, the animal being unable to rise on its own without difficulty. A significant feature is the reluctance to place any weight on the affected leg. The muscles and tissues over the fracture site are often swollen and painful and the pig is very reluctant to move unless on three legs. An examination is best carried out when the pig is lying down. Crepitus or the rubbing together of the two broken ends of the bone can often be felt.

Fractures of the spinal vertebra are common in the first litter female particularly during lactation and in the immediate post weaning period. The pig usually adopts a dog sitting position and exhibits severe pain on movement. Such animals should be destroyed.

Diagnosis

This is based upon the history, symptoms and palpation to detect crepitus.

Similar diseases

These include acute laminitis, arthritis, muscle tearing, bush foot and mycoplasma arthritis.

Treatment

☐ The affected animal should be slaughtered on the farm.

Management control and prevention

◆ If fractures are a recurring problem it is necessary to check that there are no diseases such as osteomalacia, osteoporosis or leg weakness (OCD).
◆ Check the calcium, phosphorus and vitamin D levels.
◆ Check management procedures during the period of effect.

GASTRIC ULCERS

Erosion and ulceration of the lining of the stomach is a common condition in all pigs. It occurs around the area where the oesophagus enters the stomach (called the pars oesophagea). In the early stages of the disease the pars becomes roughened and gradually changes as the surface becomes eroded until it is actively ulcerated. Intermittent haemorrhage may then take place leading to anaemia, or massive haemorrhage may occur resulting in death. The incidence in sows is usually less than 5% but in growing pigs up to 60% may show lesions at slaughter.

The causes of gastric ulceration are multifactorial. These can be categorised as nutritional and related to the physical properties of the feed, managemental, infectious causes and miscellaneous factors.

The following need to be considered as causal or contributory:

Nutritional factors:
- Low protein diets.
- Low fibre diets. (The introduction of straw reduces the incidence).
- High energy diets.
- High levels of wheat in excess of 55%.
- Deficiencies of vitamin E or selenium.
- Diets containing high levels of iron, copper or calcium.
- Diets low in zinc.
- Diets with high levels of unsaturated fats.
- Diets based on whey and skimmed milk.

Physical aspects of the diet that increase the incidence:
- Size of feed particle - the more finely ground the meal the smaller becomes the particle size and the higher the incidence of ulcers. This is still the case if the feed is then pelleted.
- Pelleting feeds in itself increases the incidence. Feed meal.
- Particle size. Where there is a problem on the farm have the feed examined to assess the varying percentages of particle sizes. This is carried out by sifting the meal through a series of 12 to 14 tiller screens and weighing the residual amounts remaining in each screen. Particle size is also affected by the type and moisture content of the cereals that are being used, the condition of the hammer mills and the screen and the rate of flow through the grinding system. The smaller the particle size the greater the incidence.
- Sometimes there can be problems in changing from pellets to meal and a compromise is to feed alternatively.
- If the feed is home-produced and is meal, then it is necessary to check the size and quality of the screen that is being used.
- Using cereals with a high moisture content.
- Rolling cereals as distinct from grinding them will often produce a dramatic drop in the incidence but the penalties of feed use have to be taken into consideration.

Managemental factors that increase the incidence:
- Irregular feeding patterns and shortage of feeder space.
- Periods of starvation.
- Increased stocking densities and movement of pigs.

Look carefully at the environment in the pens and in finishing houses. Are there undue stresses or aggressions.
- Poor management of sows in stalls and tethers.
- Transportation.
- Poor availability of food or water.

Miscellaneous factors:
- Stress associated with fluctuating environmental temperatures.
- Adverse environmental conditions that create an unhappy environment.
- Psychological stress resulting from bad or harsh stockmanship.
- The condition is more common in castrates and boars than in gilts but the reason for this is unknown. Difference in feeding patterns may be a factor.
- Split sexing may help.
- Breed. More common in certain genotypes particularly those that have low back fat measurements and a capacity for rapid lean tissue growth.

Infectious causes:
- There is a clear relationship between outbreaks of pneumonia and the incidence of gastric ulceration.
- Ulceration may occur following bacterial septicaemias such as those associated with erysipelas and swine fever.
- In the breeding sow gastric ulceration is usually confined to the individual animal and is often secondary to a specific disease.

> ***Consider changing from pellets to course ground meal.***

Clinical signs

These depend on the severity of the condition. In its most acute form previously healthy animals are found dead. The most striking sign in these cases is the paleness of the carcase due to internal haemorrhage. In the less acute form the affected pig is pale, and weak, and may show breathlessness, grinding of the teeth due to stomach pain and vomiting. The passing of dark faeces containing digested blood is often a persistent symptom. Usually the temperature is normal. When the condition becomes chronic the pig has an intermittent appetite and may lose weight. The faeces vary from normal to dark coloured depending on the presence or absence of blood. Feed intake, feed efficiency and daily gain can be affected.

> ***If ulcers are a problem then increase the screen size to 3.5mm.***

Diagnosis

Ulceration should always be considered in sows or pigs which are pale, lose body condition and develop a variable appetite particularly if the faeces are black and tarry. A sample of faeces should be examined for the presence of blood and to eliminate parasites. Although the disease is usually confined to individuals or less than 5% of sows, occasionally it can become a herd problem. In such cases poor body condition is widespread through the breeding herd.

Whenever black tarry faeces are seen gastric ulceration should be suspected and in the feeding herd an examination of stomachs at slaughter should be carried out.

Similar diseases

Haemorrhage from the bowel can also arise from the intestine in cases of bloody gut (PHE) but usually this is confined to young gilts and growing pigs.

Anaemia in pigs can also be associated with eperythrozoonosis, the stomach worm *Hyostrongylus rubidus*, chronic mange and porcine enteropathy. Nutritional deficiencies particularly of minerals and vitamins can increase the incidence.

Treatment

- Move the affected animal from its existing housing into a loose bedded peaceful environment.
- Feed a weaner type diet containing highly digestible materials.
- Inject multi vitamins and in particular vitamin E together with 0.5 to 1g of iron intramuscularly and repeat on a weekly basis.
- Add an extra 100g vitamin E / tonne to the diet for two months and assess the results.
- Cull affected pigs.

Management control and prevention

- Consider the above factors and their relevance to your situation. Make alterations and adjustments accordingly.

LAMENESS

CALCIUM AND PHOSPHORUS

Problems that may arise with calcium, phosphorus, vitamin A and D

With modern dietary formulations actual deficiencies arising due to defective diet would be unusual. Problems however occur due to faulty storage, the incorrect application of the feed or interactions that reduce the availability to the pig. The latter can result from intestinal disease, metabolic failures or adverse interactions between nutrition, the pig, management and the environment.

Calcium contributes to wide variety of functions in the body including blood clotting, muscle and nervous activity, hormone production and milk production to name but a few. Its major role however, together with phosphorus is involved in the formation of bone where on a dry matter basis it forms approximately 38% of the structure and phosphorus 20%.

Bone is a very strong and dynamic structure with minerals constantly being removed and replaced. The intestines control the rates of absorption both into the body and skeleton and these are necessary to maintain an equilibrium between demand and excretion. The ratio of calcium to phosphorus in the diet is also an important factor in this equation and this should not rise above 2:1, when it does the absorption of calcium may be impaired, likewise if the ratio drops below 1:1. The ideal is approximately 1.25:1 to 1.50:1. Vitamin D_3 is also required in calcium metabolism together with controlling hormones produced by the parathyroid gland.

OSTEODYSTROPHY

This is a general term to describe specific diseases that arise whenever there is a failure of bone structure and metabolism due to faulty nutrition. Such diseases include osteoporosis, rickets and osteomalacia, periostitis describing disease of the periosteum and osteomyelitis, disease of the centre or medullary cavity of the bone.

OSTEOPOROSIS (OP) AND OSTEOMALACIA (OM)

Both these conditions are becoming more common in modern pig producing systems particularly in the first litter gilt where the skeleton is still growing and there are heavy demands on calcium for milk production.

Bones affected with OP are quite normal in their structure but they become thinner particularly in the dense parts and shafts of the long bones. As a result they become more prone to fracture. OP can arise due to a shortage of calcium in the diet and imbalance of calcium and phosphorus, poor or inadequate absorption from the diet, heavy losses during lactation and where there is a lack of exercise. Osteomalacia is the adult form of rickets and is associated with a phosphorus or vitamin D_3 deficiency. There is a failure of the mineral to be deposited in the bones, which become soft and they either bend or fracture.

Clinical signs

These are most common in the first litter female and occasionally after the second litter.

The onset may be gradual with the pig having difficulty rising and showing pain or sudden lameness associated with complete fracture of the long bones. Spinal fractures occur in some animals and they often remain in a dog sitting position. Most pigs are affected in late lactation or shortly after weaning associated with the onset of oestrus and the trauma that results from other animals, or the weight of the boar at service.

Diagnosis

This is based on clinical signs, a history in lactating and newly weaned sows and evidence of fractures of the long bones. If the herd has a problem it is necessary to examine the bones of an affected animal by x-ray to differentiate between OP and OM.

Similar diseases
These include:
Leg weakness or osteochondrosis.
Spinal fractures.
Torn muscles at their insertions into the bones.
Mycoplasma hyosynoviae infection

Treatment
☐ In cases of bone fracture the sow is best destroyed on humane grounds.

Management control and prevention
◆ Outbreaks are often more apparent in new gilt herds. Selection of animals for good conformation is essential.
◆ Investigate the growth rates and nutrition and feeding in the gilt.
◆ Increase exercise during pregnancy if possible.
◆ Check the levels of calcium and phosphorus in the diet. They should be 10-12g/kg of calcium and 8-10g/kg of phosphorus.
◆ Only mate gilts from 220 days onwards and if the disease is a persistent problem in a particular genotype change the source.
◆ Check that floor surfaces are not slippery.
◆ The problem is less common in outdoor herds.
◆ Feed a good lactation diet during suckling and consider top dressing the diet daily with 20g of di calcium bone phosphate.
◆ Inject pregnant animals with 50,000iu vitamin D_3 three weeks prior to farrowing. Repeat again in the second week after farrowing.
◆ Maximise feed intake to appetite during lactation.
◆ Check the ratio of calcium : phosphorus in bone ash. The normal ratio is approximately 2:1 or less. In problem sows this is often 3:1 or more.

RICKETS
This arises in a similar way to OM except it occurs in young growing animals, again as a failure of mineralisation of bone and growth plate cartilage. Phosphorus and vitamin D deficiencies are the common cause but the condition today is rare.

Where it occurs young animals are often housed in dark surroundings and fed starch feed waste with no mineral vitamin supplements. It usually takes 6 to 8 weeks before symptoms become evident, by which time the disease has progressed to become irreversible.

The symptoms are similar to OM but because the growth plate and cartilage does not develop to bone the joints swell with stiffness and pain is evident. Bone fractures are also common. In the few cases treated the response to injections of vitamin D_3 has been very poor with pigs being totally uneconomical.

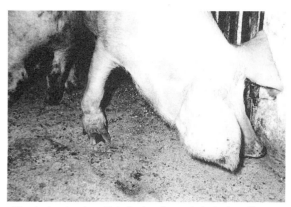

Vitamin A poisoning. Note the bending and shortening of bones (90kg pigs).
(Fig.14-15)

VITAMIN A
The classical descriptions of vitamin A deficiency are described in Fig.14-4 but in the authors experience in the field such diseases would be rare. Most if not all rations are well fortified with the vitamin, indeed in many cases to excess and gross intake leading to disease is more likely to be experienced, but not well recognised.

Two problems arise in the field. The first is where high levels of vitamin A up to 15,000 to 18,000 iu/kg are fed. This has been shown to lower the vitamin E status of the pig and therefore make it potentially more susceptible to mulberry heart disease. This depression of vitamin E may also reduce antibody production and thereby increase susceptibility to disease. This scenario has coincided with out breaks of respiratory disease in the field and lowering the vitamin A levels to around 8,000iu/kg and raising the vitamin E by 50-100iu/kg had been undertaken with improvements.

Piglets born from sows fed high levels of vitamin A may produce piglets with a low vitamin E status and this can be a fruitful line of investigation where iron dextran problems persist in sucking pigs.

The second problem arises when excessively high levels of vitamin A - 25,000 to 30,000iu/kg are fed. At these levels the growth plates of the foetus become affected with classical signs of leg weakness and grossly shortened and bent bones in pigs as young as three weeks of age.

Fig.14-15 shows a typical affected pig from a herd where such high levels produced widespread changes in the fine boned Landrace breed but were not so evident in the Pietrain. The condition disappeared four months after the levels in the sow rations were dropped to 12,000iu/kg.

Further evidence for the effects of vitamin A on growth plates was also illustrated in a severe outbreak of leg weakness in weaners and growers fed rations containing high lysine 1.5% and high vitamin A levels of 18,000iu/kg. The pigs were housed on very smooth slats the surfaces of which sloped to the edges. This resulted in the claws remaining in the gaps for long periods and by the time the pigs were 16 weeks of age the claws were completely crossed over due to a combination of pressure and weakened growth plates. When levels were reduced to 10,000iu and the lysine levels dropped to 1.1% and the slat surfaces roughened, the problem gradually disappeared.

LEG WEAKNESS OR OSTEOCHONDROSIS
- See chapter 7 for further information.

Degenerative changes in the joints and cartilage are generally described under the term leg weakness or osteochondrosis. These changes involve erosion of the articular cartilage and alterations to the normal patterns of growth at the growth plates at the ends of the long bones.

The use of both vitamins and minerals in cases of disease problems to try and prevent the conditions have been singularly disappointing and it is doubtful if specific nutrient factors are involved.

PROLAPSE OF THE RECTUM

This is a widespread condition occurring in good growing pigs from 8 to 20 weeks of age. The onset is sudden. The size of the prolapse varies from 10 to 80mm and if small it will often revert to the rectum spontaneously. In most cases however the prolapse remains to the exterior and is often cannibalised by other pigs in the pen as evident by blood on the noses of the offending pigs and on the flanks of others. The fundamental cause is an increase in abdominal pressure which forces the rectum to the exterior.

Clinical signs

At the onset the red coloured mucosa of the rectum protrudes from the anal sphincter and then may return on its own. After a short period however it remains to the exterior and becomes swollen and filled with fluid. It is prone to damage and haemorrhage and where pigs are loose housed cannibalism often results with evidence of blood on the skin.

Treatment

- ☐ Rectal prolapses must be recognised early and the pig removed from the pen.
- ☐ Replace the prolapse and retain it by a purse string or mattress suture. Return the pig to the pen. The technique for carrying this out is described in chapter 15.

If the prolapse has been badly torn still replace it, and consider moving the pig to a hospital pen and treat with a long-acting antibiotic injection. In a proportion of pigs the damaged tissues become scarred with constriction leading to rectal strictures. The incidence of this is reduced by replacing the prolapse and suturing.

- ☐ In some cases the prolapse will be completely bitten off by other pigs. Here the pig should be left in the pen as most cases will progress to slaughter although a few will develop with rectal strictures.

Management control and prevention

The following may be considered as causal or contributory when adopting control measures.

Disease
- ◆ Diarrhoea - excessive straining.
- ◆ Respiratory disease - excessive coughing increasing abdominal pressure.
- ◆ Colitis - abnormal fermentation occurs in the large bowel with the production of excessive gas increasing abdominal pressure.

The Environment
- ◆ In cold weather the incidence of rectal prolapses increases. This is associated with low house temperatures and the tendency of pigs to huddle together, thus increasing abdominal pressure.
- ◆ Wet conditions and slippery floors, particularly those with no bedding, increase abdominal pressure.
- ◆ If stocking densities reach the level whereby pigs cannot lay out on their sides across the pen the incidence may increase.

Nutrition
- ◆ Ad lib feeding - Feeding pigs to appetite results in continual heavy gut fill and indigestion. There is then a tendency for abnormal fermentation in the large bowel because undigested components of the feed arrive in greater amounts.
- ◆ High density diets and in particular lysine levels increase growth rates and outbreaks may often subside either by a change to restricted feeding or using a lower energy / lysine diet.
- ◆ Water shortage - This can lead to constipation.
- ◆ Diets high in starch may predispose to prolapse - Try adding 2-4% grass meal to the diet.
- ◆ The presence of mycotoxins in feed - If there is a problem make sure that the bins have been well cleaned out. Examine the cereal sources.
- ◆ Change of diet - By studying the timing of the problem it is sometimes possible to identify rectal prolapses not only with a change of diet but also a change of housing.
- ◆ Field evidence does not identify breed as a causal factor.
- ◆ Increases in rectal prolapses have been reported in association with the use of tylosin but the evidence for this is unclear.
- ◆ Trauma
- ◆ Tail docking - docking tails too short can damage the nerve supply to the anal ring leading to a relaxation of the anal sphincter.

Identify those factors on your farm from the above list and making changes. Consider collecting the following

information about each prolapse to see if common factors emerge:
- Age of pig.
- Comments observations.
- Days in the house.
- Diet fed.
- House and pen.
- Number of pigs per pen
- Number of rectal strictures.
- Number of prolapses sutured.
- Outcome.
- State of prolapse.
- Tail biting.
- Weight of the pig.

REPRODUCTION

It is beyond the scope of this book to discuss nutrition in detail, but you should keep in mind that the quality of the feeds and the way in which they are fed are important in the management of disease. Aspects relating to nutrition in the lactating sow are dealt with in chapter 8 "Nutrition". In the dry sow on the day of weaning three quarters of the daily lactation feed should be given prior to actual removal of the sow from the farrowing house and the remainder given later on that day. The sow should be given the opportunity to eat the same amount of food on the three days post weaning as she ate during late lactation. This will ensure that she does not become catabolic (a negative energy state) with an extended weaning to mating interval and subsequent infertility. Such diets should contain at least 14MJ DE/kg 16 % protein and 1.0 - 1.1% lysine, particularly if a lean genotype is being used. Immediately after mating, feed levels should be held at 2kg for the first 48 to 72 hours and then the sow fed to body condition. Provided energy levels are not excessive in the first 3 days post-mating then it is advantageous to feed the sow to body condition using a dry sow ration over the next 21 days with 3kg or more per day.

Many farms today feed separate lactating and dry sow rations. The latter with digestible energy ranging from 13 to 13.6MJ DE/kg and protein levels of 13 to 14%. It is beneficial from 3-21 days post mating to optimise feed intake relative to the sows demand since this will satisfy the nutritional requirements for the development of the placenta. This is pertinent where farms have variable weights and quality of piglets at birth. The development of the placenta in the first 12 to 25 days post mating helps to determine the quality of the piglet at the end of the pregnancy. A small placenta will contribute towards a small pig. The availability and intake of feed in this respect is important, for example where sows are fed in groups. If there is a shortage of trough space, nutritional insufficiencies can occur in the under-privileged females. During the pregnancy period the sow should be fed to

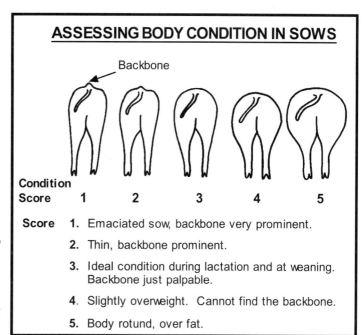

(Fig.14-16)

body condition but also to satisfy the environmental needs. Thus it is difficult to lay down specific levels of feed intake per day, they must be determined by the stockperson. The body condition of the sow can be assessed on a numerical rating of 1 to 5 and to do this the flat of the hand should be placed over the back bone just forward of the root of the tail and rolled laterally side to side. The condition of the sow can then be scored Fig.14-16.

As a guideline sows approaching the point of weaning should score around 3. This should rise to $3\frac{1}{2}$ or possibly 4 in older sows by the time of the next farrowing. Sows scoring $2\frac{1}{2}$ or less are moving into a problem area. If more than 5% of sows at any one time score $2\frac{1}{2}$ or less then feeding levels are wrong. If sows are allowed to farrow with a score of less than 3 there will be insufficient fat reserves to maintain lactation and they will use muscle as a source of energy. Such sows are then in danger of developing the thin sow syndrome, being unable to maintain body condition with the demands of lactation.

In outdoor herds it is important that all sows should score over 3 before the onset of winter. It is difficult to improve body condition in cold weather. Feed levels should be higher during winter than in spring or summer.

Key points to maintaining longevity in the breeding female

- Use the correct female, that is, one expressing maximum hybrid vigour.
- Select or purchase females with sound strong legs, good teats and not too heavy hams.

- Avoid gilts showing any signs of leg weakness e.g., standing on their toes, the back legs tucked under, the front legs bent or the pasterns dropped.
- Do not breed from a female that is too lean. Maintain at least 17mm of fat at the P2 measurement by point of mating, particularly in the gilt.
- Do not serve the gilt at less then 210 days of age. Gilts served too early will still be maturing into their second pregnancy. Equally do not serve too late (240 days) otherwise body size will increase.
- Do not allow excessive body weight to develop during the first pregnancy.
- Provide the pregnant gilt with exercise during the first half of the pregnancy if possible.
- Avoid mouldy feeds.
- Do not cull a sow if her first two litters have been poor. Review management procedures.
- Feed the sow from three days post farrowing, during lactation, and to point of mating to appetite.
- Do not serve maiden gilts or first litter gilts with heavy boars. This can precipitate leg problems.
- Identify sick or lame sows early and remove to a well bedded hospital pen. Many will simply recover in a better environment.
- Good nutrition is vital.

Remember that management, feeding, housing design and a comfortable well lit environment are under your control and they will have a major effect on the viability, health and production of the sow.

Key points to maximising reproduction

The pregnant animal

- Feed to appetite from weaning to oestrus. Use the lactating diet.
- The same amount of food eaten on the day prior to weaning should be eaten on days 1, 2 and 3 after weaning.
- For 2 days post-service feed less than 2kg per animal where feasible. 25-30MJ DE per day.
- Feed to body condition to 21 days post-service.
- Increase energy intake by 0.5-0.75kg of extra feed in the last month of pregnancy but assess this in relation to possible reduced appetite in lactation and the development of udder oedema.
- A negative energy status in the latter part of pregnancy is a major contributory factor to abortion. Always increase feed levels if the environmental temperatures are prone to fluctuation or when there are periods of low external temperatures.

The lactating animal

- Always feed a high energy (>14MJ DE/kg) and high lysine (>1%) ration.
- Intake should be at least 85MJ DE per day and preferably 100, according to the body size.

- Feed to appetite from day three post farrowing.
- Treat sows as individuals, their appetites vary considerably.
- The more dense diet will provide more energy and nutrients to the low appetite animal - invariably this is one that will have subsequent poor reproductive performance.
- Aim to maximise feed intake to maintain body weight.
- The first litter female is a particular problem because feed intake is often low. Consider feeding a grower or weaner ration as part of the diet. Where a herd has been repopulated consider a special diet for the first litter female.

The gilt

The health status and nutrition of the gilt is very important in deciding whether she will come into oestrus or not. Look at the group of gilts. Are they a good weight for age, or is growth variable or poor? If this is the case is there any clinical evidence of disease, mange for example, which may be responsible for anoestrus. Active respiratory diseases, or previous pneumonia, heart sac infection or pleurisy can inhibit puberty and the onset of oestrus. Atrophic rhinitis can destroy the sensitivity of the nose and therefore the response to pheromones (male hormones). If gilts are regularly moved into continually populated pens, heavy parasite burdens and coccidia can build up that can interfere with the digestive process. Anoestrus problems have been associated with these.

Checklists for the health of your gilts

Assess the health and disease. Do you have:
- Variable growth.
- Coughing.
- Evidence of rhinitis.
- Mange.
- Pneumonia.
- Lameness and stiffness on movement.
- Failure of the gilt to stand to the boar - Osteochondrosis or leg weakness.
- Failure of acclimatisation.
- Poor feed intake or an incorrect diet.

> *By 210 days of age good fertile gilts should have come into oestrus.*

Provide good nutrition

The methods of feeding the gilt and the composition of the diet will depend on the genotype. They will also depend on the environmental needs of the gilt relative to housing, temperature and insulation of the buildings. To determine the best system requires a degree of trial

> *If a gilt has not come into oestrus by 240 days consider culling her. She is telling you she is infertile.*

and error on the farm - the objective being to produce the second or third oestrus cycle within a predetermined time span so that the service programme can be satisfied.

Key points to success:
- Gilts should arrive on the farm at approximately 85kg and be fed a dry sow diet until 100kg. This will also allow time for acclimatisation.
- It is necessary to increase backfat in the modern genotype to 18-20mm at the P2 measurement. This is best carried out feeding a low lysine ration, such as that contained in a sow breeder ration (13.4MJ DE/kg and 0.8% lysine). Feed to appetite.
- Approximately 2-3 weeks prior to moving into the service area for mating ad lib feeding should take place. This is to maximise ovulation rate. Use a good lactator or grower diet containing 14MJ DE/kg and 1% lysine.
- Low protein, low energy, or poor quality diets in the period leading up to puberty will often produce a deep state of anoestrus that in some cases is permanent. Assess the response to the diet used.
- Do not leave gilts in a finisher house to point of service, many will never cycle and nutritional requirements may not be satisfied.

RESPIRATORY DISEASES

These are a major problem on many farms today and they usually appear at predictable times that coincide with an increased demand for energy together with a change in the environment. Of all the factors highlighted in Fig.14-5 the following three will always be important if there is a disease problem;
1. An incorrect diet during and for 7 to 10 days after pig movement that creates a negative energy situation.
2. A change in environmental temperatures associated with movement that creates negative energy state.
3. Exposure to infection and the development of disease at the same time.

A typical example would be the development of respiratory disease caused by actinobacillus pleuropneumonia. Pigs carrying these organisms will often develop acute pneumonia when they are moved from solid concrete floors onto slats. This increases the lower critical temperature for the pig and therefore more energy is required. A change in feed or system of feeding, together with a reduction in stocking density, further exaggerates the problem. The immune system does not respond efficiently, the metabolism of the pig alters and acute disease results. Energy cannot be considered alone to the exclusion of other nutrients and the following other factors need to be considered:
- Identify the time when disease first becomes evident.
- Note when nutritional changes take place. When pigs move from one house to another there is often a drop in the nutrient density of the diet. This also coincides with a drop in intake for the first 2 to 7 days.
- This reduced feed intake and change can result in catabolism and the pig dropping below the LCT.
- Maintain high energy diets at critical times. Do not change the feed for at least 5 days when pigs move from one house to another.
- Provide adequate water at all times. Look at the type of nipple drinkers, their availability and accessibility to the pig, particularly when it moves from one house to another.
- Look at the methods of feeding. Are there any features of design or feeder placement that inhibit access to the feed.
- Is there sufficient hopper space.
- Make sure there are adequate levels of vitamin E in the diet. Add an extra 50-100 gm to the tonne if there is a disease problem.

SALT POISONING - (WATER DEPRIVATION)

Salt poisoning is common in all ages of pigs and almost without exception is related to water shortage either caused by inadequate supplies or complete loss. The normal levels of salt in the diet (0.4-0.5%) become toxic in the absence of water.

Signs develop within 24 to 48 hours.

Clinical signs

The very early stages of disease are always preceded by inappetance and whenever a sow or groups of pigs are not eating always check the water supply first. The first signs are often pigs trying to drink from nipple drinkers unsuccessfully. Nervous changes are the major signs and in more advanced cases involve fits, with animals wandering around apparently blind. Often the pig walks up to a wall, stands and presses its head against it in a characteristic position. One symptom strongly suggestive of salt poisoning is nose twitching just before a convulsion starts.

Diagnosis

This is based upon the clinical signs and lack of water. Examination of the brain histologically at post-mortem confirms the disease.

Similar diseases

Aujeszky's disease, swine fever, streptococcal meningitis and glässers disease all produce nervous signs. The condition might also be confused with middle ear infection but this only affects one individual rather than a group of pigs.

Treatment

- The response to treatment is poor but involves rehydrating the animal. At a practical level this can be achieved by dripping water into the mouth of the pig through a hose pipe or alternatively via a flutter valve into the rectum where it is absorbed. (See

- chapter 15 Flutter valve).
- ☐ Discuss the possibility of administering sterile water into the abdomen with your veterinarian.
- ☐ Corticosteroids may also help.

Management control and prevention
- ◆ It must be a daily routine to check that all sources of water are adequate free flowing and available.

TORSION OF THE STOMACH AND INTESTINES

Clinical signs
There are usually none because the pig is found dead but the abdomen is grossly distended.

Diagnosis
This is the most common cause of sudden death in the growing pig and it is usually one of the best pigs in the group. The carcase is fresh the pig is very pale and the abdomen is very distended. Post-mortem examination shows the small and large intestines heavily congested and full of blood. The intestinal tract in the pig is suspended from a common point and this makes it liable to rotate and finally twist.

Management control and prevention
- ◆ Deaths are usually sporadic although they can be of significance where, for example, whey is being fed and bloat occurs.
- ◆ Over-feeding and abnormal fermentation of the contents of both the small and large intestine result in gas formation, increased pressure and a twist.
- ◆ Mortality in weaned and growing pigs should normally be less than 3% and up to a third of this may be caused by torsion. If it reaches 1% or more the dietary components should be examined closely to see if there are starch based ingredients that might cause excessive fermentation. In such cases increasing the level of the growth promoter (if allowed) or adding 100g/tonne of penicillin, OTC or tylosin will reduce the bacterial multiplication.
- ◆ If torsion's are consistent causes of death collect information about each one that includes weight, age, sex, house, stocking density, environmental temperatures and feed changes. A study of this may give guidance as to contributing causes.

UDDER OEDEMA AND FAILURE OF MILK LET DOWN

This presents itself as a failure of milk let down associated with excess fluid in the mammary tissues and is a condition seen in both gilts and sows. It is characterised by a clinically normal animal with no fever or loss of appetite. The distinguishing features are a firmness of all the glands, discomfort on high pressure but no actual pain. The oedema or fluid can be both in the skin and deep in the udder tissue. The pressure produced in the glands once farrowing has ceased prevents a good milk flow and there is a reduction in both the quantity and quality of the colostrum which means a lowered immune status of the piglet. Severe oedema, particularly in the rear glands may result in poor accessibility of teats at sucking time. Such glands often dry off. When piglets eventually find the teat they will not thrive but waste away.

Clinical signs
Usually there is a history on the farm of poor milking amongst all ages and one or two pigs per litter having to be fostered at around 5 to 7 days of age due to poor growth. Scouring problems can sometimes be related back to udder oedema and a poor intake of colostrum. Palpitation of the udder shows fluid either just beneath the skin or deep in the gland and often extending between the legs towards the vulva. The vulva is also often involved.

Diagnosis
This is based on the demonstration of oedema of the udder, by appearance and palpation and the appearance of the litter. Oedema and congestion can lead to mastitis.

Treatment
- ☐ Recognise the condition early and medicate.
- ☐ Treat the sow with small doses of oxytocin ($1/2$ to 1 ml) every 4 to 6 hours on four occasions.
- ☐ Supplement the piglets with artificial milk and make water available in dishes.
- ☐ Give a preventative injection of long-acting antibiotic either penicillin, amoxycillin or OTC if there are any signs of mastitis.

Management control and prevention
Whilst udder oedema usually occurs in individual animals it can become a problem at a herd level. If this is the case the following actions should be considered:
- ◆ Look at feed levels and the development of the udder 7 to 10 days pre-farrowing. Excessive tissue growth can be associated with high feed intake, particularly high energy levels.
- ◆ Maintain sows on the same bulk level of feed pre-farrowing and from the time of entering the farrowing house to two days post-farrowing.
- ◆ Use the same ration pre-farrowing until two days post-farrowing and then change to a lactation ration.
- ◆ Low water intake 2 to 3 days before farrowing can also predispose. Add water to dry feed.
- ◆ Constipation can be a predisposing factor. Bacterial toxins become absorbed from the gut and interfere with the circulation in the udder tissue. In some cases a response will be obtained by feeding increased levels of fibre before farrowing to increase

bulk and reduce constipation.
- ◆ Alternatively the levels of feed can be reduced but it is important to increase the fibre content with bran or other available fibre source. A typical example would be 2kg of breeding diet with 0.5 to 0.75kg of bran. This is better fed wet in the trough to improve palatability.
- ◆ A change from straw yards into farrowing houses is associated with a marked reduction in fibre intake. In such cases give the sow straw for the first 3 to 4 days pre farrowing.

WATER

The ready availability of clean fresh water is essential. Insufficient attention is given to this on many farms.
It is useful to consider the role that water plays in the normal metabolic functions of the pig.
- It helps to maintain and control body temperature, through both the intake and during exhalation when the heat is dissipated from the pig. It is lost in three ways, either by respiration, in the urine or in the faeces.
- An imbalance between water intake and loss results in dehydration and increased concentration of urine. Clinical signs include very dry dung, hollow eyes and a dehydrated skin.
- It is responsible for transporting food and waste products throughout the body. Waste products are eliminated via water through the kidneys.
- Hormones are transported around the body through the blood stream.
- Water regulates the acid alkali balance in the body through the controls exerted by the kidney.
- Water is used in protein synthesis. The digestive process will not function without it. Any restriction of water therefore will affect the above vital functions.

The piglet

Within 6 hours of birth water should be made available in a shallow dish or a trough because fluid intake is so vital at an early age. An efficient dish used for both creep and water in the farrowing pen is shown in Fig.14-17. It is interesting to note how many piglets within 24 hours will drink small amounts of water when given the opportunity. Nipple drinkers are not a very attractive method of presenting the water to the piglet. Water consumption of piglets during lactation is also influenced by the farrowing house temperature and at 28°C (82°F) in a warm creep area water requirements will increase dramatically.

The provision of water to the piglet in the first week causes no harm and is more likely of benefit. For pigs from one to three weeks of age clean water is best presented in an open type drinker rather than a nipple drinker. The water in dishes and drinkers must be clean and fresh.

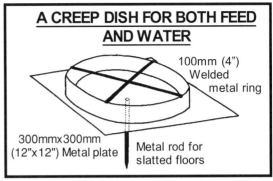

(Fig.14-17)

The weaned pig

The pig experiences dramatic changes at weaning by the sudden move from a liquid to a solid diet. The conditioned reflex, calling the pigs to suckle regularly is also lost. Dehydration associated with poor water intake and marked villus atrophy is a common occurrence

WATER REQUIREMENTS				
Guidelines For the Use of Nipple Drinkers		Water Consumption		
Weight of Pig (Kg)	Height from Floor to Drinker (mm)	Age (Weeks)	Weight (kg)	Litres Per Day
5 - 10	100 - 250	8	20	1
10 - 30	300 - 400	9	25	2.5
30 - 50	400 - 600	10	28	3.3
50 - 100	600 - 750	12	39	4.2
100 +	750 - 900	14	50	5
	750 - 900	17	70	7
	750 - 900	21	90	8.9

(Fig.14-18)

GUIDELINES FOR WATER FLOW FROM NIPPLE DRINKERS	
Pigs / Weight (kg)	Litres / minute
Piglet	0.3
Weaner 7 - 25 kg	1.0
Grower 25 - 50kg	1.4
Finisher 50 - 110kg	1.7
Dry sow	2.0
Lactating sow	2.0

(Fig.14-19)

within the first 7 days of weaning. Ensure the flow rate is at least 0.6 litres per minute from nipple drinkers. It is advisable to offer water in small open drinkers or water bowls daily for the first 5 to 7 days post-weaning. The loss of milk at weaning time and villus atrophy reduce the availability of liquid to the pig for the first 48 hours.

The sow

The changes in water intake from pregnancy to lactation are considerable. Sows that have a lower water intake during lactation generally rear poorer litters and it is important therefore to encourage the sow to drink the moment she enters the farrowing quarters. This is best carried out by giving 4.5 litres of water twice daily into the feed trough until 2-3 days post farrowing. The water flow through a nipple drinker for the lactating sow should approximate 1.5 to 2 litres per minute. Water intake in the dry sow varies from 9-18 litres per day and in lactation from 18 to 36 litres

Water quality

The variables in water quality include organisms, the physical characteristics and the mineral content. Water can become contaminated with pathogenic and non pathogenic bacteria and viruses. The presence of coliform bacteria (i.e. *E. coli* and related bacteria) is an indication of faecal contamination and a potential source of disease.

The chemical quality of water can be assessed by determining the total dissolved solids, the pH (the alkalinity or the acidity), the iron content and the presence of nitrates or nitrites. Further testing would include levels of sulphates, magnesium, chloride, potassium, calcium, sodium and manganese. The total solids in water represent the amount of matter that is actually dissolved. If this level is less than 1000ppm it is of no significance but once it reaches over 6000ppm it becomes unfit for pigs. Generally if the total solid content is low it is usually of good quality and the water is safe to drink.

The pH level of wholesome water varies between 6.5 and 8. Hardness of water is dependent on the levels of calcium and magnesium present but these have no effect on animal health. Hardness does however result in the accumulation of scale causing pipes to gradually block and the flow rate drops unnoticed. This is a common problem on farms that have metal pipes of at least four years standing.

Iron can cause problems in water, with brown coloured staining. Certain types of bacteria can grow and cause blockage of pipes.

High levels of nitrates and nitrites can interfere with the use of vitamin A by the pig and they may be responsible for high still-birth rates.

A Summary of the effects of high nutrient levels in water

Sodium and chloride
- If this is above 250-500ppm then a brackish taste may develop.
- High levels of sodium chloride (salt) affect palatability and can adversely affect pig productivity and performance.
- Sodium sulphate is a laxative and mildly irritant.

Calcium and magnesium
- There are no effects on animal health unless their are high levels of the sulphates which result in the accumulation of scale (as $Mg(OH)_2$ and $CaCO_3$) and over a period of time the diameter of pipes is reduced with the poor flow rates.

DRINKER TO PIG RATIOS *	
Type	Ratio
Nipple	1 : 15 to 1 : 10 Weaner to finisher
Bite	1 : 15 to 1 : 10 Weaner to finisher
Bowl	1: 17 finishers
Trough	300mm per 20 finishers 300mm per 15 sows

* UK welfare guidelines

(Fig.14-20)

GUIDELINES TO WATER QUALITY SUITABLE FOR PIGS	
	ppm (parts per million) Less than
Calcium	1000
Chloride	400
Copper	5
Fluoride	2-3
Hardness calcium carbonate	< 60 Soft > 200 Hard
Iron	0.5
Lead	0.1
Magnesium	400
Manganese	0.1
Mercury	0.003
Nitrites	10
Nitrates	50
Phosphorus	7.8
Potassium	3
Sodium	150
Selenium	0.05
Solids dissolved	1000
Sulphate	1000
Zinc	40
Total viable bacterial counts (TVC) per ml 37°C (99°F) 22°C (72°F)	Low but more important no fluctuation between samples. Target < 2 x 10^2 > 1 x 10^4 poor
Coliforms/100ml	None

(Fig.14-21)

Iron and copper
- High levels of copper have a catalytic effect on the oxidation of iron and if the iron levels are high precipitation of iron occurs when water is pumped, resulting in problems with the delivery system.
- Iron also supports the growth of certain types of bacteria causing foul odours and blocked water systems.

Sulphate
- High levels of sulphate in association with magnesium and sodium can cause diarrhoea.

Manganese
- High levels promote oxidation leading to a reddish tinge in the water.

Nitrates / nitrites
- Nitrites can change the structure of the haemoglobin in blood rendering it incapable of transporting oxygen. If levels are high the blood is a dark colour due to lowered levels of oxygen.
- Extremely high levels of nitrates / nitrites in water, impair the utilisation of vitamin A in pigs and a reduc-

tion in performance - such levels however are very rarely found under practical conditions but levels can be sufficiently high to increase stillbirths.

Minerals and Vitamins

BIOTIN

The role of biotin in nutrition and the changes that result when it is deficient are not clear.
Reports from studies and field observations have highlighted the following associations:

- Diarrhoea.
- Dermatitis
- Excessive hair loss
- Extended weaning to mating intervals.
- Haemorrhages on the solar surfaces of the feet.
- Lameness and laminitis.
- Poor litter size
- Reduce growth rates.
- Transverse cracks in hooves.

The fact that biotin is present in most nutrient sources used for pigs and that it is also produced by organisms in the gilt make a deficiency unlikely on most farms. This is supported by field experiences but very occasionally a herd is investigated for lameness problems that appear to be improved with biotin supplementation of the diet.

Clinical signs

Widespread lameness will be a constant feature particularly in sows. Detailed examinations should be carried out on at least 15-20 affected animals and the nature of the changes in the hooves documented. Examinations are best made when sows and gilts are at rest. The hooves will be soft over the walls and the soles will show slight evidence of haemorrhage. Dark transverse cracks will be seen on the hoof walls. If pigs have access to faeces biotin deficiency is unlikely. Assess trauma from poor floor surfaces as a cause.

Diagnosis

This is based on the clinical picture and the fact that the herd or a group of animals will be affected. The onset is usually gradual and this will distinguish the lameness from foot-and-mouth disease. Chronic lesions of swine vesicular disease could be confused with biotin deficiency.
Levels in the ration can be determined but firm recommendations are not available. 100-200μg(mcg)kg would appear adequate.

Treatment

☐ Where a herd shows widespread lesions add up to 0.5-1mg/kg to the diet. Any response will be slow, up to nine months but prevention gives more positive results.

Management control and prevention

◆ Add biotin to the diet as a routine.

CHOLINE

Choline forms part of the chemical substances that enable electrical pulses to pass between nerve endings. It is produced from the amino acid methionine. Signs include poor growth and reduced litter size. At one time it was thought that this vitamin was involved in splay-legged piglets but scientific evidence has not supported this and when it has been added to diets in cases of outbreaks there has been no response. A deficiency would be unusual.

COPPER

This, like iron, is necessary to allow red blood cells to form normally and deficiencies can lead to anaemia. Copper is also important in enzyme systems. Fortunately, nutritional deficiencies in pigs are very rare. It is added to the diet as a growth promoter at levels of up to 175ppm for pigs to 16 weeks of age and 100ppm for pigs over 16 weeks of age (EU legal requirements). It suppresses bacterial growth. There have been occasions in the field where it has been inadvertently and suddenly removed from creep diets. This has been followed by diarrhoea bacterial enteritis and poor growth probably associated with the sudden multiplication of pathogenic bacteria.

CYANOCOBALAMIN B_{12}

A deficiency of this vitamin is very unlikely because it is produced by bacteria in the gut and access to faeces provide a continual source. Synthetic sources are however usually added to diets.

FOLIC ACID

A deficiency results in anaemia, poor weight gain and loss of hair colour. It was previously thought that the intestines of the pig were capable of producing the vitamin but recent work suggests that swine diets may be deficient and that it could have a role to play in the maintenance and improvements in litter size. The addition of 1g/tonne may have a beneficial effect if litter sizes are poor and nutrition appears to be involved.

IODINE

Iodine is necessary for the production of the hormone thyroxin by the thyroid gland. This gland regulates the rate of body metabolism and if there is a shortage of iodine in the diet a condition called goitre arises. This denotes an increase in the size of the thyroid gland.

Substances called glucosinolates found in winter sown rape seeds are sometimes present in the diet and can prevent the gland using iodine.

Canola meal, an improved rape seed with low levels of glucosinolates, has enabled them to be used safely in swine diets. An iodine deficiency should be considered where large numbers of litters are born with piglets weak and hairless. With modern diets this would be rare. Iodised salt containing 0.008% of iodine provides sufficient iodine in the diet.

IRON

See chapter 8; Anaemia for further information.

Iron forms part of the haemoglobin molecule that transports the oxygen around the body. Where there is a deficiency causing anaemia the oxygen carrying capacity of the blood is greatly reduced. All pig diets should be supplemented with iron. Anaemia due to a primary deficiency of iron is unusual in pigs over six weeks of age unless they have not been administered iron in the first one to two weeks of life and had no access to a supplemented creep diet. It is usual to administer iron to the piglet by intramuscular or subcutaneous injections of 100-200mg of iron dextran between days 3 and 7 of age.

MAGNESIUM

This mineral is also found in bone but its main role is in the composition of many of the enzymes in the body. Most feed ingredients contain sufficient magnesium and it is not normally necessary to supplement the diet. Reported signs of deficiency include an abnormal gait as a result of lack of enzymes in the nervous system, incoordination and weak knees and hock joints with loss of tendon tension. If calcined magnesite is added to rations in excess diarrhoea may be caused.

MANGANESE

This is important in enzyme production and the development of bone. It is also required for normal reproductive function. Deficiencies are reported to be associated with lameness, irregular oestrus, delayed sexual maturity and weak pigs at birth.

The levels required in the diet are small at around 4g/tonne and problems likely to be experienced in the field would be rare.

NICOTINAMIDE

This vitamin, also called niacin, is involved in enzyme systems associated with metabolism. A deficiency results in reduced weight gains, poor appetite, often a very dry skin and diarrhoea. The skin may turn a yellow colour with dermatitis and loss of hair. Posterior paralysis may also occur. At post-mortem examination necrotic lesions may be seen in the intestines.

The amino acid tryptophan acts as a precursor and if this amino acid is deficient there is a greater risk of niacin deficiency. If deficiencies are suspected nicotinic acid can be added at 15mg/kg. Alternatively the levels of tryptophan could be increased. Deficiencies in the feed are rare.

PANTOTHENIC ACID

Deficiencies are associated with a high stepping gait particularly of the hind legs which is described as goose-stepping, with increasing incoordination and finally posterior paralysis. Loss of hair and diarrhoea are also seen. The condition is occasionally seen in swill fed units particularly where waste bakery foods are used. The feed can be supplemented with 5-10g/tonne of calcium pantothenate. Where modern diets are fed the condition is rare. However a condition conforming to the classical symptoms described was observed in a herd of 200 outdoor sows. Only lactating gilts were affected. Five animals were observed and each one would be grazing peacefully then suddenly the head would rise and with the nose pointed in the air the pig would walk for 10-20 minutes with a high stepping action of the hind legs. 5g/tonne of pantothenic acid was added to the ration and after three weeks the condition disappeared.

POTASSIUM

A deficiency of potassium is uncommon but it is an important mineral because of its role in maintaining water and acid balance in the body. It is also involved in maintaining a normal heart rate and in the transport of materials in and out of the cells. Clinical signs of deficiency rarely occur because nutrient sources contain adequate amounts. However when they do emaciation, reduced appetite and incoordination are seen. Excess potassium in the diet may precipitate colitis.

RIBOFLAVIN B_2

Most diets are supplemented with this vitamin because the level in basic cereal ingredients is very low. Whey however is a good source. A deficiency would be rare but anoestrus, reproductive failure, hair loss and vomiting have been reported.

SODIUM AND CHLORIDE

Although these are two individual components in the diet it is normal practice to balance them with common salt. High levels of sodium particularly in water causes scouring and poor growth rates. A low level of chloride in the ration can depress the growth rate and feed intake. Normal levels in the diet would be between 0.4 to 0.5% of salt although provided there is ad lib drinking water levels of up to 1% or more are well tolerated by the pig and often used at these levels to reduce tail biting and vice.

THIAMINE

Most cereals are good sources of thiamine and it is not normal to supplement the diet but if it is considered necessary levels of 1-2mg/kg are required. The signs of deficiency are reported to include poor appetite and daily gain, often vomiting, low body temperatures and poor heart rates. Sudden death may also occur.

VITAMIN E / SELENIUM (MULBERRY HEART DISEASE)

During the past few years problems associated with either the lack of availability of vitamin E and selenium, or absolute deficiencies have become major problems on some farms. These have arisen with the practice of using polyunsaturated fats in diets as sources of energy. The actual principles of vitamin E are called tocopherols and they are widespread in feed stuffs including vegetable oils, cereals and green plants.

Tocopherols are used in pig rations as dl-alpha-tocopherol acetate and measured in international units. The international unit (iu)1iu of vitamin E is defined as 1mg of a standard preparation of a specific tocopherol acetate.

Vitamin E is necessary for the optimum function and metabolism of the nervous, muscular, circulatory and immune systems, and the latter highlights its importance in maintaining the health of the pig.

Its function is basically to prevent the breakdown of oxygen at a cellular level (oxidation) when toxic products including hydrogen peroxide and hydroxyl radicals are produced. These oxidising agents are powerful tissue poisons.

The function of vitamin E in the pig

- To increase the efficiency of the immune system. Adequate levels must be available at critical times particularly as maternal antibody is dropping and pigs are being challenged by infectious agents. This highlights the importance of both diet quality and levels of energy lysine and vitamin E at these times.
- It acts as a tissue antioxidant. Heart muscle is particularly sensitive to oxidising agents, the reason why mulberry heart disease is so common.
- It helps to maintain the integral structure of muscles in the digestive and reproductive systems.
- It is involved in the synthesis of certain amino acids and vitamin C.
- It has a close relationship with selenium metabolism.

Selenium is an essential nutrient in its own right and part of an enzyme called glutathione peroxidase which also acts as a antioxidant and thus has a complementary role to vitamin E. The less selenium in the diet the greater is the requirement for vitamin E.

The recommended requirements to give a maximum boost to the immune system range from 75-220iu/kg. According to age of the pig and diet; this is in the first stage creep 220, the second stage 150, the grower 100, the finisher 60 and sow 50 iu/kg. These levels are probably higher than those necessary for maximum growth, which may be 50% less.

Polyunsaturated fatty acids PUFA's cause considerable oxidation at tissue levels and when added to diets 3iu of vitamin E should be added for each g of PUFA.

Vitamin E and selenium related diseases

Gastric ulcers - These are often stress oriented and the incidence increases where vitamin E levels are low.

Hepatosis dietetica (HD) - A condition where there is necrosis or death of liver cells.

Muscular or nutritional dystrophy (MD) (also called a myopathy) - This results from a degeneration of muscle fibres whether they be skeletal smooth or cardiac. Oedema or fluid is often produced around the tissues and muscles (PSE) as a result.

Mulberry heart disease (MHD) (also called a myopathy)- A specific disease of heart muscle and a common cause of sudden death.

Reproduction disorders - Vitamin E is involved in sperm production and ovarian function. The actual role of vitamin E on the farm is difficult to clarify.

Clinical signs

These vary according to the system affected. HD, MD and MHD are usually associated with sudden deaths in rapid growing pigs without any prior clinical signs, usually the best pigs in the pen are affected and they range from 15-30kg in weight. Diets being fed often contain high levels of fats and yet in many cases vitamin E levels appear within normal ranges. Post-mortem symptoms are characteristic and include:

- Large amounts of fluid around the heart and lungs.
- Haemorrhagic and pale areas in heart muscle.
- Fluid in the abdomen with pieces of fibrin.
- Pale muscle areas (necrosis) particularly in the lumber muscles and hind muscles of the leg which contain excesses amounts of fluid.
- If the liver is involved it is enlarged and mottled with areas of haemorrhage interspersed with pale areas.

Diagnosis

Histological examinations of the liver, heart or skeletal muscle will confirm diagnosis and this is the most accurate method. Serum samples should be taken from pigs at risk and tested for levels of vitamin E. Normal levels are variable from pig to pig however they should be more than 1.8mg/litre. The availability of selenium can be assessed by measuring the levels of glutathione peroxidase in the serum. If levels are less than 0.025μg/ml or 0.1mg/kg in liver a deficiency should be suspected and rations checked.

If MD is the major change stiffness and muscle trembling may be seen. If back muscle necrosis is involved sudden acute lameness occurs, particularly in gilts, especially outdoors, when they are moved into paddocks for the first time. This sudden exercise precipitates disease in association with the porcine stress syndrome (PSS).

Stress related problems include gastric ulcers and where lesions occur in more than 20% of pigs at slaughter, the addition of 50iu/kg of vitamin E should be assessed.

The role of vitamin E and selenium in reproductive performance is more difficult to quantify. Improvements have been noted in herds with persistent cases of agalactia and udder oedema by raising the levels in the lactating diet to 100iu/kg.

Similar diseases

These include:
  Actinobacillus pleuropneumonia.
  Glässers disease.
  Oedema disease.
  Streptococcal septicaemias.
Specific diseases associated with deficiencies of, or lack of availability include:
  Actinobacillus pleuropneumonia.
  E. coli diarrhoea.
  Oedema disease.
  Post-weaning respiratory syndrome.
  PRRS.
  Swine dysentery.
  and those diseases that occur during periods of immuno-suppression.

Treatment

☐ Where a population is at risk inject all the pigs with vitamin E/selenium e.g. dystocel, 70iu vitamin E and 1.5mg per 50kg is adequate, but seek veterinary advice.
☐ Sudden death in piglets following iron injection. Inject sows 14 days prior to farrowing with vitamin E/selenium.
☐ Water soluble preparations are sometimes available as alternatives.
☐ Multi-vitamins that include vitamin E and or selenium may be used. Refer to the recommended treatment levels on the bottle label.
☐ Move individual pigs to hospital pens for treatment.
☐ Increase vitamin E levels in creep and growing rations by 100-150iu/kg.

Management control and prevention

- If problems persist change to another diet with less added fats.
- Check the levels of PUFA's in the diet.
- Check the levels of vitamin E and selenium.
- Check the levels of vitamin A. If more than 10,000iu/kg this may be increasing the requirement for vitamin E.
- Rapid growth may be a contributing factor.
- Reduce stocking densities if pigs are over crowded.
- Check there are no parasite burdens.
- Grains stored with high moisture content in high temperatures and with fungal growth may have low levels of vitamin E.
- Do not breed from animals that carry the stress gene.

VITAMIN K

This vitamin is necessary to maintain normal clotting mechanisms and a deficiency causes haemorrhages throughout the tissues. Low levels of vitamin K have been implicated in navel bleeding in newborn piglets although the response to the addition of 2g/tonne of vitamin K is usually disappointing. Sulphadimidine and warfarin act as vitamin K antagonists. Oral and injectable preparations of vitamin K are available as menadione bisulphate. Treatment can be given by intramuscular injection at 2.5mg/kg liveweight. (See warfarin poisoning).

ZINC

Most of the enzymes in the pig require zinc for their normal structure and function. It forms an essential part of insulin. Pigs deficient in zinc show poor growth, poor appetite and a skin thickening called parakeratosis. Excessive calcium in the diet also reduces the availability of zinc and leads to parakeratosis but the condition in practice is uncommon. The diet should include between 50-100g/tonne. In recent years a new role has developed for the inclusion of zinc in the diet. In the period from weaning to 21 days post-weaning the inclusion of zinc oxide BP (80% zinc) at a level of 3.1kg/tonne in creep diets has been found to have a profound effect on preventing diarrhoea associated with *E. coli*. Such an inclusion provides 2.5g/kg of elemental zinc and at this level most pathogenic *E. coli* are inactivated. The mechanism by which this acts is unknown and levels less than this are often not effective. Occasionally the withdrawal of the zinc two to three weeks after weaning can result in diarrhoea and in such cases it may be necessary to continue its use for a further two to three weeks. No adverse effects at these levels have been recorded but a reduction in appetite has been suggested.

Non Nutritional Supplements

A variety of chemical and non chemical compounds and organisms are added to diets to treat or prevent disease or to enhance growth.
They include:
• Antibiotics and antibacterial compounds. (See chap-

ter 4 Fig.4-9)
- Parasecticides. (Se chapter 4).
- Growth promoters. (See chapter 4)
- Probiotics.

The addition of such substances in most countries is strictly controlled by law and the actual drugs available and the dose levels allowed also vary.

PROBIOTICS

These are live bacteria or micro-organisms that are either mixed in the feed or administered individually by mouth to produce a beneficial effect on the organism in the gut.

Under normal conditions the intestines of the pig contain a complex of 400 or more organisms which constantly protect against disease. Specific bacteria can also protect against specific pathogens.

Probiotics are believed to act in the following ways:
- Neutralise toxins in the intestinal tract.
- Prevent the adhesion of pathogens to the mucosal surface by competition.
- Stimulate local immune defences.
- Reduce the numbers of pathogens by competition.

The common organisms used include lactobacilli, yeasts, streptococci, enterococci and non pathogenic *E. coli*. Lactobacilli are the most common and at least seven have been identified as having a beneficial effect. They produce large amounts of lactic acid which creates an unfavourable environment for certain bacteria. In the piglet this creates high acid conditions in the stomach helping to prevent the establishment of pathogenic *E. coli*.

Probiotics have been available for use in pig feeds for a number of years and yet the results of their use are inconsistent and at times in the field remain unconvincing.

Oral preparations given to piglets and their response to *E. coli* diarrhoea can be difficult to assess on the farm because their use often starts with ongoing diarrhoea problems, most of which go away with better management and hygiene. A typical example was their use in a 1000 sow operation where 30% of all litters scoured. This was associated with a continual pig flow policy in the farrowing houses. This was changed to all-on all-out and at the same time probiotics were given to all piglets at birth. The problem gradually disappeared. Three months later due to costs, the probiotic use ceased. The scour problem did not return.

Probiotics appear to have little effect on piglet diarrhoea after five days of age.

Lactobacilli have been used for growth promotion but consistency of results in the field are poor and it is difficult to see large numbers of well controlled trials that give sufficient confidence for their continual use. Field experiences in the immediate post-weaning period have in a few herds shown a beneficial effect but in most an economic return could not be justified.

15 Surgical, Manipulative and Practical Procedures

Antibiotic administration into the anterior vagina post-service...................474
Blood sampling methods available...475
Castration of the normal pig..478
Castration of the ruptured pig...480
Cleaning and disinfection of buildings - see also water............................481
De-tusking a boar..482
Docking (tail clipping) piglets..483
Epidectomy 484
Feedback..485
Flutter valve and its use...486
Fumigation of houses using formaldehyde vapour 487
Hysterectomy - emergency or planned..488
Identification - tattooing, slap marking, tagging, transponders,
implants, ear notching 491
Injecting piglets with iron 493
Lancing an abscess or a haematoma..495
Libido checking - training boars to use a stool 496
Local anaesthesia 496
Lime washing concrete floors 497
Mating the sow with the boar...498
Pregnancy diagnosis..499
Penis - examination...500
Prolapse of the rectum...501
Prolapse of the cervix..503
Prolapse of the uterus (womb) 504
Prostaglandin injections to initiate farrowing..505
Recording air movement temperature and humidity in a house 506
Restraining the pig...507
Sampling air for dust levels 508
Sampling feeds for laboratory testing 509
Sampling milk from a mammary gland with mastitis 509
Sampling the air for toxic levels of gases..510
Semen collection and artificial insemination on the farm.......................511
Slaughter - humane destruction...515
Stomach tube - How to use one...517
Suturing skin and muscle...518
Swabbing the nose and tonsils for toxigenic pasteurella or other bacteria 521
Syringes and needles and their use 523
Teeth clipping..525
Temperature recording from the rectum 526
Udder - methods of examination 527
Umbilical cord applying a clamp 528
Vasectomy..529
Vulval haematoma- treating a haematoma..530
Water - cleaning and sterilising a system..531

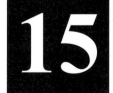

Chapter 15

15 Surgical, Manipulative and Practical Procedures

This chapter describes various surgical and practical procedures regularly carried out on the pig farm. However the regulations which govern those that can be carried out by the pig farmer and those only by the veterinarian, differ from country to country. Suggestions are made where veterinary help and advice should be sought but you should ascertain what you are allowed or not allowed to do in your country.

Some of the following procedures may require initial instruction from your veterinarian.

ANTIBIOTIC ADMINISTRATION INTO THE ANTERIOR VAGINA
POST-SERVICE

Reason

To control or eliminate endometritis or ascending infection after the sow has been mated. To improve fertility.

Materials Required

10ml or 20ml syringes and adapters to attach to the catheters.
Disposable cattle artificial insemination (AI) catheters are preferred because they have small diameters.
A sow AI catheter or a metal Neilson Catheter can also be used Fig.15-1.
The appropriate antibiotic as prescribed by your veterinarian.
A suitable AI liquid or KY jelly.
Clean paper tissues.
Disposable gloves.

Catheters used for the treatment of vulval discharges. The top one is metal and used in dairy practice (Neilson). The lower one is a disposable cattle AI catheter.

(Fig.15-1)

Procedure

1	Carry out a bacteriological examination of the prepuce and vagina secretions to determine predominating organisms and their antibiotic sensitivities. (See chapter 6)
2	Confine the sow 6 to 12 hours after the last mating, making sure she cannot back onto the catheter. Wipe the vulva clean with paper tissue. Use disposable gloves.
3	Fill the syringe with the appropriate antibiotic and attach it to the catheter with the adapter. Fill the catheter with antibiotic. Lubricate the catheter with an AI lubricant and insert gently into the vagina until resistance is felt at the cervix about 250 to 350mm inside.
4	Deposit 3-4ml of antibiotic.
5	Wipe the catheter clean with tissue before using on another sow.
6	Change the catheter every 5 sows. Discard any antibiotic left in the catheter.
7	Monitor the return rate at 18 to 22 days post service for any adverse effects.

CHAPTER 15 - Surgical, Manipulative and Practical Procedures

BLOOD SAMPLING METHODS AVAILABLE

Materials Required

Syringes - 2ml, 10ml, 30ml. Needles 20g 16mm ($^5/_8$") and 25mm (1"). 18g 38mm ($1^1/_2$") 16g 100mm (4"). Vacutainers 7-10 ml. (Fig.15-2). Surgical spirit.	Surgical blades and handle. Cotton wool. Labels. Snare. Ear muffs. Two people.

Select the Method of Sampling

Site	Method	Type of Pig	Comments
Ear Vein	Lance and collect into a container. Collect using a 20g needle and syringe.	Sow Gilt Boar	Easy. Only small samples. Sample contaminated. Haemorrhage sometimes follows, apply pressure.
Tail Vessels	a) By syringe b) By vacutainer c) Tail amputation	Sow 110kg pig Piglet	Easy access but difficult practically. Up to 0.5ml collected from piglet.
Jugular Vein	Syringe or vacutainer	All ages	Easy. Method of choice for 10-30 ml.
Anterior Vena Cava	Syringe or vacutainer	All ages from piglets to adults.	Method of choice for large samples.

Ear Vein

The veins are raised by pressure at the base of the ear. The skin is cleaned with cotton wool and surgical spirit. Use a syringe and 20g 16mm ($^5/_8$") needle. Store the blood in a glass vacutainer tube. The ear vein may be lanced and blood collected in an open tube but this is not recommended.

Tail Vessels

See Fig.15-3. Use a vacutainer or syringe with a 20g 25mm (1") needle. The blood vessels lie close to the surface. This method requires practice and probably instruction from your veterinarian.

Jugular Vein

This is the method of choice in pigs from 40 to 200kg. The position of the blood vessels is shown in the transverse section of the neck. (Fig.15-4)

NECK OF THE PIG - TRANSVERSE SECTION

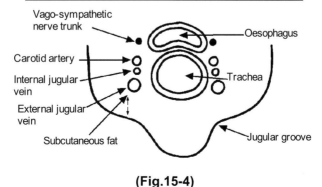

(Fig.15-4)

476 Managing Pig Health and the Treatment of Disease

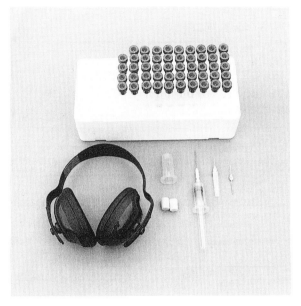

A blood sampling kit. The glass tubes are under vacuum and draw blood when pierced by the double ended needle. Ear protectors and plugs are shown.

(Fig.15-2)

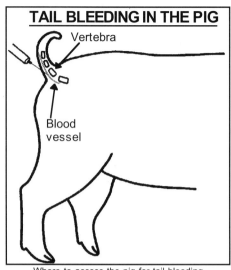

Where to access the pig for tail bleeding

(Fig.15-3)

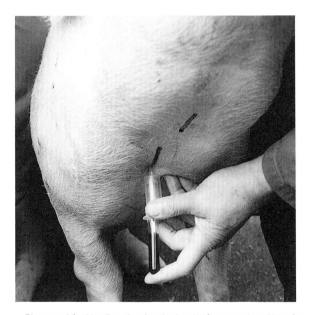

Pig snared for bleeding showing the jugular furrow and positions for bleeding.

(Fig.15-5)

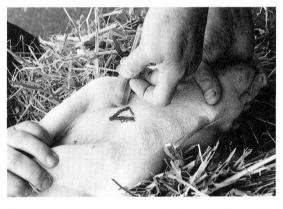

Bleeding from the anterior vena cava in pigs up to 30kg weight. The centre of the triangle indicates the point of entry on the right side of the pig as shown.

(Fig.15-6)

Chapter 15

	BLOOD SAMPLING METHODS AVAILABLE (Cont.)
	Restrain the pig with a wire noose or rope (see restraint). The external jugular vein lies 25 to 40mm below the skin. Raise the head of the pig to define the jugular groove and direct the needle slightly to the mid line 120mm above the point of the shoulder. Use ear muffs. Sixty pigs per hour can be bled by this method. Once you have mastered the technique it is easy but you may need instruction from your veterinarian initially. The secret is to snare and hold the pig in the correct position as shown to define the jugular groove.(Fig.15-5).
5	**Anterior Vena Cava**

	This is used to bleed pigs from 2-30kg weight and for adult pigs. The small pig is restrained on its back (see Fig.15-6) with the front legs held back and the chin pressed downwards. The right hand inlet of the pig between the first rib and breast bone is determined. A vacutainer or syringe can be used.
	Needle sizes:- Pigs up to 10kg 20g 25mm (1")
	                                  45kg 18g 38mm (1$^{1}/_{2}$")
	                                100kg 18g 50mm (2")
	                                Sows 16g 100mm (4")
	Older pigs and adult stock are bled in a standing position. The needle is inserted alongside the front of the breast bone directed slightly inwards towards the spine, upwards and at a slight angle backwards.
	Take care not to swing the needle, to prevent tearing of the blood vessel because you might cause haemorrhage and even death.
	Insert it straight in and slowly withdraw it in the same line with a light negative pressure on the syringe. If you have missed the blood vessel insert it again at a slightly different angle.
	You will need instruction from your veterinarian initially.

CASTRATION OF THE NORMAL PIG

Reason

In some countries entire boars are accepted at slaughter but in others castration is required.

Method

This is by surgical removal of both testicles. The best time to perform the operation is under three weeks of age.

Materials Required

A bucket of warm water, antiseptic solution and cotton wool.
A surgical blade and handle.
A marker spray.
Two people or one if a stand is used.

Procedure

1. Only commence castration after the farrowing pen has been cleaned out and the pen or creep area has been bedded with suitable dry bedding materials if applicable.
2. Hold the litter in a clean dry area or a box with no floor and covered with bedding.
3. Remove the females
4. One person holds the piglet between the legs with the testicles presented as shown or a stand may be used. Study Figs 15-7 and 15-8.

ANATOMY OF THE NORMAL AND RUPTURED PIG

(Fig.15-7)

CHAPTER 15 - Surgical, Manipulative and Practical Procedures **479**

CASTRATION OF THE NORMAL PIG (Cont.)

ENLARGED VIEW OF THE TESTICLE

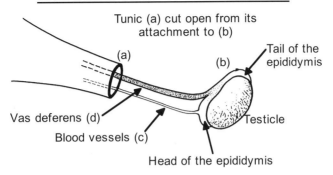

(Fig.15-8)

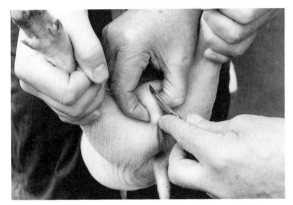

Castration. Squeezing the testicle ready for castration.

(Fig.15-9a)

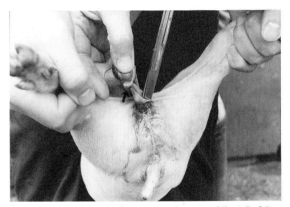

Castration. Showing the ligament attachment and the tail of the epididymus (arrow). The scalpel is placed in the tunic.

(Fig.15-9b)

	The operator must not be involved in catching pigs and at all times must keep his hands clean. He/she must scrub and wash hands before commencing.
5	The skin over the testicle is wiped clean with cotton wool and antiseptic solution.
6	Each testicle is raised to the surface with the thumb first and second fingers. (Fig.15-9a)
7	A separate incision is made into each testicle through the skin and the tunic (a) and attachment of the tunic broken (b). The testicle is either pulled away by traction endeavouring to break the blood vessels (c) and cutting the vas deferens or the complete spermatic cord (blood vessels and vas deferens) cut at (d).
8	After both testicles have been removed it is important to raise the skin incisions to make sure no strings of tissue are left behind. If so cut cleanly away. (Fig.15-9b)
9	Pigs over 5 weeks of age should only be castrated under local anaesthetic on welfare grounds. 0.5 ml should be injected into each testicle and under the skin. Castration should commence 5 minutes later.
10	Return the pig to the pen.
	Outdoor sow herds - Hygiene and sow aggravation are problems and it is wise to avoid routine castration by finding a castration free outlet for the young pigs. This is relatively easy in the UK but may be difficult in some countries.

Chapter 15

CASTRATION OF THE RUPTURED PIG

Reason

The testicle is enclosed in a sac or tunic which is a continuation of the peritoneum or lining of the abdomen. (See Figs.15-7 and 8). The blood vessels and vas deferens leave the abdominal cavity to reach the testicles via a small hole called the inguinal canal. If this is enlarged, bowel and abdominal contents enter the sac to produce a hernia, usually called a rupture but they are contained within the tunic. If a pig is castrated in the normal way and the tunic opened the bowel contents are exposed.

Materials Required

As for normal castration but include: Stresnil sedative. Local anaesthetic Syringe 21g 16mm ($5/8$") needle.	Half curved triangular suture needles 38mm ($1 1/2$)" and nylon thread or catgut. Scissors and tissue forceps. Penicillin cream or CTC powder. Two people are required.

Procedure

1	Identify the pig and prepare for the operation as for normal castration. It is best carried out at three to four weeks of age. Carry out under the guidance of your veterinarian.
2	Sedate using stresnil, inject $1/2$ml of local anaesthetic into each testicle and skin where the incision is to be made and wait for five minutes.
3	Hold the pig with its belly uppermost, identify the rupture and raise the testicle to the skin over the inguinal canal.

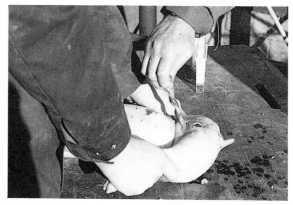

This shows the testicle held inside the tunic, and by twisting, the rupture is squeezed back into the abdomen

(Fig.15-10)

4	Carefully cut through the skin and loose tissues down to the tunic as illustrated in Fig.15-7 and 15-8. DO NOT CUT INTO THE TUNIC otherwise this will open the sack and abdominal contents will spill out. If this happens kill the piglet.
5	Twist the tunic and sac so that the ruptured contents are squeezed back into the abdomen. (Fig.15-10)
6	With the testicle held pass a curved suture needle and nylon suture through the twisted cord and sac as near to the body as possible. Wind round twice and tie.
7	Cut off the sac on the testicle side of the suture to remove the testicle.
8	Place $1/4$ml of penicillin over the suture.
9	Stitch the skin together with mattress sutures. (See suturing)
10	Return the pig to the pen. The sutures may be removed after ten days or left in.

CLEANING AND DISINFECTION OF BUILDINGS - See also Water

Reason

There are a number of important reasons for the disinfection of buildings and other areas of the farm including - reducing the numbers of organisms and risk of disease, preventing the spread of disease, maximising growth and performance, and creating pleasant working conditions.

Materials Required

A good supply of water.
A pressure washer / steam cleaner with up to 1000psi.
Waterproof protective clothing.
Eye protectors.
Detergent, disinfectants either phenol and iodine or chlorine based or organic acids. Non toxic disinfectants such as Virkon S for terminal aerosol use.

Procedure

#	
1	Remove all dirt and faeces and empty all slurry channels and tanks.
2	Disconnect all moveable equipment, feeders, lamps etc. and open all inaccessible areas e.g. channels, fan boxes.
3	Isolate the electricity supply.
4	Brush down and sweep out the house \ including fan boxes.
5	Soak the complete building, roof to floor with a farm detergent or water, leave for 24 hours if possible.
6	Soak all moveable equipment and clean down.
7	Drain and flush out the water system, bowls, nipples, water tanks etc. and fill with a detergent steriliser. Leave for two hours, empty and then refill with water.
8	Pressure wash the complete building using hot water or a steam cleaner. Use 500psi but take care not to damage concrete surfaces.
9	Visually check the building.
10	Disinfect the complete house including all equipment and surrounds using the pressure washer at 200psi or spray.
11	Follow this with fumigation using formalin gas where applicable with suitable precautions or a suitable disinfectant such as Virkon S.
12	Place a disinfectant foot bath outside the house and use prior to entry. Use an iodophor disinfectant which is brown when active and yellow when no longer active.

Do not restock the house until dry. (A minimum of 48 hours).
If you have to occupy the house before this then use a space heater to dry out the surfaces.

DE-TUSKING A BOAR

Reason

Both the upper and lower tusks of the boar become large, sharp and dangerous with increasing age. In the authors opinion all boars should have the exposed portions removed at around six months of age. The remaining stumps will not then be capable of causing such severe damage.

Method

Remove the teeth either by shears or hoof cutters or use embryotomy wire.
Carry out under the guidance of your veterinarian.

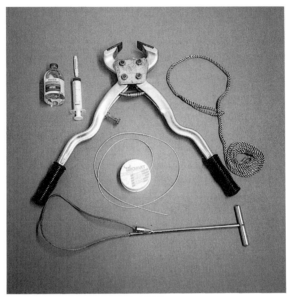

Equipment required for de-tusking a boar showing clippers and embryotomy wire.

(Fig.15-11)

Materials Required

Sedatives - Stresnil. In large boars a light anaesthetic administered by the veterinarian may be required as well.
Wire or rope noose for physical restraint.
A piece of wood to hold the mouth open.
A pair of shears or hoof cutters or embryotomy wire and handles (Fig.15-11).

Procedure

1	Heavily sedate the boar in his pen with stresnil 1ml per 10kg body weight by intra muscular injection.
2	Wait for 20 minutes.
3	Place a noose made of strong material, such as nylon calving rope, around the upper jaw and fasten to the other end to a post or bar.
4	In young boars use hoof cutters. In old boars remove the tusks with embryotomy wire. This is abraded stainless steel wire with handles attached. It is placed around the tooth which is removed with a sawing action at gum level. Do not leave any sharp edges.
5	During sedation the penis may protrude. Cover with a damp cloth or replace. Do not carry out this operation with other pigs in the same pen.

DOCKING (TAIL CLIPPING) PIGLETS

Reason

To prevent tail biting. Until the reasons for tail biting are fully understood and preventative methods can be applied with 100% success, removing most of the tail at birth causes less welfare problems in later life. Tail biting causes infection, the development of abscesses in the spine, severe pain and carcase condemnations at slaughter.

Materials Required

One of the following: teeth clippers, scissors, scalpel blade, gas cauteriser or a burdizzo instrument. A sharp surgical knife or scissors is recommended here because the cut is clean with a minimum of damaged tissue. A good blood clot is formed.
A spray or suitable marker.
A small container with water and a mild antiseptic. Iodine cow teat dip antiseptics are ideal.

Procedure

1. Wash all instruments with hot soapy water and disinfect.

2. Never remove tails at birth. Always wait until the piglet has consumed colostrum (>8 hours after birth).
Do not use the teeth clippers for this purpose but a separate pair.
The tail is best removed from 12 to 72 hours after birth. Three days is recommended - when iron injections are given.

3. Hold the piglets in the creep area or confine to a bottomless box, well bedded with either shavings or sawdust.

4. The operation is best carried out with two people but can be accomplished by one. Hold the tail into the scissors and remove with a quick cut. Leave only 16mm of tail length. Do not be tempted to leave half the tail. This is important because tail biting will occur at this length. Alternatively remove the tail by cautery or apply a burdizzo. The burdizzo crushes the tail and destroys the nerves and blood supply. The tail drops off after two to three days. In outdoor herds tetanus is a risk. (Fig.15-12a and 15-12b)

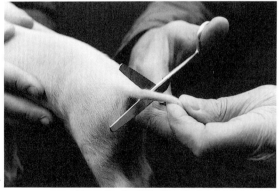

Removing the tail with scissors.
(Fig.15-12a)

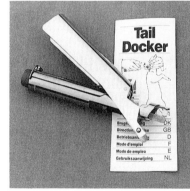

A gas cautery.
(Fig.15-12b)

5. Mark the piglet and place in a clean creep area. Any bleeding should cease in $1/2$ minute.

6. Place the instrument in the disinfectant when not in use.

7. Examine all piglets five minutes later to check that none are bleeding.

8. If bleeding does occur apply a tourniquet to the tail using a piece of string. Leave this on for 15 minutes then remove.

9. Wash all instruments with hot water and then disinfectant.

EPIDECTOMY

Reason

Epidectomy is a simple method of rendering a boar sterile but not impotent (i.e. he still wants to mate) by removing the tail of the epididymis of each testicle (see Fig.15-7). The epididymis is that part of the testicle that stores the mature sperm prior to its ejaculation. Epidectomy achieves the same objectives as vasectomy but it is much easier and simpler to perform.(Fig.15-13)

ENLARGED VIEW OF THE TESTICLE

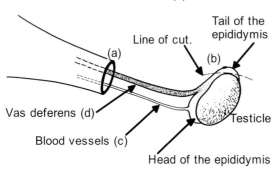

Enlarged view of the testicle showing the line of incision for epidectomy at the tail of the epididymis

(Fig.15-13)

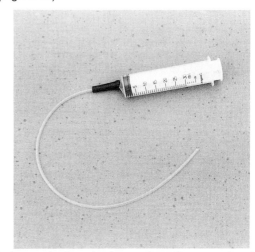

A lamb stomach tube and syringe used to collect semen from the cervix whilst the boar is mating.

(Fig.15-14)

Materials Required

As for normal castration plus a pair of surgical scissors and tissue forceps.

Procedure

These procedures should be carried out by or under the guidance of your veterinarian.

1	Proceed as for normal castration when piglets are 10 to 21 days old but use local anaesthetic. DO NOT CUT INTO THE TESTICLE ITSELF.
2	Lift each testicle up and identify the large blue swelling of the tail of the epididymis.
3	Hold the tail with the tissue forceps and cut it away making sure not to damage the testicle. The arrow on Fig.15-9b points to the tail of the epididymis and the attachment of the tunic
4	Let the testicles return into the scrotum making sure that no tissue protrudes between the skin.
5	Apply antibiotic cream into the wound and suture the skin.
6	When the boar is six months old examine a semen sample to ensure it contains no sperm. To do this allow the boar to mate a gilt and during the process slide a stomach tube to the cervix and collect a sample of fluids into a syringe. (Fig.15-14). Examine the sample for evidence of sperm. Alternatively hand collect from a stool.

FEEDBACK

Reason

To use potentially infected material to stimulate immunity prior to expected disease challenge. It is of value in rotavirus, TGE, PED, PRRS and PPV diseases. It is also used to stimulate immunity to *E. coli* in gilts, but the effectiveness varies. Do not use feedback if there is clinical swine dysentery, erysipelas or clostridial dysentery occurring in your herd.

Materials Required

Sources:
Sow faeces. Do not use afterbirth or cleansing materials they can spread diseases such as leptospirosis, endometritis, pyelonephritis and eperythrozoonosis.
Weaner faeces. This is a good source of enteric infections but do not feed back if swine dysentery exists in the herd.
Piglet scour - or in the case of TGE macerated intestines from dead piglets.

Procedure

1	Identify the disease for which feedback is to be used. Decide with the advice of your veterinarian the advisability of feedback.
2	Collect 1 to 2kg of mixed weaner faeces and mix with water in a bucket. Alternatively soak piglet scour in shavings, sawdust or meal and mix with water.
3	Expose the target group via the drinking water or feed.
4	Determine the number of occasions when feedback is to be practised, usually twice weekly.
5	In outbreaks of TGE liquidize the small intestine from piglets that have died, to harvest the virus. Expose to all pigs immediately to spread the disease and produce an immunity across the herd. However avoid sows three weeks from farrowing.

FLUTTER VALVE AND ITS USE

Reason

To drip water into the rectum in cases of salt poisoning and streptococcal meningitis.

Materials Required

A flutter valve.
500ml (1 pint) glass bottles and cord to suspend them.
Saline solution 0.5% or water warmed to body temperature. (Fig.15-15)

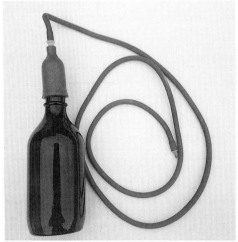

Flutter valve. The end of the tube is inserted into the rectum and bottle suspended above.
(Fig.15-15)

Procedure

1. Raise the bottle to a height and suspend it by a cord above the pig so that water slowly drips.
2. Insert the end of the rubber tube 75mm in the rectum.
3. Repeat every two to three hours.

CHAPTER 15 - Surgical, Manipulative and Practical Procedures **487**

FUMIGATION OF HOUSES USING FORMALDEHYDE VAPOUR

Reason

This is often used to disinfect the complete environment. Formalin is a toxic substance and care is necessary when it is used. The gas can be produced either by aerosol using an electric generator, from powder heated in an electric pan or by mixing formalin with potassium permanganate.

Materials Required

Face mask dampened.
Goggles.
Rubber gloves.
Electric aerosol or heat generator.
Formalin 40% solution or powder for use in generators.
Potassium permanganate crystals.
Empty metal containers - 2 litres capacity.
Two people - one as an observer from a safety aspect.

Procedure

1	Clean and pressure wash the house and fumigate whilst the building is still wet.
2	Make sure the house is sealed and gas cannot escape to other buildings or pigs. If this is not possible do not use this method.
3	Calculate the approximate cubic capacity of the building. Use 500ml formalin per $28m^3$ with 200g potassium permanganate crystals..
4	Place metal containers evenly along the centre of the house and add the crystals.
5	Add the formalin to each container starting furthest away from the door.
6	Leave the building closed for 12 hours. Place a warning sign on the door. FUMIGATION IN PROGRESS.
7	Open the building and ventilate for 24 hours before use.

NOTE: The use of formalin vapour is banned in some countries and you should be aware that it is toxic and dangerous. Great care should be taken when using it. An alternate is to fog the building with Virkon S which is non toxic and a safer and equally effective option.

Managing Pig Health and the Treatment of Disease

HYSTERECTOMY - EMERGENCY OR PLANNED

REASONS

A hysterectomy is the removal of the complete pregnant uterus from the sow at or near term. It is used routinely in organisations such as breeding companies, research institutes or SPF associations to produce piglets which are free from specified pathogens (SPF piglets), or alternatively as a remedy when a sow cannot farrow. She is destroyed but the litter is saved.

Materials Required for an Emergency Hysterectomy

Two people. A captive bolt gun, cartridges and pithing rod. A nylon rope or wire noose. A sharp knife and a 150mm nail or pair of scissors. Navel clips.	A bucket of warm water. A box to hold the piglets. Two large towels or absorbent paper to dry the piglets with.

Procedure - At the Slaughter Point.

These procedures should be carried out by or under the guidance of your veterinarian.

1	Move the sow to a clean area that can be easily washed down.
2	Restrain the sow. (See restraining the pig in this chapter).
3	Shoot and pith. Pithing involves passing the flexible rod through the hole made by the captive bolt in the skull to the back of the brain and down the spinal cord to destroy it. If this is not possible the sow should be bled by cutting her throat. The hysterectomy MUST NOT BE CARRIED OUT until the sow has been pithed or bled.
4	With the sow on her side open up the abdomen at the mid line between the udder tissue. Make a 600mm incision. Pull both horns of the womb containing the piglets completely out. Open up the womb by holding each piglet and tear the wall with the nail or scissors to prevent damage to the piglets.
5	Remove the mucus from the piglets' mouth to allow it to breathe.
6	Massage the umbilical cord back towards the piglets abdomen, squeeze the blood it contains into the piglet, apply an umbilical clip and cut the cord away. DO NOT carry this out until the piglet is breathing well and fully active or pale piglets will result.
7	Foster the litter to a newly farrowed sow. (See chapter 8).

Materials Required for a Planned Hysterectomy to Produce Specific Pathogen (SPF) Free Piglets.

This method involves removing the intact uterus from the sow to a clean area at least 50m away before the piglets are removed. Alternatively the uterus can be removed and passed through a disinfectant trap into a sealed room where the piglets are then removed. The operation is carried out on either day 112 or 113 of pregnancy. Day 113 is best. As a precaution the sow could be injected with 300mg of progesterone to delay farrowing.

At the slaughter end:
A pig free area to hold and slaughter the sow.
A captive bolt gun, cartridges and pithing rod, knife and wire noose.
A bucket of warm water, disinfectant and cloth.
One slaughter person, one operator, two bath carriers.
A two handled bath tub holding 25 litres of warm water and disinfectant -(e.g. Antec Virkon S 1% or Savlon 1%)

HYSTERECTOMY - EMERGENCY OR PLANNED (Cont.)

At the clean area:
A pig free area to receive the uterus and piglets. Three reception personnel who have had no contact with pigs for 48 hours and are wearing clean non pig contact clothing. A disinfected reception table, warm water, disinfectant, sterile towels. Scissors and a reception box containing two hot water bottles. The reception box should be approximately $0.6m^2$, insulated with a lid and hold a false bottom, beneath which two hot water bottles can be placed. Shavings make suitable bedding. Navel clips and tubular bandage. Electricians nylon ties which can be sterilised may be used instead of clamps. A pre planned reception farm with one to three newly farrowed sows. The sows can be synchronised to farrow with prostaglandin injections.

#	
1	Move the sow from the farm to isolation premises 4-9 weeks before hand. Carry out any testing procedures to confirm the disease status.
2	Move the sow to the pig-free slaughter area on day 113 of pregnancy in cleaned and disinfected transport. (In some breeds day 112 or 114 may be more appropriate). Assess the pregnancy state by examination of the udder. If the sow has started farrowing abandon the operation.
3	Fill the bath with warm water and disinfectant sufficient to cover the complete uterus.
4	Restrain, shoot and pith the sow. If pithing is not successful bleed out the sow. This operation should not be carried out by the operator. (Fig.15-16a - h)
5	Hold the sow on her back and wash the skin over the udder with disinfectant.
6	Make a careful incision into the abdomen at the sternum sufficient to pass the hand into the abdomen.
7	Place the knife with the blade uppermost into the abdomen and cut open up to the pelvis, care being taken not to cut the uterus or the intestines.
8	Hold the disinfectant bath to the edge of the abdomen and pass the uterus and piglets into it. Each horn of the uterus separates itself from the ovaries.
9	Identify the cervix, & cut through its centre. The womb must be completely covered by the warm disinfectant.
10	Carry the bath 50m away to the reception point. Piglets can survive up to 4 mins after the sow has been shot.

The Reception Point

#	
1	The uterus is placed onto the perforated metal reception table and the disinfectant allowed to drain away. The transporting personnel immediately return to the slaughter point.
2	Each piglet is grasped and the uterus torn open with blunt scissors.
3	Mucus is cleaned away from each piglets mouth and they are left until they are breathing normally.
4	The blood in the umbilical cord of each piglet is squeezed towards its abdomen and a clamp applied.
5	The cord is cut the piglet is wiped dry with the towels and tubular gauze placed over the body to hold the clamp.
6	The hot water bottles are placed beneath the false bottom then the piglets are placed in the reception box prior to transportation to a newly farrowed sow on the recipient farm.

NOTES:
Do not remove piglets until a minimum of $1^1/_2$ minutes after slaughter. Piglets will survive for up to 4 minutes after slaughter. Sometimes pithing is difficult. Shoot the sow again. If pithing cannot be carried out bleed the sow by cutting completely across the throat. Remove the uterus only when bleeding has ceased. In this case the piglets must be removed within $1^1/_2$ minutes. If a piglet breaks from the womb it must be discarded. Do not feed the piglets before they suckle the sow. Pre-feeding will close down the intestines to the absorption of colostral antibodies. Piglets can survive well in a warm dark insulated box for several hours before sucking the sow. Farrowing may be delayed for up to 24 hours by injecting progesterone, 300mg, on day 113 of pregnancy. The carcase must be condemned.

Managing Pig Health and the Treatment of Disease

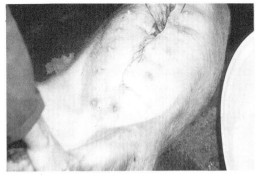

Opening up the sow.
(Fig.15-16a)

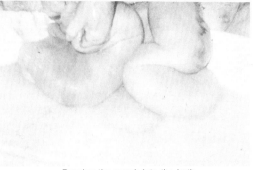

Passing the womb into the bath.
(Fig.15-16b)

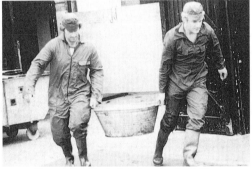

Transporting the bath to the reception table.
(Fig.15-16c)

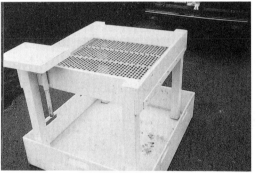

The reception table.
(Fig.15-16d)

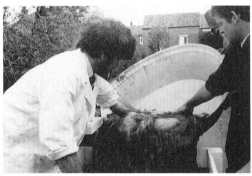

Emptying the womb onto the table.
(Fig.15-16e)

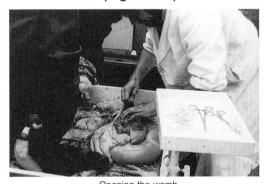

Opening the womb.
(Fig.15-16f)

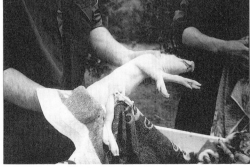

Clamping the navel.
(Fig.15-16g)

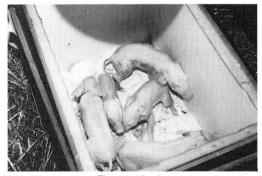

The reception box.
(Fig.15-16h)

IDENTIFICATION - Tattooing, Slap Marking, Tagging, Transponders, Implants, Ear Notching

Reason

These are the methods used for the permanent identification of pigs. They may be required for recording and management purposes, for the identification of pigs under treatments and of carcasses at slaughter.

Methods

Tattooing. Dies or spiked numbers or letters are used.
Three sizes are needed 8mm ($^5/_{16}$") for piglets for 3-21 days.
    10mm ($^3/_8$") for pigs from 10-90kg.
    16mm ($^5/_8$") for sows and slap marking.
Two sites are used. The ear, or on the neck behind the ear for use on the farm and over the shoulder or back (slap marking) on pigs destined for slaughter. Green tattoo ink shows best and is retained longer in white skinned breeds for permanent marking on the farm. Use black for pigs at slaughter.

Tagging. There are many types of tags on the market. They are used only in the ear. Positioning and hygiene are important. Infection after tagging can in some herds be a major problem. Make sure tags are stored in a clean dust proof container. Pigs can also be allergic to certain types of plastic.
If there is a problem consider the following:
Make sure instruments are clean and disinfected and tags are not contaminated.
Wipe the skin clean with antiseptic (e.g. iodine solution) before application.
Change the age when pigs are tagged.
Carry out bacteriological examinations to determine the cause.
Change the type of tag.
Assess the cleanliness of the environment - wet dirty pens predispose.
It is usual to place a tag in each ear. Use tags where possible that are numbered on both sides.

Transponders. These are electronic tags that can be read by or they respond to electronic impulses. They are used in automatic feeder systems. They can also be used to store data and be identified electronically at a distance from the pig. They are becoming increasingly common as an aid to recording and management.

Electronic Implants. These are transistors enclosed in very small non-reactive implants that are placed beneath the skin at the base of the ear. They will store a wide variety of information but are still in their early stages of development. They will ultimately become the principle method of identification.

Materials Required

Tattooing	Slap marker.
Ink - green and black.	Ink pad.
Applicators for the different dies.	Methods of restraint.
Four sets of each size of dies numbered 0 to 9.	Tags and applicators.
A clean divided box easily cleaned to hold dies.	Tissues and surgical spirit.
A container to soak and clean dies.	Recording equipment.
Disposable gloves.	Methods of restraint.
Toothbrush.	Ear notching pliers
Recording equipment.	Implanting equipment

Timing

Piglets up to 21 days old   - Are best tattooed at 3 to 5 days of age to coincide with iron injections.
Gilts at selection   - Either tattoo or tag.
Sows   - At any time with tattoos, tags or transponders.

Procedures

Tattooing

1. Restrain the pig as necessary.
Prepare the equipment and hold in a dust free clean box. Avoid external contamination.

IDENTIFICATION - Tattooing, Slap Marking, Tagging, Transponders, Implants, Ear Notching (Cont.)

2	Identify the pigs and area of application. Clean the skin with surgical spirit, unless pigs are for slaughter, when a clean area should be identified for slap marking.
3	Place ink on the dies with the toothbrush and apply the tattoo. Rub the ink into the skin with the brush.
4	Using a slap marker at slaughter press the ink pad onto the marker and slap the dies onto the skin either over the shoulder or the back near the tail. Restraint is not necessary. It will be necessary when marking breeding stock.
5	On completion of tattooing soak the dies and applicator in warm water and detergent. Clean then soak in a mild disinfectant for 15 minutes and then dry.

Tagging / Transponders / Implants

1	As in one and two above.
2	Apply the tag to the centre of the ear taking care to avoid the veins. Place the implant into the loose skin at the base of the ear, after cleaning the skin with surgical spirit.

Ear Notching

This procedure is best carried out at birth using a pair of notching pliers. Different methods are used but some breeding organisations have a specific method. One ear usually the right ear is used to identify the litter and the other to identify the individual pig. Pigs may be notched from birth to 2 weeks of age.

Each ear is divided into areas as shown and permanent numbers allotted to each. The numbers required are then identified and the notches made accordingly.

1	Clean and disinfect the pliers.
2	Clean the ear with surgical spirit. Clean the pliers between litters.
3	Tattooing is more welfare friendly and is replacing this method but for small numbers it is still useful.

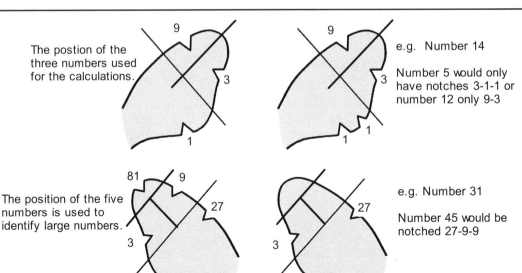

The postion of the three numbers used for the calculations.

e.g. Number 14

Number 5 would only have notches 3-1-1 or number 12 only 9-3

The position of the five numbers is used to identify large numbers.

e.g. Number 31

Number 45 would be notched 27-9-9

INJECTING PIGLETS WITH IRON

Reason

Piglets are born with minimal reserves of iron and sows' milk contains insufficient iron to satisfy their needs. They will become anaemic by ten days of age unless they have access to iron orally or are injected with an iron preparation.

Method

Iron can be given by mouth as a ferrous sulphate paste on days 4, 10 and 15. This is not a common method and it is time consuming. The best procedure is to give 150-200mg of iron dextran either by subcutaneous or intramuscular injection.
Injections are available that contain either 100mg or 200mg per ml.
If the piglets are to be weaned at less than three weeks and are provided with creep feed containing iron, the smaller dose is sufficient. A half dose may be all that is required in outdoor herds on certain soil types.

Materials Required

Marker spray.
Iron dextran 100ml, containing either 100 or 200mg/ml.
Syringes 16mm ($^5/_8$") 21g needles or an automatic syringe delivering 1 or 2ml.
Use sterile or disposable ones.
A bottle of surgical spirit and cotton wool or a surgical spirit sprayer (in outdoor herds).
A platform to hold the materials.
In outdoor herds carry the above in a small container that can be washed and disinfected between sessions.

Timing

Iron injections are best given between three and five days of age. Do not administer on day one because they cause considerable stress to the piglet.
Give iron injections at the same time as tails are removed.

Procedure

1	Collect the litter together in a bottomless box that is well bedded or hold in a clean creep area. This is a one person operation. In outdoor sow herds, routine iron injections are given when the sows' are feeding. It is best done inside the hut on clean straw and with a second person on watch outside the entrance with a pig board in case the sow returns.
2	Fill the syringe with iron solution. Use a new syringe and needle.
3	Wipe the needle clean with surgical spirit and cotton wool every third injection or in outdoor sow herds spray it with a surgical spray. Use a new needle after three litters, or before if it is damaged, in indoor units, but use a new needle for every litter in outdoor herds.
4	The site of the injection can be intramuscular into the leg or neck muscles or under the skin. The leg muscle is preferred. Follow the manufacturers recommendations.
5	Lift the piglet by the hind leg but keep the leg in line with the body as far as possible. Do not hold the pig with the leg at right angles to its body because muscle and tendon damage may occur.
6	Roll the skin over the muscle away from the mid line with the thumb and introduce the needle at a 45° angle. Inject either 1 or 2ml (200mg). 1ml is preferred. (Figs 15-17a and 15-17b)
7	Roll the skin back and apply pressure to the injection site.
8	Mark the piglet.

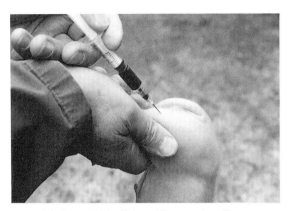

Injecting a piglet with iron. The correct position.

(Fig.15-17a)

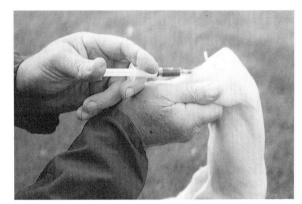

The wrong position. The leg is held at right angles.

(Fig.15-17b)

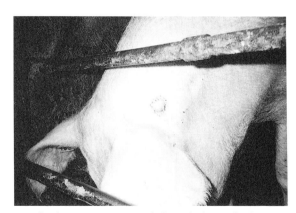

An abscess on a sows neck due to faulty vaccination

(Fig.15-18)

LANCING AN ABSCESS OR A HAEMATOMA

Reasons

A swelling that appears just under the surface of the skin is usually either an abscess or a haematoma. Haematoma commonly occur on the ears and soft tissues overlying the shoulders and sides. They are pockets of blood formed after a blood vessel has ruptured. If a swelling has appeared suddenly it is probably a haematoma, or if gradually it is possibly an abscess. If the swelling is an abscess the pus must be drained. If it is a haematoma it may be best left to repair on its own. Abscesses are common due to faulty vaccination procedures. Fig.15-18.

Materials Required

A snare or sedative for restraint.
A 10ml syringe with a 38mm (1$^1/_2$") 18g needle.
Scalpel blade and handle.
Water and antiseptic.
Saline solution (1% salt)

Procedure

1	Restrain the pig.
2	Examine the swelling.
3	Determine the softest area of the swelling and pass the needle into the mass. Withdraw fluid.
4	If the fluid is fresh blood - proceed no further. It is a recent haematoma.
5	If the fluid is clear or blood tinged it is a haematoma that has ceased bleeding and is healing. Leave it alone.
6	If the haematoma over the ear is large and causing pain open it up on the inside at the top of the ear and treat as for an abscess.
7	If the fluid is pus it is an abscess and requires opening and draining. Usually there will be evidence of skin damage and scar tissue.
8	Move the pig to a pen that can be cleaned and disinfected.
9	Make an incision 30 to 40mm long at the lowest point of the abscess and squeeze out the contents.
10	Flush out with the syringe and saline and keep the incision open with a cleaned gloved finger, or a pair of scissors, daily for three to four days.
11	Inject the pig on alternate days with either OTC, amoxycillin or penicillin (long-acting).

LIBIDO CHECKING - TRAINING BOARS TO USE A STOOL

Reason
This may be carried out to check a boar's libido before sale, in preparation for semen collection on the farm, or at an AI stud.

Materials Required
A mounting stool or dummy or a gilt on heat.
A dry pen at least 9.3m^2.   Good light.

Procedure

1	Establish a good rapport and empathy with the boars. Be quiet and patient.
2	Only test boars from six months of age onwards.
3	Young boars may be housed in groups in warm draught free accommodation but ideally in pairs. They must have visual contact with other animals.
4	Test the boar in his pen if possible in his familiar surroundings.
5	Place the stool in the pen each day early in the morning when it is cool
6	Allow the boar to make contact. Add saliva from other boars to the surface of the stool or use after another boar. Alternatively use urine from a sow in oestrus. The boar may take a few days before he will mount.
7	If there is no interest within 10 to 15 minutes remove the dummy and try again the following day.
8	See semen collection for more information

LOCAL ANAESTHESIA

Reason
Local anaesthesia in the pig is used to facilitate minor surgical techniques that include:- suturing skin and muscle, castration of older pigs, replacing prolapses and inserting retaining sutures.

Materials Required

2ml, 10ml syringes. 21g, 20g, 18g needles 0.8-1.1mm long 25 to 38mm (1-1$^1/_2$").	Local anaesthetic. Cotton wool Water and antiseptic such as Savlon or Cetrimide.

Procedure
Depending upon what procedure you intend to do you may need the help or guidance of your veterinarian.

1	Clean the tissues to be anaesthetised with cotton wool or gauze soaked in antiseptic.
2	Fill the syringe with anaesthetic and place the needle 5mm in front of the tissues to be anaesthetised.
3	Squeeze anaesthetic ahead of the needle point as it is pushed forward.
4	As a guide use 0.5ml for each 25mm of length.
5	Wait five minutes. Test the tissues by lightly pricking the area with a needle to asses the completeness of anaesthesia.

LIME WASHING CONCRETE FLOORS

Reason

Over a period of time concrete surfaces wear away and become pitted making it difficult to clean and disinfect them adequately. Bacteria and coccidia become embedded in the concrete and rise to the surface as the floor dries out after cleaning. Covering the surfaces with lime wash reduces exposure to organisms, it has a disinfectant action and the surface becomes less abrasive.

Materials Required

Builders lime or dehydrated lime powder (calcium carbonate). (Concrete cement can also be used).
Water.
A large bucket and stirrer.
A pair of eye protectors or goggles.
A soft brush and handle.
Lysol or a phenolic disinfectant.

Procedure

1	Wear eye protectors at all times. Lime wash can burn.
2	Place lime in the bucket and add water in a ratio of approximately 1:1 to form a thick consistency, sufficient to brush onto the concrete surfaces.
3	Add 30ml of a phenol based disinfectant to 5 litres of water.
4	Clean and wash the concrete surface.
5	Brush off surplus water.
6	Brush the lime wash over the surface.
7	Allow the surface to dry for at least 48 hours. DO NOT ALLOW SKIN CONTACT WITH WET MATERIAL.

	MATING THE SOW WITH THE BOAR
	Reason
	It is important to make sure the sow is at the correct time of the oestrus period before mating takes place. See chapter 5 Fig.5-20.
	Materials Required
	A large pen for mating, minimum size 3m x 3m with no projections and each side at least 2.4m. A non slip or well bedded floor. A dry floor. Good lighting. Plastic disposable gloves. A movement board for protection.
	Procedure
1	Identify the sow or gilt that is in oestrus by ear number or tattoo.
2	Examine the animal for lameness, the vulva for abnormal discharges and malformations.
3	Select a suitable boar that has not been used within 24 hours.
4	Move the sow to the boar pen or mating pen.
5	Observe the behaviour of boar and sow and check that the sow is standing firmly.
6	Allow the boar to mount. If there is no dissension by the sow allow mating to commence.
7	As the penis spirals out guide it, if necessary, into the vulva by holding the hand as a funnel against the vulva. DO NOT HANDLE THE PREPUCE. It is a heavily contaminated area.
8	Watch for the penis to lock into the cervix. The boar will stop thrusting.
9	Observe below the boar's tail for pulsation of the urethra as insemination takes place.
10	Observe that there is no leakage of semen.
11	Mating will take from five to ten minutes and observe during this period.
12	Remove the sow to a quiet area for two hours.
13	Record the mating.
	Outdoor sow herds - Some adopt individual mating so the same principles apply. Where group mating is used it is important to ensure that the boar : sow ratio is correct for the system (e.g. Danish dynamic service system) and that all boars are actually serving and serving correctly. Guard against overweight boars from overfeeding.

PREGNANCY DIAGNOSIS

Using the Döppler effect.

Reason

An early diagnosis of pregnancy indicates the efficiency of reproductive performance and also any impending management or disease problems.

Materials Required

A Döppler instrument with ear phones. (Fig.15-19)
Coupling liquid.
Marker spray and note book.
A one person job.

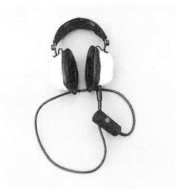

Pregnancy diagnosis. A döppler instrument showing the probe and ear phones.
(Fig.15-19)

Procedure

The döppler instrument passes high frequency sound waves from the probe into the abdomen of the pregnant sow. Any movement is reflected back with a change in frequency which is audible as a characteristic sound.

1	Sounds are produced by the uterine artery from about day 28 of pregnancy, the umbilical cord from about day 32 and the foetal heart beat by day 40.
2	Select a sow 12 weeks pregnant that is lying quietly on her side. Add coupling liquid to the surface of the probe and make direct contact on the skin. Position the probe to hear the sounds. (Fig.15-20 & 21)
3	Uterine artery - This sounds like a hand saw cutting wood and it is the first audible sound at around 28 days of pregnancy. In the heavily pregnant sow it is difficult to identify. Umbilical cord - This sound is similar but much faster with a swishing noise. Foetal heart - This is fast and sounds like the drumming of horse hooves on the ground.
4	Once familiar with the sounds select a sow 6 weeks pregnant and repeat the examinations. Apply coupling liquid at each skin contact.
5	Carry out routine pregnancy checks at 4 weeks and repeat again at 5 weeks. If there is a fertility problem in the herd check again at 6 weeks.
6	Visually check sows a 10 weeks.
7	Sows that give a negative or doubtful reading should be moved next to a boar and observed for oestrus.

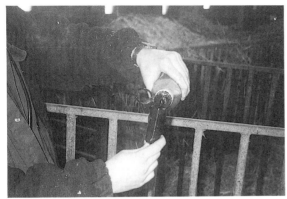
Placing coupling fluid on the probe.
(Fig.15-20)

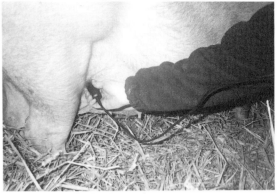
Testing the sow for pregnancy.
(Fig.15-21)

PENIS - EXAMINATION

Reason

Examination of the penis is necessary for surgical purposes, anatomical faults or where the mating procedures are suspect.

Materials Required

An empty clean pen to house the boar. Stresnil. Gauze and saline solution.	Suture materials and local anaesthetic. Surgical scissors, tissue forceps and artery forceps.

Procedure

1	Sedate the boar with stresnil 1ml/10kg. At this level the penis will protrude itself. Wait for 15 minutes and do not disturb.
2	Pull out the penis gripping it with piece of gauze and examine.
3	Carry out any procedures as necessary.
4	Return the penis to the prepuce as far as it will go and cover the remainder with wet gauze.
5	Leave the boar to recover and until the penis is fully retracted.

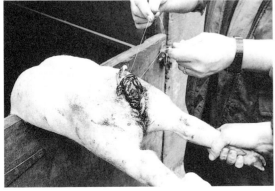
A mattress suture ready for tying
(Fig.15-22c)

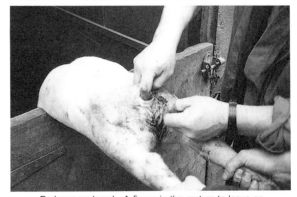
Prolapse replaced. A finger in the rectum to leave an opening as tying occurs
(Fig.15-22d)

CHAPTER 15 - Surgical, Manipulative and Practical Procedures

PROLAPSE OF THE RECTUM

Reason
This is a common condition in growing pigs and occasionally it occurs in breeding females.

Methods
There are four options for treatment, but you may need instructions from your veterinarian.
Replace and retain with a suture. This is the preferred method.
Place a piece of corrugated tube into the prolapse and apply a tourniquet to allow the prolapse to eventually slough off. Used in growing pigs.
Suture and then amputate.
Place the pig in a hospital pen and allow the prolapsed tissue to slough away. Not a preferred option.

Materials Required

A method of restraint or sedative, see page 507.	Scissors, tissue forceps.
Local anaesthetic, syringe and 21g 25mm (1") needles.	12mm diameter corrugated plastic tubing.
Curved suture needles 25 to 50mm (1 to 2") in size.	Obstetrical lubricant.
Nylon or cat gut suture for pigs up to 100kg.	Warm water, antiseptic, cotton wool.
Suture tape for sows.	

Procedures
You may need guidance or instruction from your veterinarian.

Replacing The Prolapse

1. If the pig is in a pen with others remove it as soon as possible.
2. Sedate or restrain by placing the pigs head down in a round container or hold over a wall.
3. Clean the area around the prolapse and remove all faeces.
4. Infiltrate around the rectum tissue with local anaesthetic. Usually only necessary in pigs over 60kg.
5. Select the nylon or synthetic suture material and insert around the rectum using either a mattress suture or a purse string suture. Fig.15-22a and 15-22b.

A MATTRESS SUTURE
(suitable for retaining a prolapsed rectum in pigs up to 120kg weight)

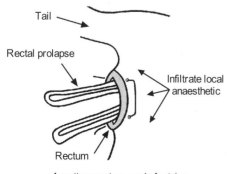

A mattress suture ready for tying

(Fig.15-22a)

A PURSE STRING SUTURE
Ideal for a Sow.

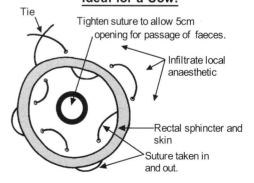

Prolapse replaced, place a finger in the rectum to leave an opening as tying occurs

(Fig.15.22b)

PROLAPSE OF THE RECTUM (Cont.)

6	Cover the prolapse with obstetrical lubricant and using fingers of both hands squeeze it into the rectum. Replace the prolapse even if torn - the pig will have a greater chance of survival.
7	Tighten the suture with a double tie to prevent it slipping and leave a finger width for the passage of faeces. See Figs.15-22c and 15-22d on page 500
8	The prolapse in sows may be swollen and full of fluid. Steady gentle pressure may then be required for 10-15 minutes to reduce it before it can be returned to the rectum. If possible the prolapse should be pushed well inside the abdomen after it has been replaced. Tighten the purse string suture allowing two fingers width. Tie leaving a bow so that it can be slackened if necessary.
9	Inject the pig intramuscularly with long-acting penicillin.
10	Mark the pig and monitor its progress. The suture may be removed after seven days or left in situ.

Using Corrugated Tubing

1	Proceed as in 1, 2 and 3 previously.
2	Insert a 75mmx18-20mm diameter piece of corrugated plastic tubing into the prolapse and place suture material or an elastic band around the prolapse next to the skin. Use electrical conduit tubing.
3	Tie tightly to restrict blood supply and eventually the prolapse will drop off.
4	Inject the pig intramuscularly with long-acting penicillin. Two injections three days apart.

Suture and Amputate

If the prolapse cannot be replaced amputation is an option. Proceed under the guidance of your veterinarian.

1	Proceed as for 1 to 4 under replacement.
2	Place two fingers into the prolapse, just past the anal ring. Insert the half curved needle and suture material 6mm from the skin into the prolapse, through to the two fingers, and out again. Place the interrupted sutures completely around the prolapse, each one over lapping the other (Fig.15-23).

AMPUTATION OF A PROLAPSE- INTERUPTED SUTURES

(Fig.15-23)

3	Once all the inter locking sutures are in place and tied the prolapsed tissue is cut off and the stump is slipped into the rectum.
4	The pig should be injected intramuscularly every other day with long-acting penicillin on three occasions.

PROLAPSE OF THE CERVIX

Reason

This occurs when the tissues that support the cervix (neck of the womb) are weak or fail. With advancing pregnancy and increased abdominal pressure the tissues are squeezed out through the vulva.

Materials Required

Sedative and / or physical restraint.
Local anaesthetic 10ml syringe and 25mm (1") 21g needles.
Large curved needles 38mm (1 1/2") and 100mm (4").
Suture tape, scissors.
Warm water and antiseptic.
Obstetrical lubricant.

Procedure

1	As soon as the prolapse is noted and if abdominal pressure is causing the prolapse, move the sow into loose housing.
2	If the prolapse ceases no further action is required.
3	Restrain the sow and infiltrate local anaesthetic under the skin and tissues down each side of the lips of the vulva. Replace the prolapse. Apply a tape mattress suture across the vulva as shown. Fig.15-24. Leave a 230mm overlap of tape and tie in a bow (not too tightly that blood supply is cut off) so that it can then be loosened if farrowing is imminent. Use a 75mm curved suture needle.

MATTRESS SUTURE ACROSS THE VULVA

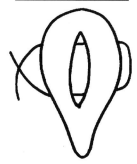

(Fig.15-24)

4	Tie the tape to hold the lips of the vulva together and prevent a further prolapse. Untie the tape at point of farrowing
5	Before the sow is moved into the farrowing crate build a wooden floor in the crate that slopes downwards to the front. Start at least 150mm high at the back. Fill in the side of the floor with straw. This slope will hold the prolapse in during farrowing.
6	After the sow has finished farrowing and passed afterbirth tie the tape sutures again to leave a small aperture.
7	Cull the sow after weaning.

PROLAPSE OF THE UTERUS (WOMB)

Reason

This occurs within two to three hours of farrowing. The uterus turns partially or completely inside out and protrudes as a large mass from the vulva. (Fig.15-25a and 15-25b)

Methods

Options: shoot the sow, replace the prolapse, or amputate it (an operation which should be carried out only by a veterinarian). In most cases shooting is the best option.

Materials Required

Sedative or physical restraint. Local anaesthetic 10ml syringe and 25mm (1") 21g needles.	Large curved needles 38mm (1$\frac{1}{2}$") and 100mm (4"). A small, clean empty bottle. Suture tape, scissors, warm water and disinfectant.

Procedure

1	If the womb has prolapsed completely and the sow is pale and anaemic shooting is the best course of action. Prior to this give the sow 1ml of oxytocin to contract the uterus and let down colostrum for the piglets, for five to ten minutes. This will ensure a better survival of the piglets for fostering.
2	If the womb is not completely prolapsed, replacement may be possible provided internal haemorrhage has not occurred.
3	Remove the sow carefully to an open pen holding the prolapse together in a clean towel or sheet during movement and taking care not to tear it.
4	Sedate the sow with stresnil 1ml/10kg and wait 20 minutes. Keep the prolapse covered with a clean towel or sheet.
5	Clean the surface of the uterus with obstetrical lubricant and place a clean towel beneath it.
6	If possible raise the sow by the hind legs to create a negative pressure in the abdomen and place a bale of straw or suitable support beneath the pelvis to elevate the prolapse.
7	Invert and replace the prolapse. This is not easy and sometimes the full bladder is within the prolapse. It maybe necessary to drain it with a large needle.

THE NORMAL UTERUS — Ovaries, Horns, Cervix, Vulva

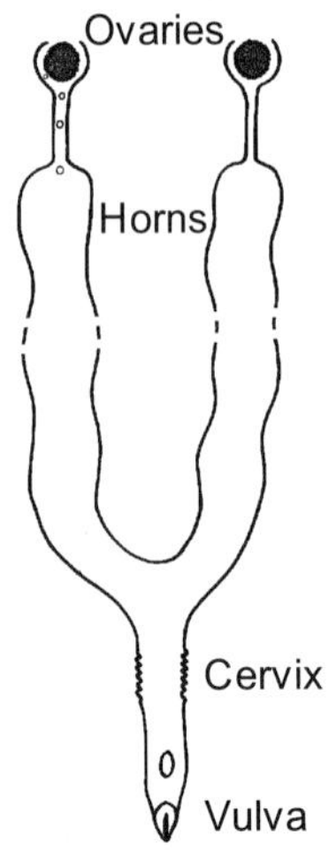

(Fig.15-25a)

THE PROLAPSING UTERUS — Ovaries (Blood vessels often rupture), Inverted horn of the uterus, Cervix, Vulva

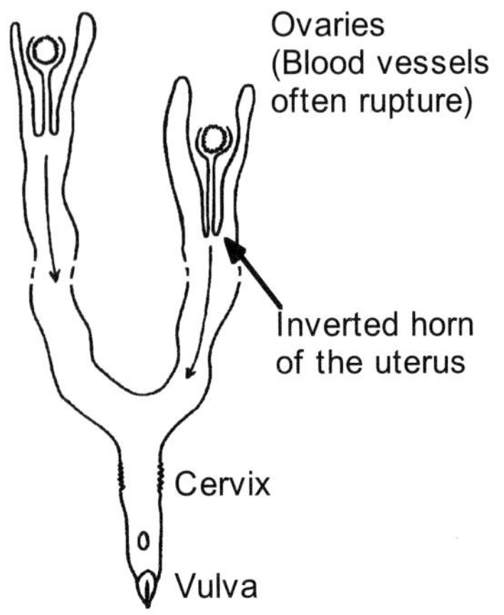

(Fig.15-25b)

CHAPTER 15 - Surgical, Manipulative and Practical Procedures **505**

8	It is essential to return both horns completely to their original position by inserting a clean arm, covered with lubricant and mild antiseptic full length into the replaced uterus. A small bottle held in the hand and covered in obstetrical lubricant will sometimes help lengthen the arm. If the uterine horns are not completely returned to their normal position they will prolapse again.
9	Place two pessaries into each horn.
10	Inject $^{1}/_{2}$ml of oxytocin. Give a long-acting penicillin injection every other day for three injections. This technique has a poor success rate.
11	Amputation - This is an operation for your veterinarian. It has a low success rate.

PROSTAGLANDIN INJECTIONS TO INITIATE FARROWING

Reason

To make the sow farrow at a more predictable time so that management procedures can be adopted to improve piglet survival.

Materials Required

Prostaglandin injection as prescribed by the veterinarian.
2ml syringe and either 38mm (1$^{1}/_{2}$") 18g (1.2mm) needle or 16mm ($^{5}/_{8}$") 23g (0.6mm).
Records of sows mating and farrowing dates.

Procedure

1	Calculate the average length of pregnancy in the herd.
2	Identify the farrowing date for each sow.
3	Examine the udder of the sow. Is it developed as expected for the farrowing date. The posterior glands always develop to maximum size last. If in doubt delay the injection
4	The sow can be injected from 112 days of pregnancy onwards but it is best at day 113. Give by intramuscular injection or using a 23g needle inject into the vulva.
5	The sow will farrow 14 to 30 hours later.
6	Dispose of the needle and syringe immediately.
7	Read the precautions for use in chapter 6.

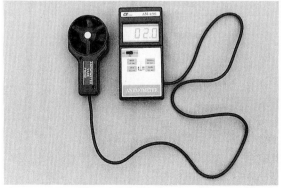

An anemometer. The vein is held in the air and the rate of flow is recorded.

(Fig.15-26a)

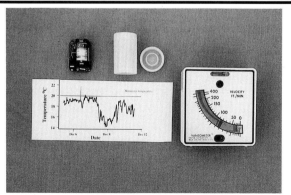

A vaneometer (right). This is placed in the air flow and a temperature recorder (left) shows a print out from a nursery.

(Fig.15-26b)

	RECORDING AIR MOVEMENT TEMPERATURE AND HUMIDITY IN A HOUSE
	Reason
	The speed and direction of air flow in a house determine the quality of the environment for the pig. This reflects on its own efficiency of growth and predisposition to disease.
	Materials Required
	Air movement can be assessed in three ways: 1. Observation of the pigs and their lying patterns. 2. The use of non toxic white vapours that are formed from compounds when they make contact with the air, (Fig.15-26d). 3. A wind vein anenometer. (Fig.15-26a and Fig.15-26b on page 505)
	Temperature can be recorded in four ways: 1. Maximum minimum thermometer. Place at pig level in a protected area e.g. behind a feeder. Read at intervals. 2. Instant reading. 3. Electronic recorders. These can be reset to record at any interval over a period of days or weeks. Using a computer programme the results can be compiled graphically. 4. A thermograph which continuously records on a revolving drum. Humidity can be recorded using a hygrometer or continuous hygrograph which records onto a revolving drum. The thermo-hygro shown in Fig.15-26c is a simple and easy method of recording both temperature and humidity. In cold weather maintain a relative humidity between 60-70%. Below 60% and in dusty conditions there is a greater predisposition to respiratory disease.
	Procedure
1	Switch on the anenometer.
2	Hold the wind in the air flow for 10 seconds and record the reading.
3	Repeat the recordings at different positions.
	The comfort zone for pigs at floor level is 0.15m/second or very little air movement. At 0.2m/s the pig may experience heat loss. At 0.5m/s the pig may experience a drop of 3ºC. At 1.0m/s the pig may experience a drop of 6-7ºC.

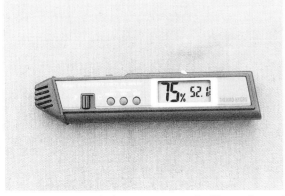

An electronic recorder for instant measurements of temperature and relative humidity.

(Fig.15-26c)

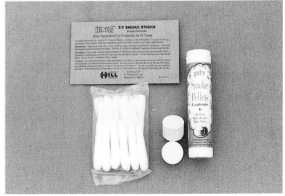

Two types of smoke generators. The sticks release vapour on contact with air. The pellets are started with a match.

(Fig.15-26d)

RESTRAINING THE PIG

Reasons

These include:
Close examination of the animal.
Lancing abscesses.
Surgical procedures, suturing, replacing prolapses etc.
Blood sampling.
Prior to anaesthesia.
De-tusking boars.
Shooting.

Methods

There are three methods of restraint, physical restraint (e.g. with a noose), sedation by injection or a combination of both.

Materials Required

Stresnil (azaperone), acetylpromazine injection or other available sedative.
10ml syringe 25 to 38mm (1-1$\frac{1}{2}$") x 16g needles.
Nylon rope with loops on each end. Cow calving ropes are ideal. Or use a wire noose. (Fig.15-27a & b)
A post or wall ring to attach the rope to.
A metal or plastic drum.

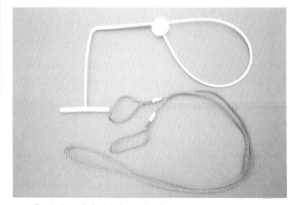

Restraint. A double looped nylon rope. A wire snare.

(Fig.15-27a)

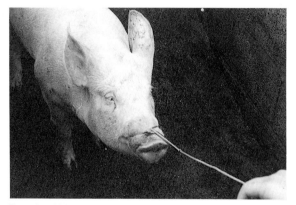

Restraint. Using a wire noose. Note the noose is behind the upper tusks.

(Fig.15-27b)

Procedure

1	Decide whether to use a rope or wire noose. The rope is better if a sow or boar is to be restrained for a period of time.
2	Stand by the side of the pigs shoulder. Hold the wire or rope in two hands and pull into the mouth behind the tusks of the upper jaw.
3	Tighten the noose with an upward movement and pull forwards to restrain the pig.
4	If a rope is used only one person is needed because the rope can be fastened to a post, bar or ring. This is ideal for restraining a sow in a farrowing crate or confinement stall. If a wire noose is used it is usually attached to a handle which has to be held.
5	To remove the noose keep the tension above the sows nose and then release downwards and allow the pig to shake it off.
6	Physical restraint can also be applied on smaller pigs <70kgs by holding the pig upside down in a plastic or metal drum with the hind legs held. Alternatively the pig can be held over the top of a wall. Both methods are useful for replacing rectal prolapses in small pigs. For some procedures, e.g. blood sampling from the anterior vena cava small pigs <30kg can be held on their backs in a trough or on a straw bale.

SAMPLING AIR FOR DUST LEVELS

Reason
Air contains 5 elements that may affect both pig and human health. They are: total dust (mg/m^3), respirable dust (mg/m^3), endotoxins ($\mu g/m^3$), toxic gases (ppm) and bacteria and fungi (cfu/m^3).

Methods
Both total and respirable dust levels are measured using pumps that draw known volumes of air through different size filters over given periods of time. The filters are weighed at the onset and on completion of the test period and from this information the levels of exposure can be calculated.

Materials
A commercial sampling kit. Fig. 15-28.
Pre-weighed filters. Access to an analytical balance.

Procedure

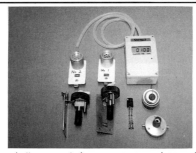

This shows a battery operated vacuum pump and pre-weighed filters.
(Fig.15-28)

1	Determine the time of monitoring usually measured over an 8 hour working period.
2	The pump is calibrated according to whether total or respirable dust is being measured.
3	Load the sampling head with a pre-weighed filter.
4	Attach the harness and pump behind the back.
5	Clip the sampling head at shoulder height.
6	Wear for the monitoring period during work.
7	The filter is removed and weighed by a specialist laboratory.
8	Calculations The weight of dust is measured and the personal exposure determined. This is usually expressed as mg/m^3 of air over an 8 hour time weighted average.
9	Interpretation. There are no universally accepted levels and many countries have their own standards. Measurements can also vary according to the type of equipment and methods used. Standard guidelines in the UK would be: Total inhalable dust - $10mg/m^3$ Respirable dust - $5mg/m^3$ Gas levels included for reference. Carbon dioxide Ammonia Hydrogen sulphide 8 hour exposure 5,000ppm 8 hour exposure 25ppm 8 hour exposure 10ppm 15 minute exposure 15,000ppm 15 minute exposure 35ppm 15 minute exposure 15ppm

SAMPLING FEEDS FOR LABORATORY TESTING

Reason

To collect representative samples for despatch to a laboratory for testing. The collection must be made in such a way that the results become meaningful both from a diagnostic and a legal stand point.

Materials Required

New polythene bags or sterile plastic or glass containers. An indelible marker pen.	Labels. A witness (independent if possible) to the sampling.

Procedure

1	Check with the laboratory to find out if there are any special requirements necessary relative to the problem.
2	Identify the material to be sampled by date received, batch number, invoice and feed bin if appropriate.
3	If a liquid take three separate samples of at least 500ml. Always use sterile glass containers. If in doubt be advised by the laboratory.
4	If sampling feed, take eight separate samples of 1kg from different parts of the material and bulk together. Mix these well.
5	Separate into 4 x 2kg samples.
6	Seal each one. Identify as 1 to 4 and label with full details. Sign and date each bag.
7	Hold samples in a refrigerator at 4°C (34°F) until despatch. Deep freeze if more than 3 - 4 days
8	Send one or two samples to separate laboratories. One to the supplier and retain one.
9	Send a full history of the problem, potential poisons suspected or test required.

SAMPLING MILK FROM A MAMMARY GLAND WITH MASTITIS

Reason

In herd outbreaks of mastitis it is often necessary to identify the organism involved and its antibiotic sensitivity.

Materials Required

Swabs in transport medium. A sterile container. Cotton wool.	Surgical spirit. Oxytocin. Needle and syringe.

Procedure

1	Identify the affected gland.
2	Inject the sow with 0.5 ml of oxytocin to release milk and wait two to four minutes.
3	Clean the teat end with cotton wool soaked in surgical spirit and then wipe dry. Wash your hands thoroughly or wear disposable gloves.
4	Squirt milk either onto the swab or into the sterile container. Place the swab into the transport medium.
5	Return the sample to a laboratory as soon as possible but within 24 hours.

SAMPLING THE AIR FOR TOXIC LEVELS OF GASES

Reasons

To assess the efficiency of the environment and ventilation systems for health and safety purposes. For the welfare of the pig.

Materials Required

These consist of an aspirating pump which draws a known volume of air through glass tubes containing reagents that are specific for the different gases. There are a number of makes on the market including Komyo Japan Kitagawa gas detectors (Fig.15-29) and Draaga tubes.
The tubes required for testing gases in the buildings should include carbon monoxide, carbon dioxide, hydrogen sulphide, methane and ammonia.

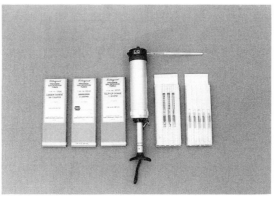

Sampling air for toxic levels of gases. Air is drawn through the glass tubes and colour changes measured.
(Fig.15-29)

Procedure

1	Read the instructions for each gas carefully and attach the glass tube to the aspirator, after removing the end of the tube.
2	Assess the environment to be tested to ensure there is no hazard to human health. Always have two people in the house.
3	Sample the air at pig level by drawing back the suction handle. Repeat the test again at human level.
4	Wait the appropriate time and record the changes.
5	Calculate from the instructions the level of the gas.
6	Interpretation. There are no universally accepted levels and many countries have their own standards. Measurements can also vary according to the type of equipment and methods used. Gas levels for reference. Carbon dioxide Ammonia Hydrogen sulphide 8 hour exposure 5,000ppm 8 hour exposure 25ppm 8 hour exposure 10ppm 15 minute exposure 15,000ppm 15 minute exposure 35ppm 15 minute exposure 15ppm

SEMEN COLLECTION AND ARTIFICIAL INSEMINATION ON THE FARM

A METHOD FOR INSEMINATION WITHIN 1-2 HOURS OF COLLECTION ONLY.

REASONS

The objective is to collect a sample of fresh semen for examination, or fresh semen samples regularly for dilution and insemination within one to two hours of collection.

Materials Required

Semen collection
A separate clean collecting area 3mx3m containing a stool or sow dummy. Collection can also be carried out in the boar pen.
Place posts 0.9m away from the wall, 0.7m high and 0.3m apart to provide a means of escape.
An environmental temperature of 21-22ºC (70-72ºF) in the collecting area.
A non-slip floor and an easy escape access from the pen.
A sow dummy preferably fixed to the floor.
A boar protection board.
A large polystyrene cup for semen collection and a 150mm diameter plastic funnel.
Fine muslin cloth or sterile gauze or milk filters.
Soft disposable polythene gloves (non toxic to sperm).
A marker pen and elastic band.

Semen preparation
A clean processing area held at 30ºC (86ºF) as shown in Fig.15-30, with an area to change into clean clothing. All bench surfaces must be smooth and easily cleaned.
Use as much disposable equipment as possible.
This reduces the risk of contamination.
Purified and distilled or de-ionised water.
Microscope glass slides and disposable pipettes.
Water bath or incubator.
Ready made packs of semen diluent.
1.5-2.5 or 5 litre semen bags.
Semen bag holder and dispenser.

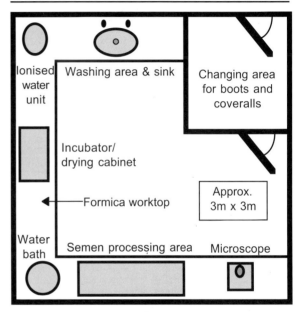

A SIMPLE ON THE FARM AI LABORATORY

(Fig.15-30)

Flat packs or collapsible semen bottles.
Disposable catheters. If flat packs use the golden rod catheter.
2 thermometers.
Tissue papers.
Polystyrene boxes for storage.

Collection Procedures

Initially you will probably need guidance from your expert in the field.

1	Place the gauze over the polystyrene collecting vessel and retain by an elastic band. Graduate the volume by previously marking with a marker pen.
2	Prepare fresh semen diluent by adding powder to water, check the temperature in the water bath and maintain at 35ºC (95ºF) for one hour before use.
3	Introduce the boar to the pen, squeeze out fluids from the prepuce and clean the area with tissues. Allow the boar to mount the stool.
4	Put on plastic gloves and clean the prepuce area again with tissues.
5	Use a clean gloved hand for collection. Wait for the penis to emerge and grasp it firmly around the spiral to lock into the hand. Relax the hand slightly as semen flows. Fig.15-31.

SEMEN COLLECTION AND ARTIFICIAL INSEMINATION ON THE FARM (Cont.)

6	Commence collecting the ejaculate of the sperm rich fraction, which is white, followed by clear fluid, into the gauze covered cup. Avoid any preputial fluids entering the semen. A tissue held in the hand will prevent this or bend the penis during collection.
7	Continue collection (5 to 15 minutes) until all fluid has ceased and the penis twitches, and then remove the sample immediately to the processing area. Approximately 100-500ml will be collected. Enough for up to 20 doses.
8	If a boar is not trained to a dummy sow and a sample is only required to check that the semen is fertile allow the boar to serve a female. Whilst he is ejaculating slide a small 5mm diameter stomach tube up the vagina to the cervix and using an attached 50ml syringe draw off semen.
9	Return the boar to his pen and feed him. Make sure to clean and wash the pen after use. Hygiene is very important.

Processing

1	Prepare the sample in the clean processing area where the above materials are kept. Maintain a room temperature 30°C (86°F).
2	Determine volume of the ejaculate. This will vary between 100-500ml. Examine its colour. It should be creamy white with no evidence of blood.
3	Determine the number of sows to be inseminated on the farm and the amount using 100ml doses.
4	Check the temperature of the semen and the diluent. They should be within 1-2°. Dilute the semen to a maximum of 1 in 4 and place in warmed disposable collapsible packs.
5	Place 2 drops of semen on a warm glass slide and check for wave motion under the microscope.
6	Inseminate within half to one hour.

INSEMINATION (Fig.15-33a - e)

1	Only inseminate after the sow has been standing firmly for 6-8 hours and preferably whilst stood next to the boar. Test by back pressure,
2	Lubricate the catheter with a small amount of special AI jelly (KY Jelly) or other recommended lubricant. Lubricant is not necessary with a foam catheter.
3	Clean the lips of the vulva with tissue and introduce the catheter in a forward and upward direction.
4	Using a spiral catheter rotate anti-clockwise after contact is made a the cervix until resistance is felt. Using the bulb catheter press the catheter firmly in until it enters the cervix. Withdraw the catheter slightly to check it is locked. Fig.15-32.
5	Bend the catheter upwards and attach the bottle after rotating it. Maintain pressure on the back of the sow and boar contact.
6	Allow the semen to enter via gravity although slight pressure may be required if a collapsible pack is not used.
7	Be prepared to take five to ten minutes over the insemination. If semen leaks out realign the catheters. BE PATIENT. Do not force the semen in.
8	If semen appears from the vulva check the catheter position to ensure that it is locked.
9	Once insemination is complete keep the sow quiet for 30 minutes and leave the catheter connected to the sow for 5-10 minutes then remove it.

The above procedures should only be adopted for immediate insemination on the farm. For longer storage and when using more diluted semen, better control procedures are necessary and you are referred to specialised books or further advice.

Outdoor sow herds: Semen collection is rarely if ever done but artificial insemination (AI), using brought in semen, is used by some outdoor pig farmers, mainly in hot days of summer, to top up on boar services when boar fertility may be adversely affected. Hygiene is one problem. Outdoor AI can result in uterine infections.

Further reading : A field and laboratory technicians' guide to artificial insemination in swine. Ed. R. Cronje. Pub. by M Morrow. ISBN 0-9640737-06. This includes a world-wide list of suppliers of AI equipment and information.

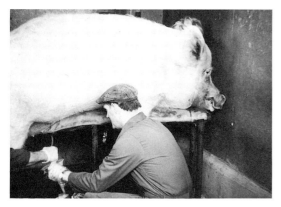

Collecting semen on the farm.
(Fig.15-31)

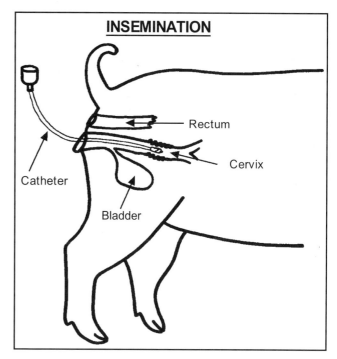

(Fig.15-32)

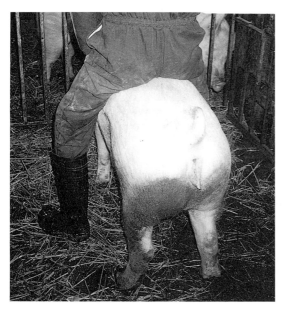

Testing the sow for oestrus.
(Fig.15-33a)

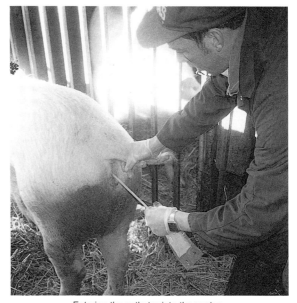

Entering the catheter into the vagina.
(Fig.15-33b)

514 Managing Pig Health and the Treatment of Disease

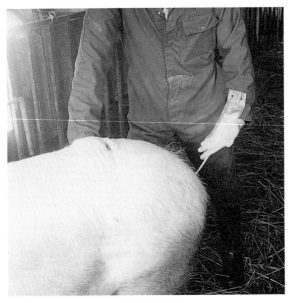

Insemination using a flat pack.
(Fig.15-33c)

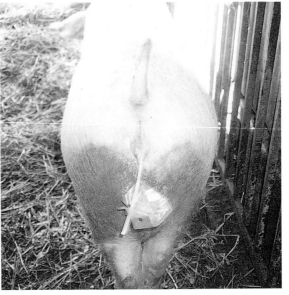

The catheter bent over is left in situ for 10 minutes after insemination.
(Fig.15-33d)

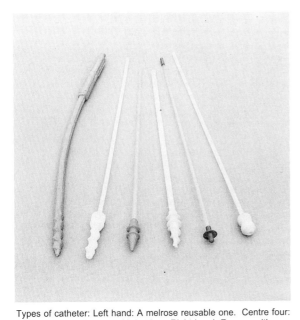

Types of catheter: Left hand: A melrose reusable one. Centre four: Disposable for use with bottles. Right hand: For use with collapsible packs. The foam end is pressed into the cervix.
(Fig.15-33e)

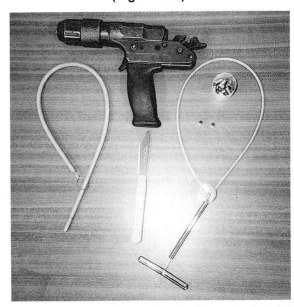

Equipment required for slaughter. Note the pithing rod on the left of the picture.
(Fig.15-34)

SLAUGHTER - HUMANE DESTRUCTION

Methods

This can be carried out in one of four ways:
1. Stunning with a captive-bolt pistol. Ideal and recommended for pigs from 6kg to adults.
2. Shooting with a shot gun; 4.10 or 12 bore. Suitable for pigs from 100kg to adults.
If methods 1 or 2 are used on pigs over 50kg weight they should either be bled or the spinal cord destroyed by pithing after stunning.
3. A sharp blow to the head. Suitable for pigs up to 6kg of weight.
4. Injecting a strong solution of barbiturate into the heart. Suitable for pigs up to 15kg weight. In most countries barbiturates can normally only be obtained and used by veterinarians. Their advice should be sought.

Materials Required

A captive-bolt pistol and blank cartridges or a shotgun. A wire snare or rope. (Fig.15-34) A sharp knife. A flexible rod to destroy the spinal cord.	A bottle of barbiturate, 20ml syringe 38 to 50mm ($1^{1}/_{2}$ to 2")18g needles. Two people. An area to hold the equipment.

Procedures

Using a Captive-bolt Gun

1	Instruction must have been given in the use and maintenance of the gun from a licensed slaughterer or a veterinarian. A licence may be required in some countries.
2	Check the gun to see that it is assembled correctly. Load with a blank cartridge in the slaughter area. Cock the gun and apply the safety catch.
3	Place the loaded gun on the platform with the other materials. Always point the gun away from the body and other people. Have a second cartridge ready in case it is required.
4	Move the pig to the slaughter area. Make sure the floor is not slippery.
5	Snare the pig and identify the point that bisects lines drawn from the base of each ear to each eye as illustrated. (Fig.15-35)

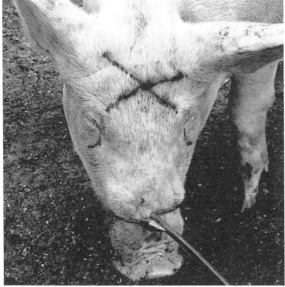

The position for shooting.

(Fig.15-35)

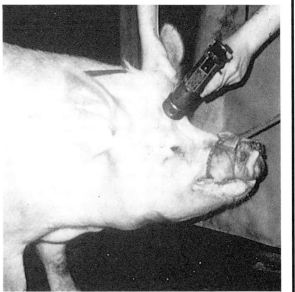

The angle of the gun.

(Fig.15-36)

	SLAUGHTER - HUMANE DESTRUCTION (Cont.)
6	The person holding the snare stands well forward and the gun is pressed firmly to the head. (Fig.15-36)
7	Remove the safety catch
8	Place the finger on the trigger at this point.
9	Shoot the pig and either bleed or pith.
10	To bleed either cut the throat transversely or stick the knife deep into the inlet into the chest on the right hand side of the pig to sever the main arteries and veins. Do not enter the chest.
11	To pith, pass the rod into the hole made in the skull by the captive bolt and push to the back of the brain and into the spinal cord to destroy it.
12	Dismantle the gun, clean and oil and return to its secure housing
	Note . Some old sows and boars have very thick skulls and a normal cartridge may not be sufficient. Always have heavy duty ones available. This problem does not arise if a shot gun is used.
	Using a Shotgun
	This is an effective method for pigs from 30kg weight up to boars. A 4.10 bore can be used up to 150kg and a 12 bore for sows and boars.
1	Remove the pig to an outside area. Do not shoot indoors.
2	Restrain the pig using a wire noose or nylon rope but with sufficient length to allow the person to stand behind the operator using the gun. Alternatively place feed on the floor and wait until the head is still and presented without restraint.
3	Once the pig is restrained stand in front of the head.
4	Load the gun and close the barrel.
5	Aim and hold the nozzle 0.5 metres from the head.
6	Release the safety catch and shoot.
	Care in the Use of a Shotgun
1	In many countries a certificate is necessary to both hold and use a gun.
2	Always keep equipment and cartridges locked in a secure place.
3	If you have not used firearms before seek expert instruction. Discuss procedures with your veterinarian.
4	Check the gun is unloaded at the onset and leave the breech open. Always point away from people.
5	Select the correct and most suitable area and restrain the pig as appropriate. Make sure that personnel involved are always behind you.
6	Only load the gun after No. 3 above.
7	If the gun fails to fire wait five seconds before opening it to replace the cartridge. Have spare cartridges available if it is necessary to shoot again.
8	As soon as the gun has been used open the breach and remove the cartridges. Dismantle, clean and return to its safe custody.

STOMACH TUBE - HOW TO USE ONE

Reason

This procedure is usually carried out at birth to give the piglet colostrum, either the natural product or an alternative source. Dextrose sugar solution can also be given to provide an instant source of energy

Materials Required

A plastic stomach tube 4mm and syringe. (Fig.15-37a)
Sows colostrum milked into a container at farrowing or
Irradiated cows" colostrum with added porcine immuno globulins or 20% dextrose solution.

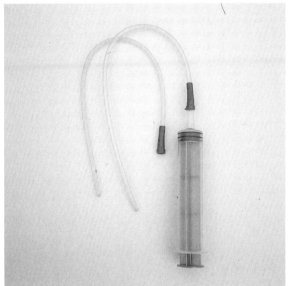

A plastic stomach tube and syringe.
(Fig.15-37a)

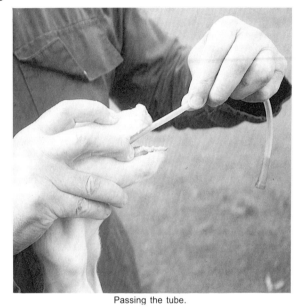

Passing the tube.
(Fig.15-37b)

Procedure

1	Fill the syringe and tube with the liquid.
2	Lubricate the tube with either colostrum or liquid paraffin.
3	Identify the piglet and place the little finger at the back of the tongue. Only carry on the procedure if there is a suckling reflex.
4	Hold the pig under the arm with the hand over the head and the third finger placed in the angle of the jaw.
5	Introduce the tube over the back of the tongue and gently push in feeling for a swallowing reflex. Accidental introduction of the tube into the trachea (windpipe) instead of the oesophagus rarely occurs. If it does the piglet will cough violently. Withdraw it and try again. (Fig.15-37b)
6	Gauge the distance from the mouth to the stomach. Resistance will be felt after the tube enters the stomach.
7	Introduce no more than 20mls at any one time. Repeat the procedure in two hours if thought necessary.

SUTURING SKIN AND MUSCLE

Reason

The common causes of skin and muscle damage arise from trauma in the case of piglets and fighting in older animals.

Materials Required (Fig.15-38a - c)

Sedative injection - stresnil (azaperone)
Local anaesthetic.
2 or 10ml syringe and either 25mm (1") 21g needle or 38mm ($1^{1}/_{2}$") 18g needles.
Curved suture needles 25 to 50mm (1 to 2") in size.
Scissors, forceps, scalpel blades and handle.
Suture materials: See below
Suture tape.
Warm water, cotton wool, mild antiseptic.
A table to hold the instruments.

Suture Materials

These are classified by diameter, using numbers. Two methods are in use.

The old system	$^4/_0$	$^3/_0$	$^2/_0$	0	1	2	3	4
The metric system		1.5	3	3.5	4	5	6	7	8
		Small			$\rightarrow$		Bigger		

Uses: (metric)
1.5, 3   Suitable for piglets skin
3.5, 4   Suitable for pigs from 30 - 100kg weight
5, 6, 7, 8   Suitable for the skin of sows and boars

Suture materials consist of: synthetic non absorbed ones, usually made from nylon or cotton tape and absorbed ones such as catgut .

Non absorbed materials are used for suturing the skin and rectal and vaginal prolapses. Catgut is used in muscle or subcutaneous tissues. Tape is used to retain a prolapse of the cervix prior to farrowing. The vulva can be easily opened and tied again.

Skin sutures would be removed after 14 days but catgut remains in the tissue and is gradually absorbed.

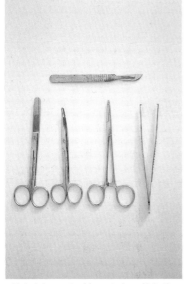

Materials required for suturing. Note the tooth or tissue forceps on the left.

(Fig.15-38a)

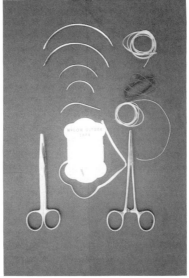

Suture materials. The tape is used for suturing the vulva.

(Fig.15-38b)

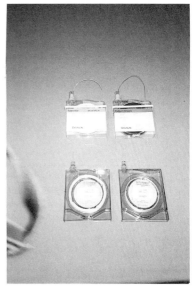

Suture holders and contents.

(Fig.15-38c)

CHAPTER 15 - Surgical, Manipulative and Practical Procedures **519**

SUTURING SKIN AND MUSCLE (Cont.)

Procedure

1	Prepare the suture materials and equipment and decide where the operation will take place.
2	Sedate the pig if over 5kg weight or if it cannot be restrained manually. Use stresnil, 1ml per 10kg. Wait for 15-20 minutes until it has taken effect.
3	With larger animals it may be necessary to restrain the pig by using a snare over the upper jaw.
4	Infiltrate local anaesthetic beneath the skin and wait five minutes.
5	Shave the skin over the wound and clean with warm water and cotton wool. Make sure all hair is removed out of the wound.
6	Pick up the skin edges with the forceps and loosen them from the underlying tissues with the scalpel blade.
7	Decide the type of suture to be used. There are three methods: (Ask your veterinarian for advice).

1. Interrupted sutures (Fig.15-39) - Used where there is plenty of loose skin and no tension. Ideal for small piglets. Place the sutures 6mm apart.

INTERRUPTED SUTURES

Skin — Skin Wound — Cross section of skin

(Fig.15-39)

2. Mattress suture (Fig.15-40) - This is used where there is tension on the skin. The suture turns the edges of the skin outwards. It is best used in pigs over 10kg weight. It is important to free the skin from underlying tissues so that it will turn outwards.

MATTRESS SUTURE

Skin edges — Suture — Cross section of skin

(Fig.15-40)

SUTURING SKIN AND MUSCLE (Cont.)

	3. Continuous suture (Fig.15-41) - This is used for suturing subcutaneous tissue and muscle and also for the skin. If used in tissue, use a cat gut which dissolves away. **CONTINUOUS SUTURE** 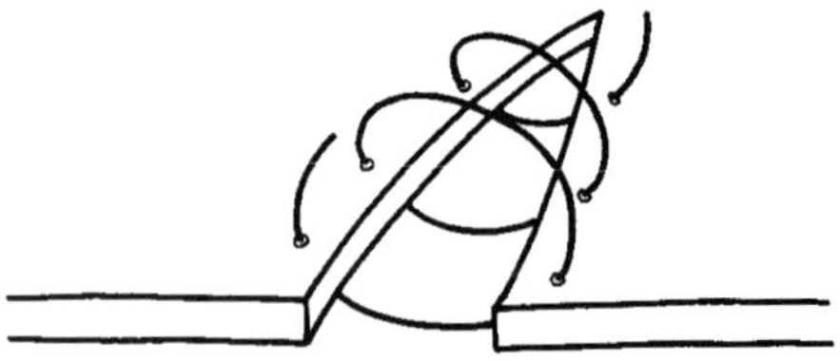 Cross section of tissue (Fig.15-41)
8	Clean the suture line after completion and apply an antibiotic cream or inject the pig with long-acting penicillin.
9	Leave the pig to recover and then return it to its pen.
10	Remove the sutures after ten days.
	Outdoor herds - Suturing may be difficult but when sows or boars suffer skin injuries e.g. after fighting it is wise to administer penicillin by injection and in hot weather to watch out for fly strike. The maggots may get into the damaged skin under the healing skin. If so use ivermectin injections.

SWABBING THE NOSE AND TONSILS FOR TOXIGENIC PASTEURELLA OR OTHER BACTERIA

Reason

If a pig herd is affected by progressive atrophic rhinitis it will be carrying toxigenic strains of *Pasteurella multocidia*. These organisms are found in the nose and tonsils.

Materials Required

Wire noose for restraint.
Mouth gag, small and large.
Wire or flexible nasal swabs in transport media.
A polystyrene box for posting swabs to the laboratory.
An ice pack for use in the box.
Identification material i.e. tags.
Torch.

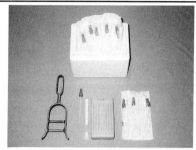

Materials required for swabbing.
(Fig.15-42)

Procedure

1. Clean the nose with cotton wool.
   Remove the swab from its container
   Pigs less than 10kg weight restrain manually otherwise use a noose.

2. Place the hand over the mouth and nose and rest the other hand on the wrist. (Fig.15-43)

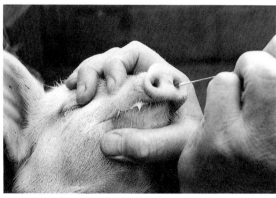

Open the pigs mouth to insert a swab.
(Fig.15-43)

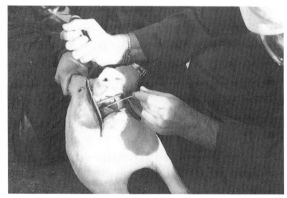

Using a mouth gag to examine the tonsils.
(Fig.15-44)

3. Insert the swab 25 to 70mm into each nostril to the back of the nose and replace in the protective cover with the end dipped in the transport medium.

4. If the tonsils are to be swabbed hold the pigs head by the ears or restrain by a noose. The operator then opens the mouth using a gag (Fig.15-44).

5. Restrain the pig with a snare if over 15kg. Open the mouth with the gag (Fig.15-46), the tongue beneath the bar. Depress the tongue and identify the tonsils using the torch.
   They are rough areas on each side of the soft palate at the back of the throat. (Fig.15-45)

SWABBING THE NOSE AND TONSILS FOR TOXIGENIC PASTEURELLA OR OTHER BACTERIA (Cont.)

	SWABBING THE TONSILS	A TYPICAL PIG GAG
	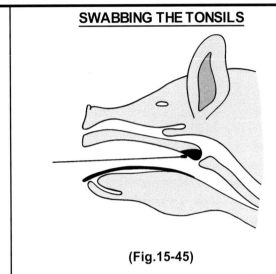 (Fig.15-45)	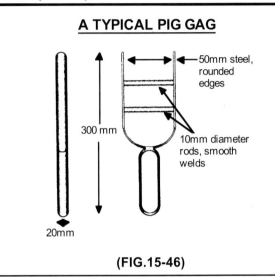 (FIG.15-46)
6	Rub the swab over each tonsil and replace in the swab case in the liquid. Label with the pig number	
7	Deliver the swabs together with the ice pack to the laboratory within 24 hours.	

CHAPTER 15 - Surgical, Manipulative and Practical Procedures

SYRINGES AND NEEDLES AND THEIR USE

Reason

Syringes can be bought already sterilised and intended for disposal after use or they may be designed for repeated usage after re-sterilisation. Disposable materials should always be used where possible.

Materials Required

Needles - These are measured by diameter in mm and standard wire gauge or g. (Fig.15-47a and 47b). Sizes are given in mm and the table below gives comparisons of measurements.

Length	gauge (g)	mm diameter	Uses	
16mm	($5/8$")	23, 21	0.6 - 0.8	Piglets
25mm	(1")	21, 20, 18	0.7 - 1.2	Piglets, weaners
38mm	($1 1/2$")	18, 16	1.4	Weaners, finishers, sows
50mm	(2")	18, 16	1.4	Sows
100mm	(4")	18, 16	1.4	Sows, boars blood sampling

Similar sizes may be used for both intramuscular or subcutaneous injections.
Syringes - multi-dose automatic syringes for vaccinating large numbers. Disposable 2ml, 10ml, 20ml, 30ml, 50ml.
Cotton wool.
Surgical spirit.
A small dish to hold needles in.

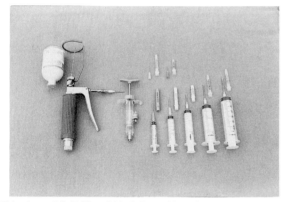

This shows 2-3-10-20 and 30ml disposable syringes and re-useable multidose ones.

(Fig.15-47a)

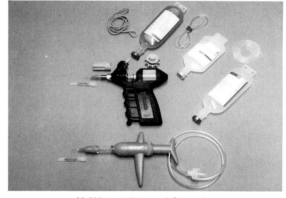

Multidose syringe and flat packs.

(Fig.15-47b)

Procedure

1	Select the appropriate syringe size for the volume to be administered.
2	Select the needle by size and length. Always use disposable ones with a protective plastic cap attached to protect needle and operator.
3	Select the bottle to be used and wipe the rubber cap clean with surgical spirit and cotton wool. Shake well and invert.
4	Draw an equivalent amount of air into the syringe, place the needle through the rubber cap into the liquid expel the air and draw liquid out into the syringe. This is not necessary with a collapsible bottle.
5	Remove the bottle. Place the protective cap over the needle after use.
6	Use a fresh needle after it has been used five times.

	SYRINGES AND NEEDLES AND THEIR USE (Cont.)
7	If a number of animals are to be injected keep a 25mm (1") 16g needle in the top of the bottle and re-attach the syringe to it each time for filling.
8	Where large numbers of animals are being injected in one period with an antibiotic or preserved inactive vaccine, wipe the needle before each use with cotton wool soaked in surgical spirit. Change the needle every five animals and hold other needles soaking in the container of surgical spirit. Shake out each needle before use. Do not use surgical spirit or disinfectant to store needles or wipe them if you are injecting sensitive substances such as live attenuated vaccines.
9	Always keep part-used bottles in a fridge, do not re-use them too often or store them too long and follow the manufacturers instructions.
10	If self inoculation occurs take the following actions: - Immediately inform someone on the farm. - Read the literature and safety sheets that should be present on the farm. - Are there any immediate actions which should be taken? - If it is on oil based vaccine seek medical advice immediately. - Ring your veterinarian, doctor or supplier for advice.
11	Disposal - Special containers should be used for the disposal of needles. These consist of special plastic boxes with a non-returnable flap. Some have facilities for cutting the needlepoint prior to entry into the box. The total contents are finally incinerated. Syringes should be placed in separate containers for incineration. Your veterinarian will have facilities for disposal.

CHAPTER 15 - Surgical, Manipulative and Practical Procedures

TEETH CLIPPING

Reason
Piglets are born with needle-sharp canine (eye) teeth at the corners of the upper and lower jaws. These traumatise both the sows' teats and the faces of other piglets. Damage to the skin can lead to greasy pig disease. The sow may become reluctant to suckle

Timing
Teeth should not be clipped until at least six hours after birth until the piglets have taken in adequate amounts of colostrum. Teeth removal at birth before suckling will predispose to joint infection.

Instruments
A sharp pair of clippers either stainless steel or piano wire cutters.
A small container with mild skin antiseptic or cow teat dip (iodine based).
Hold the clippers in the container when not in use.
A toothbrush to clean the instruments.
A marker spray.

Procedure
1. Wash the clippers in hot soapy water and disinfect before use.
2. Close the blades and hold to the light to check for any damage. If evident use a new instrument. Always have a spare pair available.
3. Hold the piglets in the creep area or in a bottomless box. Bed the creep area with wood shavings or other suitable bedding.
4. Hold each piglet with the third finger placed in the angle of the jaw and the fourth finger across the trachea to suppress squealing.
5. Place the clippers parallel to the jaw bone. Do not point the clippers into the gum. This will cause damage and infection. (Fig.15-48a-c)
6. Make sure that no sharp points of teeth left. These will predispose to skin damage around the face and the development of greasy pig disease.
7. Mark the piglet.
8. Clean the clippers on completion.

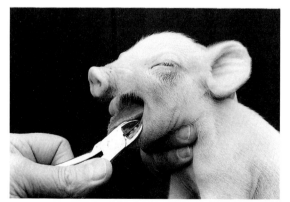

Teeth clipping. Note the holding position and angle of the clippers parallel to the gum.

(Fig.15-48a)

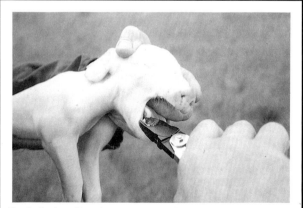

Teeth clipping. Note the wrong angle of the clippers pointing into the gum.

(Fig.15-48b)

TEETH CLIPPING (Cont.)

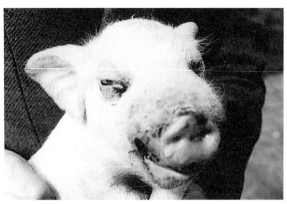

Infected gums due to faulty clipping of teeth.

(Fig.15-48c)

TEMPERATURE RECORDING FROM THE RECTUM

Reason

The temperature of the pig indicates that it is either normal, hypothermic, shocked, toxic or fevered.

Temperature °F	°C	Clinical state	Temperature °F	°C	Clinical state
99	37.2	Approaching death	101.5	38.6	Normal
99.5	37.5	Approaching death	102	38.9	Normal
100	37.7	Toxic or hypothermic	102.5	39.2	Normal
100.5	38	Toxic or hypothermic	103	39.4	Fevered
101	38.3	Toxic or hypothermic	103.5+	39.7+	Fevered
			109	42.8	Approaching death

Materials Required

Two clinical thermometers (one spare), mercury bulb type held in a metal casing.
Surgical spirit placed in the casing to sterilise the thermometer. Always use your own on-farm thermometer.
Wire noose (may be required occasionally).
Cotton wool.

Procedure

1	If the pig is in a stall make it stand, remove the tail gate if it interferes with the procedure.
2	If the pig is loose-housed it may be necessary to restrain it, or hold the tail and thermometer together.
3	Shake the mercury down the glass tube of the thermometer towards the bulb and examine to see it records below 36°C (97°F). Wipe clean with cotton wool.
4	Lift the tail of the pig place the thermometer 50mm in the rectum and angle gently into the lining or mucous membrane.
5	Record for 30 seconds, remove and read the temperature.

	UDDER - METHODS OF EXAMINATION
	Reason
	Changes in the udder can be divided into three broad areas, poor development, congestion or oedema and mastitis. It is important to differentiate these to determine cause and subsequent action.
	Procedure
1	Examine the sow lying down or standing. In outdoor herds this is best carried out when the sows are feeding and particularly when they are drying off post weaning.
2	Assess the visual appearance of the glands. Are any enlarged? - suggests mastitis or congestion. Is there evidence of trauma over the skin and teats? - suggests mastitis. Is the skin overlying the glands discoloured and red? - suggests mastitis and toxaemia or fever. Is there generalised discoloration of the skin? - suggests toxaemia or fever.
3	Palpate each gland separately.
4	To do this place the teat in the palm of the hand and firmly hold the gland with the fingers and thumb grasping it all.
5	Find a totally soft normal gland and apply pressure until the sow shows signs of discomfort.
6	Apply slightly less pressure to the remaining glands. Any reaction by the sow will indicate discomfort and pain and possibly early mastitis.
7	Press the thumb or first finger deep into the udder tissue, hold for two seconds and then feel for and look for an impression left in the tissue. This will indicate oedema.
8	If all glands are normal with no pain and poor udder development suspect agalactia possibly due to water shortage.

528 Managing Pig Health and the Treatment of Disease

UMBILICAL CORD APPLYING A CLAMP

Reason

Persistent haemorrhage from the umbilicus at birth occurs in certain herds at a high frequency and occasionally those using prostaglandins. Piglets die from anaemia. Clamps should be used on all hysterectomy derived piglets and on farms where piglets are confined immediately after birth if navels become damaged..

Materials Required

Plastic self fastening umbilical clips - those used for babies. Electricians nylon wire binders are also useful. Scissors or scalpel blade and handle. Use ones that can be reused.

Procedure

1	This is a two person operation ideally, but with practise one person can become proficient. Hold the piglet by the hind legs with the umbilicus facing the operator.
2	Place the clip across the cord approximately 6mm below the skin. Do not fasten too near the skin because this can damage the umbilicus and may cause umbilical ruptures. (Fig.15-49)

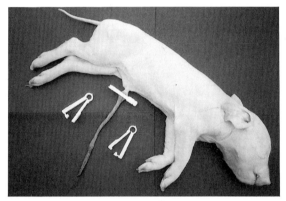

Umbilical clamp. Note the position on the cord.
(Fig.15-49)

3	Squeeze the clip to close it.
4	Cut the cord below the clip.
5	It may be necessary to place a piece of adhesive tape around the body to protect the clip. This is essential if hysterectomy derived piglets are being transported.

VASECTOMY

Reason

A vasectomy consists of cutting and removing a piece of the vas deferens (sometimes called the spermatic cord) to make the boar sterile but still capable of a normal but aspermic mating. This is a procedure that will only be carried out by the veterinarian but see also epidectomy.

Method

This involves a general anaesthetic although it is possible to perform the operation under sedation and local anaesthetic or epidural anaesthetic. It can be carried out at any time but is best from 50 to 100kg weight.

Materials Required

A surgical kit containing scissors, scalpel blade, artery forceps and suture materials.	A bale of straw or low table.
	A clean well lit pen.
Stresnil sedative and barbiturate anaesthetic.	Syringes 16mm ($^5/_8$") 23 gauge needles.
Warm water and antiseptic such as savlon.	Two people plus the veterinarian.
Cotton wool.	Penicillin cream and long-acting injection.

Procedure

1	Identify the boar by ear tag or tattoo. Starve him for 12 hours and sedate with stresnil 1ml/10kg. Wait for 20 minutes.
2	Restrain with a noose and inject anaesthetic using pentobarbitone into the ear vein. Anaesthetise until the eye reflex is just lost - and no more.
3	Place the boar on his back supported by the people at the head and the tail. The operator should not handle the pig but scrub up in preparation for the operation.
4	Wash and clean the area between the hind legs and over the testicles with warm water containing 1% savlon. Dry and finally soak in surgical spirit.
5	Identify the skin area above and just to the rear of the inguinal canal. Make a 50mm incision through the skin on one side.
6	Using the two fore fingers blunt dissect through the subcutaneous tissue until the complete cord and blood vessels are seen. It helps if the testicle is moved to highlight the structure. Pass a finger round the complete cord and pull upwards to the surface. Hold in position by passing forceps beneath.
7	Identify the vas deferens, a small white tube beneath the clear sac or the tunica.
8	Make a small incision into the tunica to expose the vas, raise it and clamp artery forceps to it approximately 40mm apart. Remove this portion.
9	Tie off each end of the vas and fold back and re-tie.
10	Return the vas into the sac and replace the complete cord.
11	Suture the skin with mattress sutures.
12	Repeat the operation on the other side.
13	Inject the boar with long-acting penicillin. Ideally tattoo the ear with a V or number for permanent identification.
14	Place the two removed pieces of the vas in liquid preservative for histological examination to confirm its structure. It can also be identified by squeezing fluid from the tubes onto a glass slide and examining each drop for the presence of sperm.
15	Do not use the boar for three weeks and then only after a semen sample has given clearance. Record the date of the operation and the boar number on the bottle containing the vas.

VULVAL HAEMATOMA - TREATING A HAEMATOMA

Reason

Vulval haematomas are common in gilts, occasionally in second-litter females and rarely in sows. If they rupture continual haemorrhage may be fatal (Fig.15-50).

Materials Required

A noose for restraint or sedative.
A 1 metre length of strong cord or bandage.
Warm water, cotton wool, and mild antiseptic.
Scissors, suture material or tape and needles.
Local anaesthetic syringe and 21 g 25mm (1") needles.
Tissue forceps, sterile artery forceps.

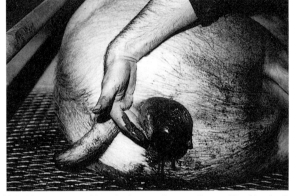

Vulval haematoma. Note the haemorrhage. gilts can bleed to death

(Fig.15-50)

Procedure

1	Sedate or restrain the sow.
2	Clean the vulva.
3	Infiltrate local anaesthetic into the skin anterior and to the front of the haematoma.
4	**Option 1** - Place the cord or bandage between the lips of the vulva, continue behind the haematoma and tie as a tourniquet. It may be necessary to keep tightening this. Observe for 2-3 minutes to see if the bleeding stops. **Option 2** - If haemorrhage continues place a mattress sutures behind the haematoma and tighten. **Option 3** - If haemorrhage continues open up the haematoma and identify the bleeding vessels. Clamp with the sterile artery forceps and tie off the bleeding points. Seek veterinary advice.
5	Place clean bedding behind the sow so that good observation can take place. If the sow is on slats use a paper bag.
6	Pad the back of the crate or alter it to prevent further trauma and crushing of the vulva.
7	Inject the sow with 10-15mls of penicillin.
8	Watch the sow every 15 minutes over two to three hours to ensure no further bleeding occurs.

WATER - CLEANING AND STERILISING A SYSTEM

Reason

Any water system with or without a header tank may become contaminated with bacteria, dirt, rodents or potential poisonous substances such as fungal or bacterial toxins or warfarin. Regular cleaning is essential and the frequency is dependent upon the degree of contamination.
Farrowing houses - clean and sterilise between batches.
Flat decks and nurseries - clean and sterilise between batches.
Water bowl and troughs - inspect and clean daily.

Materials Required

Sterilising detergent.
Spanner.
Pressure washer or piped source of water.

Procedure

1	Turn the water off or fasten the float up in the header tank.
2	Remove the last nipple drinker or bowl on the line. Periodically remove all nipples, clean and replace.
3	Drain out the system. Inspect and clean out the header tanks.
4	If water bowls are used open up, clean and wash out.
5	Open up the water supply and allow to flush through. Use a pressure washer if necessary.
6	Add a detergent steriliser or chlorine based dairy steriliser to the header tank and allow to flush through. Hold this water in the system for 30 minutes.
7	Drain the system, refill and check all nipples are flowing.
8	Periodic check list: Assess the number of pigs per drinker. Check the rate of water flow and: - The colour and quality. - The build-up of deposits in the pipes. - The pressure from the holding tank. When was the system last cleaned? - The covers over the holding tank. - The presence of vermin in the holding tank. - If there is a mastitis or scour problem carry out bacteriological examinations of the water in the pipes tanks and drinkers. Sterile containers and swabs can be used.

Chapter 15

Managing Pig Health and the Treatment of Disease

16 Welfare and Disease

Guidelines to good welfare practices 535
The 5 freedoms 535
Factors responsible for good welfare 536
Disease and welfare problems associated with indoor housing systems 539
    Sow stalls and confinement 539
    Cubicles or free access stalls 540
    Group sow housing 543
    Yards and individual feeders 544
The health and welfare of lactating sows and sucking piglets 546
The health and welfare of newly weaned sows indoors 546
The health and welfare of weaned and growing pigs 548
The health and welfare of sows outdoors 550

Chapter 16

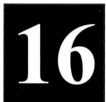

16 Welfare and Disease

Guidelines to Good Welfare Practices

This chapter discusses the important factors that are necessary to ensure good animal welfare on the farm. The guidelines are based upon the requirements of UK legislation and in many respects these give a lead to future developments across the world.

Many of the factors associated with good welfare on the farm are discussed at the beginning of the relevant chapters in this book and in particular the management and control procedures specific to particular diseases. The reader will be referred to these throughout.

Different countries have different attitudes towards standards of welfare and the points raised here should be considered in relation to the accepted standards and legal requirements in your country. Guidelines to pig welfare in the UK are found in The Codes of Recommendations for the Welfare of Livestock, Pigs, published by the Ministry of Agriculture Fisheries and Food, London. The statutory requirements are The Welfare of Livestock Regulations 1994.

The Welfare codes state:

The basic requirements for the welfare of pigs are a husbandry system appropriate to health and as far as practicable the behavioural needs of the animals and a high standard of stockmanship.

Stockmanship is a key factor because no matter how otherwise acceptable a system may be in principle, without competent and diligent stockmanship the welfare of animals cannot be adequately cared for.

The 5 Freedoms

Freedom from hunger and thirst
Ready access to fresh water and a balanced ration which maintains full health and vigour.

Freedom from discomfort
Provision of a suitable environment and a comfortable resting area.

Freedom from pain, injury and disease
Prevention where possible and prompt diagnosis and treatment when injuries or disease occur.

Freedom to express normal behaviour
Provision of sufficient and appropriate space, interest and the company of other pigs.

Freedom from fear and distress
Sympathetic stockmanship, constant environmental conditions and freedom from aggression by other pigs.

These represent the ideal which can rarely be achieved fully within the practical constraints of an efficient pig farm. Nevertheless they provide a comprehensive starting point from which to assess your own pig farm.

Freedom to express normal behaviour

This is the most difficult one to provide on intensive units. It is also the most controversial, beset by strong emotional and anthropomorphic opinions. It implies freedom of movement, so that all pigs should be able to turn round and carry out their normal bodily functions. This is a contentious issue with respect to the confinement of sows in stalls or tether systems. In the UK dry sow stalls (confinement) and tethers will be illegal from 1st January 1999. The other countries of the EU are partly following this lead by the Council Directive 91/630/EEC. This states that no new sow tethers or conversions to sow tethers should be constructed from the 31st December 1995 but those already in use can continue to be used until the year 2005. Council Directive 91/630/EEC is reviewed by the EU in 1997. Individual pig farmers in countries such as Denmark and the Netherlands, who sell pork products into the UK, are removing sow stalls and tethers so that their products will remain acceptable to UK supermarkets.

Changing from stalls and tethers to loose housing replaces one set of welfare problems with another, particularly in relation to individual sow feed rationing and aggression. Good pen or yard design is required combined with skilled stockmanship if freedom from fear, distress, pain and injury are to be achieved. Housing must be such that animals can stand and lie down without difficulty, have a clean place in which to rest and have visual contact with other pigs.

> ***Good welfare conditions result in less disease, better production and greater profits.***

Other aspects which are not spelt out by the 5 freedoms but which may be implied by them are:
- The provision of a caring and knowledgeable management team.
- The provision of light during the hours of daylight.
- The avoidance of unnecessary mutilation.
- The provision of emergency arrangements to cover disasters such as fire, the breakdown of mechanical services and the disruption of supplies.
- Humane slaughter.

Factors Responsible for Good Welfare

These are outlined so that they can be used as a checklist across your farm.

Quality of the management

As already stated this is crucial. People should be selected for their standard of stockmanship which includes a caring nature and ability to establish empathy with their pigs. (See chapter 3 Staff training). Leadership on the pig farm starts with the manager motivating his staff. He must ensure that all the disciplines required on the farm are achieved. Attention to detail and the monitoring of daily routines are vital.

Education and understanding

There should be an on going process of education as part of the management system. Young people entering the farm should be trained by more experienced stock people and in particular to recognise what is normal and abnormal. To do this requires a recognised training programme on the farm that is continually reinforced.

> **Poor welfare of the growing pig leads to inefficient growth and feed conversion.**

Observation

Each day a detailed examination of all the pigs on the farm should be carried out. Sick animals should be identified and procedures adopted to ensure that they are comfortable and not victims of aggression from other pigs. This may require movement to a hospital pen. Whilst this statement may seem simple, nevertheless it is most important. A typical example would be the failure to identify a tail bitten pig. The consequences of this are considerable, not only for the welfare of the pig but also because excessive tail damage invariably results in abscesses of the spine and a condemned carcase. The procedures for carrying out clinical observations on the farm have been documented in chapter 3. It is strongly recommended that these formats are used daily by each person responsible for a section or part of the farm and for the supervision of trainees.

The mixing of pigs

Whenever pigs are mixed there are varying degrees of fighting and trauma. This is a constant problem on most pig farms. The adverse effects on growth are often unrecognised but growth rates may be reduced by as much as a week, and welfare aspects must also be considered. The use of injectable sedatives such as stresnil and the use of industrial scent sprays at the time of mixing help to reduce fighting. Reducing the light intensity for 24 hours after mixing also helps.

A GUIDE TO STOCKING DENSITIES. SLATTED SYSTEMS

Weight of Pig		Area		Pig weight	
Kg	lbs	sq.m	sq.ft	Kg/sq.m	lbs/sq.ft
5	11	0.09	1	55	11
10	22	0.15	1.5	66	15
20	44	0.2	2.5	100	17
30	66	0.3	3.0	100	22
40	88	0.34	3.6	115	24
50	110	0.4	4.3	125	25
60	132	0.45	5.0	133	26
70	154	0.5	5.6	140	27
80	176	0.55	6.0	145	29
90	198	0.6	6.6	150	30
100	220	0.65	7.0	153	30
200(sow)	441	2.8	30	74	15
Boar mating pen		9.3	100		
Boar housing only		7.5	80		
Sow loose-housed		2.8	30		
Sow confined		1.5	16		
Gilt housing during oestrus		2.8	30		
Farrowing crate		4.6	50		

As a guide 0.1sq.m / 10kg liveweight or 1sq.ft / 10kg liveweight
For straw based grower systems add 30%

(Fig.16-1)

SLAT AND GAP SIZES FOR PERFORATED / SLATTED FLOORS

Weight of Pig kg	Width of Slat (concrete) mm	Width of gap mm
5	Not suitable	10
50	75	18
140	100	25
200	115	30

(Fig.16-2)

TROUGH LENGTHS, LIVEWEIGHT AND FEEDING METHODS

Weight of Pig kg	Trough Length Per Pig	
	Restricted feeding mm	Ad lib feeding mm
5	100	33(at weaning)
10	130	33
20	175	38
40	200	50
60	240	60
90	280	70
120	300	75

Single space feeder (350mm wide) 1 per 10 pigs

(Fig.16-3)

WATER REQUIREMENTS

Guidelines For the Use of Nipple Drinkers		Water Consumption		
Weight of Pig (kg)	Height from Floor to Drinker (mm)	Age (Weeks)	Weight (kg)	Litres Per Day
5 - 10	100 - 250	8	20	1
10 - 30	300 - 400	9	25	2.5
30 - 50	400 - 600	10	28	3.3
50 - 100	600 - 750	12	39	4.2
100 +	750 - 900	14	50	5
	750 - 900	17	70	7
	750 - 900	21	90	8.9

(Fig.16-4)

Stocking densities

It is important to work within recognised and accepted standards for various ages and weights of pigs. This is to ensure optimum growth rates, good welfare and a low level of disease and mortality. The total square feet or metres of accommodation required for growing and finishing pigs needs to be determined from the mating programme, farrowing rates, litter sizes and pigs weaned. This is needed to ensure adequate capacity to maximise production. Fig.16-1 gives stocking density levels that would provide acceptable welfare conditions.

Floor and wall surfaces

The floors should be free from projections, well maintained, easily cleaned and if solid with good drainage towards the exterior of the pen. Slats should be well maintained and of a suitable size for the age of the pig to prevent trauma and disease. (Fig.16-2). Where bedding is used there should be provision for dry lying areas. All solid floors should be well insulated.

The walls and partitions should be constructed and maintained so that there are no sharp edges or protrusions likely to cause injury or distress. All surfaces should be capable of being cleaned and disinfected.

Automatic equipment

This should be thoroughly inspected on a daily basis. Where breakdowns occur provision should be made to ensure that the welfare of the pigs is not compromised.

Food and water

Food should be presented in a manner that allows all pigs to eat without distress or fear. Feed hoppers or dispensers should be examined daily for failure of supply. This is to ensure any automatic delivery systems are functional and are working efficiently. Pigs should be fed at least once a day. If fed only once a day all the pigs in a group should have access to food at the same time. Guidelines for trough space are given in Fig.16-3, and water flow rates and drinker ratios in Fig.16-4 though to Fig.16-6.

All pigs should have an adequate supply of fresh clean water daily. There must be a sufficient number of accessible drinkers per pen for every pig to drink readily, including the underprivileged pigs at the bottom of the pecking order. Every drinker should be checked daily to ensure adequate flow rate. All header tanks should have a lid to prevent contamination by debris, dust and vermin. This also helps to prevent pipework blockages. If necessary pipes should be insulated to prevent freezing. An inadequate flow rate from partially blocked drinkers is one of the commonest management faults found in commercial piggeries. As well as being a welfare issue water shortage leads to poor productivity and predisposes to disease. This is particularly serious when single nipple drinkers with poor flow rates are incorporated into farrowing pens. This results in low milk yield, loss of appetite and sow condition and poor piglet growth. It is a wise precaution to have a single tap system on the water line over the sow's trough which can be turned on twice a day to let the sow have a good drink. The trough must of course be watertight to prevent wet floors, a common predisposition to mastitis and piglet diarrhoea. A single space hopper with an integral nipple drinker should not be the only source of water to a pen of growing pigs.

GUIDELINES FOR WATER FLOW FROM NIPPLE DRINKERS	
Pigs / Weight (kg)	Litres / minute
Piglet	0.3
Weaner 7 - 25 kg	1.0
Grower 25 - 50kg	1.4
Finisher 50 - 110kg	1.7
Dry Sow	2.0
Lactating Sow	2.0

(Fig.16-5)

DRINKER TO PIG RATIOS *	
Type	Ratio
Nipple	1 : 15 to 1 : 10 Weaner to finisher
Bite	1 : 15 to 1 : 10 Weaner to finisher
Bowl	1: 17 finishers
Trough	300mm per 20 finishers 300mm per 15 sows

* UK welfare guidelines

(Fig.16-6)

Management and housing systems

Housing systems for pigs from birth to weaning and for lactating and weaned sows should be used on an all-in all-out basis, keeping pigs of similar age within a common environment. There should be provision for the cleaning and disinfection of each section between each batch of pigs. This is a major component in disease control and hence good welfare. The adoption of this principle on a number of breeding finishing farms has, together with other management methods resulted in significant improvements in feed efficiency (up to 0.4) and improved daily liveweight gains (up to 120g). Segregating one age group of pigs from another is now the

ENVIRONMENTAL TEMPERATURES COMFORT ZONES (Lean Genotype)		
Weight (kg)	Range	
	°C	°F
Piglet 1 - 7	31 - 28	88 - 82
Weaner 7- 10	30 - 25	86 - 77
Weaner 10 - 20	25 - 22	77 - 71
Grower 20 - 50	22 - 21	71 - 70
Finisher 50 - 95	21 - 18	70 - 64
Weaned sow	22	71
Dry sow	20	68
Lactating sow	22 - 19	71 - 66

(Fig.16-7)

> *The importance of feed and water in disease is grossly underrated and experiences over the years in the investigation and control of disease outbreaks constantly reinforces this. Access, availability and quality are the three important components.*

most important aspect of disease control. These procedures and principles are discussed in detail in chapter 3.

The environment

Temperature

Pigs should be maintained within their thermo-neutral zones at their comfort level. Guidelines for different ages of pigs are given in Fig.16-7

Even with these guidelines the pigs may not be comfortable. You can assess this by their lying patterns either huddled together or separated. Past experiences have shown that the failure to maintain a stable comfortable temperature is one of the most important trigger factors to the development of disease. This is particularly so in post-weaning diarrhoea and respiratory disease. (See chapter 9).

Humidity

Relative humidity should be maintained between 60 and 80%.

Ventilation

This should be maintained at a controlled level so the pigs remain within their thermo-neutral zone and to ensure toxic gases are adequately removed. However, a light draught e.g. an increase in air movement from 0.15m/sec to 0.5m/sec can lift the lower critical temperature (LCT) by 4°C (7°F) or more. Mechanically ventilated systems must have an alarm to identify when a failure occurs and have provision for alternative means of ventilation under these circumstances. Alarm systems should be tested at least every seven days, and a backup system should be available when electricity supplies fail. Losses of 500-800 pigs have been experienced where such systems fail.

Light

Pigs should not be kept in darkness but have sufficient light to satisfy their behavioural and physiological needs. The period of light should be at least that of natural light. Sufficient light should also be available to allow adequate daily inspections. Adequate light has an important role in maximising reproductive efficiency as discussed in chapter 5.

Hospital pens

There must be adequate provision to cope with the number of sick pigs that have to be moved from their normal environment during periods of illness and treatment. Aspects of this are discussed in detail in chapter 3 "The management and treatment of the sick pig".

Any ill pig that cannot fend for itself must be moved immediately to a hospital pen e.g. tail bitten, severely lame, acutely ill etc.

The failure to provide adequate well managed hospital pens is a cause of serious economic loss on many farms. The experiences on one large farm are worthy of consideration. No ill pig was ever treated in its pen but moved to one of a series of small hospital pens. The owner often remarked that many of the pigs reached slaughter weight before their contemporaries - a rather sobering thought.

Vice (Abnormal behaviour)

All efforts should be made to ensure the environment satisfies the pig's physiological and behavioural needs. This is particularly important in the prevention of tail biting and other behavioural disorders. Vice is the traditional term used by stockpeople, but it is now discouraged by welfare and behaviour authorities who use the term abnormal behaviour. (See chapter 9).

Electrical installations

These must not be accessible to pigs and should be correctly earthed with trip out switches. They should be protected against damage and contamination by water during cleaning and disinfection.

Mutilations

Mutilations include nose-ringing of sows kept outdoors, tattooing, ear tagging or notching, tail docking, tooth clipping, castration and boar tusk removal. It is accepted that some of these procedures are necessary in some intensive environments to avoid behavioural problems but you should consider carefully whether it is necessary in your pig farm to carry out each of these. For example, modern genetically-improved pigs now reach slaughter weight before they are sexually mature so that castration is less important to reduce boar taint. Castration has virtually ceased in the UK and other countries may follow. The procedures that you deem necessary on your pig farm should be carried out by well-trained operators, at the correct age, and in a manner that minimises pain and distress to the animal. Clipping the eye teeth and tail docking should be carried out within seven days of birth, preferably under three days. Castration

TYPES OF HOUSING SYSTEM
Dry Sow Housing
Tethers
Stalls (confinement)
Free access stalls
Cubicles
Straw yards
Slatted / concrete yards
Yards and individual feeders
Paddocks and huts (outdoor)

(Fig.16-8)

should also be carried out under three weeks of age, preferably under one week. All equipment should be well maintained and kept clean and disinfected. Older pigs should not be castrated or tail docked without a local anaesthetic and where necessary by a veterinarian.

Disease and Welfare Problems Associated with Indoor Housing Systems

There are many different types of housing available for dry sows, lactating sows and weaning, growing and finishing pigs. Fig.16-8 shows the different types of sow housing and Fig.16-9 the feeding systems, both manual and mechanical that are in use.

The following is a résumé of these different systems to illustrate the welfare and disease problems that may arise. It is not however intended to provide details of housing designs but only sufficient information to highlight the interactions between the structure, management, welfare and disease. Please refer to publications on pig housing for precise details. (See appendix).

Sow Stalls and Confinement

Design requirements

Size - Width 0.5-0.68m. The smaller width of stall is used for gilts to prevent them turning around and defecating in the trough at the front. If this occurs enteric diseases then become a risk particularly porcine enteropathy and salmonella.

Length - 2.28m. If the rear part of the stall is slatted, gilts housed in long stalls will tend to defecate on the solid concrete area leading to sore legs and other leg problems.

A short stall side 1.2m long is used for tethers, the width the same as the stall.

Rear gate - Ideally this should be made of vertical bars so that faeces and urine can spill away from the back of the slats. Care is required however to make sure that the bars do not cause pressure sores. Where solid rear gates are used their bottom edges should be raised 80mm above the slats so that faeces cannot build up, contaminate the vulva and lead to vaginitis and endometritis (but not too high to cause pressure sores). The height of the rear gate should be sufficient to prevent the sow from sitting on top of it. Out breaks of rectal prolapse and abortion have been associated with this.

Floors - These may be totally slatted, part slatted or totally solid. Totally slatted floors are not recommended. They are uncomfortable for the sow and create difficulties when the sow stands, increasing the incidence of leg weakness. On part-slatted floors the solid area should be approximately 1m at the front and the remainder slatted. The slats should be 80-100mm wide and with a gap of 10-25mm and run parallel to the sow to provide a better less traumatic surface for the feet. If sows are housed on solid floors there should be a 1:20 fall in the last 300mm of the floor. This allows drainage of urine and easy removal of faeces. If the whole length of the floor slopes to the back it may predispose to vaginal prolapse and in gilts and second litter females a predisposition to osteochondrosis or leg weakness. All the accessible concrete edges should be round and not sharp and the surfaces of the slats flat and not sloping to the gaps.

Bedding - If bedding is used the faeces and urine soiled material must be removed from behind the sow daily.

Water - Fresh water should be made available to the sow in a trough at the front after each feed. If this is supplied manually, it may be necessary to provide extra in hot weather. A drinker may also be provided but it can leak producing wet floors that result in skin sores. A shortage of water will predispose to cystitis pyelonephritis and increased sow mortality.

Feeding - Sows may be fed once or twice daily, preferably once a day to prevent agitation and anticipation in sows awaiting their second feed. From a welfare point of view automatic dispensers held in front of each sow are best so that all animals can be fed at the same time. This will reduce the risk of torsion of the intestines, trauma due to excitation and stress associated reproductive failure.

Group size - There are no constraints on the numbers of animals held in any one building.

Temperature requirements - 18-20°C (64-68°F).

Management, welfare and disease (Fig.16-10)

If you keep a sow in a stall or tether she is totally confined and has no control over her environment. It is therefore important the stall is long enough, (some modern-day prolific sows grow too long for standard stalls), the floor is comfortable to lie on, she has sufficient feed to satisfy her appetite, the environmental temperature remains constant day and night and there are no draughts. You can tell whether you are achieving these if you quietly open the door to the dry-sow house when no pig persons have been present for a period. Over 95% of the sows should be lying down on their sides.

The majority of sows lie down most of the time and will only rise to drink, urinate, and defecate at feeding time. This leads to problems such as cystitis and

TYPES OF FEEDING SYSTEM
Dry Sow Feeding Systems
Individual / mechanical
Trickle feeding
Manual into a trough or onto the floor
Dump or drop feeders - floor feeding
Spin feeders onto the floor
Ad lib feeding
Electronic sow feeders (ESF)
Wet Feeding

(Fig.16-9)

pyelonephritis. If they are only fed one main meal a day, the ration should contain sufficient fibre to satisfy appetite and keep the faeces soft. It is advisable to stimulate all sows to rise at least once a day by walking the boar round or sprinkling small quantities of feed into the water in the troughs.

All animals should be examined daily in a standing position to detect any signs of lameness or leg weakness. Additionally feet, legs, shoulders and hips should be examined for any sores, swellings or granulomas. At least twice a week neck or girth tethers should be checked and adjusted as necessary. Every two to three weeks an assessment of body condition and body score should be carried out. The skin should be examined for evidence of lice or mange. A frequent examination should be carried out of the slats, to check that they are not worn and causing trauma to feet and legs. All metal work and rear gates should be examined regularly to check there are no parts likely to cause trauma. A maximum and minimum thermometer should be checked daily to ensure that the sows are being maintained within their comfort zone. A minimum of 14 hours of light should be available to maintain a constant photo period and reduce the predisposition to abortion. If sows are weaned into stalls or tethers, both feed and water should be available at all times and the floor must be kept very clean and well drained. If straw is used keep surfaces well bedded to prevent udder contamination and the development of mastitis. A combination of the above factors can often be responsible for embryo reabsorption, abortion and heavy culling rates, resulting in persistent low farrowing rates.

Arguments for and against confinement

Sow stalls and tethers provide 4 of the 5 freedoms. They also allow individual sow examination, controlled feeding, and handling (e.g. treatment). The criticism levelled against them is that they deny the freedom to express normal behaviour and can lead to abnormal stereotypic behaviour such as bar biting. Thin sows can develop "bed-sores", leg bones can become softer and more readily broken than those of loose-housed sows and being less fit they farrow more slowly. In addition, tethers can result in neck or girth sores if not regularly checked and adjusted. They can however serve a welfare-friendly purpose if used for short periods e.g. to hold aggressive sows at weaning and during oestrus or to hold a sow for treatment for a short period.

Cubicles or Free Access Stalls

Design requirements

Size - Width of stall 0.68 m. Length 2.28m to the front of the trough. The sow lies in its own stall but it has free access behind to a defecating passage and it can move around. Some designs have self opening and closing tail gates and are often referred to as free access stalls.

The width of the dunging passage will be determined by the width of each cubicle and whether they are in groups of three or four. In a group of four the passage widths would be approximately 2.74m.

DISEASE PROBLEMS IN STALLS AND TETHERS ASSOCIATED WITH WELFARE FAILURES
Condition/Problem and Welfare Failures

Abortion
  Badly maintained concrete. Pools of urine
  Decreasing daylight length
  High air flow
  Lack of boar contact
  Lameness
  Low feed levels
  Low intensity of light
  Low variable temperatures
  Poor hygiene
  Stressful environment

Abscess
  Arthritis
  Bad slats
  Bursitis / trauma
  Bush foot / trauma
  Environmental trauma
  Faulty vaccination
  Poor concrete
  Stalls too small

Arthritis
  Leg weakness (OCD)
  Slippery floors
  Stalls to small
  Trauma
  Worn slats

Bursitis
  Poor concrete surfaces
  Trauma

Cystitis pyelonephritis
  Frozen pipes.
  Infrequent urination.
  Lameness.
  Once a day feeding.
  Poor access to water.
  Water shortage.

Hygroma
  Poor concrete surfaces
  Pressure sores
  Trauma   (Cont.)

DISEASE PROBLEMS IN STALLS AND TETHERS ASSOCIATED WITH WELFARE FAILURES (Cont.)
Condition/Problem and Welfare Failures

Inability to express natural behaviour

   Total individual confinement

Leg weakness (OCD) Lameness

   See arthritis
   Bush foot
   New concrete or slats
   Poor muscle tone
   Poor selection of gilts
   Poor slippery floor surfaces
   Thin weak bones from lack of exercise
   Worn slats
   Young animals

Mastitis

   Bad drainage
   Poor hygiene
   Solid gates in stalls
   Trauma
   Udder contamination

Neck and girth sores

   Old worn-out or dirty tethers
   Poor management
   Tethers too tight, poor design

Overgrown distorted claws

   Lack of exercise
   Leg weakness factors
   Slats wrong way, gaps too wide
   Smooth surfaces

Prolapse rectum or vagina

   Badly designed tail gates
   Short standing area and a deep step
   Slippery floors
   Sloping floors

Shoulder sores

   Poor concrete surfaces
   Slippery floor surfaces
   Thin animals

Slow farrowing

   Lack of muscle tone
   Old sows

Stereotypic behaviour

   Boredom

Thin sow syndrome

   Bullying
   Disease (Cont.)

DISEASE PROBLEMS IN STALLS AND TETHERS ASSOCIATED WITH WELFARE FAILURES (Cont.)
Condition/Problem and Welfare Failures

   Draughts
   Low feed intake
   Mange
   Parasite burdens
   Poor environments (cold)
   Poor nutrition

Vulval discharge

   Build up of faeces behind the sow at the bottom of the tail gate
   Dirty weaning pens
   Dirty wet boar pens

(Fig.16-10)

Floors - These should consist of solid concrete well insulated lying areas and not too smooth defecating areas. This type of housing is not conducive to totally slatted systems.

The cubicle divisions may be barred or solid, preferably the former. Slats may be used in the dunging area but there could be a higher incidence of lameness.

Bedding - A minimum amount can be used or the lying areas can be deep bedded. The manure in the solid dunging area should be removed three times per week. This area should also be well drained.

Water - This must only be provided in the dunging area either by a nipple drinker, bowl or trough. If water is placed in the feeding troughs sows tend to defecate and urinate in the lying areas resulting in lameness, sores on the feet and legs and a predisposition to leg weakness.

Feeding - Feed is put into the trough once daily. Feed levels required may be higher than in stalls to satisfy the sow's environmental requirements.

Group size - These are usually three or four sows but can be up to ten in free access stalls depending on the size of herd. Sows of similar size should be grouped together.

Temperature requirements - Because of the low stocking density and mating system well insulted buildings are advised. In temperate climates such housing is best ventilated naturally. In very cold climates heating will be required.

Management, welfare and disease (Fig.16-11)

The total lying and defecating area per sow ranges from 2.23 to 2.29m^2. In such confined spaces however sows should not be mixed together for the first time but rather in large open pens for 24 hours, because severe trauma fractures and lameness may result from fighting. The lying areas should be raised above the defecating passage but not by a kerb, since this increases the incidence of foot and leg damage and mastitis. Furthermore, with a kerb faeces and urine tend to be retained in the lying bed. If the cubicles are covered, observation and management become difficult. If free access stalls close automatically behind the sow there is no need to confine them during feeding, however with the cubicles it may be advisable to close the gate at feeding time to prevent aggression and bullying. Sows should be fed and examined from a central feed passage..

Arguments for and against cubicles and stalls

From a welfare viewpoint cubicles would appear to be an improvement on stalls since they retain many of the advantages of stalls but have the added benefits of freedom to express some degree of natural behaviour and the exercise results in stronger bones and better muscle tone. Unfortunately, part of the natural behaviour of sows is aggression to establish a pecking order and this is particularly marked in a confined space. Not only can they damage each other physically and cause fear and distress, thus denying 2 of the 5 freedoms, but also because the aggression occurs in the early weeks of pregnancy it can cause pregnancy failure and raise the rate of regular and irregular returns to oestrus. The sows that return can be mated again but at some point they then have to be mixed into another group. If this is done in the first six weeks of pregnancy aggression may result in more returns and so on. It is best to move sows to this type of accommodation in the second half of pregnancy when pregnancy is more secure and sows are more docile but this is often not possible. Generally however well managed cubicles can provide very successful and welfare friendly housing.

DISEASE PROBLEMS IN CUBICLES AND FREE ACCESS STALLS ASSOCIATED WITH WELFARE PROBLEMS
Condition/Problem and Welfare Failures

Abortion
Decreasing daylight length
High air flow.
Lack of boar contact
Lameness
Low feed levels
Low intensity of light
Low temperatures
Low stocking density
Poor building insulation
Stress
Trauma

Abscess
Arthritis
Bad slats
Bullying
Bursitis from trauma (Cont.)

DISEASE PROBLEMS IN CUBICLES AND FREE ACCESS STALLS ASSOCIATED WITH WELFARE PROBLEMS (Cont.)
Condition/Problem and Welfare Failures

Bush foot from trauma
Environmental trauma
Faulty vaccination
Fighting
Poor concrete

Aggression
A feature of cubicle houses
Establishment of pecking order
Uneven group mixing of sows

Arthritis
Bullying
Bush foot - poor concrete
Fighting
No bedding
Leg weakness (OCD)

Bursitis
Fighting
Bullying
Trauma

Bush foot
Bad slats
Concrete kerbs
Poor concrete surfaces
Trauma

Cystitis pyelonephritis
Frozen pipes
Leg weakness
Poor access to water
Slippery concrete surfaces
Sows reluctant to drink
Water shortage

Erysipelas
Straw systems
Wet feeding
Wet pens

Fear and distress
From bullying
Mixing sows

Haematoma
Vulval biting

Hygroma
Pressure sores
Trauma (Cont.)

DISEASE PROBLEMS IN CUBICLES AND FREE ACCESS STALLS ASSOCIATED WITH WELFARE PROBLEMS (Cont.)
Condition/Problem and Welfare Failures

Infertility
  High return rate and "not in pig" from aggression

Leg weakness (OCD)
  Poor slippery floor surfaces
  Water available at the front
  Wet dunging areas
  Wet lying areas
  Young animals

Mastitis
  No bedding
  Poor concrete
  Poor hygiene
  Trauma
  Wet pens

Parasites
  Continuous access to faeces.
  Inability to remove faeces adequately

Prolapse rectum or vagina
  Badly designed tail gates
  Slippery floors

Shoulder sores
  Poor concrete surfaces
  Thin animals
  Trauma as animals rise

Thin sow syndrome
  Disease
  Draughts
  Low feed intake
  Low house temperatures
  Parasite burdens
  Poor environments
  Poor nutrition

Vulval biting
  Occurs towards the latter end of pregnancy

Vulval discharge
  Dirty weaning pens
  Dirty wet boar pens
  Wet defecating areas

(Fig.16-11)

Group Sow Housing

Design requirements

Pens - Allow $2.7-2.8m^2$ per sow for lying and defecating. Do not house groups of sows in long narrow pens. These will increase the incidence of vulva biting.

Yards - Allow $3.4m^2$ per sow. At the recommended stocking density there is a marked reduction in fighting episodes when sows are mixed.

Floors and bedding - Solid concrete floors bedded with straw or other suitable materials are best. Totally slatted floors are not recommended due to the high levels of lameness, arthritis and the foot problems that occur. Solid floors can be bedded with a minimum amount of straw but in all cases the floors should be well insulated. If minimum amounts of straw are to be used the floors should be laid on a 1:20 slope so that the straw bedding is walked "towards the defecating area". Solid defecating areas should be well drained and the manure removed three times weekly.

Water - This should be provided ideally by a self levelling small trough or one bite drinker per 15 sows.

Feeding - This can be provided by feeders suspended above the lying area and the feed dropped to the floor (dump feeders) or alternatively a single feeder that spins the feed out across the lying area. Wet feeding systems are also being used successfully feeding the sows from troughs placed down the sides of large straw yards or along the front of the pens. Electronic sow feeder systems (ESF) are common. Here the sow is individually fed a maximum daily amount when it enters the feeder station in response to a transponder placed in the ear or around the neck. One feeder station will accommodate 20 to 30 sows. Trickle feeder systems have been developed whereby the feed is dispersed in small amounts at a time, sufficient to keep the sow feeding continuously. The troughs are divided by short divisions to separate each animal during feeding. They are suitable for groups of up to 12 sows.

Group size - This should ideally be no more than 30 sows per pen, unless electronic sow feeders are used when the size may be increased. Some farmers keep up to 150 sows in a dynamic group but this is not recommended because with an increasing number of sows there is a tendency for more welfare problems to occur. In spite of this the recently introduced Danish Dynamic Mating System, which has group sizes of up to 80, works very well if the stockmanship is good. Small numbers of sows are introduced into the group weekly when they are on heat and are less aggressive and they are naturally mated by the boar.

Temperature requirement - This depends on the amount of bedding and floor insulation and ranges from 16 to 20°C (61 to 68°F).

Management, welfare and disease (Fig.16-12 and Fig.16-13)

Welfare problems and disease arise due to the aggressive nature of sows in group housed systems. Furthermore this aggression creates problems of varied feed intake and predisposes the individual under-nourished sow to disease.

The ideal management system should allow newly weaned sows to mix in a large pen together with a boar for the first four days. He should be then removed and the sows held in stalls for a period of 48 hours over the mating period after which they are returned to the group. The boar is introduced again for the next 21 days. Sows should be maintained in the same group throughout the whole of pregnancy. Alternatively, the sows can be weaned into stalls mated in boar pens and kept in stalls or cubicles for the first half of pregnancy before being group-housed. If pregnant animals are mixed together between 2-21 days post-service there is a risk of higher embryo mortality and more variable litter size. Wet feeding ESF and trickle feeding systems give a more even feed intake compared to group feeding systems. If aggression is a problem, particularly when sows are mixed, a series of soft rubber mats (1.2m x 1.2m) suspended vertically, 500mm above the floor, over the lying area in large pens provides a means of separating one sow from another when a fighting episode commences.

Sows fed in electronic feeders have the advantage of individual feeding but aggressive behavioural patterns can develop, particularly when they are waiting to enter the feeders. This can cause considerable stress particularly to animals that have just joined a large group. Severe bullying with trauma and skin damage can take place and poor hygienic conditions and wet areas often develop around the feeder stations.

ESF systems require careful design and skilled experienced stockmanship. It is best to use feeders with a separate front or side exit door so that sows do not back out and be confronted by sows which are eager to feed. Some sows tend to lie in the feeder thus blocking others. If the design of the layout is not well thought out and the stockperson not properly trained there may be an unacceptably high level of vulva biting and badly scratched and bruised skin.

If you decide to construct an ESF system you should first visit and study successful established ones and get competent training in ESF management. Training gilts to ESF systems is necessary.

If possible the stockperson working the system should be involved in the selecting of the equipment and the design of the yards. He should be enthusiastic, committed to making the system work and should understand the computer technology. He should be competent to undertake every day maintenance. In areas of frequent power failure, a standby generator will be necessary.

Yards and Individual Feeders

Design requirements

The yards may be of variable size housing from six sows to large groups. They resemble a cubicle system in that sows are fed in individual stalls.

Size - The lying area $1.4m^2$. Defecating area $0.93m^2$. Total $2.33m^2$ per sow..

Floors - The lying area is insulated concrete with minimum bedding or deeply bedded with straw. Slats in the defecating area are not common and tend to result in high levels of lameness.

DISEASE PROBLEMS IN GROUP HOUSING ASSOCIATED WITH WELFARE FAILURES
Condition/Problem and Welfare Failures

Abortion
- Inadequate access to food
- Lack of bedding
- Lack of boar contact
- Low feed
- Low temperatures
- Poor body condition
- Reduced daylight length
- Stress
- Wet bedding

Abscess
- Fighting
- Trauma

Aggression
- Adding new sows
- High stocking density
- Mixing

Anaemia
- Gastric ulceration
- Haemorrhage - vulva
- Trauma

Arthritis
- Environmental trauma
- Damage at oestrus
- Leg weakness (OCD)

Bursitis
- Shortage of bedding
- Trauma

Bush foot
- Trauma due to poor concrete surfaces

Erysipelas
- Dirty bedding (Cont.)

Water - Provide a trough drinker or nipple drinker placed in the dunging area.
Feeding - Feeder stalls should be 0.6m wide and 2m long.
Temperature requirements - Temperatures are well maintained usually because the lying areas consist of small pens with solid sides and a well insulated roof.

Management, welfare and disease

Due to the individual feeding many of the problems associated with group housing are avoided. There are still problems from mixing, particularly at weaning, but bullied animals should be able to escape into stalls.

It is important to ensure that a minimum of 14 hours of light are available in the lying areas.

DISEASE PROBLEMS IN GROUP HOUSING ASSOCIATED WITH WELFARE FAILURES (Cont.)
Condition/Problem and Welfare Failures

Ease of spread from clinically ill animals
Stress

Foot rot
 Dirty wet bedding
 Poor management

Fractures
 Leg weakness
 Slippery floors
 Trauma

Haematoma
 Fighting

Hygroma
 Trauma

Infertility
 Stress induced embryo losses

Leg weakness (OCD)
 Poor floor surfaces
 Trauma

Mastitis
 Permanently bedded yards
 Poor hygiene

Internal parasites
 Access to faeces
 Wet dirty areas

Prolapse rectum or vagina
 Abdominal pressure
 Nutrition

Thin sow syndrome
 Bullying
 External and internal parasites
 Poor environment
 Variable feed intake

Vulva biting
 Feeding methods
 Pen design
 Stocking density

(Fig.16-12)

PROBLEMS IN ELECTRONIC FEEDER SYSTEMS ASSOCIATED WITH WELFARE FAILURES
Condition/Problem and Welfare Failures

Aggression
 Adding sows to an established group
 Group systems
 Shape of yard

Infertility
 Stress after feeding
 Stress at feeding

Loss of sow identification
 Lost transponder tags / collars
 Thin sow
 Education - understanding
 Poor design and maintenance

Skin abrasions
 Aggression

Stress at mixing
 Badly designed ESF system

Variable litter size
 Embryo reabsorption / stress

Vulva biting
 Feeder design
 Poor pen/yard design
 Queuing for feed

(Fig.16-13)

The Health and Welfare of Lactating Sows and Sucking Piglets.

Design requirements

The majority of sows in indoor units are farrowed in crates, although a few are loose-housed in pens, usually with wall bars, rounded corners and other structures to reduce piglet crushing. Outdoor sows are farrowed in arcs.

The farrowing pen - There are a wide variety of designs but they should be approximately 2.4m in length. In some designs the pen width is only 1.68m in which case the pen has to be longer with a forward creep. The creep lying area should be about $0.6m^2$ and be either in front of or beside the head of the sow.

The crate should be a minimum length of 2.3m preferably with a moveable rear bar or gate for shorter gilts. The width between the bottom bars of the crate should be 730mm to allow for ease of suckling and at a height 230mm from the floor.

Modifications in design are largely aimed at preventing the sow crushing the piglets as she stands up and lies down or moves suddenly. They include angled projections on the bottom bars, or bottom bars which move in when the sow stands' and move slowly out when she lies down again. Cold air fans which automatically blow across the floor when she stands can be used to encourage the piglets to retreat to their warm creep.

Tail gate - This should be designed to prevent trauma to the vulva (parallel retaining bars at right angles to the crate are likely to cause this) and yet allow the sow room to farrow. A good design consists of two "D" shaped bars that project into the crate and hold the sow from the tail gate itself.

Floor - This may be either totally perforated using metal or plastic slats or part solid, the front half of the crate floor being insulated concrete. Alternatively the complete floor may be insulated concrete. The floor may be raised slightly to provide good drainage if slats are used with bedding. Make sure that the area where the front feet make contact with the floor is not slippery otherwise the sow has great difficulty standing (causing trauma to the piglets) and this increases levels of leg weakness and shoulder sores.

Water - This is best provided through a mono-flow nipple drinker delivering a minimum of 2 litres per minute, that projects into a trough either at head height or at floor level, with an over-flow to drain away surplus water. Alternatively bite drinkers can be used. Some crates also have a tap to fill the trough after feeding, an excellent procedure. Welfare codes recommend that all pigs should have access to clean water at all times. Sucking piglets drink little water during the first two weeks, but to comply with the codes a small drinker should be attached to the crate or pen wall for the piglets. Water should be made available in small dishes for the first 48 hours after farrowing.

Feed - This is fed in the trough to appetite throughout lactation.

Group size - The numbers of farrowing pens in any one house or section should be restricted to the numbers of sows that farrow in any one week up to a maximum of twelve.

Bedding - This should be available in the creep area for the first 10 - 14 days after farrowing.

Temperature - Creep area - This should be capable of being maintained at between 20 - 34°C (68 - 93°F). The farrowing house should be maintained at 22°C (72°F) during farrowing and between 20 - 21°C (68 - 70°F) during lactation although some houses are operated much lower.

Management, welfare and disease (Fig.16-14)

The welfare and management requirements in the farrowing house are many both during farrowing and throughout the sucking period. You are referred to chapter 7 for further details. There is pressure from elements of the welfare lobby for farrowing crates to be banned because they deny sows freedom to express natural behaviours (i.e. to make a nest, hide away, and move freely). This pressure should be resisted strongly by the industry. In the farrowing house the sow is not the only concern. The welfare of the piglets and of the stockpeople must also be considered for the following reasons:

- Trials carried out on free choice farrowing accommodation in the UK resulted in piglet mortality levels of 25-50%, which is totally unacceptable considering mortality in crates should be less than 8%.
- The attendants are at risk from protective sows some of which can be highly dangerous at or just after farrowing.
- It is difficult to examine and treat the piglets with iron injections or anti scour remedies etc. and the sows for mastitis or metritis.

The Health and Welfare of Newly Weaned Sows indoors

Design requirements

These need to satisfy the change in ambient temperature, feeding patterns and psychological and physiological stress that are associated with the process of weaning. The following methods of housing can be adopted:

- House sows individually in sow stalls or tethers from weaning.
- House sows in groups of two or three in spacious pens.
- Mix all sows into one group at weaning.
- Group sows from the day of weaning together with a boar and then remove to confinement during the mating period. Sows are then regrouped with the boar within 48 hours after mating.
- Use a dynamic group system.

DISEASE PROBLEMS IN FARROWING AND LACTATING SOWS AND SUCKING PIGS ASSOCIATED WITH WELFARE FAILURES
Condition/Problem and Welfare Failures

SOWS

Agalactia / udder congestion
  A change from straw to no bedding
  Constipation
  Frozen pipes
  Incorrect feeding
  Poor nutrition
  Poor water supply

Leg weakness (OCD)
  Leg stresses
  Particularly first litter animals
  Poor nutrition
  Slippery floors or slats

Loss of condition
  Cold / draughts
  Failure to foster piglets from large litters
  Poor nutrition
  Under feeding

Mastitis
  Failure to clip teeth of piglets
  Poor hygiene
  Poor management
  Shortage of water
  Wet pens

Metritis
  Ascending infection from the vulva
  Dead piglets
  Problems at farrowing
  Unhygienic manual assistance

Prolapse: vagina / uterus / rectum
  Difficulty in the sow rising
  Obstructed or prolonged farrowing
  Faulty tail gates in the crates
  Increased abdominal pressure
  Old age
  Slippery surfaces
  Sloping floor

Vulval haematoma
  Crushing of the vulva by the tail gate or crate projections
  Previous damage in yard (Cont.)

DISEASE PROBLEMS IN FARROWING AND LACTATING SOWS AND SUCKING PIGS ASSOCIATED WITH WELFARE FAILURES (Cont.)
Condition/Problem and Welfare Failures

PIGLETS

Arthritis
  Joint infections
  Faulty teeth clipping
  Lack of colostrum
  Poor hygiene. Dirty udders
  Rough floors
  Starvation
  Trauma to teeth and tails
  Sore knees from rough concrete surfaces

Atrophic rhinitis
  High humidity
  High levels of dust

Coccidiosis
  Poor pen hygiene

Diarrhoea
  Wet draughty dirty pens
  Lack of colostrum
  Lack of sow immunity

Greasy pig disease
  Poor pen maintenance
  Poor teeth clipping
  Skin trauma

High mortality
  Badly designed crates
  Cold
  Damp
  Draughts
  Excessive disturbance
  Failure to obtain colostrum
  Lack of supervision in first 24 hours
  Overweight sows
  Poor management

Hypoglycaemia
  Agalactia
  Badly designed crates
  Chilling
  Cold
  Failure to suckle
  Poor management
  Poor teat access
  Slippery floors
  Splay legs

(Fig.16-14)

DISEASE PROBLEMS IN NEWLY WEANED SOWS ASSOCIATED WITH WELFARE FAILURES
Condition/Problem and Welfare Failures
Abscess
Trauma - loose-housing
Fighting
Bruising and skin abrasions
Fighting
Heavy boars
Trauma
Variable sizes of sows
Fracture
Fighting
Mixing different sizes of pigs
Slippery floors
Trauma - loose-housing
Haematoma
Fighting
Trauma
Lameness
Activity at oestrus
Foot damage
Heavy boars at mating
High stocking densities
Inadequate bedding
Poor bone strength
Slippery floors
Leg weakness (OCD)
Gilt rearing and selection
Inadequate nutrition
Poor body condition
Poor crate design
Poor slippery surfaces
Trauma
Muscle tearing
Damage during suckling
High stocking density
Lack of exercise
Poor floors
Mastitis
Poor hygiene
Trauma
Wet floors

(Fig.16-15)

Size - In loose-housed weaning accommodation allow approximately $3.4m^2$ of floor area per sow.

Floors - Keep these as dry as possible at all times and ensure that they are comfortable and well drained. Ideally use straw bedding but if this is not available use other materials. Replace bedding daily. Soiled wet bedding can cause mastitis, vaginal infections and infertility.

Water - Site nipple drinkers or troughs in a well drained area.

Feed - Feed to appetite from day one after weaning through to the day of mating, preferably from an ad lib feeder. If your sows are group-housed allow a minimum of two separate feeders spaced well apart to reduce stress at feeding time and prevent anoestrus developing in disadvantaged sows.

Group size - Ideally 6 - 15 sows.

Temperature - For the first 4-5 days post-weaning this should approximate that being used in the farrowing houses at the time of weaning.

Management, welfare and disease (Fig.16-15)

The weaning to mating period is a critical time for the group housed sow because there can be a considerable amount of disturbance and aggression. Good non slip floor surfaces and smooth walls are essential to prevent trauma and injury. Where practicable, sows should be grouped by size. Particular care should be taken with the weaned first litter gilt and thin sows to ensure adequate food intake and reduce any fighting and aggression.

The Health and Welfare of Weaned and Growing Pigs

Design requirements

Weaned and growing pigs are usually group-housed in pens of 5 to 200 pigs per pen..

Size - This is dependent on the numbers of pigs per pen, their weight, the type of floor surface, the bedding used if any and the shape of the pen. Fig.16-1 gives guidelines to stocking density requirements on either solid or part slatted systems.

Floors - These can be totally solid, insulated and drained towards the defecating area, part solid and part slatted, totally slatted or straw based. If the quality of the slats is good and they have a round edge, a totally slatted area provides the best performance and welfare conditions provided that the temperature, air flow and humidity are controlled within the pigs' requirements. Welfare codes favour bedding but for this to be satisfactory it must be available, clean, dry and deep enough to provide warmth and comfort. This is often not the case and pigs are better without it.

Water - This can be provided either through nipple drinkers, automatic bowls or troughs. The water requirements for pigs are given in Figs.16-4 to 16-6

DISEASE PROBLEMS IN WEANED AND GROWING PIGS ASSOCIATED WITH WELFARE FAILURES
Condition/Problem and Welfare Failures

Abscess
    Faulty injections
    Fighting
    Lameness factors
    Mixing of pigs
    Tail biting
    Trauma

Bursitis
    Badly designed slats
    Foot problems
    Incorrect slat: gap ratio
    Lameness
    Poor floor surfaces
    Trauma
    Weight too heavy for slats

Colitis
    Disease
    Faulty nutrition
    Poor building hygiene

Erysipelas
    Dirty wet conditions in finishing pens
    High exposure in straw based systems

Enteric diseases in growing pigs
    Infections such as those that cause PE, swine dysentery, salmonellosis
    Poor hygiene
    Poor nutrition
    Poor environments

Greasy pig disease - Exudative epidermitis
    Faulty teeth clipping
    High humidity
    High stocking densities
    Infection
    Skin abrasions

Gastric ulcers
    Faulty nutrition
    Feed too finely ground
    Stress

Haematoma and haemorrhage
    Fighting
    Mange
    Trauma from the environment

Lameness
    Fat sprayed diets
    High stocking densities (Cont.)

DISEASE PROBLEMS IN WEANED AND GROWING PIGS ASSOCIATED WITH WELFARE FAILURES
Condition/Problem and Welfare Failures

    Poor nutrition
    Slippery floor surfaces (fat sprayed diets)
    Increasing gap size between slats caused by wearing

Leg weakness (OCD)
    Gilts served too young
    Heavy stocking densities
    Poor floor surfaces

Pneumonia
    House not split into modules
    Permanently populated housing
    Poor management
    Poor environment
    Poor nutrition
    Specific infections

Post-weaning diarrhoea
    Excess feed
    Failure to clean and disinfect between batches
    Fluctuating temperatures
    Poor environment
    Stale feed

Rectal prolapse
    Poor environment
    Poor nutrition
    Respiratory disease

Respiratory disease
    Fluctuating temperatures and humidity
    High stocking densities
    Permanently populated houses
    Poor nutrition

Vice (Abnormal behaviour)
    An unhappy pig
    Poor environment

(Fig.16-16)

Water should be available at all times.

Feed - This can be presented to the pig by a wet feeding system three to four times daily, restricted feeding or ad libitum through feed hoppers. Wet feeding systems have several advantages. Within a group all pigs tend to drink at about the same speed whereas there is a wide variation between pigs in the amounts of dry feed they can eat. Feeding space requirements are shown in Fig.16-3.

Group size - The optimum size varies depending upon the type of system and the availability of feed. For example in indoor totally slatted pens 20 pigs may be the maximum for efficient production. In straw yards this could rise to 60 pigs or more per pen.

Temperature - A guide to requirements is given in Fig.16-7 but always adjust to maintain the pigs in a comfortable lying pattern.

Management, welfare and disease (Fig.16-16)

If the pigs' requirements are not satisfied, disease problems are created particularly if a catabolic state develops. Housing should be managed on an all-in all-out basis with a total depopulation, cleaning and disinfection between groups. This is important for both respiratory and enteric disease control.

Reduced feed availability, lower temperatures or poor quality food will also lead to stress and an increased predisposition to enteric and/or respiratory disease as well as behavioural abnormalities.

The Health and Welfare of Sows Outdoors

The general welfare requirements to maintain healthy outdoor pigs are similar to those required for indoor production, but are often more difficult to control when they occur. However a greater management input is required during extremes of weather, for example the provision of water during periods of freezing. During wet periods extra bedding is essential in both the dry sow and farrowing huts. Huts should be sited on higher ground during periods of snow and heavy rainfall. Adequate shade and wallows must be provided in the summer.

Design requirements

Site - It is vital that the ground used is light, free draining and flat. Ideally the soil should be sandy but chalk and gravel are also satisfactory. The site should be low lying in a valley rather than on a hill, be in an area of low wind and have good vehicular access. The huts for dry sows should be approximately 2.5-3m, hold four to six sows and face away from the prevailing wind.

Water - This should be available in troughs which should be no more than a short walking distance for suckling sows.

Feed - This should be presented on the ground in the form of cobs dropped along a line. Feeding lines should be at least 3m apart and change frequently.

Stocking rate - There should be 15 to 20 sows per hectare (6 to 8 sows per acre).

Bedding - Farrowing huts should be placed on the higher parts of the land and bedded twice weekly with straw. They should also be checked daily for draughts and wet floors.

Temperature - Outdoor pig breeding can only be carried out efficiently in temperate climates and ideally all the huts should be insulated. However due to the small cubic capacity of dry sow huts and the heat given off by groups of sows there are usually less problems here in maintaining adequate temperatures.

WELFARE AND DISEASE PROBLEMS - OUTDOORS
Condition/Problem and Welfare Failures

Abortion
  Cold wet conditions
  Draughts
  Feed intake
  Heat stress
  Parasites
  Poor nutrition
  Season
  Sunlight

Agalactia
  Faulty nutrition
  Frozen or inadequate water supplies

Clostridial infections
  No vaccination

Erysipelas
  Exposure to the organism and failure to vaccinate

Infertility
  Fighting
  Hot weather
  Lack of adequate wallows
  Lame boars
  Overuse of boars (especially young ones)
  Shortage of shade
  Trauma to the boar's penis

Haemorrhage from the penis
  Associated with the sandy soils

Lameness
  Bad feet
  Flint land
  Mycoplasma
  Leg weakness (OCD)
  Wet land

Leptospirosis
  Associated with the constant exposure of sows to contaminated wallows or water
  Exposure to rodents

Loss of body condition
  Associated with the leaner genotype that is used as a terminal sire
  Inadequate feed
  Poor feed presentation
  Poor parasite control

Mortality (piglets)
  Bad management   (Cont.)

WELFARE AND DISEASE PROBLEMS - OUTDOORS (Cont.)
Condition/Problem and Welfare Failures
Cannibalism Crows Foxes Poor bedding Poor environment Sloping floors
Parasites 　Continual exposure to eggs and larvae particularly the stomach, nodular and lung worms 　No worming programme 　Old pastures
Sunburn 　Lack of shelter 　No wallows 　White breeds

(Fig.16-17)

Wallows - There should be two in each paddock near the fence line so that they can be used alternatively to allow drying for disease control. Not only do they help to cool sows in hot weather but they also allow sows to cake their skins with mud to prevent sunburn.

Shade - This must be provided to lessen the effects of strong direct sunlight.

Management, welfare and disease (Fig.16-17)

Outdoor systems have a major disadvantage in that the sows can only be managed as groups rather than individuals. Generally if there is a welfare problem it is due to climate and therefore involves the group as a whole. Feed intake and quality of feed are important in relation to disease, the maintenance of body condition and reproductive performance. It is very important to feed sows well in summer and autumn to provide good fat cover for the winter. Routine control of lice, mange and worms is essential in maintaining the health and welfare of the group. In periods of inclement weather piglets suffer due to cold and wet conditions and increased trauma by the sow. Foxes, crows and other large birds often cannibalise piglets. Three strand electric fences will deter foxes.

Fortunately disease problems in outdoor herds tend to be less but parasite burdens can become a problem on permanently grazed pastures. The identification and treatment of sick piglets can be difficult.

Chapter 16

17 Health and Safety

Introduction 555
The management of health and safety 555
The cost benefits 557
How to develop a health and safety management system for your farm 558
    Step 1 - Identify the people involved on your farm 558
    Step 2 - Understand your national regulations 560
Policy statements and policy organisation 561
    Step 3 - Produce your policy statements 561
    Step 4 - Assign responsibilities for health and safety 561
Risk assessments 562
    Step 5 - Plan your risk assessments 562
    Step 6 - Carry out your risk assessments 568
    Step 7 - Devise and apply your control measures 570
    Records 572
Safe systems of work (SSW's) 572
    Step 8 - Document your safe systems of work (SSW's) 572
    Step 9 - Document your accident, first aid, fire and emergency procedures 573
    Step 10 - Review your system periodically 575

Chapter 17

17 Health and Safety*

Introduction

There are three reasons why a chapter on health and safety should appear in a book dealing with the management control and treatment of pig diseases.

The first is perhaps obvious, some of the environmental hazards commonly associated with pig production, such as dust and slurry gases, can affect the health of both people and pigs. The need to assess and control these environmental factors is therefore a health and safety issue as well as being an integral part of disease control.

The second is often overlooked. A positive proactive approach to health and safety, just as with disease control, can help you maximise production, reduce costs and increase profitability.

The third is the most important. Good management practice is now as applicable to health and safety as it is to other business activities such as finance, personnel management and the control of pig diseases.

Over the last twenty years health and safety legislation has been changing in many countries. In the past employers could achieve compliance simply by following specific directives; however these directives were often retrospective, reactive and prescriptive. They were introduced as a result of accidents that had already occurred in an attempt to prevent them from happening again. They placed the same constraints on all employers regardless of individual circumstances or the levels of risk involved.

Now, in many countries, the emphasis of modern legislation is more on self regulation. This requires employers to set their own safety standards within minimal legal requirements and to define and implement the controls necessary to achieve them. The most effective way for the employer to approach this is to carry out **Risk Assessments** and national regulations may make it a legal obligation to do so.

To achieve full compliance however, employers have to show that they have addressed all aspects of health and safety that apply to their operations and everything that should be done is being done. The legal term "due diligence" may be used to describe this.

This view is now so widely accepted that in many countries it has (or is likely to) become a legal requirement for all employers to implement a health and safety management system. An example of such legislation is

---

* *Mark Enright, Salus (Quality Partnerships) Limited. See appendix.*

"The Management of Health and Safety at Work Regulations 1992", which came into force in the UK in January 1993 in compliance with a European Council Directive.

This chapter explains methods of risk assessment and health and safety management that are straightforward and appropriate for pig farms, large or small.

Study the outline given so that an appreciation of the structure can be understood. Steps 3, 6 and 8 are the key stages.

The Management of Health and Safety

Several books have been written on the subjects of health and safety management and risk assessment and there are many different ways to approach them. Pig farmers are free to adopt or devise any system that suits them provided that the end results comply with their national legislation and their own requirements.

> *A pro-active, structured approach to health and safety is what you should aim for.*

The following approach, developed by Salus QP Ltd., is to consider risk assessment as one key component of health and safety management and to devise methods whereby all of the components can be combined in an overall working system.

The resulting management system shown in Fig.17-1 revolves around the development and implementation of **Safe Systems of Work** (SSW's). These incorporate both the work instructions (how to do a job safely) and the management procedures whereby you can ensure and demonstrate that:

- The relevant Regulations, Approved Codes of Practice and Industry Standards are being addressed appropriately.
- The work areas and activities are being fully assessed.
- The methods of work are safe and without risk, so far as is reasonably practicable.
- The methods of work are adhered to.
- The persons carrying out the work have received sufficient training instruction and information, that they are aware of any associated hazards and can carry out the work safely.
- The necessary personal or environmental monitoring is carried out.

- The necessary building, machinery and equipment safety checks and routine services are carried out.
- The necessary occupational health checks are carried out.
- The necessary records are kept.
- The necessary safety audits and reviews are carried out.

The SSW's are the hub of the working system and you should have them for every aspect of health and safety that applies to your operation. The way in which you should document them will depend on the size and type of your farming operation. The aspects of health and safety applicable to you as a pig producer and appropriate ways to compile and present SSW's are discussed later.

Fig.17-1 illustrates the components of health and safety management. Clearly a considerable amount of health and safety knowledge is required in order to develop a workable system and regulations may state that employers must appoint competent persons to assist in their development.

Large pig organisations may have the necessary expertise in house to fulfil these obligations but the majority of pig farmers will not. It is possible to gain the necessary expertise yourself or to send a member of your staff on a health and safety management course but first consider the cost benefits of this approach. As with other management operations requiring expert knowledge, such as accounting, building design, veterinary medicine and legal matters, it is usually more cost effective to seek outside advice or to appoint a professional agency. Choosing the right partner can bring savings in your time and in insurance premiums. (See the cost benefits).

You should appoint a safety professional with a proven track record and considerable first hand experience of pig farming operations. The person should be competent to:
- Advise on the hazards and safety risks associated with pig production systems.
- Advise on the regulations, industry guidelines and standards in your country - and how to observe them.
- Devise safe working systems that are applicable to your situation.
- Draw up policy statements and organisation arrangements that are workable.
- Carry out risk assessments and report the findings in a way that will satisfy you, your employees, and health and safety inspectors.
- Advise on maintenance and safety of machinery and buildings.

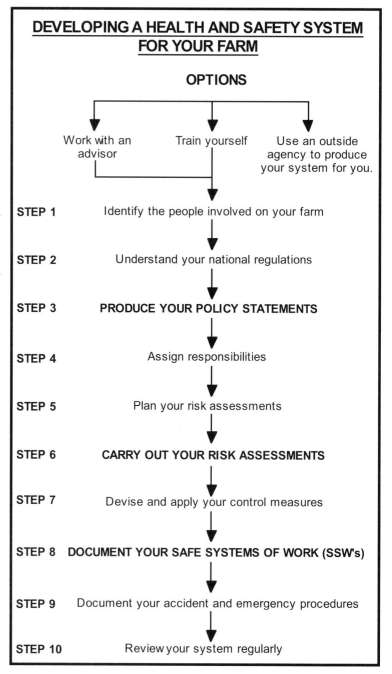

Good health and safety management depends on effective risk assessment.

- Advise on personal protective clothing and equipment.
- Advise on and help with appropriate training.
- Organise monitoring of environmental hazards such as dust, noise and gases and advise on methods to reduce them or control exposure to them.

CHAPTER 17 - Health and Safety

MANAGING HEALTH AND SAFETY AT WORK

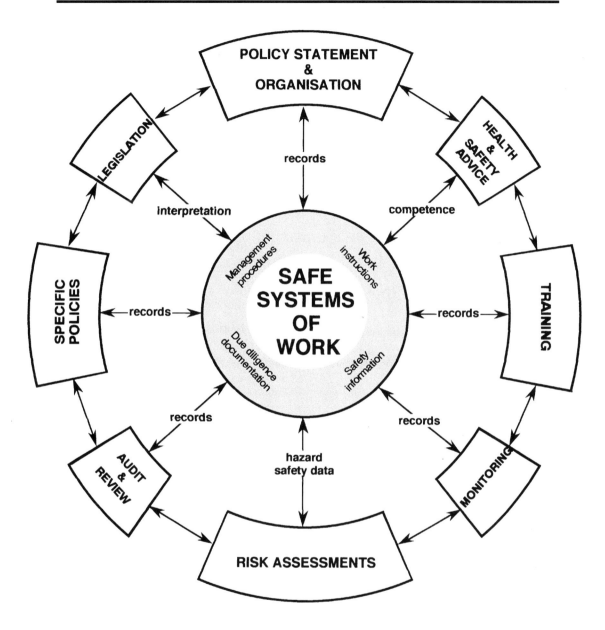

(Fig.17-1)

The Cost Benefits

Few pig farmers are fully aware of the cost implications of poor health and safety systems or of the benefits that can be associated with good management.

Agriculture is a dangerous industry. In many countries it ranks second only to the construction industry for the highest numbers of deaths, accidents and working days lost each year. In the UK and the USA it is top of the list.

The figures that are officially reported are only the tip of the iceberg. (Fig.17-2).

In addition to the suffering caused to the individuals and their families, accidents can seriously harm a business. In addition to the insured costs there can be a number of hidden, uninsured costs which include:

> **The Responsibility for Health and Safety is YOURS.**

- Plant and building damage.
- Tool and equipment damage.
- Legal costs.
- Spending on emergency supplies.
- Loss of expertise / experience.
- Pig disease problems due to loss of management expertise.
- Pig production problems due to loss of management expertise.
- Overtime and temporary labour requirements.
- Investigation time.
- Supervisor's time.
- Clerical paperwork.
- Fines.

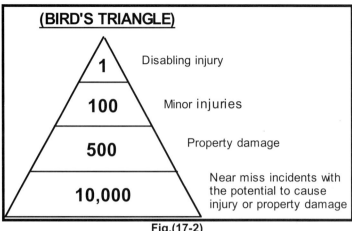

Fig.(17-2)

The investment needed to generate extra profits to cover accidental losses could be much greater than the investment needed to reduce those losses. The principles of loss control should therefore be applied to health and safety, just as they are to other aspects of business.

In addition to controlling the losses described, an effective management system can also result in:-
- Lower insurance premiums.
- Proof of due diligence, reducing the likelihood of civil claims.
- Higher efficiency / productivity / less pig disease.
- Higher staff health, morale and motivation.
- Better utilisation of plant and equipment.
- Better legislative compliance.
- Better cost control.
- A better image for your organisation.

Many insurance companies now offer reduced premiums to businesses that can demonstrate a positive commitment to health and safety.

Further reductions in premiums may be achieved in one of three ways:
1. By individual pig producers demonstrating a reduction in their accident rates and the number of successful claims against them.
2. By groups of pig producers or organisations with several farms implementing the same management system so that combined accident and claim statistics could be used.
3. By individual pig producers adopting and implementing a well recognised management system that was already being used by a number of other businesses, whose combined accident and claim statistics already showed significant, measurable results.

How to Develop a Health and Safety Management System for Your Farm

When planning your health and safety management system, and before writing policy statements, conducting risk assessments and developing safe systems of work, you will need to be fully aware of two things.

1. The categories of people that you have a duty to protect.
2. The health and safety regulations that apply to you and your farming operations in your country.

The remainder of this chapter deals with setting up the safe systems of work.

Step 1 - Identify the People Involved on Your Farm

All employers have a duty to protect the following categories of people:
- Employees
- Employees with known disabilities
- Trainees/agricultural students/temporary workers
- Visitors and the general public
- Contractors
- Trespassers

The points to address for each of these categories are:

Employees

Before asking an employee to carry out a task:
- You must take account of their capabilities.
- This should include consideration of the employees age, sex, physical strength, size, experience and competence, in relation to the tasks that you will expect them to perform.
- You must provide them with adequate training:
  - When they are first appointed.
  - As and when there are changes in procedures, systems of work etc.
  - On a routine refresher basis.
- You must provide them with information regarding:
  - The risks to health and safety associated with their jobs.
  - The health and safety control measures in place.
  - Their obligations regarding health and safety.

A poor health and safety record leads to increased insurance premiums.

- The safe systems of work to be observed.
- The accident, fire and emergency procedures.
- The results of any monitoring and health surveillance.

Employees with known disabilities

In addition to the above
- You must ensure that employees are not asked to perform tasks or handle substances that may, for them, present particular risks. Examples of this would be asking a pregnant female worker or a known asthmatic to administer prostaglandin to sows. Other examples of disabilities that may be relevant to pig farm workers include dermatitis, a history of back or joint weakness, hypersensitivity to certain antibiotics and respiratory problems.
- You may be obliged to implement a staff health surveillance scheme. This will depend on the regulations that apply to you (seek advice). Even when it is not a specific requirement, it is good practice to implement a health surveillance system anyway. This should include pre-employment health checks (questionnaires) and on-going records of employee absence, sickness and complaints or requests to do with health and safety. This can be used to identify existing disabilities and also to spot any health effects associated with particular tasks and individuals. Respiratory disease would be a typical example

Trainees / students / temporary workers

Because of their inexperience and unfamiliarity with your work environment trainees are a particularly high risk group.
- You must provide the same degree of protection as for full employees (see above).
- You must stipulate the special provisions made for the trainees regarding your systems of work etc.
- You must be able to demonstrate, on record, the point at which trainees no longer require special provision (i.e. are deemed to be competent) for each system of work.

Visitors and the general public

You have a duty to ensure that your premises and activities do not present a risk to visitors or the general public.
- You should not leave visitors unaccompanied or allow them access to hazardous areas un-necessarily.
- You should ensure that appropriate directions, instructions and safety notices are displayed
- You must ensure that areas such as changing rooms, toilets, showers and offices that may be used by visitors are kept as clean and tidy as practicable.
- You must ensure that visitors are provided with sufficient safety information, for example, regarding dust, noise, fumes, electrical safety and fire precautions.
- You must ensure that sufficient protective clothing is available for use by visitors and that it is kept clean and in good order.
- You should have a plan of the premises available for the emergency services (in the event of fire) which shows the positions of hazards such as high voltages, gas cylinders, dangerous chemicals, slurry tank covers and dangerous animals (e.g. boars). How many farms have this available?
- You must consider your impact on the general public with regard to environmental hazards such as dust, noise and fumes and also physical hazards such as concealed farm exits, heavy works traffic at certain times and mud on the road.

Contractors

Although to some extent you share health and safety responsibility with contractors it will remain primarily with you as the pig farmer.

You have a duty to ensure that the contractor is not exposed to hazards as a result of your acts or omissions and that your employees are not exposed to hazards as a result of the acts or omissions of the contractor.

The points regarding visitors will also apply to contractors. In addition
- You must ensure that all contractors are competent and that they and their equipment comply with statutory provisions.
- You must ensure that contractors are fully informed of the hazards and risks to health and safety which they may be exposed to on your farm.
- You must inform contractors of the measures that you have taken and of those that they must take, in order to ensure compliance with legislative requirements and your systems of work.

A practical way to ensure that the above points are covered is to use a "contractors declaration" record form. This can be a standard form that specifies what you require of contractors (i.e. that they comply with the appropriate statutory provisions and levels of competence) and has a section for you to give details of the hazards present at the work site, the accident fire and emergency procedures, location of the nearest first aid box, the name of their contact on the farm, etc. The contractor and the farm safety manager should both sign the form and each retain a copy. The record can then be kept as proof that you complied with your obligations - should such proof be needed at any time.

Trespassers

The law regarding pig farmers duties towards trespassers is different in each country but it is generally the case that unless you are certain that trespassing will never occur you must take steps to offer some protection against risks which you know to be present. In most cases the repair of any unsafe or damaged items such as loose hand rails and missing slurry tank covers or the provision of warning signs and measures to deter entry may suffice.

Step 2 - Understand Your National Regulations

These may include specific regulations, approved codes of practice (ACOPs), industry standards, local authority by laws, duties of care, etc.

Each country has its own health and safety regulations and how they apply to pig farmers can depend on a number of variables. It is therefore not appropriate here to cite specific regulations and ACOPs etc. However, Fig.17-3 lists the topics that may be applicable to your pig farm and that are likely to be covered by regulations in most countries. The list is by no means complete and you should use it as a guide to compile your own comprehensive register. For your management system to

TOPICS TO WHICH REGULATIONS, ACOPs AND INDUSTRY STANDARDS ARE LIKELY TO APPLY	
Health And Safety Topic	Regulation / ACOP / Duty Of Care Industry Standard /Guidance
Abrasive wheels	
Accident/fire/emergency	
Asbestos (roofing & insulation)	
Confined spaces	
Construction	
Contractors	
Electrical safety	
First aid	
Hazardous substances	
Ladders	
Liability insurance	
Lift trucks	
Management of health and safety	
Manual handling	
New employees / trainees	
Noise	
Occupational health (health surveillance, working hours, rest rooms)	
Overhead power lines	
Permits to work	
Personal hygiene (toilets, washing facilities)	
Personal protective equipment	
Pesticides	
Pregnant women	
Pressure systems	
PTO shafts	
Roof work	
Safety signs	
Stairways	
Tractor safety	
Vehicles	
Veterinary medicines	
Waste disposal	
Work environment (heat, lighting, ventilation)	
Work equipment (machines, hand tools)	
Working alone	
Young people/children	

(Fig.17-3)

CHAPTER 17 - Health and Safety **561**

be effective you must be aware of the regulations etc., know how they apply to you and what you must do to comply with them. You may need outside help with this.

Policy Statements and Policy Organisation

Step 3 - Produce Your Policy Statements

The need for you to write down a policy statement and to make it available to all employees may or may not be compulsory but it is a good practice to do so.
In its most basic form your policy statement can simply be that you:

'undertake to do all that is reasonably practicable to ensure the health, safety and welfare of all employees, contractors and visitors'.

However, it should ideally also show your commitment to health and safety in that you have addressed all of your obligations under the prevailing legislation and have made your employees aware of theirs.

An example of a policy statement is shown in Fig.17-4.

In addition to the general policy statement you will need to adopt and possibly document policies on specific aspects of health and safety. To further define these policies and the associated SSW's you will need to carry out risk assessments. Once defined these specific policies should be coupled with, or cross referenced to the SSW's.

Step 4 - Assign Responsibilities for Health and Safety

It is at this stage that you must decide who is to be responsible for what, giving due consideration to competence, training needs, available time, etc.. The titles (e.g. safety manager) and names of the designated persons should be stated on the policy and if the designated person is an employee you may also wish to include their health and safety duties in their job descriptions. See

---

THE MANAGEMENT OF HEALTH & SAFETY AT WORK
Statement of Policy

In compliance with the Health and Safety at Work Legislation it is our policy to do all that is reasonably practicable to ensure the health, safety and welfare of all employees, contractors and visitors.

To this end we will adopt policies on all matters of Health and Safety that are compatible with the provisions of all relevant Health and Safety Acts, Regulations, ACOPs, Industry Standards and Duty of Care.

All personnel will receive appropriate information and training to ensure that they:
- are aware of the hazards at their workplace.
- are familiar with all relevant Safety Rules, Procedures & Safe Systems of Work.
- know where and how to access all necessary safety data.
- know where to find and how to use first aid and fire fighting equipment.
- are familiar with the procedures for reporting accidents and for reporting or raising other health and safety issues.

We also undertake to ensure that:
- staff will be supervised until fully trained and assessed as competent.
- machinery, equipment and safety devices are regularly maintained and inspected and are safe and suitable to use.
- the workplace is safe and suitable in terms of comfort, space, heating, lighting, ventilation, cleanliness and freedom from unnecessary hazards.
- working practices are regularly reviewed to improve health and safety.
- accidents and incidents are investigated and appropriate actions taken to prevent recurrence.
- individual members of staff will not be expected to perform tasks that may present risks to them specifically due to their age, sex or health status.
- an on-going health surveillance scheme is in operation and that the records are regularly reviewed to check for possible links between working practice and ill health and that any such links are fully investigated and appropriate action taken.

Signed ....
On behalf of

Fig.(17-4a)

GENERAL DUTIES OF EMPLOYEES
It is the duty of every employee:

- To take reasonable care for the health and safety of himself or herself and of other persons who may be affected by his or her acts or omissions at work.
- To co-operate with their employer and Safety Manager so far as is necessary to enable them to comply with any duties or requirements imposed on them under any of the relevant statutory provisions.
- Not to intentionally or recklessly interfere with, or misuse, anything provided in the interest of health, safety or welfare.

Detailed in .... are the Rules, Procedures and Safe Systems of Work which are to be followed by ALL personnel.

All employees must sign the declaration to indicate that they have read and understand them.

The four key points regarding our Health and Safety Policy are listed below.

1. All staff will receive formal instruction and training in the relevant health and safety aspects pertaining to them.
   Written records of this training will be retained by the employer and by the individual staff members.
2. Staff must not perform any tasks for which they have not received formal instruction or training detailing the health and safety procedures involved.
3. Staff must not perform any task or handle any equipment or hazardous substance if they know that the required health and safety procedures cannot be complied with.
4. When authorisation, training, advice or health and safety information / equipment is needed for specific purposes, staff must approach the Safety Manager or his/her deputy.

Your own Health and Safety policy should be:

IF IN DOUBT.......DON'T DO IT

Fig.(17-4b)

Fig.17-5
The policy statements should be prepared by the employer in consultation with the designated people. Individuals must be fully aware of their duties and must have the chance to voice their opinions. The whole system will be more likely to work if the employer is seen to be taking it seriously and if it is not considered to be just a paper exercise. It will almost certainly fail if people do not know what is expected of them or they do not feel competent to discharge their responsibilities or if they think that aspects of the policy are impractical or irrelevant.

Risk Assessments

Step 5 - Plan Your Risk Assessments

Risk assessment is now a legal requirement of health and safety regulations in many countries and it has become the subject of many conferences, workshops, articles and even regular journals. Only the basic requirements are covered here but hopefully enough to enable you to carry out assessments of the major aspects of your pig farm. You should check the specific requirements of your regulations, particularly with regard to the extent of the assessment required and the need to appoint a 'competent person'.

Risk assessment is a key stage towards the development of SSW's and the implementation of a health and safety management system. To satisfy the legal requirements it must involve these five stages:

1. Careful consideration of what in your pig farm could cause harm to people.
2. Careful consideration of which people might be affected.
3. An evaluation of whether you are taking enough precautions or should do more to prevent or reduce the likelihood of harm.
4. A record of your findings (depending on the regulations) and informing your employees.
5. A periodic review and revision (from time to time or when significant changes take place).

It should also involve an evaluation of the risks to the key aspects of your management systems and the measures necessary to control them.

For example, if an assessment determines that a risk of injury and/or damage is associated with a specific procedure and it can only be controlled by a specific working practice, then the risk assessment should not only identify the need for a detailed written work instruction (how to do the job safely) but also for appropriate staff training, instruction and information, an inspection/monitoring regime, suitable records, specific responsibility for the process and an assessment review date. All of these controls (management and work process) should then be incorporated into the appropriate SSW.

POLICY - ORGANISATION

Our policy with respect to all matters concerned with health, safety and welfare is formulated and carried out by:

The SAFETY MANAGER ....
who undertakes to:
- maintain an up to date knowledge of all relevant Health & Safety legislation.
- ensure the implementation of the policy throughout.
- organise the staff training and instruction in methods of safety.
- keep staff aware of the problems of safety and of their responsibility for the safety of themselves and of those around them.
- advise those responsible for the design and construction of new buildings and the modifications of existing buildings on all matters which affect safety, and to ensure that the necessary safety features are included in all designs.
- ensure the provision of first aid materials, occupational health supervision and monitoring, where appropriate.
- compile and review data concerning accidents, incidents and staff health issues and ensure that all are recorded, reported and investigated in accordance with the Safe Systems of Work and legislative procedures.

The AREA SAFETY OFFICERS ....
who undertake to:
- disseminate information on safety matters within their areas.
- advise on and check procedures to ensure the safety of work within areas.
- ensure that new employees are fully aware of the safety policy and standards, and all area safety arrangements and procedures.
- ensure that all employees and the Safety Manager are made aware of any special or new hazards about to be introduced into areas.
- ensure that the first aid boxes and the safety and fire equipment are checked regularly and that any deficiencies or faults are made good.
- ensure that all accidents, incidents and staff health issues are reported promptly to the Safety Manager in accordance with procedures.

The FIRE OFFICER ....
who undertakes to:
- supervise, or arrange for, the routine inspection and maintenance of fire fighting equipment, fire escapes, fire detection/alarm systems and any fixed systems e.g. sprinklers.
- undertake the posting of appropriate warning signs and notices.
- provide instruction in the use of emergency fire fighting equipment.
- ensure that appropriate fire drills are carried out.
- ensure that the proper liaison is maintained with the Local Authority Fire Protection Officer and that all architects drawings are submitted for approval.
- provide advice on any topic related to the fire precautions.
- maintain liaison with outside inspectors e.g. fire officers and insurance company assessors and ensure that the appropriate licences and fire certificates are obtained and their conditions observed.
- maintain a record of all fires reported and of the steps taken to ascertain their cause.

The FIRST AIDER ....
who undertakes to
- maintain an up to date knowledge of current accepted first aid practices.
- carry out or witness all initial first aid treatments in the event of accidents and / or act as first call when medical advice is sought by a member of staff.
- maintain an up to date knowledge of the approved first aid box contents as recommended by the HSE and report any deficiencies or discrepancies to the Area Safety Officers.
- check the contents of first aid boxes and eye wash bottles and to re-stock or renew as necessary.
- ensure that all accidents are reported promptly in accordance with procedures.

(Fig.17-5)

Before conducting risk assessments you will need to be familiar with the following:
- Hazards and safety data
- Risk rating
- Acceptable risks
- Record keeping requirements

Hazards and safety data

A hazard is anything that has the potential to cause harm and can include substances, machines, methods of work or a situation. Hazards on the pig farm can be categorised as follows:
- Physical - (noise, lighting, heat, fire, electricity).
- Chemical - (dust, drugs, chemicals, gases).
- Biological - (bacteria, fungi, viruses, parasites).
- Mechanical - (machines, equipment, tools).
- Ergonomic - (design, layout, manual handling).
- Psychosocial - (work load, personal security).

You will see from Fig.17-6 that the hand feeding of pigs may be more than just a dusty job!

Identifying the hazards present on your farm is the first step in conducting risk assessments. Not many farmers have the expertise to identify all the hazards which is partly due to their familiarity with their own pig farms. The fresh eye of an independent specialist or that of a friend with experience of risk assessment and pig production can make a useful contribution at this stage.

The checklist Fig.17-7 gives some examples of common hazards on pig farms. It is a memory jogger to refer to when you are conducting risk assessments. The list is not exhaustive and you should add other hazards known to be present on your farm.

The fourth column on the check list is headed Safety Data. The person conducting the risk assessments must have a knowledge of the harm that each hazard can cause. For some hazards you may need to refer to additional information. For example, you should obtain safety data for all of the drugs and chemicals used on your farm. In some countries it is a legal obligation to have such data available on site so that the information can be used in assessments and referred to for first aid advice in the event of exposure. The safety data that may be required for other hazards include such things as plant and machinery operating instructions and specifications that detail the machine operating performance limits, maximum load capacities, service requirements, safety test parameters, personal protective equipment required, and operator training requirements.

You will also need to know the legislative requirements regarding personal exposure limits for dust, noise and the various slurry gases, the required lighting levels for work areas and store rooms (the absence of light can constitute a hazard) - and anything else that would contribute to the assessment of the risks associated with the hazards identified.

THE FOLLOWING EXAMPLES ILLUSTRATE THE DIVERSE NATURE OF HAZARDS		
Hazard	Potential	Harm
Lifting a sack of feed.	Muscular stress.	Back injury / Hernia.
Work from a gantry.	Gravity.	Fall to ground.
Dust from feed.	Respiratory sensitiser.	Bronchitis / respiratory distress.
Penicillin in feed.	Hypersensitivity.	Breathing difficulty / collapse.
Noise from squealing pigs.	Sound energy.	Hearing damage.
Rotating auger.	Friction of moving surface.	Entanglement.
Hectic work schedule.	Mental stress.	Hypertension / depression / suicide.

(Fig.17-6)

Zoonoses safety data

Zoonotic organisms are a special type of biological hazard. They are the infections (bacteria, fungi, parasites and viruses) that may be present in animals or their products which can cause disease in people.

Information on the zoonotic organisms associated with pigs is given in Fig.17-8. Each one is a specific hazard with different properties and potential to cause harm. They should be evaluated individually.

To help you put each in perspective the more common or serious ones are dealt with here. Fortunately there are relatively few serious zoonotic organisms in pigs and some of these are limited to particular regions.

Salmonella - Food poisoning is the most common world-wide, mainly *Salmonella typhimurium* but also from time to time other serovars including *Salmonella enteritidis* and *Salmonella derby*. The host adapted serovar in pigs, *Salmonella cholerae-suis*, rarely causes food poisoning in people but when it does it is serious. Food poisoning derived from pig meat products results from unhygienic handling and inadequate cooking and is not directly related to what you do on the farm unless you are selling pig products through a farm shop. From the viewpoint of health and safety salmonella are likely to be present on most pig farms but the levels are so low that they do not normally present a hazard to farm workers. If clinical cases of salmonellosis occur in your pigs then the levels rise and become high enough to cause human disease. Everyone on the farm must then take hygienic precautions particularly before eating.

Campylobacter - Derived from animals are also a common source of food poisoning in people. Fortunately the majority of campylobacter found in pigs are not the same types that cause human disease (although some are) and pig products are not usually implicated. Nevertheless, you should be aware that they might be present in your herd and you should insist on strict hygiene when eating and drinking.

Leptospira - Some of the leptospira serovars in pigs, particularly *Leptospira pomona*, can cause a serious generalised infection in man, with fever and meningitis,

> *Provide an eating room for your pig workers and insist on cleanliness and hygiene when they are using it.*

564 Managing Pig Health and the Treatment of Disease

\multicolumn{3}{c}{HAZARD CHECK LIST}		
\multicolumn{3}{l}{The list below describes hazards that are commonly found on pig farms. It is not exhaustive. It is intended as a memory jogger for you to use when conducting risk assessments. Make a note of those hazards which apply to your farm.}		

No.	Hazard	Nature Of Harm	Safety Data
1	Adhesives.	May harm skin, eyes, lungs.	Product safety data sheet.
2	Ammonia (slurry gas).	Respiratory problems. Watering eyes.	Chemical safety data sheet.
3	Asbestos (roofing / insulation).	Respiratory problems. Carcinogenic.	Official H&S information.
4	Carbon monoxide (exhaust gas).	Toxic by inhalation.	Chemical safety data sheet.
5	Compressed gases.	Explosion. May also be harmful.	Product safety data sheets.
6	Conveyor belts.	Entanglement.	Official and supplier information.
7	Damaged electrical cables.	Electrocution, burns, death.	-
8	Debris.	Trips. Hinder escape.	-
9	Diesel.	Skin and respiratory problems.	Product safety data sheet.
10	Disinfectants.	May harm skin, eyes, lungs., body.	Product safety data sheets.
11	Drugs.	May have serious health effects.	Product safety data sheets.
12	Dung, urine, tissue, body fluids.	Zoonotic diseases.	Zoonoses safety data.
13	Dust	Respiratory problems.	Official and industry information.
14	Faulty wiring / earth.	Electrocution, burns, death.	-
15	Flame / Arc.	Ignition source; burns; Arc Eye.	-
16	Flammable gases.	Burns.	Product safety data sheets.
17	Flying debris.	Puncture; cuts; impact; eye damage.	-
18	Fragile roof covering.	Falls.	-
19	Gantries/ scaffold/ stairs.	Falls, manual handling problems.	-
20	Hand tools (knives / hammers).	Cuts, impact injury, trapping injury.	-
21	Heat / cold.	Exposure, hyperthermia, heat stroke.	-
22	Heating oil.	Burns. Harm eyes, skin, lungs, body.	Product safety data sheet.
23	Herbicides.	Potentially toxic.	Product safety data sheets.
24	Hydraulic equipment.	Entrapment. Crushing.	Manufacturer's information.
25	Hydrogen sulphide (slurry gas).	Toxic by inhalation (fast acting).	Chemical safety data sheet.
26	Hypodermic needles.	Puncture. Effects of drugs / body fluid.	-
27	Insecticides.	Potentially toxic or very harmful.	Product safety data sheets.
28	Insecurity.	Stress effects. Depression.	-
29	Lack of oxygen.	Asphyxia.	-
30	Machinery (general).	Cuts, entrapment, entanglement.	Manufacturer's information.
31	Marker sprays.	Harmful by inhalation.	Product safety data sheets.
32	Methane (slurry tank gas).	Highly flammable. Burns. Explosion.	Chemical safety data sheet.
33	Moving vehicle.	Cuts, crushing, entrapment.	-
34	Noise.	Hearing damage. Lose concentration.	Official H&S information.
35	Overhead power lines.	Electrocution, burns, death.	-
36	Paints.	May harm skin, eyes, lungs., body.	Product safety data sheets.
37	Paraffin.	Burns. Skin & respiratory effects.	Product safety data sheet.
38	Pesticides (crops).	Many are highly toxic. All harmful.	Product safety data sheets.
39	Petrol.	Burns. Skin & respiratory effects.	Product safety data sheet.
40	Pigs (or other animals).	Physical injury. Zoonotic diseases.	Specific zoonoses safety data.
41	Poor lighting.	Eye strain. Cannot see other hazards.	-
42	PTO shafts.	Entanglement.	-
43	Restricted access / egress / space.	Can't avoid hazards. Hinders escape.	-
44	Rodenticides.	Toxic / harmful by mouth, skin, lungs.	Product safety data sheets.
45	Rotating parts (fan blades; auger).	Cuts, amputation, entanglement.	Manufacturer's information.
46	Solvents.	Harmful by mouth, skin, lungs, eyes.	Product safety data sheets.
47	Steam.	Burns.	-
48	Trailing cables.	Trips.	-
49	Uneven / slippery floors.	Slips, trips.	-
50	Unstable stacks (bales; stores)	Injury, crushing by falling objects	-
51	Used engine oils.	Carcinogenic.	-
52	Vermin (rats, mice & their urine).	Zoonotic disease (esp Weil's disease).	Zoonoses safety data.
53	Welding fumes.	Respiratory problems.	-
54	Wet plugs / sockets.	Electrocution, burns, death.	-
55	Work - pressure, harassment, abuse.	Stress effects. Depression.	-

(Fig.17-7)

called "Swine herds disease" or "Weil's disease" (caused by *L. icterohaemorrhagiae*). In pigs the main clinical signs are abortion, stillbirths and infertility. Fortunately *L. pomona* is now relatively rare in Northern Europe and North America and pig-derived disease in humans is uncommon but you should still be aware of it. The main source of infection to people is pigs urine or vaginal discharges contaminating cuts (e.g. on the hands) or mucous membranes (e.g. the eyes or lips). Cuts should be covered and pigs urine kept away from the face. The disease is amenable to prompt antibiotic therapy so if a person working on the farm comes down with fever, depression and headache call a doctor quickly.

Brucella suis - This is now rare in Northern Europe and North America but is more common in some other parts of the world. The main clinical effects are abortions, swollen testes and joint problems particularly of the spine. It causes a very serious disease in people and if it is suspected the greatest care should be taken not to contaminate cuts in the skin or mucous membranes such as the mouth or eye when dealing with aborted materials, vaginal discharges or cutting up a dead pig.

> **Wear protective clothing and rubber gloves when doing post-mortem examinations.**

> **If a farm worker develops an acute skin lesion, or an acute fever with a headache, or severe diarrhoea call a doctor promptly.**

If your farm is in a region where *Leptospira pomona* or *Brucella suis* are prevalent then it would be a wise precaution to blood test your herd routinely to check that it is not infected and to get prompt veterinary diagnosis and advice if suspicious clinical signs occur.

Streptococcus suis serotypes 2, 4 and 14 - These are widespread in pig populations around the world and sometimes cause fever, joint problems, meningitis and deafness in people. Most people who become affected are people who handle meat. Cases in farm workers are rare. The number of people affected is tiny relative to the exposure rate that must take place so infection cannot be regarded as a high risk. Nevertheless, protective clothing, particularly rubber gloves should be worn when carrying out post-mortem examinations and a doctor should be sought promptly if anyone should develop fever, dizziness and a headache. The disease is amenable to antibiotic therapy if treated early.

Some strains of the influenza virus can cross-infect between pigs and people sometimes causing clinical disease in both.

\multicolumn{3}{c}{PIGS ZOONOSES}		
Source	Organism / Disease	Symptoms In People
Most common or most serious to human health		
A, P	*Brucella suis*	Recurrent fever, weakness, sweating, headache, backache, joint pain.
R	Influenza - some serotypes	Typical influenza symptoms - pneumonia fever and malaise.
I	Japanese B. encephalitis	(S.E. Asia only). Viral encephalitis and fever.
A, U, P	Leptospira (pomona mainly)	Fever, influenza-like symptoms, headache, muscle ache.
F, D, P	*Salmonella typhimurium* and others.	Watery diarrhoea, dehydration, abdominal pain and fever.
Uncommon in people (from pigs) may be common in pigs.		
S, F, U, B	Bacteria, various, mainly faecal	Contaminated wounds becoming septic and possibly necrotic.
S	Erysipelothrix - human erysipeloid	Local skin lesions usually on hand. Mainly fish and meat handlers.
S	Ringworm	Typical superficial circular skin lesions.
S	*Streptococcus suis* type 2, 4, 14	Fever, arthritis, sometimes meningitis and deafness.
Rare in people or unimportant		
D	Anthrax	Skin lesions (black scab), pneumonia, diarrhoea with blood.
F	Ascariasis	Asthma, coughing, pneumonia, possible abdominal pain.
A	Chlamydia	Rarely isolated from pigs. No reports of pig to man transmission.
F	Clostridia	Tetanus, gas gangrene, diarrhoea. Rarely from pigs.
F	Cryptosporidium	Diarrhoea, vomiting, headache, abdominal pain. (Immuno-suppressed people).
A, F	Listeria	Fever, headache, vomiting, PREGNANT WOMEN ABORT. (Pigs unlikely source).
F, S	Swine vesicular disease	Vesicles on skin and fever.
D	Taenia and Trichinella	In meat. Not direct from pigs. Muscle cysts.
A	Toxoplasma	Theoretically possible but no cases from pigs.
D, P	Tuberculosis (avian)	In meat. Not direct from pigs. Immuno-suppressed people.

A = Abortion, still birth, discharge
B = Bites and scratches
D = Dead animals and carcasses
F = Faeces and dirty bedding
I = Biting insects, mosquitoes
M = Mastitis
P = Doing a post-mortem examination
R = Respiratory disease - inhalation of aerosols
S = Skin contamination, wounds, abscess
U = Urine and soiled bedding

(Fig.17-8)

Japanese B. encephalitis - This is the most serious zoonotic infection of pigs. It is spread from pigs to people by mosquitoes. It is confined to herds in South East Asia and does not occur in Europe or the Americas. People working with pigs in endemic areas should be vaccinated.

Disease in people caused by other potential zoonoses listed in Fig.17-8 is extremely rare and they warrant only brief mention here.

Anthrax - This is rare in pigs outside anthrax incubated areas. In such areas the disease is well understood and controlled.

Erysipelothrix rhusiopathiae - This is wide-spread in pigs everywhere causing the common pig disease erysipelas. The organism can (rarely) cause skin lesions in people usually on the hands but mainly in fish and meat handlers. (Note that the disease "erysipelas" in people is unrelated and is caused by a streptococcus).

Clostridium perfringens **type A** - This is common in pig faeces but poses little direct threat to pig workers. Food poisoning results from poor food preparation.

General safety precautions

If a pig is exhibiting clinical signs of disease or it is in contact with diseased pigs and may be infected take the following precautions:-
1. Cover cuts and abrasions with waterproof dressing.
2. Wear gloves and coveralls.
3. Disinfect gloves and coveralls after use.
4. Always wash your hands after handling the animal or its products even if gloves were worn.

All staff involved with handling pigs or their excreta should be vaccinated against tetanus.

Risk rating

Determine whether the level of risk associated with each of the hazards identified is high, moderate or low. For risk assessments to be of greatest value you should adopt a risk rating and priority system.

Risk has two components the likelihood of a harmful event occurring and the degree of damage if it should occur. If these two contributory factors are given numerical values, say from 1 to 3, the risk rating is the product of these values multiplied together.

From this it can be seen that the risk ratings will be 1, 2, 3, 4, 6 or 9 with **1** representing very high risk (very likely to happen. with severe consequences) and **9** representing negligible risk (unlikely to happen, slight consequences if it did). These risk rating values can be used to set priorities for actions. With **1** requiring immediate decisive action to eliminate or reduce the risk (i.e. very high priority and **9** requiring little or no action (i.e. very low priority).

Using a risk rating/priority system in your assessment will make it less likely that you ignore what you consider to be trivial risks. They may indeed turn out to be so but to show due diligence it is better that your assessment is recorded.

In order to determine the likelihood of a harmful event you have to make informed judgements based on:
- What hazards are present?
- What harm could they cause?
- Under what conditions they would be present in a form to cause harm and who would be affected (number of people, sex, health status)?
- What precautions are already in place to prevent exposure?

The task of moving sacks of feed can be used to illustrate this point:

It is highly likely that a back injury will result if a slightly built person with no manual handling training has to carry a full sack of feed several times a day along a slippery walkway, up narrow steps to an unstable gantry and then raise the sack above the shoulders to tip it into the auger.

It is unlikely that a back injury will result if a strongly built person, trained in manual handling techniques, has to slide a sack of feed from a pallet, across a stable gantry then open the top of the sack and let the contents empty into the auger.

You should also consider your past accident/incident record and those of the pig farming industry in general. If you judge an event to be unlikely and yet such events have occurred on your farm or are common in the industry you should think again.

PIGS ZOONOSES SAFETY PRECAUTIONS

Source	Precautions
Abortion, stillbirth and vaginal discharge	Take care not to get vaginal discharges in cuts or near your mouth, nose or eyes. Pregnant women must not work with farrowing sows.
Diarrhoea	Take special care with animals suffering from diarrhoea not to get faeces near your mouth.
Urine	Take care not to inhale or swallow urine or splash it in your eye.
Skin disease	Avoid skin contact.
Respiratory disease	Take care not to get the pigs' nasal discharges or sputum near your lips or nose e.g. if it has been rubbed onto your clothing or boots. Wear a face mask.
Dead pigs	Carcasses should be removed and disposed of promptly. Disinfect the area occupied by the carcass.
Bites	Take care with unrestrained pigs. Disinfect bites quickly. See a doctor if you think the wound is infected.

Likelihood of event	X	Consequences
(i.e. exposure to a hazard, that causes harm)		(i.e. severity of harm)
1. = Highly likely		1. = Severe (death/major injury)
2. = Moderately likely		2. = Serious (off work more than 3 days)
3. = Unlikely		3. = Slight (off work less than 3 days)

Statistics show that within any organisation there are likely to be many near miss incidents. These are accidents waiting to happen and many organisations now accept that risk assessments must also take account of these near misses.

Once you have decided on the likelihood of an event you can consider the consequences if that event should occur. When doing this you will need to take into account the number of people that could be affected and whether certain individuals would be more seriously affected than others because of an existing disability or medical condition. For example, the consequences of damage to an eye as a result say of using a grinding tool would be far greater for a person who is poorly sighted in one eye than it would be for a person with two good eyes.

In addition to the harm done to a person, consequential loss should also be included. For example if the person at risk is a key employee whose absence from work even for a short period would affect production, the risk rating should be higher than it would otherwise be.

You can see from these examples that this form of risk rating is not an exact science and you may need to modify it in order to give yourself more flexibility. For example, with certain hazards you may want to multiply in a third component by splitting up "consequences". Thus you could have three columns i.e.

Likelihood of event
Degree of harm to people
Consequential loss / cost

You would then have a wider range of scores, namely, 1 (the worse risk) 2, 3, 4, 8, 12, 18, 27 (the lowest risk).

It is important to recognise that this method of risk rating is not intended to give an objective quantitative measure of risk but rather to create a list of priorities and to provide a record that shows you have carefully considered likelihood and consequences.

Acceptable risks

Although the ideal situation would be to eliminate all risks or reduce them to a trivial level this is obviously not possible. Pig farming is a physical occupation involving manual handling, potentially dangerous machines, potentially hostile environments and large strong unpredictable animals. There will always be some risks associated with it. With the emphasis now on self regulation, the onus is on you if you are the employer to determine what the acceptable levels of risk are in your situation and to be able to justify them.

This is summed up by your legal obligation (and policy) "*to do all that is reasonably practicable to ensure the health, safety and welfare of all employees, contractors and visitors*". The implications of the term "*... do all that is reasonably practicable ...*" are significant here.

Most employers appreciate that they are entitled to take cost and inconvenience into account when considering what actions would be required to reduce a risk unless the risk is high. Perhaps less well appreciated are other criteria that must also be taken into account.

The term "do all that is reasonably practicable" applies to both legislative and industry standards which means that you have to ensure that the levels of risk in your pig farm are at least within any specified legal limits and also that they are not significantly higher than those on other similar pig farms.

If other pig farmers are achieving fewer accidents and incidents than you, you cannot claim that it is not reasonably practicable for you to reduce risks also.

Therefore, before you can finally determine the appropriate control measures you have to find out what the legislative and industry standards are. This type of information may be available in Government publications and agricultural information bureaux or from the farmers trade association / union. You may have to compare notes with other pig producers and / or take advice from a consultant. You have an over-riding duty to exceed legislative and industry standards if it is reasonably practicable for you to do so.

The following three examples will hopefully put these points into context:

Example 1. <u>Noise</u> is a hazard that many pig producers consider 'goes with the business' and is therefore to be expected and accepted. Furthermore, because the effects of noise can take years to develop many farmers are not aware that the levels of noise on their farms may pose a significant risk to health. Consequently, the majority of farmers do not have a policy to reduce personal exposure to noise. The result, as surveys have shown, is that 25% of indoor pig workers have a noticeable hearing loss by the age of 30 and 50% have significant hearing loss by the age of 50.

Given these statistics it would be difficult for you to claim that it is not necessary or reasonably practicable for you to reduce it, particularly since control measures (using ear plugs at noisy times) would be simple and cheap to implement.

You probably do not have this option anyway because in many countries it is a legal requirement for employers to assess noise at work and if they think that there may be a risk to hearing, to measure the level of personal exposure to noise and if necessary apply controls to ensure that it is kept below legally defined limits. In this case you <u>must</u> control the risk. Cost and inconvenience only have a bearing on your choice of control measures.

Example 2. **Back injuries** are common in the pig industry and a certain level of risk is to be expected. But what level? Some countries have regulations stipulating that all manual handling activities must be assessed and that if risks are identified appropriate controls must be implemented. But they do not specify the levels of risk to be achieved other than that they must be as low as is reasonably practicable.

In this situation you must look to industry standards and your own records to provide a baseline for assessment. The pig industry may have set standards for, or national statistics may show, the average number of days lost per employee per year due to back injuries. If your record is worse than the standards or the national average, your employees and the enforcement agencies would be entitled to expect you to reduce the manual handling risks on your farm.

<u>Example 3.</u> **Dust** is another hazard associated with intensive pig production and not an easy one to cope with. The high levels present in many farms constitute a health and safety issue. More than 60% of all pig farmers suffer from dust induced respiratory problems during their working lives and in many cases these continue after they retire. The effects can be debilitating.

Research has attempted to determine the safe levels of exposure to dust and practical ways to control it. However, the complex make-up of piggery dust and the lack of long term clinical data make this a difficult task. Consequently, although occupational exposure limits (OELs) are specified in many countries they not only vary widely between countries but also refer to dust in general rather than to piggery dust specifically. Piggery dust has many potentially harmful components such as animal and feed proteins, bacteria and viruses, fungal and bacterial spores, mycotoxins and endotoxins. The reality is nobody knows the safe exposure levels for piggery dust which has implications for you as an employer. Although you may be able to achieve and demonstrate (by dust monitoring) levels of exposure to dust that are below the specified OELs (and any industry standards that apply), if any of your existing or past employees exhibit signs of respiratory problems (persistent cough, chest tightness, wheezing, shortness of breath, constantly runny nose, or sore throat) that are thought to be associated with the dust on your farm, you have to implement additional controls to further reduce the levels of personal exposure. Alternatively you must be able to justify why it is not reasonably practicable for you to do so.

All three of these examples highlight the need for you to keep abreast of the legislation, pig industry standards and general health and safety information. They also underline the importance of pre-employment and on-going health checks.

In the event of a criminal or civil claim being made against you, ignorance of the law is no defence.

Step 6 - Carry out Your Risk Assessments

The risk assessment procedures described here involve systematic appraisals of all of the areas in and around the pig farm and the procedures that take place in them.

Before conducting the assessments it will be necessary to compile the following information.

A list of the areas to be assessed. For example:
- Barns.
- Drying sheds.
- Feed bagging rooms.
- Feed milling rooms.
- Feed stores.
- Fields.
- Grain stores.
- Hospital pens.
- Loading bays.
- Muck heaps.
- Offices.
- Pig houses.
- Rest rooms.
- Silos.
- Tractor sheds.
- Workshops.
- Yards.

It is important not to ignore any areas. A field may look harmless enough but several farmers are killed each year when raised tractor shovels touch overhead power lines.

A sketch map of the site is useful to help list the areas in a logical sequence in preparation for a walk round inspection. It can also be used to mark safety features and hazards such as the positions of first aid boxes and fire extinguishers, fuel stores and power lines etc.

A list of the Procedures to be assessed. For example:
- Feed / grain silo management.
- Feed milling / mixing / bagging.
- Grain handling / drying.
- Hand feeding.
- Hazardous chemicals - handling / storage / use.
- Maintenance / repairs.
- Pest control - rodents / vermin / flies / mites.
- Pressure washing.
- Sick pigs - handling / treatment / carcase disposal.
- Slurry channel drainage.
- Straw handling.
- Use of mechanical scraper.
- Veterinary medicines - handling / storage / use.
- Weighing pigs.

All hazards on the farm need to be assessed. The lists of areas and procedures should therefore be as comprehensive as possible. However, there will be some hazards associated with general items and activities that cannot be described as areas or specific procedures (e.g. equipment and machinery, animal handling). You must ensure that these are also assessed and that the relevant points are addressed and covered in the appropriate SSW's.

Human factors. You should compile a list of all employees and others who may be affected by the hazards present. Include contractors and maintenance personnel who may be on site occasionally or at specific times. Alongside each name (or category of people) include any information that will help you to evaluate the risks to their health and their contribution toward reducing or increasing risks to themselves and others. For example:

- Levels of training.
- Competence.
- Responsibilities.
- Specific skills.
- Disabilities.
- Health status.
- Health record.
- Accident / incident record.
- Attitude to health and safety.

Management practices. Make a note of any existing health and safety systems. For example:
- Accident / incident records and reviews.
- Health and safety policy statements.
- Monitoring of hazards (dust, noise, fumes).
- Occupational health surveillance.
- Organisation and health and safety responsibilities.
- Previous assessments (for hazardous substances, manual handling, etc.).
- Safety checks / audits.
- Work instructions.

You should also give an indication of the current standards of health and safety on the farm and what priority is given to improving them.

These lists can now be used to provide information for the assessments.

Although it may not be a legal requirement for you to record the assessments, it is your duty to conduct them and to inform employees of the findings. It is therefore sensible to record them so that you can prove your due diligence if necessary.

Area assessments

For each area to be assessed you should compile a record sheet with 12 columns. For the first 10 column headings, the information to be considered and the points to record are as follows:

1. **What is the identity of the area?**
   Simply record the name and basic description of the area e.g. Farrowing House 1. 10 crates, slatted floors at rear, slurry channel under slats. Mechanical ventilation.
2. **What procedures are carried out here?**
   Consult the list of procedures to be assessed and note those that apply to this area. It may be useful to number all of the procedures and simply record the relevant numbers here.
3. **What hazards are present?**
   See hazards and safety data. Carefully consider all categories of hazards. Use the hazard check list. List all the hazards (significant and trivial) associated with the area, i.e. those that are always, usually or sometimes present here.
   Include the hazards associated with the procedures that take place here.
   Include any hazardous substances that are stored here, even if they are used elsewhere. They may seem to present no risk but breakage, spillage or fire could result in personal exposure to them.
4. **What harm could they cause and how?**
   Refer to the hazard check list and Safety Data. Specify the nature of the harm and how it could occur e.g. a chemical could be strongly irritant if splashed into eyes. A wobbly gantry could cause serious injury if a person fell from it.
5. **To whom could they cause it?**
   List the people who work in the area regularly or occasionally. Specify the length of time that they are present in the area. Refer to the human factors for consideration and record any significant points.
6. **What precautions are currently taken?**
   See control options. List the physical and personal control measures and the management practices. If risk assessments have already been carried out for particular aspects of health and safety you do not need to repeat them but can refer to them e.g. Noise assessment carried out. Results recorded. Assessment is ear plugs must be, and are worn by all personnel present when hand feeding of the pigs takes place.
7. **What is the likelihood of harm occurring?**
   See risk rating. In the cases of dust, noise and slurry gases you will probably need to carry out personal monitoring to determine the levels of these hazards in order to assess likelihood.
8. **What would be the degree of the harm?**
   See risk rating. You will possibly need to refer to the hazard Safety Data and occupational health information to be able to judge this.
9. **What would be the consequential loss / cost?**
   See risk rating and cost benefits.
10. **What is the level of risk (priority for actions)?**
    See risk rating.

You have now identified and assessed the risks. The remaining two columns on the record sheet are for you to specify what you will do in order to eliminate or reduce those risks.

Procedure assessments

For each procedure to be assessed you should compile a record sheet of 12 columns with headings similar to those above except for questions 1, 2, 3 and 6. The information to be considered here and the points to record for each procedure are as for the area assessments with the exception of:

1. **What is the identity of the procedure?**
   Simply record the name of the procedure e.g. slurry channel drainage.
   If there is a written work instruction for the procedure you must refer to it here.
   If no work instruction exists you should include

2. **Where does this procedure take place?**
   Consult the list of areas to be assessed and note those where this procedure is performed. It may be useful to number all of the areas and simply record the relevant numbers here.
3. **What hazards are present?**
   See hazards and safety data. Carefully consider all categories of hazards. Use the hazard check list. List all the hazards (significant and trivial) associated with the procedure.
6. **What precautions are currently taken?**
   See control options. List the physical and personal control measures and the management practices.
   Specify whether any written work instructions are available for this procedure, and if so refer to them.

If risk assessments have already been carried out for particular aspects of health and safety you do not need to repeat them but can refer to them e.g. Hazardous substances assessment carried out. Results recorded. The assessment record and the work instructions specify the control measures.

They must be, and are always implemented by persons performing this procedure.

Self assessment by employees

No matter how thorough you are with your assessments, there will always be some situations that you cannot fully address until they arise and you cannot always be there when they do. Therefore, if you want the system to work you must also be able to rely on your employees to look out for the well-being of themselves and the well-being of the business as a whole. To achieve this you will need to demonstrate a positive, pro-active commitment to health and safety and encourage all employees to conduct their own risk assessments before carrying out any new activities. If they think that there is a risk to themselves or to others they should not continue with the activity but should inform you of their concerns so that you can fully assess the situation. This self assessment need not involve them having to write anything down but should be a simple 'stop and think' exercise.
For example:

1. What am I about to do? Where will I be doing it? How long will it take?
2. Do I know what hazards are present or will be produced?
3. Do I know what harm they could cause - and how?
4. Are sufficient safety precautions in place?
5. Is it safe for me (and those around me) if I continue?

If they cannot answer yes to all of the points 2-5, they should not continue.

Step 7 - Devise and Apply Your Control Measures

Control options

You must now decide how to eliminate or reduce the risks identified by your assessments and legislative and industry standards are likely to have a bearing on your selection of the appropriate control measures. There are a number of ways to control risks but legislation may, and often does, require you to adopt a hierarchical approach when deciding which control option to use. In other words you must consider the best (safest) option first and if that is not reasonably practicable you should consider the next best - and so on. Once again, if other pig producers are controlling specific risks by using control measures higher up the hierarchical scale than you are, you should review your situation.

Some aspects of health and safety are governed by regulations that state precisely what controls measures must be applied. You must be aware of any that apply to you (see step 2) and must obviously comply.

For other aspects of health and safety several regulations may apply which have their own specific hierarchy of control measures to be considered. It is not possible to list all of the variations here but the general principles are explained below. Control measures are divided into two categories: physical controls, which are directed against the hazard itself, and personal controls, which apply to the people at risk of exposure to the hazard.

Physical Controls
These are usually the most effective and should be considered first.
In order of priority they are:
- Remove.
- Replace.
- Restrict.
- Reduce.

Remove the hazard completely by eliminating the task or making design or organisational changes. This is the most effective control measure. For example:
- Mechanise an activity to eliminate manual handling.
- Re-design a loading bay to avoid having to reverse vehicles.
- Repair floors to eliminate the trip hazard.
- Replace a flammable solvent based paint with a non-flammable water based paint.
- Replace an electric pressure washer with a diesel powered one to eliminate the risk of electric shock.
- Replace a diesel powered pressure washer with an electric one to eliminate hazardous exhaust fumes.

This last example is to illustrate the point that eliminating one hazard may mean that a different one will have to be assessed.

Replace the hazard with one that is less hazardous. This is different from removal (and less effective) as the same type of hazard is still present but the likelihood of an event or its consequences are reduced. For example:

- Replace a disinfectant that is highly caustic to skin and eyes with one that is only a mild irritant.
- Replace a highly flammable solvent based paint with one that is less flammable.
- Replace an aggressive sow with one that is docile.

Restrict access to the hazard by physical means. For example:
- Put guards on dangerous parts of machinery.
- Put barriers around hazards such as machinery and slurry pit openings.
- Put guard rails on raised gantries.
- Fit an automatic lock out so that the auger cannot be accessed until it has stopped rotating.

Reduce the level of the hazard or the duration of exposure to it by physical means. For example:
- Use dust extracted straw for bedding to reduce dust levels.
- Fit a residual current device to electrical equipment.
- Store sacks of feed closer to the points of use to reduce the amount of carrying involved.
- Fit baffles or box-in noisy machinery (feed milling and bagging plant) to reduce the level of noise.

Personal Controls

These will be required in all cases in addition to the physical controls.

Such personal controls may include:
- Training.
- Instructions.
- Information.
- Supervision.
- Permits to work.
- Protective devices.
- Personal protective equipment.

Training, instructions and information - must be provided for all employees by law in most countries but many employers are unsure of the distinction between the three terms.

Training can be considered to have been sufficient once a person is judged to be competent to perform a task safely without supervision.

Instructions may be written or verbal and usually consists of a list of the steps to take to complete a task (i.e. work instructions) or a statement that a specific control must be implemented (e.g. switch off the power before opening the cover of the auger).

Information must be given regarding the hazards and risks that the employees may be exposed to in an area of the pig farm or when performing particular tasks. For example the nature of any hazardous chemicals involved (caustic, irritant, toxic, etc.), how the chemicals can cause harm (by ingestion, inhalation, skin contact, etc.), what level of risk is associated with the chemicals in particular areas or situations, how to prevent or minimise exposure to them and what to do in the event of accidental exposure.

Employees must also be provided with information regarding accident, first aid, fire and emergency procedures.

When assessing risks and evaluating control measures the existing standards of employee training, instruction and information must be considered.

Supervision - of all new employees and of existing employees undertaking new tasks must be carried out and must be sufficient for the employer to determine whether the procedures arc always performed safely, or whether additional training, instructions, information and supervision is needed.

Permits to work - are documents that must be obtained by an employee or contractor before certain works can be carried out. The permit must state that the necessary controls have been implemented and that it is safe to proceed with the work. In many countries it is a legal obligation to operate a permit to work system for certain activities. You must check how your regulations apply to you.

Even if it is not a legal requirement it is sensible to operate your own permit to work systems for high risk activities. These need not necessarily be written documents but could include, for example, a stipulation in the work instructions that the employee must obtain permission before starting a given job so that somebody is aware that the activity is about to take place and can implement the appropriate controls or simply be standing by e.g. fumigation using formalin. Other situations where such a permit system may be required are high voltage electrical work and entry into confined spaces e.g. slurry pits and feed silos.

Protective devices - can be used by a person to reduce the likelihood of a harmful event. An example is the use of a pig board.

Personal protective equipment (PPE) - includes such items as ear defenders, hard hats, dust masks, respirators, eye shields, gloves, boots, coveralls, waterproof aprons and washing facilities.

Coveralls, boots and gloves are obviously essential items for pig farmers and should be used routinely which they generally are. Other items of PPE are often used inappropriately, incorrectly or insufficiently.

Each situation needs to be carefully assessed. The important points to consider are:
- Legislation usually demands that PPE must be the last control option and should only be used if exposure to hazards cannot be controlled by any other reasonably practicable means.
- PPE can itself be a hazard. Dust masks for example make breathing laboured and can put unnecessary strain on the heart and lungs. Ear plugs may mean that audible safety warnings such as fire alarms are less effective.
- The item of PPE used must be appropriate for the level and type of hazard. Nuisance dust masks afford little protection. A mask that is adequate for general piggery dust is unlikely to be adequate for dust that could contain antibiotics (medicated feed). Different types of mask will be required for aqueous mists (e.g. from

pressure washers), slurry gases and welding fumes - all common hazards. Ear plugs and ear defenders come in grades appropriate for the level and type of noise.
- PPE can be used as a stop gap to reduce a known risk until it is reasonably practicable to implement a more effective control.
- Only use PPE that has official approval (all PPE in Europe must be CE marked).
- PPE can lead to a false sense of security. Employees must be instructed to continue to take due care.
- PPE is ineffective and possibly hazardous if badly fitted. Dust masks and ear plugs must be close fitting.
- Oversize gloves can result in clumsy handling of hazards. Oversize boots are a potential trip hazard.
- PPE is ineffective and possibly hazardous if damaged, dirty or worn out. Employees must be instructed in the use and care of PPE.

Once you have considered the control options you can complete the last two columns on your assessment record sheets i.e.:

11. **What measures will be implemented to control the risk?**
    Specify the physical and personal controls you think are appropriate.
12. **What management procedures are needed to ensure the controls are maintained?**
    This section should specify, what if anything, is needed in terms of a staff training programme, spot checks. machinery, service contracts, health surveillance schemes, assigning responsibilities, safety audit and review systems, etc.

Records

Record keeping requirements can arise in relation to a wide range of health and safety issues. In many cases specific risk assessments must by law be documented but a number of other records should also be kept. They are an additional control measure in that they serve as reminder that things need to be done, they facilitate auditing and reviews and demonstrate your due diligence.

You therefore need to decide what records are applicable to your situation.

Some examples of the types of records that may be needed are given below. This list is by no means complete and you should compile your own up to date version.

1. Organisation / administration - appointment of competent persons; policy changes.
2. Training - official health and safety qualifications; in-house training (re: SSW's, risk assessment procedures); assessment of competence for tasks; specific health and safety instruction courses e.g. pesticides, tractors, forklift trucks, etc.
3. Employment and occupational health records - pre-employment and on-going health surveillance; permits to work e.g. confined spaces.
4. Monitoring survey results - dust, noise, slurry gases.
5. Personal protective equipment (PPE) - PPE issue notes; examination records; test certificates.
6. Fire and emergency - alarm tests; fire drills; fire extinguisher / sprinkler system checks; staff training.
7. Work equipment - machinery and equipment inventories; routine safety checks; certification; guard checks
8. Buildings and services - inspection of electrical installation; water treatments; construction and design safety plans; assembly / removal by competent persons e.g. asbestos work; contractors declarations.
9. Risk assessments - hazardous substances, noise, manual handling; management of health and safety.
10. Accidents and incidents - accidents and incident reports (official and in-house); first aid treatments; follow up actions.

Safe Systems of Work (SSW's)

All of the components of your risk assessments and management procedures can now be combined into a series of working documents - the Safe Systems of Work (SSW's).

Step 8 - Document Your Safe Systems of Work (SSW's)

The assessment process should have identified the things that need to be done. The management procedures should ensure that they are done. This combined health and safety working system is therefore designed to ensure your due diligence. In the event of an accident, if you cannot prove due diligence you will have little or no defence against legal action or civil claims.

The key points that should be incorporated into the SSW's are as follows:

The regulations

Each SSW should include a note of the Specific Regulations, ACOPs Industry Standards, etc. that apply to the particular aspect of health and safety covered (e.g. noise) and a brief description of what you are obliged to do to comply.

Policy statement

Your policy on the particular aspect of health and safety should be stated, along with who is responsible for ensuring that the policy is implemented.

Risk assessment

The significant findings of the risk assessments with regard to the specific topic should be noted and attention should be drawn to the detailed assessment records that are on file and who is required to read them. This will only apply to those employees who work in areas or carry out procedures that were assessed as presenting risks. The assessment records will mention any specific controls but the SSW should specify whether any general control measures are required (such as the provision of safety notices), when they will be implemented (priority rating) and what interim measures must be adopted. It should also specify any control measures already in place that must be complied with.

Instructions

The work instructions for specific procedures are not usually included on the same page but are referred to elsewhere - such as in a separate file of work instructions, on the assessment records or as laminated sheets that are on permanent display at the points of use. The work instructions specify the actual steps to take to perform a task safely. General safety points are usually included on the SSW and specify the codes of practice that all employees must adhere to in order to ensure that risks remain adequately controlled.

Records

The SSW should specify what records are to be kept e.g. personal monitoring records, work equipment inventories and inspection records, staff training in the correct use of PPE etc. and who should keep them, how, when and where.

Hazard and safety data information

Together with the information regarding legal obligations, responsibilities and employee duties, the nature of the hazard e.g. noise and how it can cause harm damage hearing, affect concentration, should also be described on the SSW. It should also contain references to any other information or safety data that is relevant or which may be needed for assessment purposes e.g. machinery and equipment literature that gives details of noise levels under different conditions.

The overall aim of this type of management system is to have a series of single documents, each one of which provides all of the key information about one aspect of health and safety. Everyone must be familiar with all of the SSW's.

Each SSW should clearly state where individual employees can find other information of relevance to them, for example specific work instructions, risk assessment records and safety data. In this way employees only have to read what directly applies to themselves.

Each SSW should also state when, how and by whom the necessary on-going safety checks, reassessments and audits will be carried out and the information updated and reviewed. These details should also be noted in a diary or on a year planner so that the people responsible can be reminded.

This type of system ensures that all aspects of health and safety have been appropriately addressed and enables you to demonstrate that they have been. It also makes safety inspections and audits very simple for you, external safety consultants and inspectors.

The UK example SSW for noise Fig.17-9 shows the type of information to be included. It is in a format that can be used for most health and safety topics and easily adapted to suit large or small organisations.

You should have SSW's for all aspects of health and safety that directly impact on you.

A list of farm topics for which you should have SSW's is given in Fig.17-10. This list is not exhaustive and you will need to compile your own.

Step 9 - Document Your Accident, First Aid, Fire and Emergency Procedures.

Most countries have their own regulations concerning these including the assessment, staff instruction, recording and reporting duties of employers.

In effect, safe systems of work are also needed for these topics but because of their importance and to comply with the regulations, the information needs to be presented in a different format.

Accidents

Legislation sets out an employer's legal obligations for reporting accidents and dangerous occurrences to the Enforcing Authorities. In the UK this is covered by the **Reporting of Injuries, Diseases and Dangerous Occurrences Regulations 1995 (RIDDOR).** As defined in your policy statement, it is a key function of the safety manager to ensure that these obligations are fulfilled.

It is also important to compile your own accident and incident statistics and to review these periodically to determine what steps, if any, should be taken to prevent recurrence in the future. These reviews should also be coupled with health surveillance and be incorporated into risk assessments so that any control measures needed can be identified and given the necessary priority.

You should document and prominently display "The procedures to be followed in the event of an accident at work". The information should include:

- Accident reporting procedures to inform the safety manager and the enforcement authority and to record all accidents even minor ones, in the accident book.
- How to summon first aid assistance.
- The location of the first aid boxes.
- The telephone numbers of local doctors, hospitals and emergency services.

First aid

You may need to seek advice regarding what you are obliged to provide in terms of first aid facilities. Some authorities stipulate that there must be a qualified first aider on site (no matter how few people you employ) and there may be specific requirements concerning the number and location of first aid boxes, eye wash stations, signs, posters and rest room facilities.

Fire

You must obviously ensure that your fire precautions and procedures are adequate in terms of:

- Building construction.
- Access and egress.
- Emergency exits.
- Emergency lighting.
- Fire fighting appliances (sufficient, appropriate and maintained).
- Fire drills and alarm checks.
- Storage of flammable/combustible materials (gas cyl-

> **EXAMPLE SAFE SYSTEM OF WORK**
> **for**
> **NOISE**
> The Management of Health and Safety at Work Regulations 1992 - Regulation 3
> The Noise at Work Regulations 1989
>
> - Prolonged exposure to loud noise can damage hearing (hearing loss, tinnitus, etc.) but the effects are often not apparent until much later in life. Continual exposure to "nuisance" noise can cause stress and/or affect concentration. This may result in risks to individuals and also to those affected by their actions.
> - To comply with the above regulations we have a duty to assess the levels of noise to which staff are exposed, and to take steps to reduce or control the noise or exposure if necessary.
> - Any areas and procedures on the farm that have been identified as presenting a possible risk to health from noise will be fully assessed.
>   - Any noise monitoring required will be carried out by
>   - The results of any noise monitoring surveys will be recorded and filed in
>   - The results of the assessments will be recorded and made known to all relevant staff.
>   - Any remedial actions considered necessary will be implemented as soon as is practicable.
>   - Assessments will be reviewed annually, or as necessary, by
> - The noise contributed by machinery and equipment must be included in the assessments (worn machinery may become noisier and new machinery must meet noise specifications).
>   - For further information regarding machinery assessors must see the Work Equipment SSW.
> - Listed below are some specific areas and procedures associated with the farm which can expose staff to high or nuisance noise levels.
>
> **If any of them apply to you, you must read:**
>   - the specific **Area or Procedure Assessment** record (filed in ....)
>   - the relevant procedure **Work Instructions** (in the Work Instructions Manual and on display).
>
> | **AREAS** | **PROCEDURES** |
> |---|---|
> | Feed Mill | Feed Mill Operation |
> | .... | Hand Feeding of Pigs |
> | .... | .... |
> | .... | .... |
>
> **IN GENERAL** - all staff must adhere to the following Codes of Practice:
> 1. If normal conversation is difficult to hear across a distance of two metres, for significant periods of time, the background noise levels may be above acceptable limits and may present a risk of damage to your hearing.
>   - If in doubt consult the Area Safety Officer. Ear protection will be made available if needed.
> 2. Repetitive background noise (maintenance work etc.) can result in loss of concentration and is therefore a safety hazard.
>   - Individual staff and particularly Area Safety Officers should assess the potential risks in each situation and implement control measures (turn off the noise if possible, stop maintenance work for set periods, use ear protection) as necessary.
> 3. The pigs can create high noise levels a certain times (feeding, weighing, bleeding).
>   - Staff exposed to these conditions for significant periods should assess the situation and use ear plugs or defenders as necessary. Seek advice if you are unsure.
> 4. All situations will be assessed at least annually, but if you consider any area, equipment or procedure on the farm to be 'noisy' you must inform the Area Safety Officer so that an assessment can be made sooner and the appropriate controls implemented.
> 5. Some areas of the farm present a definite risk to hearing and have been designated as **"Hearing Protection Zones"**. Safety signs are displayed on the doors to these areas.
>   - **All persons MUST wear hearing protection in these areas - at all times or as instructed.**
>   - Ear defenders are available in these areas. Extra ear plugs are kept in
> 6. Before using ear protection you must be familiar with the SSW for Personal Protective Equipment.

(Fig.17-9)

inders, fuel oils, wood and paper waste).
- Identification of fire / explosion risk areas and instructions for isolating power, fuel, gas etc.
- Evacuation procedures and responsibility for roll calls.
- Employee training in procedures and general fire safety practices.

It is wise to obtain guidance from your Local Authority fire service on these matters. Once you have established appropriate facilities, systems and procedures you should document them and have the notice prominently displayed. As mentioned earlier, it is also useful to have a plan of your premises which clearly shows the sites of fire hazards (fuel stores etc.), fire extinguishers and escape routes.

Your fire procedures can also include details of the arrangements for evacuation or protection of the pigs but it must be made clear that personal safety must be the primary concern of all employees.

Emergencies

Similar procedures to those for accidents and fire are required for emergencies, to cover such events as gas leaks, explosions, pressure vessel rupture, building collapse and chemical leaks.

Step 10 - Review Your System Periodically

Once your health and safety working system has been developed and implemented you will need to review it periodically. The more comprehensive your written SSW's and records are, the easier this will be. Reviews serve three important purposes:

1. To comply and keep up to date with legislation

Many health and safety regulations stipulate that risk assessments, monitoring results and equipment checks etc. must be reviewed at specific intervals and whenever you make any significant changes. You will need to be aware of those that apply to you. Changes in the legislation or hazard safety data may also mean that assessments will have to be amended. For example, the significance of endotoxins in piggery dust is being investigated and the findings may result in lower occupational exposure limits being set.

In general you should review your risk assessment records at least annually and as and when you introduce changes such as new areas, procedures, staff or hazards. Once your initial assessments have been revised to take account of any new control measures most records will hopefully not require further amendments, but you should still document the fact that you have checked them and that they are still valid.

If you have introduced any changes you must re-assess the relevant areas and procedures, and revise the existing records or compile new ones. For example, if you have an outbreak of salmonella in pigs in the finisher / grower house, you may need to introduce additional controls to minimise the risk of employees contacting or transmitting the disease. The new controls must be documented on the assessment record and brought to the attention of the employees.

You must also review your risk assessments if circumstances suggest that problems are occurring. For example, you may have assessed the risks associated with dust in the pig houses to be low (providing your specified control measures are implemented) but find that employees still suffer from, or begin to suffer from, respiratory problems. This may be due to an incorrect assessment originally, or because a change has gone unnoticed e.g. a different type of feed or bedding perhaps. Whatever the reason you will need to investigate and re-assess.

2. To monitor and improve the system

As with all management practices it is necessary to check whether the system is working effectively, or if it should be improved.

For example, your SSW's may specify that something is to be inspected by somebody at given times and

FARM TOPICS YOU SHOULD HAVE SSW's FOR	
Abrasive wheels	Personal hygiene.
Accident prevention	Personal monitoring.
Animal handling	Personal protective equipment.
Asbestos (roofing & insulation)	Personal safety and security.
Cleaning	Pesticides.
Compressed gas cylinders	Post-mortems.
Confined spaces.	Pregnant women.
Construction.	Pressure systems.
Contractors.	PTO shafts.
Dust.	Public access.
Electrical safety.	Roof work.
Environmental monitoring.	Safety signs.
Fire prevention.	Slurry gases.
Handling of animals.	Stairways.
Hazardous chemicals.	Tractor safety.
Hostile environments.	Training.
Ladders.	Vehicles.
Lift trucks.	Veterinary medicines.
Manual handling.	Visitors.
New employees / trainees.	Waste disposal.
Noise.	Work environment.
Occupational health.	Work equipment.
Overhead power lines.	Working alone..
Pathological specimens sent by post.	Young people/children
Permits to work.	

(Fig.17-10)

that the results are to be recorded. If your review of the system shows that the inspection is not being carried out or that the results are not being recorded you will need to revise the system. It may be that the person is not aware of their responsibility to perform the task, does not appreciate the importance of it, or does not have enough time to do it.

The solution may be to leave the SSW unchanged but to re-train the individual concerned, emphasise the importance of the task and / or make more time available for them to do it.

Alternatively the responsibility for the task may have to be assigned to somebody else and the SSW should be re-written accordingly.

3. To demonstrate your commitment to health and safety

If you want the system to work and for everyone to play their part you must convince all concerned that you will continually check it and make changes as necessary. Formal reviews will achieve this. If however, it is seen as simply a one off paper exercise with no follow up, it will not be taken seriously and the time and effort spent developing the system will have been wasted.

If you think all of this is too much (and for the small business it invariably is) use the services of a competent organisation that specialises in health and safety in your country. It will save you considerable time and effort and allow you to concentrate on what you are good at - pig production. Salus QP Ltd can provide this service.

Chapter 17

Managing Pig Health and the Treatment of Disease

CHAPTER 17 - Health and Safety

Chapter 17

APPENDIX

Quick References and Useful Information

Further reading - references and information 580
Product references 582
Equipment, materials, medicines and chemicals you may require on the
farm for maintaining health and controlling disease 583
    Equipment and materials 583
    Chemicals 583
    Antibiotics and antibacterial substances 584
    Sedatives 584
    Anti-inflammatory injections 584
    Anthelmintics 584
    Coccidiostats 584
    Hormones 584
    Action on the uterus 584
    Nutrition and metabolism 585
    Parasecticides - topical use 585
    Miscellaneous substances 585
    Mating to farrowing date indicator 585
Physiological data 586
    Blood sampling requirements for serological tests 586
    Semen 586
    Urine 586
    Haematology SI (standard international) 586
    Temperature, respiration, pulse rates 586
    Enzyme tests in serum or plasma. International units (i.u.) 586
    Biochemistry 586
    Sampling herds to detect evidence of infection 587
        95% confidence limit 587
        99% confidence limit 587
Units of measurement used in biological science 587
    Metric units and relative values 587
    How to convert units of measurements 588
Quick conversion tables 588
    Length - inches - millimetres - centimetres 588
    Length - miles - kilometres 589
    Length - feet - yards - metres 589
    Weight - pounds - kilograms 589
    Area - square feet - square metres 589
    Volume (imperial) - pints - gallons - litres 590
    Temperature conversion °C - °F 590
Growth 591
    Calculating days to slaughter (growth rate unknown) 591
    Effect of variable growth rate on days to slaughter 591
    The possible effects of feed changes on the growing pig 591

Further Reading - References and Information

A Colour Atlas of Disease of the Pig, Smith, Taylor and Penny. Wolf Publishing Ltd, London, UK.
A Handbook of Breeds of the World, Porter, Valerie. *Pigs*: Helm Information, E. Sussex, UK.
Anaporc, Prodive, S.A. Adpo 140 28820 Coslada, Madrid, Spain
Animal Breeding and Infertility, Meredith, M. J., Blackwell Science Ltd, Cambridge, USA.
Control of Pig Production, Foxcroft Hunter Doberska, The Journals of Reproduction and Fertility Ltd, Henry Ling Ltd, Dorset, UK.
Depopulation and Repopulation, 5M Enterprises, PO Box 233, Sheffield UK.
Diseases of Swine, Iowa State University Press, Ames, Iowa USA.
Effects of Draughts as Climatic Stress on the Health Status of Weaned Pigs, Schaepens, C., Faculty of Veterinary Science, University of Utrecht, Netherlands.
Essentials of Pig Anatomy, Sack Veterinary Text Books, New York, USA.
Feed Compounder, HGM Publications, Derbyshire, UK.
Feed International, Watt Publishing Co. Illinois, USA.
Growth of the Pig, Hollis, G, CAB International, Oxon, UK.
Housing the Pig, Brent, G. Farming Press Books Ipswich UK.
Intensive Pig Production Environmental Management and Design, Baxter, Granada Publishing Ltd, London, UK.
International Pig Veterinary Proceedings, Biannual Congress, 1984 Ghent, 1986 Barcelona, 1988 Rio de Janeiro, 1990 ,Lausanne 1992 The Hague, 1994 Bangkok, 1996 Thailand, 1998 Birmingham,UK, 2000 Brisbane.
International Pigletter, Pig World Inc. Owatanna, Minneapolis 55060, USA.
Manual of Pig Production in the Tropics, CAB International, Oxfordshire, UK.
Meat and Livestock Commission Pig Year Book 1997, Milton Keynes, UK.
National Hog Farmer, Intertec Publishing Corporation, USA.
Nutrient Requirements of Swine, National Academy Press, Washington D.C., USA.
Outdoor Pig Production, Thornton, Keith. Farming Press Books, Ipswich, UK.
Outdoor Pigs. Principles and Practice, Stark, Machin and Wilkinson. Chalcombe Publications, Bucks, UK.
Pet Pigs. Advice on Management Training and Health Care, Walton, Carr and Duran. Liverpool University Press, Liverpool, UK.
Pig Diseases, Taylor D, St. Edmundsbury Press, Bury, St. Edmunds, Suffolk, UK.
Pig Farming, Farming Press, Ipswich, UK.
Pig Industry British Pig Association, BC Publications, Suffolk, UK.
Pig International, Watt Publishing Co. Mt Morris, Illinois 61054, USA.
Pig Management Yearbook, PIC UK. *Easicare and Pigtales Data*, Oxfordshire, UK.
Pig News and Information, CAB International, Oxon, UK.
Pig Production in Australia, Gardner Dunkin Lloyd, Butterworths, Sydney, London, Boston, Toronto.
Pig World, Lincoln, UK.
Pigs, Misset International, The Netherlands.
Pork Journal, Milne, Richard. Pty Ltd, Pyrmont, NSW, Australia.
Pork Producer, Ontario, Canada.
Pork Report, National Pork Producers Council, Des Moines, Indianapolis, USA.
Swine Housing and Equipment Handbook, Watt Trade Press, Mt Morris, Illinois 61054
Swine Nutrition Guide, Patience, J.F., and Thacker, P.A., Prairie Swine Centre, University of Saskatchewan, Canada.
Swine Production and Nutrition, Pond and Manner. AVI Publishing Co. Inc., Connecticut, USA.
The Economics of Pig Production, Ridgeon, R., Farming Press Books, Ipswich, UK.
The Growing and Finishing Pig. Improving Efficiency, Baxter, S., English, P., Fowler, V., Smith, W., Farming Press Books, Ipswich, UK. Diamond Farm Enterprises, New York, USA.
The Nutrient Requirements of Pigs, Commonwealth Agricultural Bureaux, Slough, UK.
The Pig Journal, The Grove Centre, Malmesbury, Wiltshire, UK.
The Science and Practice of Pig Production, Whittemore, C. Longman Group UK Ltd, Essex, UK.
The Swine AI Book, Morrow, Morgan., Department of Animal Science, North Carolina, USA.
Welfare Aspects of Pig Rearing, Marx Grauvogi Smidt, Commission of the European Communities, Luxembourg.
Wild Pigs in the USA, Mayer and Brisbin. University of Georgia Press, Georgia, USA.

You are now reading one of the best sources of information you'll find anywhere. Care to see another?

The International Pigletter, the swine industry's leader for objective, cutting edge, practical information, is now even better. Recently redesigned and expanded, Pigletter gives you information you won't find in any other pig publication. Access the latest insights of industry leaders from around the world, our articles are written by the experts themselves. Join us and you too, will have access to exclusive information that will make a difference. Published monthly.

Pigletter is pleased to offer a variety of educational tools to help you achieve your objectives. From Australia, we bring you comprehensive training packages (video, audio, print, diskette). Ask us about "The Good Health Manual", "Mating and Reproduction", or "The Managers Toolbox" and we'll send you more information. For on-farm training, we offer "The Basic" video series. For the latest in swine health management on audiotape, our "Conversation Series" brings you lively discussion from the experts. To subscribe to the Pigletter or receive more information about our educational tools, fax us a 507-444-9520. Be sure and ask about PigCHAMP® and Growthmaster or visit our web site at http://www.holoweb.com/pigworld

201 North Oak Avenue, #312, Owatonna, MN, USA 55060
Ph/Fax 507-444-9520   email: pigworld@ic.owatonna.mn.us

International PIGLETTER

Facts and opinions from around the world

Now you have a wealth of expert advice and information - All you need is the time to implement it!

But when you are working 25 hours a day some things get put off until tomorrow... and tomorrow..

Looking after the health of your pigs and profits will be taking up most of your time, so its likely that even with the best intentions taking care of your own health and safety is way down you list of priorities. But after talking to Salus many pig farmers and veterinarians have found that managing health and safety doesn't have to be a time consuming no return activity - it can be straight forward and bring real benefits.

If you would like to know more contact us at the address below.

While you are taking care of your pigs,   whose taking care of you?

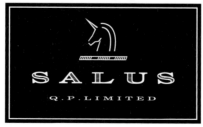

Salus (Quality Partnerships) Limited
97a Main Street, Beeford, East Yorkshire, UK, Y025 8AY
Tel: +44 (0) 1262 488 175, Fax: +44 (0) 1262 488 635 e-mail: garth@garth.demon.co.uk

Product References - as Noted in the Book

Many companies have subsidiaries or agents world wide. Most products are trade marked.

AI equipment Tail docker	Kruuze Byvej 35, DK-5290, Marsler, Denmark.
Anenometer	Hyper-Per-Graph Ltd. Unit 8, West End Industrial Estate, Bruntcliffe Road, Morley, Leeds UK LS27 0JZ.
Breeding equipment	Roteck Breeding Equipment Ltd. Appledram Barns, Birdham Rd, Chichester, W. Sussex, UK PO20 7EQ.
Burdizzo castrator	Cox Equipment Surrey, UK.
Carbon dioxide smoke tablets	Smoke Products Ltd Glen View Road, Eldwick, Bingley, West Yorkshire UK BD16 3EF.
Döppler pregnancy testing equipment	Medata Systems Ltd Old Bilsham Farm, Bilsham Lane, Yapton, Arundel, West Sussex, UK BN18 0JX.
Dust monitoring equipment	Cassella Ltd. London UK.
Ear tags	Ketchum Manufacturing Co. Tadworth, Coulsdon, Surrey, UK KT20 5RE.
Fly control - Biological Health and Safety	Salus QP Ltd. Salus House, Beeford, Driffield, UK YO25 8AY.
Fly control products Alfradex, Alfracon, Neporex, Nurvanol	CIBA-GEIGY Ltd. Basle, Switzerland.
Fly control products Methomyl (Golden malrin)	Sanofi Animal Health. 7 Awberry Court, Hatters Lane, Watford, UK WD1 BYJ.
Fly control products Pyrethrins, Turbair	Pan Britannica Industries Ltd. Waltham Cross, Herts, UK
Gas detectors - Kitagawa	Komyo Nikagaku Kogkokk, Japan.
Hibiscrub	Zeneca Ltd. Macclesfield, Cheshire, UK.
Injector - automatic	Simcrovac Automatic Injector. Solvay Duphar Veterinary. Southampton, UK.
KY Jelly	Johnson and Johnson Airlington, Texas 76004
Lice Control Deltamethrin (Coopers spot-on)	Pitman Moore Ltd. Crew Hall, Crew, Cheshire, UK CW1 1YR
OO-CIDE	Antec International Ltd. Windham Road, Chilton Industrial Estate, Sudbury, Suffolk, UK CO30 6XD.
Pig breeding calendar - Bray	Cox Equipment Surrey, UK
Savlon	Zeneca Ltd. Macclesfield, Cheshire, UK.
Surgical blades	Swan Morton Ltd. Sheffield, UK S6 2BJ.
Suture materials - Braun	B. Braun. Melsungen AG, Melsungen D43709, Germany.
Sutures - Catgut	SMI AG. 4784, Hunnigen 37, Belgium.
Sutures - Supramid	Ethicon Ltd. PO Box 408, Bankhead Avenue, Edinburgh, UK EH11 4HE.
Syringes - metermatic	Alstoe Animal Health. Alstoe Ltd PO Box 5, Oakham Road, Leicester, UK LE15 7ZU.
Syringes - monoject, needles	Sherwood Medical. St Louis, MO 63103, USA
Tags - Allflex	Cox Equipment Edward Road, Coulsdon, Surrey, UK CR5 2XA.
Tags - Jumbo, Rota	Dalton Supplies Ltd. Nettlebed, Henley-on-Thames, Oxon, UK RG9 5AB.
Tattooing equipment and inks.	Ketchum Manufacturing Co. Tadworth, Coulsdon, Surrey, UK KT20 5RE.
Temperature data loggers -Tiny Talk.	Gemini Data Loggers (UK) Ltd. Orion Companies Chichester, West Sussex, UK PO19 2UJ.
Vacutainers and needles.	Becton Dickinson UK Ltd, Cowley, Oxon OX4 3LW.
Virkon S Virudine	Antec International Ltd. Windham Road, Chilton Industrial Estate, Sudbury, Suffolk, UK CO30 6XD.

Appendix

Equipment, Materials Chemicals and Medicines you may Require on the Farm for Maintaining Health and Controlling Disease

EQUIPMENT AND MATERIALS	
AI catheters disposable.	Nasal swabs.
AI cattle catheters disposable.	Navel clips.
AI equipment.	Needles 20g 16mm, and 25mm, 18g 38mm, 18g 50mm, 16g 100mm.
Antiseptic for skin use - Savlon, Cetrimide.	Paper tissues.
Bandages - tubular, elastoplast, white and adhesive tape.	Paper towels.
Capture bolt pistol or 12 bore shot gun.	Pithing rod.
Corrugated plastic tubing for treating a prolapsed rectum.	Plastic bags.
Cotton wool.	Post-mortem knife.
Detailing equipment - knife, scissors, burdizzo or gas.	Pressure washer.
Detergent.	Rectal thermometers.
Disinfectant for aerosal use.	Rubber gloves.
Disinfectant for surfaces.	Scissors - pair tissue forceps, 2 pairs artery forceps.
Disinfectant or foot baths.	Snare or wire noose.
Disposable gloves.	Surgical blades (handle).
Döppler pregnancy tester and coupling liquid.	Surgical spirit.
Dust masks.	Suture materials.
Ear muffs.	Suture needles.
Embryotomy wire.	Suture tape.
Eye protectors.	Swabs in transport medium.
First aid box.	Syringes 2 - 5 - 10 - 20 - 30ml.
Flutter valve.	Tattoo equipment - slap marker, tattoo pastes, tags, ink pad, ear notchers
Hoof cutters.	Teeth clippers.
Indelible marker pen.	Temperature electronic recorder.
KY jelly.	Thermometer - maximum minimum.
Labels self adhesive.	Tissues.
Liquidiser.	Vacutainers.
Marker sprays, wax crayons.	Water steriliser.
Mouth gag.	

CHEMICALS	
Aerosol disinfectant (Virkon S)	Obstetrical fluid
Dehydrated lime powder	OO-CIDE
Detergent	Organophosphorus (Alfracon)
Fenitrothion (Durakil)	Potassium permanganate
Fly control	Pyrethrins (Alfradex, Turbair)
Foot bath disinfectants (Virudine)	Savlon or cetrimide skin disinfectant
Formaldehyde 40%	Surface disinfectants
KY or AI lubricants	Surgical spirit
Methomyl (Golden Malrin)	Water steriliser

Medicines

(As advised by your veterinarian)

The active or generic names are given and an example of a commercial product (™). There are many similar products available.

ANTIBIOTICS AND ANTIBACTERIAL SUBSTANCES	
Injectable	Oral and / or in-feed
Amoxycillin (Amoxypen). Ampicillin (Penbritin). Apramycin (Apralan). Baquiloprim (Zaqualan). Ceftiofur (Excenel). Cephalexin (Ceporex). Enrofloxacin (Baytril). Erythromycin (Erythrocin). Framycetin (Framomycin). Gentamycin (Pangram). Griseofulvin (Griseovin). Lincomycin (Lincocin). Neomycin (Neobiotic). Oxytetracycline (Terramycin). Penicillin (Depocillin). Spectinomycin (Spectam). Streptomycin (Devomycin). Sulphadiazine. Sulphadimidine (Vesadin). Tiamulin (Tiamutin). Trimethoprim / Sulpha (Borgal). Tylosin (Tylan).	Chlortetracycline (Aureomycin). Enrofloxacin. Griseofulvin. Lincomycin spectinomycin (Lincospectam). Lincomycin. Neomycin. Nitrofurans (Neftin). Oxytetracycline. Phenoxymethyl penicillin. Sulphonamides. Tilmycosin (Pulmotil). Trimethoprim sulphonamides. Tylosin.

SEDATIVES	
Acetyl promazine - injection. Azaperone (Stresnil) - injection.	Primidone (Mysoline) - tablets.

ANTI-INFLAMMATORY INJECTIONS	
Betamethasone (Betosolan). Dexamethasone (Dexafort).	Flunixin (Finadyne). Phenylbutazone (Phenyzene).

ANTHELMINTICS	
Doramectin (Dectomax). Fenbental (Bayverm). Fenbenazole (Panacur). Flubendazole (Flubenol). Ivermectin (Ivomec).	Levamisole (Many). Oxibendazole (Loditac). Piperazine (Same). Thiophanate (Nemafax).

COCCIDIOSTATS	
Amprolium (Amprol) Dimetridazole (Emtryl). Monensin (Elancoban).	Salinomycin (Salocin). Sulphonamides (Same). Toltrazuril (Baycox).

HORMONES	
Altrenogest (Regumate). Gonadotrophin (PG600).	Oestradiol benzoate (Same). Testosterone (Androject).

ACTION ON THE UTERUS	
Antibiotic pessaries (Many). Buscopan - pain relief. Monzaldon assists farrowings	Oxytocin - contraction. Pituitary extract - contraction Prostaglandins - induction of farrowing.

NUTRITION AND METABOLISM	
Calcium boroglucinate 40%. Dextrose. Electrolytes (Lectade, Iron-aid). Glucose 40%. Iron dextran (Leodex).	Multivitamins (Duphafral). Respirot - oral respiratory stimulant. Vitamin E / selenium (Dystosel). Vitamin minerals (Duphasol).

PARASECTICIDES - TOPICAL USE	
Amitraz (Taktic, Topline - mange). Deltamethrin (Coopers spot-on lice).	Diazinon - mange. Phosmet (Porect - mange)

MISCELLANEOUS SUBSTANCES	
Liquid paraffin.	

MATING TO FARROWING DATE INDICATOR

Date of Service	Expected Date of Farrowing	Date of Service	Expected Date of Farrowing
Jan 1	Apr 25	Jul 5	Oct 27
6	30	10	Nov 1
11	May 5	15	6
16	10	20	11
21	15	25	16
26	20	30	21
31	25	Aug 4	26
Feb 5	30	9	Dec 1
10	Jun 4	14	6
15	9	19	11
20	14	24	16
25	19	29	21
Mar 2	24	Sep 3	26
7	29	8	31
12	Jul 4	13	Jan 5
17	9	18	10
22	14	23	15
27	19	28	20
Apr 1	24	Oct 3	25
6	29	8	30
11	Aug 3	13	Feb 4
16	8	18	9
21	13	23	14
26	18	28	19
May 1	23	Nov 2	24
6	28	7	Mar 1
11	Sep 2	12	6
16	7	17	11
21	12	22	16
26	17	27	21
31	22	Dec 2	26
Jun 5	27	7	31
10	Oct 2	12	Apr 5
15	7	17	10
20	12	22	15
25	17	27	20
30	22		

Physiological Data

BLOOD SAMPLING REQUIREMENTS FOR SEROLOGICAL TESTS

Test	Sample Required	Minimum Sample Required	Anticoagulant Required
Bilirubin	Serum or plasma	1 ml	Heparin
Calcium	Serum or plasma	1 ml	
Chloride	Serum or plasma	1 ml	
Copper	Serum or plasma	1 ml	
Cortisone (cortisol)	Plasma	2 ml	Heparin or EDTA
Creatinine	Serum or plasma	1 ml	
Glucose	Blood	0.2 ml	Oxalate-fluoride
Haematological tests (PCV, Hb, RBC, WBC)	Blood	3 ml	EDTA
Inorganic phosphate	Serum or plasma	1 ml	Oxalate-fluoride or heparin
Iron	Serum or plasma	1 ml	
Lead	Blood	7-10 ml	Any lead free container
Magnesium	Serum or plasma	1 ml	
Platelets	Blood	1 ml	EDTA (not a Vacutainer)
Potassium	Serum or plasma	1 ml	
Protein (total, albumin or globulin)	Serum or plasma	5 ml per test	
Selenium	Blood	2 ml	Any
Enzymes	Serum or plasma	5 ml	For the (GSH-Px-test use whole blood - heparin)
Sodium	Serum or plasma	1 ml	
Urea	Serum or plasma	1 ml	
Zinc	Plasma	1 ml	Any one but avoid contact with rubber materials

SEMEN

Volume	50 - 400 ml - mean 250 ml
Colour	White cloudy
Consistency	Clear/Cloudy/gel
Motility	Active some wave motion
Sperm density	10^6 /100ml
pH	7.3 - 7.8

URINE

Volume l/day	2 - 6
Specific gravity	1.020 - 1.040
pH	6 - 8
Bilirubin	None
Blood	None
Glucose	None
Protein	None

BIOCHEMISTRY

Normal Ranges

		SI Units
Total Protein	g/l	60 - 80
Albumin	g/l	15 - 40
Globulin	g/l	25 - 50
Bilirubin	µmol/l	0.9 - 5.0
Calcium	mmol/l	2.0 - 3.8
Copper	µmol/l	10 - 30
Glucose	mmol/l	3.5 - 7.5
Inorganic phosphate	mmol/l	1.4 - 3.2
Iron	µmol/l	17 - 26
Lead	µmol/l	0.5 - 2.4
Magnesium	mmol/l	0.8 - 1.2
Potassium	mmol/l	4.0 - 5.5
Selenium	µmol/l	> 1.5
Vitamin E	µmol/l	> 2.3

HAEMATOLOGY SI (Standard International)

		Units	Normal Range
Red Cells	Numbers	$\times 10^{12}/l$	6.0 - 9.0
	Haemoglobin	g/dl	11.0 - 17.0
	Packed cell volume	l/l	0.37 - 0.5
White Cells	Numbers	$\times 10^9/l$	10 - 23
	Lymphocytes	$\times 10^9/l$	9.8 - 11.4
	Monocytes	$\times 10^9/l$	1.0 - 2.5
	Eosinophils	$\times 10^9/l$	0.8 - 1.0
	Basophils	$\times 10^9/l$	0.1 - 0.2
Platelets		$\times 10^9/l$	100 - 900

ENZYME TESTS IN SERUM OR PLASMA
INTERNATIONAL UNITS (i.u.)

Enzyme	Normal Range
ALT (GPT)	10 - 18
AP	10 - 50
AST (GOT)	10 - 50
CK	< 200
GSH - P x (iu/ml red cells)	> 10
Gamma GT	8 - 50
LD (LDH)	40 - 700
SDH	< 5.0

TEMPERATURE, RESPIRATION, PULSE RATES

Age/Weight	Rectal Temperature		Respiratory Rate	Pulse Rate
	°C	°F	(per minute)	(per minute)
At birth	39.0	102.0	40 - 50	200 - 250
During suckling	39.2	102.5	30 - 40	80 - 110
At weaning	39.3	102.7	25 - 35	80 - 100
25 - 45 kg	39.0	102.5	30 - 40	80 - 90
45 - 90 kg	38.8	101.8	30 - 40	75 - 85
Pregnant sow	38.6	101.6	15 - 20	70 - 80
During farrowing	39.0 - 40.0	102.0 - 104.0	40 - 50	80 - 100
During lactation	39.1	102.5	20-30	70 - 80
Boar	38.6	101.5	15 - 20	70 - 80

Appendix - Quick References and Useful Information

SAMPLING HERDS TO DETECT EVIDENCE OF INFECTION							
95% Confidence Limit							
Herd Size	Sample Size to detect > 1+ve Sensitivity (= % = +ve) = Prevalence						
	0.1	0.2	0.5	1	2	5	10	20
50	50	50	50	50	48	35	22	12
100	100	100	100	95	78	45	25	13
150	150	150	148	130	95	49	26	13
200	200	200	190	155	105	51	27	14
300	300	300	260	189	117	54	28	14
500	500	475	349	225	129	56	28	14
750	750	648	412	246	135	57	28	14
1000	950	777	450	258	138	57	29	14
1500	1279	947	493	271	142	58	29	14
2000	1553	1054	517	277	143	58	29	14
5000	2253	1294	564	290	147	59	29	14

| 99% Confidence Limit ||||||||
| Herd Size | Sample Size to detect > 1+ve Sensitivity (= % = +ve) = Prevalence |||||||
	0.1	0.2	0.5	1	2	5	10	20
50	50	50	50	50	50	42	29	17
100	100	100	100	99	90	59	36	19
150	150	150	150	143	117	68	38	20
200	200	200	198	180	136	73	40	20
300	300	300	286	235	160	78	41	20
500	500	495	420	300	183	83	42	21
750	750	715	530	343	197	85	43	21
1000	950	890	601	368	204	86	43	21
1500	1430	1177	687	395	212	88	44	21
2000	1800	1367	737	410	216	88	44	21
5000	3008	1844	840	438	223	89	44	21

Courtesy of J.T. Done.

Units of Measurement used in Biological Science

There are two methods used; the imperial system, also called the Foot Pound Second and the metric system, based upon the Centimetre Gram and Second. The metric system was modernised in 1960 and an international system of units (SI) agreed. This is now used throughout the world.

Most pig producing countries use the metric system but in some, part metric and part imperial are also used, for example in the USA.

This book uses the metric system throughout in the text but for ease of reference, some tables include imperial measurements.

| METRIC UNITS AND RELATIVE VALUES ||||
Weight	Volume	Length	Relationship
Gram (g)	Litre (l)	Metre (m)	1
Kilogram (kg)	Kilolitre (kl)	Kilometre (km)	1,000
Decigram (dg)	Decilitre (dl)	Decimetre (dm)	1/10
Centigram (cg)	Centilitre (cl)	Centimetre (cm)	1/100
Milligram (mg)	Millilitre (ml)	Millimetre (mm)	1/1,000
Microgram (ug or mcg)	Microlitre (ul)	Micrometre (um)	1/1,000,000
Nanogram (ng)	Nanolitre (nl)	Nanometre (nm)	1/1,000,000,000
Picogram (pg)	Picolitre (pl)	Picometre (pm)	1/1,000,000,000,000

( ) = abbreviations

Managing Pig Health and the Treatment of Disease

HOW TO CONVERT UNITS OF MEASUREMENTS

Imperial to Metric			Metric to Imperial		
To convert	into	multiply by	To convert	into	multiply by
Length			**Length**		
inches	millimetres	25.4	millimetres	inches	0.0394
inches	centimetres	2.54	centimetres	inches	0.0397
feet	metres	0.3048	metres	feet	3.2808
yards	metres	0.9144	metres	yards	1.0936
miles	kilometres	1.6093	kilometres	miles	0.6214
Area			**Area**		
square inches	square centimetres	6.4516	square centimetres	square inches	0.155
square feet	square metres	0.093	square metres	square feet	10.764
square yards	square metres	0.836	square metres	square yards	1.196
acres	hectares	0.405	hectares	acres	2.471
square miles	square kilometres	1.6093	square kilometres	square miles	0.386
Volume			**Volume**		
cubic inches	cubic centimetres	16.387	cubic centimetres	cubic inches	0.061
cubic feet	cubic metres	0.0283	cubic metres	cubic feet	35.315
cubic yards	cubic metres	0.7646	cubic metres	cubic yards	1.308
fluid ounces	millilitres	28.41	litres	pints	1.760
pints	litres	0.568	litres	gallons	0.220
gallons	litres	4.55			
Weight			**Weight**		
ounces	grams	28.35	grams	ounces	0.0352
pounds	kilograms	0.45359	kilograms	pounds	2.2046
tons	kilograms	1016.00	kilograms	tons	0.000984
tons	tonnes	1.016	tonnes	tons	0.9842

Quick Conversion Tables

LENGTH - Inches - Millimetres - Centimetres

Approximate 1 in = 25 mm (25.4 mm) 1 mm = $^1/_{32}$ in (0.039 in)
= 2.5 cm (2.54cm) 1 cm = $^2/_5$ in (0.393 in)
(Exact values)

Inches	↔	Millimetres	Inches	↔	Centimetres
	$^1/_4$	6.4		$^1/_4$	0.6
	$^1/_2$	12.7		$^1/_2$	1.3
	$^3/_4$	19.0		$^3/_4$	1.9
0.04	1	25.4	0.39	1	2.5
0.08	2	50.8	0.79	2	5.1
0.12	3	76.2	1.18	3	7.6
0.16	4	101.6	1.57	4	10.2
0.20	5	127.0	1.97	5	12.7
0.24	6	152.4	2.36	6	15.2
0.28	7	177.8	2.76	7	17.8
0.31	8	203.2	3.15	8	20.3
0.35	9	228.6	3.54	9	22.9
0.39	10	254.0	3.94	10	25.4
0.43	11	279.4	4.34	11	27.9
0.47	12	304.8	4.72	12	30.5

LENGTH - Feet - Yards - Metres

1ft = 0.3 m (0.3048)   1m = 3ft $^3/_8$in (3.2808 ft)
1yd = 0.9m (0.9144)   1m = 1yd 3in (1.0936 yds)

Feet	↔	Metres	Yard	↔	Metres
3.3	1	0.3	1.1	1	0.9
6.6	2	0.6	2.2	2	1.8
9.8	3	0.9	3.3	3	2.7
13.1	4	1.2	4.4	4	3.7
16.4	5	1.5	5.5	5	4.6
19.7	6	1.8	6.6	6	5.5
23.0	7	2.1	7.7	7	6.4
26.2	8	2.4	8.7	8	7.3
29.5	9	2.7	9.8	9	8.2
32.8	10	3.0	10.9	10	9.1
49.2	15	4.6	16.4	15	13.7
65.6	20	6.1	21.9	20	18.3
82.0	25	7.6	27.3	25	22.9
98.4	30	9.1	32.8	30	27.4
114.8	35	10.7	38.3	35	32.0
131.2	40	12.2	43.7	40	36.6
147.6	45	13.7	49.2	45	41.1
164.0	50	15.2	54.7	50	45.7

LENGTH - Miles - Kilometres

1 mile = 1.6 km (1.6093km)
1 km = $^5/_8$ mile (0.6214 mile)

Miles	↔	Kilometres
0.6	1	1.6
1.2	2	3.2
1.9	3	4.8
2.5	4	6.4
3.1	5	8.0
3.7	6	9.7
4.3	7	11.3
5.0	8	12.9
5.6	9	14.5
6.2	10	16.1
12.4	20	32.2
18.6	30	48.3
24.9	40	64.4
31.1	50	80.5

AREA - Square feet - Square metres

1 sq ft = 0.1 m^2 (0.0929 m^2)
$1m^2$ = $10^3/_4$ ft^2 (10.764 sq ft)

Square Feet	↔	Square Metres
10.8	1	0.09
21.5	2	0.19
32.3	3	0.28
43.1	4	0.37
53.8	5	0.46
64.6	6	0.56
75.3	7	0.65
86.1	8	0.74
96.9	9	0.84
107.6	10	0.93
118.4	11	1.02
129.2	12	1.11
139.9	13	1.21
150.7	14	1.30
161.5	15	1.39
172.2	16	1.49
183.0	17	1.58
193.8	18	1.67
204.5	19	1.77
215.3	20	1.86

WEIGHT - Pounds - Kilograms

1 pound - 0.5 kg (0.454 kgs)
1 kg = $2^1/_4$ lbs (2.205 lbs)

Pounds	↔	Kilograms
2.2	1	0.45
4.4	2	0.91
6.6	3	1.36
8.8	4	1.81
11.0	5	2.27
13.2	6	2.72
15.4	7	3.18
17.6	8	3.63
19.8	9	4.08
22.2	10	4.54
24.3	11	4.99
26.5	12	5.44
28.7	13	5.90
30.9	14	6.35
33.1	15	6.80
35.3	16	7.26
37.5	17	7.71
39.7	18	8.16
41.9	19	8.62
44.1	20	9.07

VOLUME - Imperial / Metric

1 imperial pint = 0.5 litre (0.568 litres)
1 litre = 1³/₄ pints (1.7598 imp pints) = ¹/₄ gallon (0.22 gallon)
1 gallon (8 pints) = 4.5 litres (4.546 litres)

Imp. Pints	↔	Litres	Imp. Gallons	↔	Litres
1.76	1	0.57	0.22	1	4.55
3.52	2	1.14	0.44	2	9.09
5.28	3	1.70	0.66	3	13.64
7.04	4	2.27	0.88	4	18.18
8.80	5	2.84	1.10	5	22.73
10.56	6	3.41	1.32	6	27.28
12.32	7	3.98	1.54	7	31.82
14.08	8	4.55	1.76	8	36.37

Note:
1 US gallon = 0.833 Imperial gallons = 3.785 litres
1 Imperial gallon = 1.2 US gallons = 4.546 litres

TEMPERATURE CONVERSION °C - °F

$°F = (°C \times 1.8) + 32 \qquad °C = (°F - 32) \div 1.8$

°C	↔	°F	°C	↔	°F	°C	↔	°F
-32.8	-27	-16.6	-17.2	+1	33.8	-1.7	29	84.2
-32.2	-26	-14.8	-16.7	2	35.6	-1.1	30	86.0
-31.7	-25	-13.0	-16.1	3	37.4	-0.6	31	87.8
-31.1	-24	-11.2	-15.6	4	39.2	0	32	89.6
-30.6	-23	-9.4	-15.0	5	41.0	+0.6	33	91.4
-30.0	-22	-7.6	-14.4	6	42.8	1.1	34	93.2
-29.4	-21	-5.8	-13.9	7	44.6	1.7	35	95.0
-28.9	-20	-4.0	-13.3	8	46.4	2.2	36	96.8
-28.3	-19	-2.2	-12.8	9	48.2	2.8	37	98.6
-27.8	-18	-0.4	-12.2	10	50.0	3.3	38	100.4
-27.2	-17	+1.4	-11.7	11	51.8	3.9	39	102.2
-26.7	-16	3.2	-11.1	12	53.6	4.4	40	104.0
-26.1	-15	5.0	-10.6	13	55.4	5.0	41	105.8
-25.6	-14	6.8	-10.0	14	57.2	5.5	42	107.6
-25.0	-13	8.6	-9.4	15	59.0	6.1	43	109.4
-24.4	-12	10.4	-8.9	16	60.8	6.7	44	111.2
-23.9	-11	12.2	-8.3	17	62.6	7.2	45	113.0
-23.3	-10	14.0	-7.8	18	64.4	7.8	46	114.8
-22.8	-9	15.8	-7.2	19	66.2	8.3	47	116.6
-22.2	-8	17.6	-6.7	20	68.0	8.9	48	118.4
-21.7	-7	19.4	-6.1	21	69.8	9.4	49	120.2
-21.1	-6	21.2	-5.5	22	71.6	10.0	50	122.0
-20.6	-5	23.0	-5.0	23	73.4	10.6	51	123.8
-20.0	-4	24.8	-4.4	24	75.2	11.1	52	125.6
-19.4	-3	26.6	-3.9	25	77.0	11.7	53	127.4
-18.9	-2	28.4	-3.3	26	78.8	12.2	54	129.2
-18.3	-1	30.2	-2.8	27	80.6	12.8	55	131.0
-17.8	0	32.0	-2.2	28	82.4	13.3	56	132.8

Growth

Calculating Days to Slaughter (Growth Rate Unknown)

Information Required	Example
Weaning age in weeks	= 3
Average sold per week over the last 3 months	= 90
Average number of weaners, growers and finishers over past 3 months	= 1900

$$\frac{\text{month end figures}}{3} \quad \frac{(1800 + 1900 + 2000)}{3} = 1900$$

Growth rate : -

$$\frac{\text{Average No. pigs on farm}}{\text{Nos sold / week}} + \text{weaning age} \times 7 = \text{days to slaughter} \quad \frac{1900}{90} + 3 \times 7 = 168 \text{ days}$$

If the sale weight is 100kg

Daily live weight gain = $\frac{100}{168}$ = 595g from birth to slaughter

$\frac{100}{147}$ = 680g from weaning to slaughter.

EFFECT OF VARIABLE GROWTH RATE ON DAYS TO SLAUGHTER

Growth Rate per Day (g)	Weight Gain (kg)												
	30	35	40	45	50	55	60	65	70	75	80	85	90
	Days to slaughter												
450	67	77	88	100	111	122	133	144	155	166	177	188	200
500	60	70	80	90	100	110	120	130	140	150	160	170	180
550	54	63	72	81	90	100	109	118	127	136	145	154	163
600	50	58	66	75	83	91	100	108	116	125	133	141	150
650	46	53	61	69	76	84	92	100	107	115	123	130	138
700	43	50	57	64	71	78	85	92	100	107	114	121	128
750	40	46	53	60	66	73	80	86	93	100	106	113	120
800	37	43	50	56	62	69	75	81	87	93	100	106	112
850	35	41	47	52	58	64	70	76	82	88	94	100	105
900	33	38	44	50	55	61	66	72	77	83	88	94	100
950	31	36	42	47	52	57	63	68	73	78	84	89	94

The Possible Effects of Feed Changes on the Growing Pig

Increasing the lysine intake by 1 g per day:-
DLWG (daily live weight gain) is increased by up to 10g per day.
Feed efficiency is improved by up to 0.05.
Fat depths (P2) are reduced by up to 0.1.

Increasing energy intake by 1MJ/DE per day:-
DLWG is increased by up to 16g per day.
Feed efficiency is improved by up to 0.06.
Fat depths (P2) increase by up to 0.6mm.

Increasing the liveweight at slaughter by 1kg:-
DLWG is increased by 2.5g per day.
Feed efficiency deteriorates by up to 0.01.
Fat depths (P2) increase by up to 0.2mm.

Increasing feed intake by 100g per day:-
DLWG is increased by 30g per day.
Feed efficiency is virtually unchanged.
Fat depths (P2) increase by up to 0.6mm.

Appendix

INDEX

A

Abbreviations. *See* back page
Abdomen
    atresia ani, 261
    distended, 298, 458
    peritonitis, 297, 315
    rectal stricture, 328
Abnormal behaviour. *See* Vice
Abortion, 10
    African swine fever, 398
    Aujeszky's disease, 168, 398
    boar, 151
    brucellosis, 180, 402
    checklist, 152
    classical swine fever, 169
    cost, 150
    diseases, 178
    encephalomyocarditis, 169
    factors causing, 151
    fever, 168
    infections, 152
    investigation, 150
    management, 153
Abscess, **199**
    treatment, **495**
Acclimatisation, **140**
    gilt, 140
Acetyl promazine, 122
Actinobacillus pleuropneumonia, **299**
    control, 300
    management, 300
    treatment, 119, 300
Actinobacillus suis, **258**
Acute stress syndrome, **218**
Adenomatosis. *See* Porcine enteropathy
Adenovirus, 22
Adjuvant, 9
Adrenal glands, 8
Aflatoxin, 432
    infertility, 160, 434
African swine fever (ASF), **394**
Agalactia, **239**, 10
    mastitis, 237, 241
Age
    sow, 229
Aggression. *See* Vice
Air, **34**
    checklist, 92
    dust, 508
    humidity, 506
    movement, 506
    pathogens, **34**, 23
    quality, 91
    temperatures, 506, 294
Airborne disease, 23, 34, 37
Aldehydes, 47
Aldrin poisoning, 429
Algae poisoning, **426**
All-in all-out systems, 95
Amino acids, **446**
Aminoglycosides, 111
Amitraz poisoning, 429

Ammonia, **436**, 510. *See also* Poisons
Amoxycillin, 112
Ampicillin, 112
Amprolium, 264
Amputation
    tail, 483
    rectum, 501
Anaemia, **199**, **259**
    aflatoxin, 432
    coal tar, 427
    copper, 427
    Eperythrozoonosis, 185
    gastric ulcers, 207
    Hyostrongylus rubidus, 377
    iron, 259
    lice, 385
    mange, 385
    parasites, 367
    proliferative enteropathies, 218 252
    thin sow syndrome, 222
    thrombocytopenia purpura, 277
    vitamins, 264
    warfarin, 438
Anabolism, **446**
Anaesthesia, **121**
    local, 121
    general, 121
Analgesics, **122**
Anatomy, **3**
    bladder, 203
    bones, 16
    brain, 10
    cartilage, 16, 211
    cervix, 10
    joint, 16
    reproduction, 12
    skin, 114
Anal atresia, **261**
Anoestrus, **137**. *See also* Oestrus
    acclimatisation, 140
    gilt, 139
    key factors, 140
    light, 142
    management, 139
    nutrition, 141
    sow, 142
    summary, 142
Anoxia, 4
    stillbirths, 242
Anthelmintics, 122
Anthrax, 200, 301
Antibiotics, **111**. *See also specific diseases*
    disease uses, 116
    dry sows, 224
    growers, 345
    growth promoters, 127
    in-feed, 108, 117
    injectable, 112, 116
    lactating sow, 280
    residues, 114, 115
    scour, 116
    trade names, 121

    vagina, 181, 474
    water soluble, 115
Antibody, 9, **63**
    intestine, 331
    maternal, 331
    mucosal, 60
    respiratory disease, 329
Antigen, 9
Antiserum, 49
Apophyseolysis, 211
Apramycin, 111. *See also* enteric diseases
Arsenicals, **117**
    poisoning, 427
Arthritis, **260**, 301
    actinobacillus, 258
    erysipelas, 205
    Haemophilus parasuis, 315
    Mycoplasma hyosynoviae, 321
    osteochondrosis, 211
    piglets, **260**
    streptococci, 334
Artificial insemination, **511**
    mating, 160
    on-farm techniques, 157
Ascaris suum, **375**
Ascarops, **377**
    thick stomach worm, 377
Aspergillus. *See* fungus
Asymmetric hindquarter, 9
Ataxia
    aujeszky's disease, 396
    copper, 427
    glässers disease, 315
    oedema disease, 324
    poisons, 424
        insecticides, 429
        herbicides, 428
        metals, 424
        plants, 435
        salt, 435
    swine fever, 403
Atresia ani, **261**
Atrophic rhinitis, **301**, 248, 261
    control, 303
    snout section, 302
    treatment, 118, 302
Atropine, **429**
Aujeszky's disease(AD), **167**, **396**
    eradication, 399
    infertility, 167
    piglets, 262
    skin lesions, 354
    sow, 200
    weaners, 303
Autogenous vaccines, **6**, **124**
Azaperone, **122**. *See also* Vice
    stresnil, 122

B

Back muscle, **201**
    necrosis, 9
Bacteria, **24**

disease, 24
   sensitivity test, 112
Bacterin, 64. See also vaccination
Back fat, 150, 459
   body condition, 459
   infertility, 150
   nutrition, 446
Bacitracin, 127
Balantidium coli, **379**
Bambermycin, **127**
Bar chewing, **209**
Baquiloprim, **112**
Baycox, **380**
B cells, **5**
Bedding, **237**
Behaviour, 342. See also Vice
Biochemistry, **586**
Biopsy, **148**
   pregnancy
Biosecurity, **40, 417**. See also infection
   birds, 34
   disinfection, 44
Biotin, **464**
   deficiency, 201
   nutrition, 464
   reproduction, 465
   sow, 201
Birds, **34**
   disease, 34
Birthweight, 244
Bladder, **203**, 12, 17
Blindness, 424
   lead poisoning, 430
   salt poisoning, 435
   vitamin A, 445
Blood, **34**
   cells, 4
   circulation, 5
   composition, 3
   diarrhoea, 218, 252
   hypocalcaemia, 271
   plasma, 5
   poisoning, 4
   sampling, 475, **586**
   serum, 5, 9, 62, 180,
   terminology, 5
   values, **586**
Bloody gut, **324,** 7, 218, 252,
Blue ear disease. See Porcine reproductive respiratory syndrome (PRRS)
Blue eye disease, **400**
Boar, **154**
   age, 155
   anatomy, 155
   detusking, 482
   disease transmission, **167**
   fertility, 156
   lameness, 157
   libido, 157
   litter size, 155
   management, 197
   mating, **157**
   semen, 156
Body condition, **459**
Bone, **15**
   anatomy, 16
   crepitus, 207
   diseases, 16

   skeletal system, 15
   terminology, **16**
Bordetella bronchiseptica, 304
Borrelia suis, 364
Bovine viral diarrhoea, **168**
   infertility, 168
Bowel oedema. See oedema
Brain, 10
Breeding
   age, 134
   heterosis, 133
   selection, 40
   teats, 235
Brucella-suis, 179
   serum tests, 180
   yersinia, 180
Brucellosis, **401**
   sow, 201
Bursitis, **202**
Bush foot, **202,** 305
Button ulcers, 405

C

Calculi, 204
Calicivirus, 23
Calcium, **456,** 442
   bones, 456
   injection, 247
   milk fever, 249
   parakeratosis, 468
   phosphorus deficiency, 444, 456
   porcine stress syndrome, 218
Callous, 304
Campylobacter, 563
Canine teeth, **482, 525**
Cannibalism. See Vice and Savaging
Carbadox, 430
Carbamate, 429
Carbohydrate, **446**
Carbon dioxide, **437**
Carbon monoxide, **437**
Cartilage, 16, 211
Castration, **478**
   normal, 478
   rupture, 480
Catabolism, 289
Catheter, 474
   artificial insemination, 511
Cattle
   diseases, 36
Cats
   diseases, 36
Ceftiofur, 111
Cell mediated immunity, **61,** 59
Central nervous system, **10**
Cephalexin, 111
Cephalosporins, **111**
Cervix, 12
Check lists
   abortions, 152
   air quality, 92
   anoestrus, 142
   biosecurity, 41, 73
   dry sow, 69
   equipment, 583
   farrowing area, 68
   feed efficiency, 295
   fertilisation, 144
   growing / finishing, 70

   low litter size, 154
   mating, 68, 159
   medicines, **579**
   outdoor dry sow, 72
   outdoor farrowing, 71
   outdoor health, 70
   outdoor weaning, 72
   ovulation, 143
   piglet viability, 245
   safety hazards, 564
   sick pigs, 74, 75
   stillbirths, 244
   weaning, 69
Chemicals, **583**
Chlamydia, 24
Chloramphenicol, 112
Chlordane, 429
Chlorinated hydrocarbons, 429
Chlortetracycline, 112. See also *specific diseases*
Choline, **465**
Circovirus, 28
Circulatory system, 3
   terminology, 4
Citrinin, 160
Classical Swine Fever (CSF), **403,** 168
Clay pigeons, 427
Clostridia, **203**
   growers, 305
   piglet, 263
   sow, 203
Clostridium perfringens, 263
Coal tar poisoning, 427
Coccidiosis, **263**
   amprolium, 264
   Baycox, 264
   flies, 264
Coecum, 7
   diseases, 6
Coliform infections, **306.** See also Diarrhoea
   enteritis, 306
   mastitis, 237
Colitis, **307**
Colostrum, **63**
   intake, 242
Commensals, 56
Conception, **143, 146**
Concrete. See also Trauma
   welfare, 533
Congenital abnormalities, **28**
   tremor, 28
Congenital tremors, **264**, 10, 398
   circovirus, 10
   classical swine fever, 403
   Landrace, 264
Conjunctivitis, 244, 273
Constipation, 197
   agalactia, 239
   prolapse, 254
   vomiting wasting disease, 279
Consultant, 76. See also Veterinary services
   role 79
Convulsions. See Nervous signs
Copper, **465**
   anaemia, 465
   deficiency, 465
   poisoning, 427

Coronary band, 406
Coronavirus, 23, 326
Corpus luteum, 10, 505
Corticosteroids, 345
Coryne bacteria. *See Eubacterium suis*
Costs, **48**
   breeding and feeding herds, 83
   depopulation, 50
   disease, 49
   disinfectants, **44**
   growth, 48
Creep, **242**
   area, 240
   environment, 240
   feeding, 287
   water, 102
Crepitus, 207
Cross fostering, **242**
Cryptosporidiosis, **265**, 380
Cubicles, **540**
Culling, **194**
Cyanocobalamin, **465**
Cyanosis, 5, 354
Cysticercus, 368
Cystitis **203,** 17, 248
   control, 205
   sow, 204
   terminology, 17
   treatment, 204
Cytomegalovirus 22
   infertility 170

D

Death. *See also* Mortality
   anthrax, 198, 301
   Actinobacillus pleuropneumonia, 297
   carbon monoxide, 437
   clostridia, 203
   cystitis, 203
   E. coli, 306
   electrocution, 249
   gastric ulcer, 207
   mulberry heart disease, 320
   pleuropneumonia, 297
   poisons, 424
   porcine stress syndrome, 218
   purpura, 277
   streptococcal meningitis, 344, 336
Dehydration, 127
Defects. *See* Congenital
Defined high health status, 39
Demodectic mange, 385
Density. *See* Stocking density
Depopulation, **50**
   costs, 50
   planning, 52
Dermatitis, **349**
   allergic, 359
   erysipelas, 355
   exudative epidermitis, 356
   foot and mouth disease, 406
   nutritional, 358
   pityriasis, 361
   pustular, 362
   ringworm, 362
   swine fever, 403
Detergents, 46
De-tusking, 482, 525
Diarrhoea, 265, 297

   aflatoxins, 432
   anthrax, 198
   antibiotics, 266
   antibodies, 331
   bloody, 263, 324
   citrinin, 160
   clostridial diseases, 263
   coccidiosis, 263
   coliform infections, 306
   colitis, 307
   cryptosporidiosis, 265
   malabsorption, 128
   monensin, 430
   mycotoxins, 431
   nutritional, 265, 306
   organophosphates, 424
   parasites, 369
   piglet, 265
   poisons, 423
   porcine enteropathies, 324
   porcine epidemic diarrhoea, 265, 273, 323
   post weaning, **306**
   pre weaning, 265
   recording, 87
   rotavirus, **333**, 274
   salmonellosis, **334**
   secretary, 128
   sow, 197
   spirochaetal, **336**
   strongyloides, 378
   swine dysentery, 338
   swine fever, 403
   transmissible gastro-enteritis, 277
   Trichuris suis, 378
   weaner, 306
Diazinon, 387
Dieldrin, 429
Diet, **446**
Digestive system, **5, 286**
   systems, 6
   diseases, 6
   terminology, 5
Disease
   bacteria, 24
   biosecurity, 40
   causes, 21
   changing patterns, 296
   chlamydia, 24
   control/spread, 88
   costs, 49
   digestive system, 6
   environmental factors, 33, 94, 329
   eradication, 66
   exotic, 395
   finisher, 298
   flies, 35, 383
   fungi, 26
   gastric, 207
   growth, 289, 293
   health, **39**
   immunosuppression, 65
   infectious agents, 329
   management, 58
   medicines, 116
   mortality, 216, 227, 298
   mycoplasma, 25
   pathogens, 56
   recognition, 197, 247, 298

   recording, 84, 88
   respiratory, 329
   segregation, 94
   sow, 191
   sucking pig, 259
   transmission, **31**
   understanding, 19
   vice, 343
   virus, 22
   weaner, 289, 296
   weaning, **96**
Dimetridazole, **339**
Disinfection, **44**
   compounds, 47
   costs, 46
   fumigation, 45
   houses, 45, **481**
   vehicles, 32
   vehicle dip, 41
Disposal
   dead animals, **76**
   needles, 109
   syringes, 109
Docking tails, 483
Doramectin, 373
Drugs. *See* Medicines
Due diligence, 555
Duodenum, 7
Dust, 508
Dysentery. *See* Swine dysentery

E

Ear
   biting, 343
   cyanosis, 5, 354
   haematoma, 357
   infections, 270
   necrosis, 343
Earth worms, 376
Eclampsia, **249**
E. coli, **306**
   bowel oedema, 322
   cystitis, 203
   enteritis, 306
   immunity, 62
   mastitis, 237
   nephritis, 203
   vaccination, 129
Economics. *See also* Costs
   health, 56
   viability, 55
Ectoparasites, 382
Eczema, 270. *See also* Skin diseases
Edema. *See* Oedema
Education, 77. *See* training
Electrocution, **249**
Electrolytes, **127**
Embryo. *See also* Infertility
   mortality, 172
   terminology, 11
Encephalitis, 10
   erysipelas, 205
   haemagglutinating virus, 279
   pseudorabies, 396
   salmonellosis, 335
   salt poisoning, 335
   streptococci, 334
   swine fever, 403
Encephalomyocarditis virus, **169**

Endocarditis, 5, 205
Endocrine system, **7**. *See also*
  Hormones
  terminology, 8
Endometritis, **180**. *See also* Vulva
  control, 184
  discharge type, 181
  infection, 182
  infertility, 182
  leptospira, 181
  records, 181
  terminology, 11
  treatment, 184
Endoparasites, 369
Endotoxin, 299
Energy, **446**
  deficiency, 446
  megajoule, 446
Enrofloxacin, 112
Enteritis, **308**. *See also* Diarrhoea
  diseases, 6
Enterocyte, 7
Enterotoxin, 322
Enteroviruses, **169**
  infertility, 169, 170
  SMEDI, 169
Environment, **90**
  air, 23, 91, 92
  disease, 31, 40
  humidity, 506
  temperature, 92
Enzyme tests, **586**
Enzootic pneumonia, **308,** 267
  control, 310, 311
  growth, 309
  lung changes, 309
  treatment, 118, 309
Eperythrozoonosis, **184, 311** 267
  infertility, 184
  piglet, 267
  sow, 187
Epidectomy, **484**
Epidermis, 114
Epididymis, 484
Epiphyseal plates, 16
Epiphyseolysis, 211
Epitheliogenesis imperfecta, **269,** 355
Equipment, **583**
Eradicating disease, **66**
Ergot, **433**
Erysipelas, **205,** 250, 269, 312
  diamonds, 355
  infertility, **185**
  mummified pigs, 148
  sow, 205
  treatment, 206
  vaccination, 207
Erythema, 355
Erythrocytes, 5
Erythromycin, 111
Ethylene glycol, 428
Eubacterium suis, 203
Euthanasia, 315
Exotic diseases, **391**
  biosecurity, 418
  distribution, 395
  terminology, 393
Exudative epidermitis. *See* Greasy pig disease

Eyes, 400
  lids, 244, 273

F

Faeces, 31, 277, 372
False pregnancy, 145 -152
Farm visit, 77, 79-80
Farrowing, **230, 240**
  acclimatisation, 242
  crates, 240
  dates, **585**
  environment, 24, 237
  fostering, 242
  induction, 233
  management, 241
  pen, 240
  piglet mortality, 227
  problems, 231
  process, 230
  prostaglandin, 233
  rate, 11
  stillbirths, 153
Fat, **446**
Fatty acids, 442
Fear, 533
Febantel, 373
Feed
  additives, 127
  contaminants, 421
  creep, 242
  efficiency, 295
  feed back, 62
  intake, 242, 287
  medication, 117
  mycotoxins, 432
  nutrition, 439
  sow, **459**
  troughs, 294
  ulcers, 207
  weaner, 287
Feed back, **62 485**
Fenbendazole, 373, 374
Fenitrothion, 384
Fever, **250**
Flavomycin, 127
Flubendazole, 127
Flutter valve, 486
Fertility 144. *See also* Reproduction *and* Infertility
Finishing
  diseases, 296
Flank biting, 355. *See also* Vice
Flies, **383**
  coccidiosis, 264
  control, 384
  disease spread, 35, 383
  treatments, 384
Floor, 27, 235, 276
  bursitis, 202
  lameness, 211
  skin necrosis, 235
  trauma, 27
Flunixin, 345
Fluothane, 218
Fluorine poisoning, 428
Flutter valve, **486**
Foetus. *See also* Infertility
  mummified, 145
  terminology, 11

Folic acid, **465**
Follicle stimulating hormone, 139
Food poisoning, **563**
  campylobacter, 563
  salmonella, 563
Foot
  biotin, 464
  rot, 202
  trauma, 27
  vesicles, 406
Foot and mouth disease (FMD), **406**
Foot rot. *See* Bush foot
Formalin. *See* Fumigation
Fostering, **242**
  methods, 243
  procedure, 243
  reasons, 243
Fracture, **207**
Framycetin, 111
F-2 toxin, 432
Fumigation, **46, 487**
Fumonisins, 432
Fungus, **431**
  aspergillus, 432
  ergot, 433
  fusarium, 432
  microsporum, 362
  mycotoxins, 431
Furazolidone, 4
  poisoning, 430
  treatment, 112
Fusarium, 432

G

Gall bladder, 7, 334
Gangrene, 203
Garbage, 418
Gases, **436**
  sampling, **510**
Gastric torsion, **341**
  nutrition, 341
  sow, 251
Gastric ulcers, 207
  growers, **314**
  management, 208
  nutrition, 207
  sow, 207, 251
Gastritis, 7, 277
Genetics
  artificial insemination, 44
  defects, 28
  embryo transfer, 44
  gene movements, 43
  lameness, 211
  rectal prolapse, 327
Gentamycin, 111
Germ free pigs, **38**
Gilt, 140
  acclimatisation, 140
  anoestrus, 139
  health light, 142
  management, 139
  nutrition, 141
  selection, 227
Gingivitis, 525
Glands, 8, 125
Glässers disease, **315**
Glutathione peroxidase, 320
Gnotobiotic, **38**

Goose stepping, 466
Grain
  bin storage, 321
  mycotoxins, 160
Granuloma, **356**
  ulcer, 364
Greasy pig disease, **270**
  skin, 356
  vice, 344
Greasy skin, **357**
Growth
  calculating, **590**
  curves, 291
  differential diagnosis, 291
  disease, 294
  efficiency, 295
  environment, 294
  feed effects, **591**
  finishing period, 290
  immunity, 63, 94
  nutrition, 293, 294
  osteochondrosis, 211
  post-weaning, 290
  records, 290
  targets, **293**
  variability, **591**
Growth promoters, 127
Growing pig
  disease control, 63, 94
  environment, 91
  growth, **290**
  sickness, 75
  targets, **293**

H

Haemagglutinating encephalomyelitis.
  See Vomiting wasting disease
Haematology, **586**
Haematoma, 209, 256, 298
  ear, 357
Haematopinus suis. See Lice
Haematuria, 5
Haemoglobin, 5
Haemolysis, 5
Haemophilus parasuis. See Glässers
  disease
Haemorrhage
  bleeding navel, 272
  gastric ulceration, 207
  gilt, 209
  mycotoxins, 432
  parasites, 377
  porcine enteropathy, **324**
  purpura, 277
  sow, 197
  ulcers, 208
  vitamin K, 468
  warfarin, 438
Haemorrhagic bowel syndrome, 324
Hazards, 563
  checklist, 564
Health
  control, **55**
  definition, **21, 38**
  diseases, 53
  high, **39**
  maintenance, 31-40
  management, 55
  normal, 38

selecting stock, 40
status, **38**
terminology, 38
weaner, 285
Health and safety, **553**
  accidents, 573
  management, 557
  policies, 561
  risk assessments, 562
  safe systems work, 575
  systems, 556
  zoonoses, 563
Heart
  mulberry heart disease, 320
  myocarditis, 5
  pericarditis, 5, 14
  swine erysipelas, 205
Heat stroke, 363, 538
Hepatosis dietetica, 320
Herbicide poisoning, **428**
Herd
  check list, 67
  clinical examination, 67
  disease, 21
  health, 53
  size, 88
Heritability, 27
Hernia, **334**
  inguinal, 480
  umbilical, 334
Herpes virus, 22
  aujeszky's disease, 396
Heterosis, 133
High health. *See* Health
Hog cholera. *See* Swine fever
Hormones, **8, 125**
  corpus luteum, 11
  follicle stimulating, 139
  glands, 8
  luteinising, 139
  oestrogens, 8
  oestrus, 126
  PG600, 126
  progesterone, 8, 39
  prostaglandins, 125
  regumate, 126
Hospital, **74**
  management of dead pigs, 76
  pen, 75
  sick pigs, 74
Housing systems, **537**
Humane destruction, **516**
Humidity, 506
Hybrid vigour, 133
Hydrogen sulphide, **437**
Hygiene, 44. *See also* Disinfection
  dry sow 196
Hyostrongylus rubidus, **377**
Hyperkeratinization, **358**
Hyperthermia, 218
Hypoglycaemia, **271**, 5
Hypothalamus, 8
Hypothermia, 271
Hysterectomy, **488**
  emergency, 488
  planned, 488

I

Identification, **491**

implant, 491
slap mark, 491
tagging, 491
tattooing, 491
transponders, 491
Ileitis. *See* Porcine enteropathy
Immunity
  antibodies, 61
  antiserum, 62
  acquired, 60
  compliment system, 58
  growth, 63, 94
  humoral, 57
  immuno suppression,65
  immunoglobulins, 8
  inherited, 58
  passive, 62
  respiratory disease, 327
  response, 56
  serology, 62
  system, **8**
  terminology, 9,
Immunisation. *See* Vaccination
Immunoglobulins, 8
Immunosuppression, 65
  aflatoxin, 432
Implantation, **145**
Inclusion body rhinitis, **170**
Infection, **31**
  abortion, 178
  aerosol, 34
  birds, 34
  disease, 23-26, 329
  faeces, 33
  feed, 33
  flies, 35
  immunity, 56
  people, 37
  pig, 32
  respiratory, 329
  rodents, 35
  spread, 31
  understanding, 21
  vehicles, 32
  water, 34
Infertility infectious, **165**
  aujeszky's disease, **167**
  bacteria, 168
  border disease, 167
  bovine viral diarrhoea, **167**
  brucellosis, **180**
  classical swine fever, **167**
  endometritis, **181**
  enterovirus, 169
  eperythrozoonosis suis, 184
  erysipelas, **185**
  identification, 166
  leptospirosis, **186, 409**
  porcine parvovirus, **170**
  porcine reproductive respiratory
   syndrome, **174**
  swine influenza, **177**
  viruses, 167
Infertility non infectious
  abortion, **4**, 150
  anoestrus, 135
  areas of loss, 138
  boar, 151
  catabolism, 150

cystic ovaries, 149
embryo loss, 137, 138
endometritis, 180
farrowing loss, 136
fertilisation, 144
foetal death, 147
foetal loss, 137, 138
light, 151
mummies, 147
mycotoxins, 160 434
records, 135
seasonal, 150
summer, 150
Injections
medicines, 108, 113
methods, 114
self inoculation, **113**
sites of bacteria, 114
syringe/needles, 113
Inoculation
self, **113**
Insecticides, **429**
carbamates, 429
organophosphorus, 429
poisoning, 429
Intagen, 117
Intestine. *See* Diarrhoea
Iodine, **465**
deficiency, 465
Iron
deficiency, 259
dextran, 279
injecting, **493**
toxicity, 279, 428
Isolation
segregation, 94
weaning techniques, 96
Isospora suis. See Coccidiosis
Isowean. *See* Segregation
Ivermectin, 373, 387

J

Japanese B. encephalitis, **408**
Jaundice, 409
Jaw deviation, 209
Joint
anatomy, 16
arthritis, 258, 301, 321
Jugular vein, 475

K

Kidneys
cystitis, 204
Kidney worm, **373**
Klebsiella, **237**
bedding, 237
mastitis, 214
metritis, 180
vaginitis, 180

L

Lactation, **235**
failure, 235
length, 154
litter size, 154
Lactogenic immunity, 62
Lameness, **209**, 298, 317
back muscle necrosis, 201
bowel oedema, 322
brucellosis, 401
bursitis, 202
bush foot, 202
causes, 197, 210
clostridia, 203, 263
conformation, 211
diseases, 210
epiphyseolysis, 211
erysipelas, 205
foot and mouth disease, 406
foot rot, 202
fractures, 207
glässers disease, 209, 269
identification, 318
laminitis, 209
leg weakness, **211**
muscle, 216
mycoplasma arthritis, **321**
nutritional deficiencies, **443, 456**, 444
osteochondrosis, 211
osteomalacia, 456
poisons, 424
rickets, 457
sow, 209
splay leg, 275
streptococcal infections, 334
swine vesicular disease, 411
tail biting, 342
tetanus, 277
tissue changes, 210, 317
trauma, 27
vitamin deficiencies, 464
Laminitis, 16, 211
Large white worm. *See Ascaris suum*
Lead poisoning, **430**
Leg weakness, **211**, 16, 251, 318
confirmation, 212
management, **213**
osteochondrosis, 211, 16
Leptospirosis, **409**
control, 188
discharges, 181
infertility, 186
treatment, 188
types, 186
Leucocytes, 5
Levamisole, 373
Libido, 155
problems, 155
testing, 496
Lice, **358, 385**
Life cycle, 370
Light, **142**
anoestrus, 142
gilt, 142
lactation, 142
puberty, 142
Lime washing, **497**
Lincomycin, 112
Lindane, 429
Litter size
boar, 154
embryo loss, 317
low, 153
nutrition, 154
ovulation, 143
problems, 153
recording, 87
solutions, 154
Liver
abscess, 342
milk spot, 375
necrosis, 320
parasites, 375
Local anaesthetic, 496
Low viable piglets, 244
colostrum, 63
managing, 242
Lung
anatomy, 309
Lung worm, **376**
Luteinising hormone, 139
Lymph nodes, **5**
lymphocytes, 5
terminology, 5
Lymphocytes, 5, 61
Lysine, 446

M

Macrolides, **111**
Macrophage, 5, 59
Magnesium, 466
Malabsorption, 7, 286
Malignant hyperthermia, 218
Mammary gland. *See also* Udder
mastitis, 214, 237
Management, **55.** *See also specific diseases*
abortion, 153
disease, 55
dry sow, **193**
environment, 89
functions, 79
health, **55**
hospital pen, 74
sick pig, 74
Manganese, **446**
deficiency, 446
toxicity, 446
Mange, **385**
control, 387
eradication, 387
skin, 359
sow, 214
Mastitis, **214, 237**
E. coli, 237
epidemiology, 215, 238
feeding, 236
klebsiella, 237
metritis/agalactia, 239
prevention, 238
pseudomonas, 237
treatment, 215, 238
Mating, **157**
age, 155
boar usage, 155
disease, 88
environment, 159
failure, 228
fertilisation, 156
indicator, **585**
key points, 159
management, 88, 228
multiple, 159
planning, 88, 228
procedures, **498**
programme, 89
repeats abnormal, 146, 147

repeats normal, 146, 147
single service, 157
single, 157
skip, 158
terminology, 12
timing, 145
Meat products, **418**
Medicated early weaning, **95**
Medicines, **107**, **584**. *See also*
  Antibiotics
  administration, 108, 111, 116
  anaesthetics, 121
  antibacterial, 111
  check list, 584
  continuous use, 120
  control, 108
  data sheet, 110
  disposal, 109
  dose levels, **108, 224, 281**, 345
  dry sow use, **224**
  electrolytes, 127
  growth promoters, 127
  hormones, 8, 125
  in-feed, 117
  injection, 112
  lactating sow, **281**
  maximum residue limit, 114
  poisoning, **430**
  prescription, 107
  pulse, 120
  recording, 109
  sedatives, 121
  storage, 109
  strategic use, 118
  vaccines, 129
  water, 115
  withdrawal times, 114
Meningitis 10. *See also* Streptococcal
  infection
  piglet, 276
  sow, 215
  weaner, 338
Mercury poisoning, **431**
Metaldehyde, **431**
Metastrongylus, 376
Methane, **437**
Methionine, 446
Metric system, **587, 589**
  conversion, 588
Metritis, **252**. *See also* Endometritis
Mice, 35
Middle ear infection, **319**, 272
Milk, 62
  failure, 239
  let down, 239
Milk spot, 375
Minerals, **465**, 464
Minimal disease, **38**
Monensin
  poisoning, **430**
  swine dysentery, 338
Mortality. *See also* Death
  causes, 216
  piglet levels, 228
  post-weaning, 298, 301. 319
  pre-weaning, **227**
  sows, 215
Monocytes, 5
Mosquitoes, 408

Mucous
  mucosa, 7
Mulberry heart disease, **320**. *See also*
  Selenium *and* Vitamin E
Multiple site production, 100
Mummified pigs, **145**, 167
  age, 148
  aujeszky's disease, 167
  blue eye disease, 400
  diseases, 145
  encephalomyocarditis virus, 169
  enterovirus, 169
  Japanese encephalitis virus, 408
  parvovirus, 172
  porcine reproductive and respiratory
    syndrome, 174
Muscle, **9**
  atrophy, 9
  dark firm dry, 9
  haemorrhage, 277, 438
  myocarditis, 169
  myopathy, 9
  myositis, 10
  necrosis, 9
  pale soft exudative, 218
  suturing, 518
  system, 9
  tearing, 216
  terminology, 9
  tremors, 264
Muscle worm, 376
Mycobacteria, 342
Mycoplasma, **25, 217,** 267. *See also*
  Enzootic pneumonia
  arthritis, 216
  hyopneumoniae, 25
  hyosynoviae, 25, 216
Mycotoxins, **432**
  disease, 433
  feed, 160
  infertility, 160, 179
  prolapse, 160
  reproduction, 434
  types, 431
Myocarditis, 169
Myoclona congenita. *See* Congenital
  tremor
Myopathy, 10, 320

N

Nasal discharge. *See* Atrophic rhinitis
Navel
  bleeding, **272**
  umbilical hernia, 334
Necrosis, 359
  ears, 360
  knee, 260
  muscle, 9
  pneumonia, 297
  tail, 359
  teats, 235, 276, 360
Necrotic enteritis, 324
Needles, **523**
  disposal, 524
  suture, 518
  use of, 523
Nematodes, 373
Neomycin, 111
Nephritis, 203

Nervous signs
  ammonia, 436
  anatomy, 10
  aujeszky's disease, 167, 396
  blue eye disease, 400
  bowel oedema, 322
  clostridia, 203
  congenital tremor, 10, 264
  epiphyseolysis, 211
  glässers disease, 315
  haemagglutinating encephalomyelitis, 279
  heat stroke, 218
  hydrogen sulphide, 437
  inorganic poisons, 424
  meningitis, 334
  mortality, 298
  plant poisons, 435
  salmonella, 334
  salt poisoning, 335
  streptococci, 334
  terminology, 10
  tetanus, 277
  vomiting wasting disease, 10
Nicotinamide, **466**
Nitrate / Nitrite poisoning, **434**
Nitrofurans, **112**
No rectum, 261
Nodular worms, 376
Non-productive days, 12, 136
Nutrition, **441**
  abortion, 448
  anoestrus, 141
  colitis, 450
  deficiencies, 30, 444
  diarrhoea, 452
  disease, 101, 447
  energy, 453
  excesses, 444
  feed composition, 442
  feed levels, 453
  gastric ulcers, 454
  lactation, 246
  lameness, **456**
  litter size, 459
  problems, 443
  rectal prolapse, 458
  reproduction, 459
  requirements, 442
  vice, 343
Nystagmus, 337

O

Obstetrics, **230, 240**
Ochratoxin, 432
Oedema, **322,** 11
  disease, 322
  pulmonary, 433
  udder, 11, 236
  vulva, 365
Oestrus, 12
  abnormal cycle, 145-147
  anoestrus, 137
  detection, 139
  failure, 139
  gilt sow, 137
  hormone changes, 139
  management, 139
  normal cycle, 145

signs, 139
sow, 143
Oesophagostomum, 376
Oesophagus, 7
Oestrogen, 139
Olaquindox, 431
Ontario encephalitis. See Vomiting wasting disease
Orchitis
   blue eye disease, 400
   brucellosis, **401**, 201
Organophosphates, **429**
Osteochondrosis, 16, 211
Osteomalacia, 16, 456
Osteomyelitis, 16, 456
Osteoporosis, 456
Ovulation, **143**
Oxibendazole, 373, 374
Oxfendazole, 373, 374
Oxyhaemoglobin, 5
Oxytetracycline, 105, 112
Oxytocin, 12

P

Palate, **521**
Pale pig syndrome, 270
Pathogen, **56**
   commensal, 56
   opportunist, 56
   primary, 56
   virulence, 58
Pantothenic acid, 446
Papules, 349
Parakeratosis, 361, 468
   calcium toxicity, 456
   zinc deficiency, 468
Paramyxovirus, 23
Parasecticides, **123**
Parasites, **367**
   egg counts, 372
   control, 371
   external, 382
   internal, 369
   parasecticides, 123
   treatment, 123, 373, 374
Parity, **134**
   distribution, 134
   farrowing rate, 134
   litter size, 134
   mastitis, 214, 237
   mortality, 86
   stillbirths, 153
   terminology, 12
Pars oesophagus, 6. *See also* Gastric ulcer
Parturition. *See* Farrowing
Parvovirus. *See also* Porcine parvovirus
   immunity, 172
Pathogen, 56
Pasteurellosis, 323
   atrophic rhinitis, 301
Penicillin, **112**
   vomiting, 66
Penis
   examination, 500
   injuries, 500
   prepuce, 11
Pentobarbitone, 121
Pericarditis, 5, 15, 315, 297, 309

Periostitis, 17
Peritoneum, 7
Peritonitis, 7, 297, 315
   sow, 217
   terminology, 7
Peroxides, 47
Peroxygen compounds, 48
Personnel. *See* training
PG600, 126
pH 17, 204
Phagocytes, **59**
   macrophages, 59
Pharynx, 5
Phenols, 47
Phenylbutazone, 122
Phosmet, 387, 388
Phosphorus, **456**
   deficiency, 444
   osteoporosis, 456
   rickets, 457
Photosensitisation, 178
Pietrain creeper syndrome, 10
Piglets
   acclimatisation, 242
   diarrhoea, 267, 268
   disease from sow, 95, 96
   diseases, **225**
   environment, 90
   fostering, 242
   low viable, **244**
   mortality, **227**
   problems, 257
   rhinitis, **301**
   stillbirths, 153
   trauma, 28
Pig pox. *See* Swine pox
Pigs
   dead/disposal, 76
Pituitary gland, **8, 125**
Pityriasis rosea, **361**
Placenta, 231
   infection, 180
Plant poisoning, **435**
Plasma, 5
Pleurisy, 15, 315, 297
   actinobacillus, 297
   glässers disease, 315
   influenza, 177
   pasteurellosis, 323
Pleuropneumonia. *See* Actinobacillus pleuropneumonia
Pneumonia. *See also* Respiratory system
   actinobacillus pleuropneumonia, 297
   actinobacillus suis, **299**
   African swine fever, 394
   ammonia, 436
   ascarids, 375
   aujeszky's disease, 303
   blue eye disease, 400
   causes, **309, 328**
   control, **328**
   enzootic, 308
   lung worm, 376
   pasteurella, 323
   porcine reproductive and respiratory syndrome, 325
   salmonellosis, 334
   sow, 217

swine fever, 403
swine influenza, 341
treatment, 105
Poisons, **423**, 29
   salt, 335
Porcine cytomegalo virus, **170**
Porcine enteropathy, **324**, 218, 252
   bloody gut, 324
   haemorrhagic bowel (PHE), 324
   necrotic enteritis (NE), 324
   porcine intestinal adenopathy PIA, 324
   regional ileitis (RE), 324
Porcine epidemic diarrhoea, **273, 323,** 410
   sow, 218
Porcine intestinal adenopathy. *See* Porcine enteropathy
Porcine parvovirus, **170**
   immunity, 171
   records, 171
   titres, 171
   vaccination, 172
Porcine reproductive and respiratory syndrome, **173, 177**
   boar, 175
   control, 175
   elimination, 177
   growers, 325
   immunity, 176
   infertility, 173 - 177
   piglet, 273
   respiratory, 325
   serology, 176
   skin, 361
   sow, 173, 253
   spread, 173
   treatment, 175
Porcine respiratory coronavirus, 274, 411
Porcine stress syndrome, 218
   back muscle necrosis, 201
Potassium, **466**
Pregnancy, **148**
   diagnosis, **499,** 149
   loss, 149
   maintenance, 146
   resorption, 145
Premix, 108
   feed supplement, 108
Prepuce, 12
   diverticulum/sac, 12
   ulcers, 362
Prescription medicines, 107
Primidone, 122
Probiotics, **468,** 59
   lactobacillus, 59
Production. *See also* Reproduction
   planning, 89
   targets, 88
Products, **582**
Profitability, 55, 56, 78, 79, 83
Progesterone, 8, 231
   abortion, 10
   anoestrus, 139
   endometritis, 180
   pregnancy, 144
Prolapse
   bladder, 253

cervix, **503**
rectum, **501**, 160, 219, 253, 458
uterus, **504**, 254
vagina, **220**
Prostaglandins
control, 233
uses, 125, 505
Protein deficiency, 446
Protozoa, 379
Pseudomonas, 237
Pseudopregnancy, 138
Pseudorabies. *See* Aujeszky's disease
Puberty, 137
Pulmonary oedema, 433
Pulse rates, 586
Pustules, 349
Pyelonephritis, 17

Q
Quaternary ammonia compounds, **47**
Quinalones, **112**

R
Rats. *See* Rodents
Reading, 580
Rectal prolapse. *See* Prolapse
Rectal stricture, 328. *See also* Prolapse
haemophilus, 328
salmonellosis, 328
Records, **82**
disease formats, 84, 88
endometritis, 181
farrowing house, 227
farrowing rate, 136
forecasting, 83
growth, 290
reproduction, 135
targets, 82
types, 82
use of, 82
Red stomach worms, **377**
References, **582**
Regional ileitis. *See* Porcine enteropathy
Regumate, 126
Reovirus, **274**
Repeat breeding **143-148**. *See also* Mating
diseases, 166, 168, 175, 178, 184
irregular, 11
regular, 12
Repeat matings. *See* Mating
Repopulation, **49**
Reproduction, **133**, **165**
age/parity, 134, 230
anatomy boar/sow, 137
anoestrus, 137
boar effects, 156
breeding, 133
failure, 135, 138
farrowing rates, 136
fertilisation, 144
foetal death, 145
infertility, **133**, **163**
libido, 157
nutrition, 246 459
planning, 228
pregnancy, **148**, **499**
records, 135

system, 10
targets, 84, 88, 96, 134 ,136
teats, 234-236
terminology, 10
Respiratory disease, **309**, **328**. *See also* Pneumonia
control, 328, 332
immunity, 330
infection, 329
nutrition, 461
segregated weaning, 332
vaccination, 333
Respiratory system, **14**. *See also* Pneumonia
anatomy, 14
antibiotics, 108
atrophic rhinitis, 14
diseases, **309**, **328**, 14, 96
epidemiology, 99
feed medication, 108
immunity, 329
respiration rates, 586
segregated weaning, 96
system, 14
terminology, 14
turbinates, 14
Restraint, **507**
Return to service. *See* Repeat breeding
Rhinitis. *See* Atrophic rhinitis
Riboflavin deficiency, **466**, 445
Rickets, **457**
Rigor mortis, 218
Ringworm, **362**
Rodenticides, 438
Rodents, **35**
atrophic rhinitis, 301
aujeszky's disease, 396
encephala myocarditis, 35
leptospirosis, **186**, 409
pasteurellosis, 35
salmonella, 35, 334
swine dysentery, 35
Ronidazole, 339
Rotavirus, **333**
Roxarsone, 117
Rupture. *See* Hernia

S
Salinomycin, 127
Salivation, 66. *See also* Vesicular disease
Salmonella choleraesuis, 334
Salmonellosis, **334**
piglet, 275
sow, 220
zoonoses, 335
Salt, 221
poisoning, 335
requirements, 466
Sampling
air, **508**, **510**
blood, 475
dust, 508
feed, 509
herd requirements, **587**
laboratory, **509**
milk, **509**
semen, **511**
Sanitation. *See* Disinfection

Sarcoptes scabei. See Mange
Savaging of piglets, **255**
Sawdust
klebsiella, 237
mastitis, 214, 237
tuberculosis, 342
Scour. *See* Diarrhoea
Season infertility, **150**
Sedatives, **122**
Segregation, **94**
disease control, **96**
isowean, 96
medicated early weaning, 95
multi-site, 100
segregated early weaning, 94
segregated disease control, 96, 97
Selenium, **467**
deficiency, 467
gastric ulcers, 468
immunity, 467
mulberry heart disease, 320
toxicity, **436**
Semen
collection, 511
disease spread, 168
sampling, 511
Seminal vesicles, 13
Sensitivity test, 112
Sensory system, **15**
Septicaemia, 5
Serology, 9, 62
acute, 63
brucellosis, 180
convalescent, 63
Serpulina hyodysenteriae. See Swine dysentery
Serpulina pilosicoli. See Colitis
Service. *See* Mating
Serum, 9
hyperimmune, 9
Shoulder sores, **221**, 362
Sick pig, **74**
hospital pen, 75
management of, **75**
Sight, 66
Site, **100**
two site, 100
three site, 100
multi-site, 100
Skeletal system, **15**
terminology, 15
Skin
diseases, **347**
identification, 351
observations, 352
suturing, 518
Slatted floors, 211, 457
Slaughter, **515**
checks, 371
destruction, 515
lungs, 309
SMEDI, **170**
enterovirus, 171
parvovirus, 171
porcine reproductive respiratory syndrome, 175-178
stillbirths, 244
mummification, 145
Smell, 67

Snare, 507
Sneezing. *See* Atrophic rhinitis
Snout, 302
   bent septum, 302
   infection, 301
   scoring, 302
Sores
   callous, 304
   flank, 342
   shoulder, 221
   trauma, 27
Sow
   age, 229
   anoestrus, 142
   breeding, 194
   culling, 194
   death, 86
   diseases, 85, 193, 197
   environment, 90
   feeding, **459**
   lameness, 209
   mating, 86
   mortality, 215
   nutrition, 195
   parity effects, 134
   piglet mortality, 229
   records, 85, 86, 193
   reproductive tract, 12
   sick pig ,75
Sow stalls, **539**
   problems, 194, 229, 539
Specific pathogen free, **38**
Spectinomycin, 111
Sperm, 152-155
Spine, 10
Spirochetes
   diarrhoea, 336
Spiromycin, 127
Splay leg, **275**
Staphylococci
   abscesses, 199
   arthritis, 260
   greasy pig disease, 270
   mastitis, 237
   necrosis of ear, 360
Starlings, 34
Stephanurus dentatus, 373
Sterilisation, 113
   syringes, 113, 523
   water, 531
Stillbirths, **242,** 153
   age, 153
   aujeszky's disease, 68
   blue eye disease, 400
   carbon monoxide, 153
   enterovirus, 170
   Japanese B. encephalitis, 408
   leptospirosis, 152
   poisons, 424
   porcine parvovirus, 170
   porcine reproduction respiratory syndrome, 273
   sow, 242
   toxoplasma, 381
Stocking density, **93**
   weaner, 288
Stomach
   diseases, 6
   haemorrhage, 207
   tube, **517**
   ulcers, 7, 207
   worms, 377
Straw, **98**
Streptococcal infections, **334,** 221
   arthritis, 260
   meningitis, 334, 276
   metritis, 182
   suis, 336
   treatments, 119
Streptomycin, 111
Stress
   causes, 29
Strongyloides, 378
Sulphonamides, **112**
   poisoning, 431
   residues, 112
Summer infertility, **150**
   light, 142
   energy, 459
   pheromones, 151
Sunburn, 363
   abortion, 178
   embryo absorption, 178
Suturing, **518**
   anaesthetic, 497
   materials, 518
   methods, 519
   muscle, 518
   needles, 523
   skin, 518
Swab
   nasal, **521**
   transport, **522**
Swine dysentery, **338**
   control, 338
   eradication, 339
   grower, 338
   piglet, 276
   sow, 221
   treatment, 119, 339
Swine erysipelas. *See* Erysipelas
Swine fever, **168, 403**. *See also* African swine fever
Swineherds disease, **409**
Swine influenza, **177,** 222
   grower, 341
   infertility, 177
   piglet, 276
   sow, 222
Swine pox, 363
Swine vesicular disease, **411**
Synovial fluid, 16
Synovitis, 17
Syringe, **113, 523**
   disposal, 109
   self inoculation, 113
   sizes, 523
   use, 113

T

T cells, 5
Tail, **342,** 363
   biting. *See* Vice
   blood collection, 475
   docking, **483**
   necrosis, 359
Talfan disease. *See* Teschen disease
Tape worms, **378**
Targets. *See* Records
Tattooing, 490
Teats, **234**
   anatomy, 235
   inverted, 235
   necrosis, 235, 276
   placement, 236
   selection, 235
Teeth, **525**
   clipping, 525
   de-tusking, 482
   infection, 526
Temperature, **526**
   ages, 526
   body, 526
   conversions, **590**
   energy intake, 466
   environment, **92**
   fluctuation, 90
   heat stress, 538
   lower critical, 538
   recording, 506
   rectal, 526, 586
   upper critical, 538
Tenosynovitis, 17, 321
Terminology, **3**
   immunity, 56
   systems, 3, 17
Teschen disease, **413**
Testicle
   castration, 478
   haematoma, 209
   infection, 179
   rupture, 480
Tetanus, 277
Tethers, 539
Tetracycline, 111
Therapeutics. *See* Medicines
Thiamine, **446**
Thin sow syndrome, **222**
   body condition, 222
Thorny-headed worm, **377**
Thread worms, **378**
   strongyloides, 378
Three site production, 100
Thrombocyte, 5
   Thrombocytopaenic purpura, **277**
Thrombosis, 355
Thyroid gland, 8
Tiamulin, 111
   respiratory disease, 308
   toxicity, 431
Ticks, 388
Tilmycosin, 112
   erysipelas, 187, 206
   parvovirus, 171
Titre, 58
   erysipelas, 186, 206
   parvovirus, 171
Tonsil, 7, 521
Torsion, **341**
   intestine, 341
   stomach, 341
Touch, 67
Toxic gases, **436**
Toxins. *See* Poisons
Toxoids, **124**
Toxoplasmosis, **381**
Trachea, 14

Transit erythema, 355
Transmissible gastro-enteritis, **277**, 414
   grower, 342
Training, **77**
   education, 77
   employees, 78
   management, 81
   manager, 79
   programmes, 81
   topics, 80
Transport, 32
   disease control, 32, 41
Trauma, **27**
   diseases, 28
Treatment, **105**. *See also* Medicines *and* Specific diseases
   diarrhoea, 114
   hospital pen, 75
   in-feed, 113
   injection, 110
   principles, 106
   sick pig, 74
   strategic, 116
Trichinella, 376
Trichocethenes. *See* Mycotoxins
Trichostrongylus. *See* Parasites
Trichuris suis, 378
Trimethoprim, 112
Tuberculosis, 342
Turbinate bone, **302**
   atrophy, 302
   structure, 302
Tylosin, 112
T2 toxin, 432

U

Udder, **234**. *See also* Mastitis
   agalactia, 236
   conformation, 234
   examination, **527**
   hypoplasia, 237
   nutrition, 239
   oedema, 236, 462
   teats, 234
Ulcers. *See* Gastric *and* Shoulder sores
Umbilicus
   clips, **528**
   haemorrhage, **272**
Units measurement, **587**
Ureter, 17
Urethra, 17
Urine
   composition, 586
   diseases, 17
   system, 17
   terminology, 17
Uterus
   discharge, 180
   inertia, 231
   infection, 180
   placenta, 231
   prolapse, 504
   rotation, 232

V

Vaccination, **63, 125**
   adjuvant, 9
   application, 129
   autogenous, 64
   availability, 129
   diseases, 65
   effectiveness, 65
   failure, 65
   respiratory disease, 333
Vagina. *See also* Prolapse
   discharge, 180, 223
   haematoma, 530
   infections, 474
   trauma, 223
Vasectomy, **529**
   vas deferens, 479
Vehicles
   cleaning, 32
   disinfection, 32
   loading, 33
Vena cava, 4
   bleeding, 477
Ventilation, 89, 91, 94
   fluctuation effects, 538
   gases, 436
   respiratory disease, 328
Vesicles, 364
Vesicular diseases, **406**, 364
Vesicular exanthema, 415
Vesicular stomatitis, 415
Veterinary services, 76-79
   on farm training, 80
   profit, 78
   role, 79
   visits, 80
Viability piglet, **244**
   causes, 245
   treatment, 246
Vice, **342**
   control, 343
   ear biting, 343, 359
   environment, 343
   flank biting, 355
   management factors, 343, 3345
   sow vulva, 223
   tail biting, 343
Villus atrophy, 7, 286
   villus, 7
Virginiamycin, 127
Viruses, **22**
   diseases, 23
   clinical signs, 24
   DNA, 22
   RNA, 23
   survival, 23
   viraemia, 5
Vitamins, 464
   A, 457
   B12, 465
   biotin, 464
   choline, 465
   D3, 456
   deficiencies, 30 466
   E, 279, 467
   excesses, 30
   folic acid, 465
   K, 438, 468
   nicotinamide, 466
   pantothenic acid, 466
   requirements 442
   thiamine
Vomiting, 297
   aujeszky's disease, 167
   E coli, 306
   gastritis, 7, 277
   penicillin, 66
   plant poisons, 424, 435
   porcine epidemic diarrhoea, 273
   toxic substances, 421
   transmissible gastro-enteritis, 66
   vomiting wasting disease, 279
   vomitoxin, 432
Vomiting and wasting disease, **279**
Vulva. *See also* Endometritis
   biting, **223**
   discharges, 87
   haematoma, **256, 530**
   haemorrhage, **256**
   oedema, 365
Vulval discharges, **180**
   bacteriology, 183
   control, 183, 184
   treatment boar/sow, 183

W

Warfarin poisoning, **438**
Wart hog, 394
Water, **102**
   consumption, 103
   medication, 115
   metabolism, 102
   piglet, **102**
   quality, **103**
   requirements, **103**
   shortage, 335
   sow, 102
   sterilisation, **531**
   weaner, **102**
Weak piglets. *See* Viability
Weaner, **283**
   age, 286
   diseases, 88, 289, 296
   growth, 287
   management, 283
   mortality, 88
   nutrition, 287
   segregation, 97
   straw kennels, 98
   temperature, 288
   trauma, 28
   villi, 286
   weight, 286
Weil's disease, **409**
   outdoors, **549**
Welfare, **535**
   confined sow, **539**
   cubicles, **540**
   farrowing, **545**
   freedoms, 535
   group housing, **543**
   at weaning, 547
Whipworms, 378
Withdrawal times, 110

Y

Yersinia, 344
   brucellosis tests, 180

Z

Zearalenone, **434**. *See also* Mycotoxins
   infertility, 160
   prolapse, 160

splay leg, 275
Zinc, **468**
   deficiency, 468
   enteritis, 306
Zoonoses, 563
   anthrax, 198
   ascarids, 375
   brucellosis, 565
   campylobacter, 563
   chlamydia, 24, 297
   Clostridia, 263, 566
   cryptosporidium, 380
   erysipelas, 566
   external parasites, 382
   foot and mouth disease, 406
   internal parasites, 565
   Japanese B. encephalitis, 408
   leptospirosis, 409, 563
   ringworm, 362
   salmonellosis, 563
   Streptococcus suis, 565
   swine influenza, 565
   swine vesicular disease, 565
   taenia, 378
   toxoplasmosis, 381
   trichinella, 376
   tuberculosis, 344

Index

ABBREVIATIONS USED IN THE BOOK

App	Actinobacillus pleuropneumonia.	**FCE**	Feed conversion efficiency.
ACOP	Approved codes of practice.	**FSH**	Follicle stimulating hormone.
ASF	African swine fever.	**GSL**	General sales list. Relates to the availability of medicines.
AI	Artificial insemination.		
AR	Atrophic rhinitis.	**HC**	Hog cholera, synonymous with classical swine fever.
AD	Aujeszky's disease(AD) also called Pseudorabies (PR).	**HD**	Hepatosis dietetica.
BE	Blue eye disease.	**HEV**	Haemagglutinating encephalitis virus. Also called vomiting and wasting disease and ontario encephalitis.
BVD	Bovine viral diarrhoea.		
CFT	Compliment fixation test. A laboratory test for detecting antibody.	**HI**	Haemagglutinating inhibition test.
		Hps	*Haemophilus parasuis*. The cause of glässers disease.
CL	Corpus luteum.		
CRD	Chronic respiratory disease.	**HSE**	Health and Safety Executive.
CSF	Classical swine fever. Also called Hog cholera (HC) or just swine fever.	**IFA**	Indirect fluorescent antibody test.
		IM	Intramuscular.
CTC	Chlortetracycline. A broad spectrum antibiotic.	**IPMA**	Immunoperoxidase monolayer assay.
		IV	Intravenous.
DFDM	Dark firm dry muscle.	**JBE**	Japanese B. encephalitis.
DHHS	Defined high health status.	**LH**	Luteinising hormone. The hormone that causes eggs in the ovaries to be released.
DNA	Deoxyribo nucleic acid - genetic material.		
		MD	Muscular dystrophy.
ED	Epidemic diarrhoea. A virus disease sometimes called Porcine Epidemic diarrhoea (PED).	**MH**	Malignant hyperthermia or PSS.
		MHD	Mulberry heart disease.
ELISA	A laboratory test to detect antibodies.	**MJ**	Megajoules a unit of energy in feed.
EMCV	Encephalomyocarditis virus.	**MMA**	Mastitis metritis agalactia.
EP	Enzootic or mycoplasma pneumonia.	**MRL**	Maximum residue limit. Defines the maximum legal amount of drug residue in a tissue.
Epe	Eperythrozoonosis. A blood disease caused by the bacterium. *Eperythrozoon suis*.		
		NE	Necrotic enteritis. Dead tissue on the surface of the small intestine. Part of the proliferative enteropathy complex.
ESF	Electronic sow feeding.		
FMD	Foot and mouth disease.		
FAT	Fluorescent antibody test used for diagnosing disease.	**NIP**	Not in pig.
		NPD	Non productive days.

OCD	Osteochondrosis. Joint and bone changes occurring in young growing pigs, also called leg weakness.	**PRCV**	Porcine respiratory coronavirus. A respiratory virus.
OD	Oedema disease.	**PRRS**	Porcine reproductive and respiratory syndrome.
OEL	Occupation exposure limit.	**PSE**	Pale soft exudate. Describes changes in muscle at slaughter associated with the porcine stress syndrome.
OTC	Oxytetracycline. A broad spectrum antibiotic.		
P2	A point over the last rib 6-5cm from the spine at which fat depth measurements are made.	**PSS**	Porcine stress syndrome. A gene based stress condition.
		PTO	Power take off.
PCR	Polymerase chain reaction. A diagnostic test used for identifying viruses.	**RNA**	Ribo-nucleic acid.
		RI	Regional ileitis. Part of the porcine enteropathy complex.
PCV	Packed cell volume. A measure of the volume of red and white cells in the blood.	**RIDDOR**	Reporting of injuries diseases dangerous occurrences regulations.
PD	Pregnancy diagnosis.	**SDC**	Segregated disease control.
PE	Porcine enteropathy. Describes conditions associated with *Lawsonia intracellularis* infection of the intestine i.e. PHE, PIA, RI, NE.	**SD**	Swine dysentery. A bacterial disease of the large bowel.
		SEW	Segregated early weaning. Weaning pigs early into totally isolated premises.
PED	Porcine epidemic diarrhoea (or just epidemic diarrhoea). A virus disease of the intestines.	**SI**	Swine influenza.
		SM	Streptococcal meningitis. Meningitis caused by *Streptococcus suis* type 2.
Pen V	Phenoxymethyl penicillin an oral form, of penicillin.	**SMEDI**	Stillbirths, Mummification's, Embryo, Death, Infertility.
PHE	Porcine haemorrhagic enteropathy. Commonly called bloody gut associated with infection by *Lawsonia intracellulare*. Part of the porcine enteropathy complex.	**SN**	Serum neutralisation test.
		SSW	Safety system of work.
		SVD	Swine vesicular disease. An entero virus infection.
PIA	Porcine intestinal adenomatosis. Describes a thickening of the small intestine. Part of the porcine enteropathy complex.	**SW**	Segregated Weaning. Weaning pigs at the normal weaning age (or earlier) into isolated premises.
		TGE	Transmissible gastro-enteritis. A highly infectious enteric disease.
PMCV	Porcine myocarditis virus.		
PML	Pharmacy merchant list. A list of medicines dispensed by a pharmacy or a licensed Agricultural Merchant.	**TMS**	Trimethoprim sulpha. Synthetic antibacterial compounds
		TPs	Touch preparations.
PMt	Toxin producing strains of *Pasteurella multocidia*.	**VES**	Vasicular exanthema of swine.
		VS	Vasicular stomatitis.
POM	Prescription only medicine. Medicines only available by authorisation of a veterinarian.	**VWD**	Veterinary written directive or prescription for medicaments
PPE	Personal protective equipment.		
PPV	Porcine parvovirus.		
PR	Pseudorabies. Synonymous with Aujeszky's disease.